PRINTED IN THE UNITED STATES OF AMERICA

DER CHIRURG WIDMET SICH DEM GÖTTLICH-
STEN ALLER GESCHÄFTE: OHNE WUNDER ZU
HEILEN, UND OHNE WORTE WUNDER ZU TUN.

GOETHE.

EDITOR'S PREFACE

The first American edition of Kirschner's work, based upon the first German edition, includes many manuscript additions, with a number of new illustrations, all generously provided through the courtesy of the author and publisher prior to the appearance of a second edition in the German.

A work so skillfully conceived and so beautifully illustrated with large detailed original drawings, mostly in color, fills a definite need in surgical literature. The illustrations are so well done that very little is left to the surgeon's imagination.

While this volume may not be designated a complete surgical treatise, it does cover many important phases of surgery which have heretofore been to a large extent neglected. The book discusses the preoperative investigation of the patient by systems and gives the methods which can be employed to make a "bad risk" patient a better operative risk. It discusses the general contra-indications to operation, but the author rightly maintains that if there is a chance of favorable outcome by operation this chance should be accepted.

The position of the patient on the operating table, the general principles of operative technic, the control of pain, the various methods of anaesthesia, the control of infection and hemorrhage, and operations on the skin, subcutaneous tissues, muscles, fascia, tendons, blood vessels, nerves, bones and joints, including amputations, are discussed thoroughly.

Kirschner has described the operations which he finds most useful and has amplified this by adding other operative procedures for the same condition. In each instance the text is carefully illustrated. Throughout the text one is conscious that the author is thinking of the alteration in function which may result from operation and that he is attempting by the methods which he employs to restore normal function as closely as possible.

The editor has attempted to construe faithfully the author's ideas, while at the same time he has avoided a literal translation, which only too frequently makes the translated text cumbersome and impairs its usefulness. In some sections the German material has been added to, but where inserted material in any way differs from the author's viewpoint, such additions have been indicated by the use of parentheses and the editor's initials. Several illustrations have been remade where this seemed necessary, and a few have been added.

The editor wishes to express his deep debt to his wife, Dr. Elizabeth Glenn Ravdin, without whose help this translation would not have been possible. The publishers have been most considerate and patient during the many delays which occurred in the preparation of the material.

I. S. Ravdin.

Philadelphia,
April, 1931.

CONTENTS

OPERATIVE SURGERY

GENERAL AND SPECIAL CONSIDERATIONS

CHAPTER I

INTRODUCTORY CONSIDERATIONS

The most dramatic part of surgical therapeusis is the operative interference, but this is only part of the science of surgery. Preoperative preparation and the postoperative care are of equal importance. The operation may have been performed skilfully, and yet due to poor postoperative management the patient may succumb. The surgeon is able in a very brief period to perform the most impressive act in the art of healing, but by Surgery one does not mean simply the mechanical interference.

Every operation, in addition to the local involvement, entails changes and damage to body tissues, as well as associated physiologic changes, subjecting the individual to a continuous strain before, during, and after operation. In view of these changes, the surgical interference proper, which is after all the hope of the patient for recovery or improvement, constitutes the maximal danger. The outcome of this critical situation depends on the one hand upon the resistance of the patient, and on the other hand, upon the extent, degree and duration of the operation to which the patient is subjected.

The effect of surgical procedures can not be judged from operations on the cadaver since these can be carried out with accuracy. In the living we can only superficially estimate, and imperfectly judge, the resistance and the reaction to surgical interference.

Many external factors and conditions influence the outcome; these, we can prognosticate and control only in part. The surgeon must always consider the unforeseen. He can not guarantee the outcome of any operation. Short and Fraser have reported that in 16,000 operations there occurred 116 unexpected deaths. The combination of these incalculable forces may be referred to luck by some and to God by others. Ambroise Paré said: "I have operated upon him, God will cure him!"

However, we are in the position of being able to influence considerably conditions and incidents in many operations, so much so, that we may predict the outcome with a certain degree of probability. This justifiable sense of security in the ultimate outcome of our surgical procedures is the result of the technical observance of the recognized laws of modern surgery. This certainty of operative success has not only advantages, but it has at times led to abuse and misfortune. Operative Surgery has fallen more and more into the hands of the less skillful, and to an extraordinary number of varying personalities, whose surgical work does not always conform to the highest standards. The increasing number of surgeons of this type and the apparent safety of operative work have led further to various operative procedures, recommended and applied, which can not withstand serious criticism. Finally, the ease and the lack of danger with which many operations can be undertaken have led too often to surgical interference when neither evident necessity existed nor benefit to the patient could be expected.

Against this implied impropriety, error and abuse, one must take a firm stand. There should be a definite indication for every operation. The question should be, not that which *can* be operated upon, but that which *must* be operated upon. When doubt exists the surgeon should ask himself whether he would subject himself or a member of his family to operation for a similar condition and, if so, which procedure he would elect.

A critical estimate of the value of an operation can in reality be made only through the exercise of one's own conscience. By presentation in the surgical literature or before surgical societies, the evaluation of various procedures and end results can be obtained, as for example, before the forum of the German Surgical Society, or the American Surgical Association.

"The purity of Surgical Science is entrusted to you."

(v. Bergmann).

A. THE OPERATOR AND HIS ASSISTANTS

The outcome of an operation depends upon certain factors, and of these the personality of the operator takes first place. Knowledge, conscientiousness and skill are indispensable qualities which the surgeon must have. He must master general surgery in all its aspects. He must learn self-discipline. The acquisition of the necessary broad and many-sided knowledge and judgment requires years of application and for the most part, tedious apprenticeship in an outstanding school of surgery.

The formation of such a school with its own character and traditions for the development of successful independent students is the rarely attained goal to which every surgical teacher strives. Such students will have a just pride in the school from which they have come. It is necessary to develop in the student his talent for surgery, in a spiritual as well as in a physical sense. While this is rare at this time, it is nevertheless an absolute essential for the outstanding surgeon. Therefore, in spite of the zealous efforts of the many, who have been led to surgery by chance or inclination, it remains for the few to achieve success in the practice of surgery and to become masters of surgery in the highest sense of the word.

A number of factors are responsible for the development of the outstanding surgeon. He must have a forceful personality which can inspire his assistants and his patients; he must have a real enthusiasm for the surgical art, and a solid foundation upon which his surgical knowledge has been built. He must have the ability to correlate the history of the case with the results of the laboratory investigations, and after considering the personal and social conditions of the patient, to decide upon the best method of treatment, for the patient's welfare. Often at a glance, which encompasses much in the trained observer, a decision must be made as to the type of surgical interference which will give the best end results. Success rests upon a highly developed sense of responsibility in formulating broad and bold plans for the operation, carrying them steadily to their goal, or in changing them rapidly in the presence of unexpected findings. It lies in the ability to meet difficulties, which may suddenly develop; it lies in the complete mastery of technic, in detailed attention to minor as well as major surgery; it lies in the art to combine, through care and foresight, rapidity and efficiency of management.

A man endowed with such qualities will understand how to avoid friction, and how to promote co-operation among the surgical assistants and the rest of the operating personnel. The responsibility for this, as well as the ability to harmonize all other factors concerned with the operation, brings to the patient all the surgeon has to give, conscience, precision and honesty. He must therefore be granted unlimited power in his domain, and he must use this power intelligently so that the entire clinical staff will respect his authority and be impressed by his personality. In such a frictionless, well organized clinic he is in command of the situation not only in the general run of surgical cases but he can carry through the more difficult cases calmly and with confidence. By his own excellence he fills his associates with faith and spurs them on to bring forth their best efforts for the stake involved. On the other hand, an operator who loses his natural calm and self control in a difficult situation, and thereby surcharges the operating room atmosphere with nervous tension, and who, because he does not obtain the highest degree of efficiency from his assistants during the operation, gives way to noisy exhortations or even resorts to physical measures, is not a competent surgeon. He shows clearly that he lacks ability and that under his leadership the operating team fails to co-operate and thus cannot obtain the best results.

It is essential in operative clinics that orders be given accurately, and concisely. Polite phrases, such as "please", "pardon", etc. are not only superfluous, but a waste of time and often misunderstood. At the operating table orders must be promptly obeyed. The democratic, parliamentary system has no place in surgery.

There are often a number of different surgical methods for treating certain surgical conditions. The decision as to which method should be used depends partly upon the peculiar characteristics of the lesion and partly upon the preference of the surgeon. The latter depends upon theoretical considerations as well as upon practical experience.

The surgeon must choose between equally successful operations, having in mind, above all, consideration for the utmost safety of the patient's life. All other considerations such as the reduction of time, the difficulty of the operation itself, as well as the discomfort, or pain temporarily suffered by the patient, should be of secondary importance. As a rule, the individual operator and the individual schools of surgery employ certain operative procedures and use other methods only in the presence of special indications. The evaluation of these methods belongs clearly to a research department.

However there is nothing more disadvantageous for uniform success or for the reputation of a school, than the surgeon's capricious use first of one method, then of another, in the treatment of similar lesions. Accordingly, I do not consider it to be within my province to describe here every method, especially since many carry plainly the imprint of a passing fancy. The procedures which I shall discuss are those with which I have had personal experience and which are used routinely in my clinic. I will describe other important ones so that the experienced surgeon may exercise his own judgment in selecting methods for his particular use. No attempt will be made to describe the many methods now in use for the preparation for different operations. These various procedures more often than not have nothing new to commend them. Many times they are merely due to the whims of a non-critical author who believes that he has originated something when in reality the variation is superfluous. Modern surgery has made it possible to treat a lesion in one of a number of ways. The surgeon need not know every method that can be used but he must know the procedure that is most desirable, and at least one other as an alternative.

Each operation should be performed as rapidly as possible. The slower the operation the more the patient's strength is taxed through shock, from general anesthesia, or from nervous strain in local anesthesia, from traumatism and the greater danger exists of an infection of the wound. Thus slowness in operating is usually a grave mistake. Rapidity in operating must be limited by the care needed in surgical work. Surgery of the human is work of precision in which each careless error is avenged. For this reason, thoroughness in surgery ranks ahead of rapidity. An operator who takes pride in establishing a record for speed in an operation, shows that he has not fathomed the significance of surgery. This applies also to the surgeon who boasts of the smallness of his incision.

Time can be conserved without prejudice to operative safety by increasing the rapidity in placing ordinary ties and sutures, in tying unimportant knots, in cutting the suturing material, in sponging, or in the handling of instruments. In everything of importance, such as preparing the operative site, in adequate exposure, in placing of important sutures and ligatures, in searching for concomitant lesions, the thoroughness of surgical work should not be prejudiced by speed. It is only natural, however, that one surgeon may produce work of the same quality but in less time than another; such superiority is a matter of temperament, dexterity and practise.

The assistants play an important part in the rapidity and efficiency of conduct of the operation. This is just as true of the preoperative and postoperative care of the surgical patient, as of the operation itself. The assistants must remain, of course, mental and manual subordinate aids to the operator. Just how far the operator may grant independence to the individual assistant in general, or in a special case, depends upon the agreement of the operator and his assistant. In general, the activity of the assistant surgeon during the operation will be limited to the holding of retractors, sponging, the application and removal of hemostats, to the cutting of sutures, to the holding of the suture material in continuous suture and similar simple assistance. Every operator must be in the position to carry on his work with any man who has earned the name of assistant. It is only through the long association of technically gifted persons that surgery can be performed with silent understanding and great rapidity—where movements of the operating team seem to be the expression of a single will. An operator can work best with assistants that he himself has selected. The number of assistants plays a part, also, in the success and speed of operating. I am of the opinion, that for every major operation, including appendectomy and herniorrhaphy, there should be available two operating assistants in addition to the surgeon and a person handling the instruments. I believe that the possible increase in the chance of infection from the greater number of hands is outweighed by the gain in rapidity and clearness of exposure.

The handling of the instruments is of decided importance in the speed of the operation; intelligent nurses are admirably adapted to such work. It makes a great difference whether a surgeon has a trained, intelligent person to hand him the proper instruments unasked, or whether he has to ask a poorly trained instrument nurse for each instrument, ligature or suture and then has to wait for them.

Rapidity in passing instruments can be increased by a sign code, which the operator may convey through his outstretched hand. I have become accustomed to make certain motions and signs with my hand, unconsciously at first, for the most frequently used instruments, scalpel, scissors, hemostats, forceps, ligature-needle, etc., which my nurses understand immediately.

It is of the utmost importance that the instruments always be arranged in the same way on the instrument table, so that the operator and his assistants may reach and find a desired instrument without looking up, just as a pianist or typist finds the proper keys by touch (see page 261). The initial arrangement of the instruments must be maintained throughout the entire operation and for this the instrument nurse is responsible, though the surgeon and his assistants must also aid in keeping it so. I have on my instrument table a small rubber tray, similar to a change tray in stores. The operator always places the used instruments on this tray, and it is the duty of the instrument nurse to remove them immediately, to cleanse them and redistribute them to their proper places if they do not need resterilization. It is possible to prevent in this way scattering of the instruments over the covers where they may not even be found. Through orderly arrangement of his instruments the surgeon gains time. The remainder of the necessary personnel in a clinic is discussed in the section: "The Set-up for the Aseptic Operation." (Page 256.)

Besides those taking part in the operation and the various other doctors of the clinic, there may be outside physicians and students who are present for the purpose of study. The number of these permitted on the operating floor must be governed by the space necessary to maintain asepsis, and the possibility of observation of the field of operation. I believe that in order to make my entire treatment freely accessible to others in the profession, that it is my duty to permit them to witness the operation but never, because of my duty to the patient, to permit them to assist.

In general, I have no scruples in permitting physicians who are friends or relatives of the patient to be present, as long as they pledge themselves in advance to discretion. Visitors must submit unconditionally to the general customs of the clinic and regulations of the operator, otherwise they forfeit the privileges of a guest. The surgeon must always keep uppermost in his mind his duty to his patient.

The surgeon should limit himself in the number of instruments he uses.

This is true also with regard to the different kinds of instruments; the skilful surgeon needs but a few kinds, while the unskilful must have a special instrument for each manœuvre in each operation. Newly discovered instruments are in great demand among beginners in surgery. The limitation should further prevail in the number of instruments in readiness each time; it is not necessary to use dozens of hemostats, scissors, tissue forceps, etc., even for a major operation.

In limitation one detects the Master!

To operate successfully it is essential to have a good exposure. Visibility and accessibility are actually the foundation of modern operating. In order to obtain these conditions the position of the patient on the table must be considered, as well as the widest possible exposure of the site of operation and careful hemostasis.

B. GENERAL EXAMINATION AND MANAGEMENT OF THE PATIENT

The most skilful operator will not be consistently successful even with the best operative technic, if he fails to estimate properly his patient's resistance to the different demands of the operation, to forestall the development of obviously threatened complications and to treat them quickly and expertly should they develop.

The efforts of surgeons to prognosticate, to gauge, as it were, the recuperative power of an organism and to express this by a mathematical equation, have not thus far reached beyond the beginning stages.

The ability to judge the resistance of a patient to withstand the operation depends to a large extent upon judgment, upon a thorough and systematic examination of the individual, upon the ability to visualize the entire pathology and from these to evaluate the functional capacity of each important organ. Because of the severe strain to which the cardio-vascular system is subjected during and after operation and because the condition of this system is an index of the patient's resistance, the methods for examination, which are described in the section on the examination of the heart, should be employed. These tests are moderately accurate but they are open to question, so that although we accept them we do not rely upon them entirely.

Very often the estimation by various tests of a patient's ability to withstand operation is less accurate than the observation of a trained clinician. Spare, sinewy individuals are more suitable for operation, partly because of their regional absence of fat, than are the soft, obese individuals. In general, women withstand operations, particularly abdominal operations, better than men. Children under one year should not be operated on except when absolutely necessary. In senile individuals only life saving operations should be considered, for the benefits to be expected are few and may last for only a very short time.

Short and Fraser have reported that the unexpected deaths after operation were due to pulmonary complications in 27.5 percent; kidney complications in 14 percent; hemorrhage and shock in 24 percent; cardiac failure in 11 percent and peritonitis and intestinal obstruction in 8 percent.

The maximum resistance, according to our clinical investigations (Zwerg), was found to be between the ages of 11 and 15 years (see Fig. 1). The operative mortality, as Fig. 1 shows, increases in the very young and in the aged. The increase is rapid as the age decreases and gradual as the age increases. One should therefore postpone to the second half score of years non-urgent operations, while for operations in other ages, one must exercise judgment.

One should in no case fail to make a careful preoperative examination of the entire body, even though the results give only an incomplete picture of the functional capacity of the organs, yet the conclusions which can be drawn from them form the most dependable basis for the judgment of the ability of the patient to withstand operative interference. The omission of a

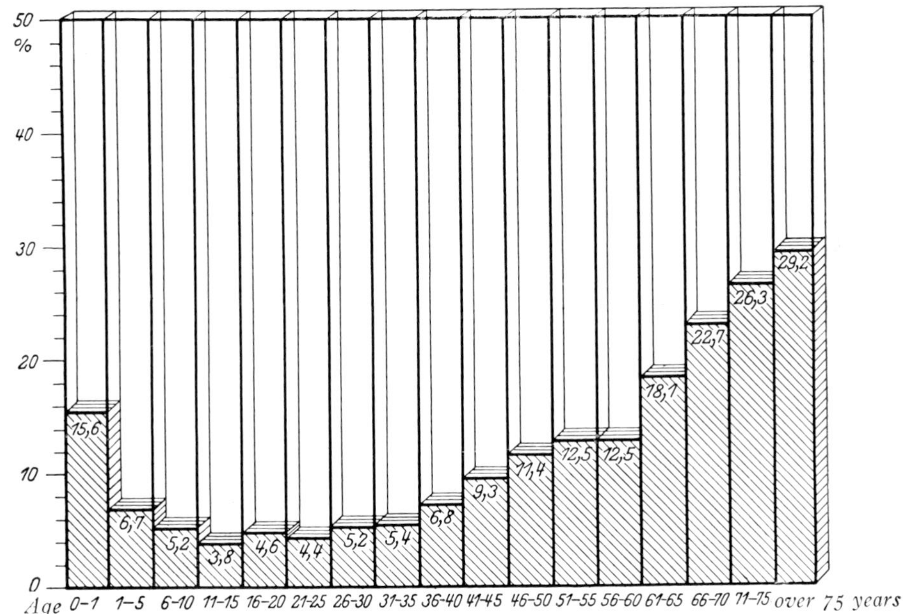

Fig. 1. Graphic illustration of the resistance of different age groups to surgical interference. The columns show the percentage of patients in the different age groups that has died after being operated upon at the Surgical Clinic at Königsberg in the last 8 years.

thorough physical examination, except in an emergency, should be judged an error of management.

The choice of the operative procedure will often depend not only upon the actual surgical lesion, but, upon the general state of the patient's health and the presence of coincidental pathological changes. Occasionally it is necessary to abandon consideration of operation, since we treat not only the local condition but the body as a whole. On the other hand there should be no hesitancy in operating on cases where, although a fatal outcome seems nearly inevitable, we feel that the operation offers some chance for success. The risk may be great. As for the operation's chances for success, on the one side stands certain, impending death; on the other side, even when chances of saving life are uncertain, there is the hope of prolonging life and relieving suffering. Only cases in which there is no doubt as to the outcome should be refused operation. "I do not operate on moribund human beings!" (v. Bergmann).

In those conditions which are not an immediate source of danger to life, but which carry merely a relative or latent danger, pain, discomfort, a reduction in the earning capacity or a disfigurement, the question of the progress of the disease and a lowering of resistance if operation is deferred, must be considered. The decision rests upon the relative dangers of the operation, on the one hand, and the probable benefits to be derived from it on the other hand.

In many instances, through careful preliminary examination and the knowledge thus gained of the insufficiency of individual organs, we are enabled through preoperative preparation, through measures adopted during the operation (*i.e.* the choice of anæsthetic, etc.), and through suitable postoperative care, to meet threatening complications. Even though the various systems show no evidence of disease, it is the better part of wisdom to use every available precautionary and prophylactic measure to offset the possible development of complications in those organs which we know from experience are most susceptible.

It is therefore necessary that besides the special examination and special care of the presenting surgical lesion, a detailed systemic examination be made. Even if each system is found to be normal, we must institute prophylaxis, and, if an organ is found to be diseased, it must be managed according to the extent and seriousness of the disease.

1. Heart and Vascular System

The **capacity of the heart for work,** which, as mentioned above, may to an extent be looked upon as a measure of the resistance of the body as a whole, may be superficially determined in several ways: by graduated physical exercise (Geisböck, Lehrnbecher); or by introducing resistance in the peripheral circulation through constriction of both femoral arteries (Katzenstein). Certain superficial conclusions may be drawn from such studies in regard to the capacity of the heart and the power of resistance of the individual. Geisböck says concerning this: "Climbing steps at a moderate rate raises the blood pressure by 5 to 10 mm. of Hg., in a heart that is functionally sound, and in a somewhat irritable heart by 20 mm. of Hg. The blood pressure at the end of the exercise returns to its initial level within 1 to 2 minutes. As a result of minor disturbances in the circulation, physical exercise gives rise to a greater increase in the blood pressure. After the exercise is discontinued, the blood pressure returns to normal; in some cases it may even drop lower. In serious cardiac disease there occurs no rise, but the blood pressure drops during physical activity."

The length of time a patient can hold his breath has been used as an indication of his cardiac capacity. Stande questions the operative prognosis of a patient who can not hold his breath for 20 seconds. As a result of investigations in my clinic, I believe that these tests give little or no indication as to the capacity of the heart or of other organs to withstand operative procedures.

The presence of **latent edema** is, according to my experience, of distinct value in determining the condition of the circulatory system. The investigation is based upon the following facts: A healthy body eliminates in a short time the same amount of fluid which has been introduced into it, if this does not exceed its fluid balance. In certain diseases the body can not immediately rid itself of a surplus of fluid, but retains it. Retention of large amounts of fluid results in incipient edema; retention of small amounts of fluid remains unnoticed as a rule and has received the name of latent edema or pre-edema. According to Widal's experiments, as much as six liters of fluid can be retained pathologically, without showing any gross evidence of its presence. Determining the presence of latent edema is a rational means for the estimation of cardiac and renal capacity. Its presence should be a factor in the decision for or against elective operations.

The presence of latent edema has been determined by Kauffmann in a unique manner. Beginning at seven o'clock in the morning while the fasting patient is still lying flat in bed, he receives 150 cc. of fluid at hourly intervals for four hours. The patient voids at the end of each hour, and the specific gravity of each specimen of urine is determined. This is the "preperiod" and lasts until 11 o'clock. The foot of the bed is then raised on blocks about 30 cm. In this position (Quincke) the patient remains under the same conditions for two hours, or until 1 o'clock, the "postperiod."

Healthy individuals and patients with marked cardiac or renal edema eliminate the same quantity of fluid hourly during the preperiod and the postperiod. In patients with moderate cardiac or renal edema the elimination in the postperiod may be greater than that of the preperiod or it may remain the same. Individuals with moderate cardiac or renal disease who, however, do not have any manifest edema, eliminate hourly in the postperiod more urine than in the preperiod. In these cases when the body is in the horizontal position the circulation is not able to handle adequately the extra load, but when the lower extremities are elevated the load is lightened. Patients who give evidence of latent edema are not considered good operative risks.

The degree of latent edema present may be expressed by a simple formula. The amount of urine excreted in the last two hours of the "preperiod" is taken as the numerator, and the amount of urine excreted in the "postperiod" is the denominator of a fraction. This fraction may be reckoned by assuming that the denominator is 100. A healthy person without manifest edema has the fraction 100/100, that is, he eliminates in the last two hours of the preperiod and in the two hours of the postperiod the same quantity of urine. The formula 50/100 signifies that the patient eliminates in the postperiod twice as much urine as he eliminated in the last two hours of the preperiod. The smaller the numerator, the greater is the amount of latent edema, and the more marked is the derangement of the circulatory capacity. It has frequently been observed that careful preoperative preparation will improve the cardiac reserve and frequently convert an unfavorable risk to a favorable one. (Frey, Surg. Congress, 1925.)

A very simple method for determining the presence of latent or pre-edematous states is the comparison of the morning and evening weight of a patient. Should the difference be over 1 kg. one should suspect latent edema (v. Gönczy). It has been my experience that as a rule patients with marked arteriosclerosis, especially when associated with hypertension, do not tolerate operative procedures well. A systolic pressure of 160 or over creates an unfavorable factor in the prognosis.

Of course the presence of **organic cardiac disease** is of the greatest importance in the estimation of cardiac capacity. The presence and extent of a valvular defect, myocardial changes, cardiac dilatation, endocarditis or cardiac displacement and the degree of resulting decompensation must be determined in deciding the effect that such lesions may have on the prognosis. Also, the experienced clinician can frequently draw certain deductions from the rate, regularity, tension and the form of the pulse, and from the degree and extent of peripheral vascular sclerosis.

Compensated cardiac disease is in itself no contra-indication to operation. Through proper preparatory treatment, it is possible to overcome a decompensated heart and establish a condition of cardiac compensation. The best preparatory treatment is rest in bed with elevation of the legs, limitation of fluids, and the administration of a potent preparation of digitalis. The amount of digitalis necessary varies in the individual case and it is wise to consult an internist during its administration. Treatment should be continued following the operation, keeping the patient digitalized during the period of stress and strain. This preparatory treatment, however, is not to be used in patients who are debilitated but have no cardiac disease. The administration of digitalis when no real indication exists may produce decidedly unfavorable results. However, it is believed by some that by this means the number and the severity of postoperative cardiac and pulmonary complications and thrombosis can be lessened. In functional cardiac disease, that is in the simple arrhythmias, and effort syndrome hearts, digitalis is not indicated. Pleural or pericardial effusions which mechanically affect the heart action should be aspirated, if possible, some time before the operation. Special care must be taken when there is cardiac displacement from adhesions.

Should cardiac failure suddenly and unexpectedly occur during or after an operation, it is not possible to wait 36 hours, more or less, for digitalization. The most rapid action is obtained by intravenous therapy, though its action is not so prolonged. Intramuscular and subcutaneous injections act more slowly but are more lasting. (The idea is becoming more prevalent that digitalis is of use chiefly in auricular fibrillation. I. S. R.)

In cases where rapid action is desired, large doses (15 to 20 grams) of digitalis may be administered in 24 hours. If a still more rapid response is desired ¼-½ mg. of strophanthin intravenously, twice daily, is a vigorous whip to a tired heart, though it is not without danger and should not be used after a course of digitalis. Strychnin, .001 gm., and 1 c.c. adrenalin (1:1000) are also at times effective. Caffeine sodium salicylate, 0.2 gm. per dose, to 1.0 gm. per day, has also been used with some success. These drugs may be given by mouth or subcutaneously. In acute cardiac collapse, I give immediately 5 c.c. of camphorated oil, subcutaneously.

By far the most valuable therapy for improving a disturbed circulation following operation, excluding true cardiac disease, is intravenous infusion. It may be given in one injection or by a slow continuous drip. Hypodermoclysis is also useful. Transfusion of blood is especially valuable after hemorrhage. Intravenous injection is the most rapid, but also the most temporary way of introducing large amounts of fluid. Hypodermoclysis and continuous intravenous injection are slower but more uniform. Continuous intravenous infusion is the most flexible method and can be adapted to any condition. Large amounts of fluid can be given quickly; small amounts can be given by the drop method over a longer period and the flow can be interrupted for a period, if this is desired. It can not be too highly recommended in serious cases.

The risk of an intravenous infusion lies in overfilling the vascular system, throwing an unnecessary amount of work on the heart. When fluid is given by this method the amount should be controlled by constant observation of the blood pressure. Too much fluid may give rise to water intoxication with its attendant symptoms, but in my experience this can be controlled if one watches the 24 hour urinary output. This output should not as a rule exceed 1500 to 2000 cc.

Instead of the customary physiologic salt solution, or Ringer's solution, it is preferable to use a 4.5 percent solution of glucose made up in normal saline or distilled water. This will provide nourishment as well as fluid.

It is important in choosing the anæsthetic, in a patient with insufficiency of the heart, that chloroform be avoided. In advanced arteriosclerosis and hypertension, one should not use nitrous oxide and oxygen which raises blood pressure. In these cases I have also been warned against spinal anæsthesia, a warning which in view of my own experience I can not accept.

Patients with poor circulation are inclined to **decubitus** if confined to bed. Such lesions may be avoided by regularly changing the position of the patient so that different portions of the body are subjected to pressure for only short periods. One should remember that patients can be comfortable when turned on the abdomen. In the recumbent position the limbs should be supported under the calf by a pillow and so allow free play of the tendon of Achilles and the heels. Thick hair mattresses, rubber sponge and kapok cushions are as serviceable as water cushions and air rings. Meticulous care of the skin areas predisposed to decubitus, through frequent washing, massaging, the application of zinc ointment and powder, is essential.

Status Lymphaticus. Of considerable general surgical importance is the frequently observed cardiac failure in status lymphaticus. It is mainly encountered in children and consists in a constitutional anomaly, the exact etiology of which is not known. A constant enlargement and histologically demonstrable change in the thymus gland are as a rule present. Besides the hyperplasia of other lymphoid organs, changes occur in the spleen, tonsils, and tongue follicles. Characteristic also are the pasty appearance, the subcutaneous accumulation of fatty tissue, and muscular atony. Clinically, these patients show a lowering of their resistance to all demands made during the operation, above all, however, to anæsthesia. There is diminished ability of the heart to withstand stress and strain, which after the brief administration of chloroform, ether, ethyl chloride, or other anæsthetic substances may lead, immediately or several days after the anæsthesia, to a sudden fatal termination. "Death of the heart in seconds" (Hering). The presence of status lymphaticus is therefore a relatively serious contra-indication to the administration of anæsthetics and operation. Unfortunately the diagnosis is frequently not established until the patient reaches the autopsy table.

The value of prophylactic Roentgen-ray treatment of the hyperplastic thymus is doubtful, although it is considered useful in America. When there is no time for prolonged dietetic and hygienic preparatory treatment, we depend upon the cardiac stimulants, which can be used in sudden heart failure. Occasionally a hyperplastic thymus may lead to sudden suffocation through pressure upon the trachea. Removal of a section of the thymus affords relief, as does also tracheotomy.

Amyloid Degeneration. A special contra-indication to operation, except in an emergency, is the presence of amyloid disease. In this condition, the resistance against anæsthetic substances and surgical procedures is very much impaired. Chronic tuberculosis, chronic suppurative disease, malignant tumors associated with suppuration, malaria, late syphilis, etc., lead to amyloid degeneration particularly in the spleen, kidneys, liver, and intestinal mucous membrane.

Clinically, the following signs point to this disease: enlargement of the spleen and liver; albuminuria; obstinate, uncontrollable diarrhea; and wasting cachexia with pallor. However all these signs are uncertain. Amyloid disease can not be demonstrated with certainty, even in the urine; it is true one may find many waxy cylindroids and much albumin, but in the amyloid shrunken kidney the urinary findings are often insignificant. Because of this, the diagnosis is often made only at the operating table, or perhaps at the autopsy table.

In investigating cases presenting signs of this disease the Congo red test is advocated by Bennhold (Dtsch. Arch. f. Klin. Med. 1923, Vol. 142) as a certain method for its determination. The dye which is introduced into the blood is absorbed in the body by the amyloid substance, in amount and in rapidity relative to the degree of degeneration existing. From the quantity of coloring matter retained in the tissues and the time of its removal from the blood stream, the presence and the degree of the amyloid degeneration is supposedly determined.

In the morning before breakfast the patient is catheterized and a specimen of urine is withdrawn. Immediately, about 5 c.c. of blood are drawn from a vein of the arm and through the same cannula are injected 2 c.c. of a 0.6 percent Congo red solution in sterile distilled water for each 10 kg. of body weight. One hour after the injection of the dye, the patient urinates, and 5 c.c. of blood are again withdrawn. The serum is allowed to separate in each blood specimen. The two specimens of urine and of serum are compared. If in the second urine there appears but little red coloring matter and the second serum is not red, the test is positive for amyloid disease. If the second urine and the second serum are red in comparison with the first, there is supposedly no amyloid disease. To eliminate any interference in the color reaction in the serum from hemolysis a drop of concentrated hydrochloric acid may be added to the serum, which produces an ivory-white precipitate; this precipitate, in the presence of even a trace of Congo red, becomes deep blue.

Careful **examination** should be made **of the blood** of all patients before operation. This includes the usual determination of the hemoglobin content, red and white blood cell count, and a microscopic examination of a stained blood smear. In secondary anemia the etiologic factor should be searched for. Patients weakened through acute and chronic blood losses may be made better operative risks by blood transfusion. Leukemic individuals can sometimes be prepared for operation by irradiating the spleen; in such cases, however, one would decide on operation only when it is absolutely necessary. Local anæsthesia is decidedly preferable to general anæsthesia in these cases.

Hemophilia makes the prognosis of any operation very grave. The rarity of the disease is no excuse for not attempting to determine its presence or absence before operation. Bleeders should be operated upon only in extreme necessity. If interference can not be avoided, it is an absolute rule to do a blood transfusion immediately before or at the time of operation. This is also the best remedy for beginning hemorrhage. Other existing medicinal

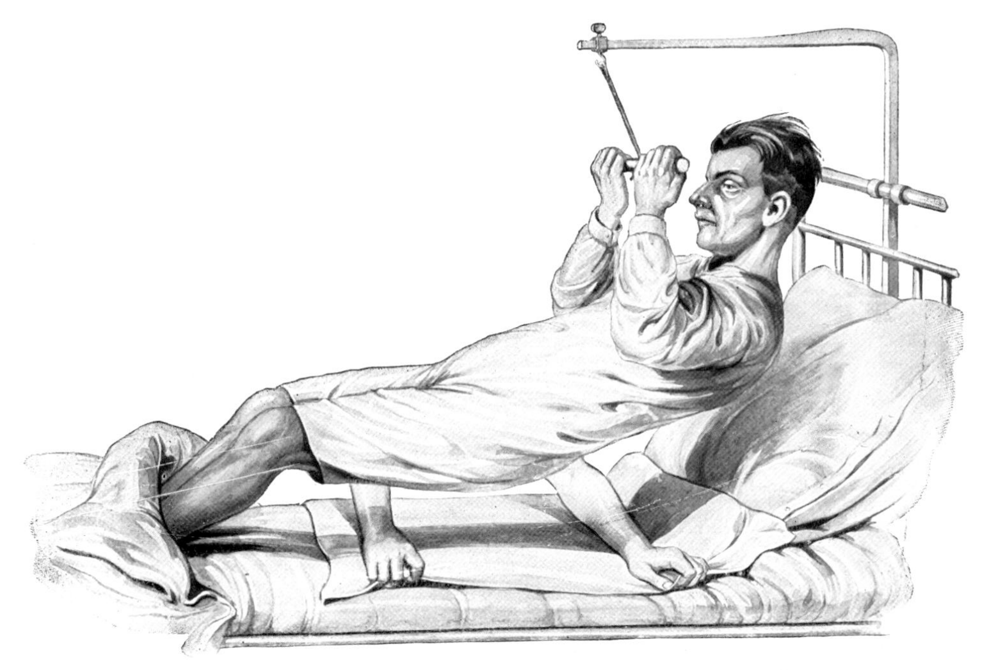

Fig. 2. Overhead bar for use by the patient in raising himself.

remedies may be employed as well. In operating on these cases we should avoid local anæsthesia and ischemia on account of the temporary stoppage of blood to the part, which makes it impossible to determine whether the bleeding points have been properly ligated. The most careful attention must be given to hemostasis. I believe that the management of the hemophiliac has entered a new stage through the preparation "Nateina." My experience with its use in these cases, has been very satisfactory. This drug should be administered to the hemophiliac for several days previous to operation. The preparation is given in ascending doses of from 16 to 36 tablets daily and can, if necessary, be increased. These are taken about ten minutes before each meal, thoroughly chewed and swallowed with a sip of water.

One disease of surgical convalescence that increases in frequency with the patient's age is **Venous-Thrombosis.** It is usually seen in a branch of the inferior vena cava, chiefly the left femoral vein. One of the many causative factors is the necessary rest in bed after major operations and the resulting slowing down of the blood stream which accompanies the decrease in metabolism. At the head of each bed in my clinic there is suspended a cross bar (Fig. 2) with which the patient as soon as possible after operation may raise himself many times a day. This bar makes it easy for the nursing personnel to adjust the pillows and to raise the upper part of the body.

In order to reduce to a minimum unnecessary jarring of the patient the bed is made easily transportable in the following manner: the legs at the head of the bed are equipped with rubber tired wheels, while at the center of the foot of the bed is a device to which can be attached a small four wheeled wagon by raising the bed. In this way the bed is changed into an easily movable wagon with a pole and rubber tired wheels. The bed is also equipped for the application of various types of extension, and half of the foot board can be removed while the other half is provided with an appliance to support the legs.

An outcome of this conception of thrombosis is Kroenig's precept: "Rest in bed after operations and childbirth is to be reduced to a minimum where no contra-indication exists. The patient on the afternoon of the day of operation should begin exercise." The opinion on the value of such radical measures is divided, although the value of certain types of motion is recognized. It is hoped through early, systematic, passive and active free movements (Henles "Promenade in Bed"), massage, through alternately shifting the position of the upper part of the trunk and of the legs from the horizontal to the upright position, through turning from side to side, through respiratory exercises, etc., to bring about an acceleration of the blood flow. As a prophylactic measure against thrombosis thyroid extract appears to be useful. Three days before the operation the drug is begun and is continued until the tenth day after operation. Care must be taken to observe the early signs of hyperthyroidism.

Pulmonary Embolism. Not infrequently postoperative thrombosis leads to pulmonary embolism, even when there is no clinical evidence of thrombosis. This may happen particularly as a result of the first efforts at active movement during the period of convalescence. The clinical picture of pulmonary embolism falls into two symptom groups: in one of the groups small emboli lodge in the smaller ramifications of the pulmonary artery. This complication begins as a rule without the stormy onset which characterizes the larger emboli. It occasionally sets in with more or less violent pain in the chest, which is followed later by the typical signs of infarction, infiltration of a circumscribed area, a limited bronchopneumonia and localized pleurisy associated with bloody expectoration. The treatment consists mainly in rest, and the administration of morphine.

In the second group where larger emboli obstruct the main stem or the larger branches of the pulmonary artery, the patients become extremely ill within a few moments. They sense a catastrophe and are conscious of impending death. They exhibit great fear, and rapidly become dyspneic and cyanosed. Cardiac weakness is soon manifest and they succumb in the majority of instances after a few minutes or hours from anoxemia and cardiac failure. Excepting the appearance of severe infection after an operation performed under supposedly careful asepsis, nothing so shakes one's faith in the surgical art as this unfortunate complication. Only one who practices surgery knows how devastating it is to the surgeon with a conscience, when suddenly, as though from the clear sky, he has before him the corpse of a man who had entrusted himself to him for an operation which was not of immediate necessity. Until a few years ago the surgeon stood powerless at the deathbed of these unfortunates. In 1907, Trendelenburg evolved a plan, with his great ingenuity, which permits us to attack even this supposedly unapproachable lesion. I have operated on one such case by his method with complete success.

The possibility of successfully carrying out the Trendelenburg operation, the favorable outcome of which depends upon the expediency with which it is performed, is in general limited to the large, fully equipped hospital, with a well organized surgical staff. In any hospital where major surgery, especially abdominal surgery, is done, there should be facilities for immediate embolectomy should the necessity arise. The decision for or against operation is difficult, since a patient apparently moribund occasionally recovers after expectant treatment, and since a patient may present a similar clinical picture with acute cardiac failure without embolus. Only those patients are to be considered for such an operation, who have not passed middle life, who are in a good general condition, and who in spite of their primary disease may be expected to live for another ten years. For the technic of embolectomy, see the section entitled "Operations on the Heart." **Fat-embolism** is discussed with "Operations on Bones."

Air-embolism. The introduction of air into a blood vessel, during an operation is possible only when there exists a subatmospheric, or so-called negative, pressure in the vessel. This is found under certain conditions both in the systemic and in the pulmonary circulation. As a rule, a negative pressure develops in the veins of the systemic circulation only during the act of inspiration and when the elevation of the opened vein is above that of the heart. In an injury of a vein, air enters more easily and in greater amount, the larger the opening, the greater the size of the opened vessel, and the nearer the vessel is to the heart. Fortunately, it is seldom that air enters an incised vein, for its thin walls are easily collapsed, mainly by atmospheric pressure. When the vessel walls, however, are passively held apart by their attachment to fixed tissues, by their firm attachment to fascial margins through adhesions, by direct pull with a tenaculum or small forceps or indirectly through pull on a tumor adherent to a vein, the air can find its way into the lumen of the vessel. One's attention is attracted in such cases by a swishing, sucking noise within the region of the wound. In other instances the occurrence of air embolism is first manifested by the appearance of a condition of collapse, and the gaping vein is only subsequently perceived as the reason for the threatening symptoms. In doubtful cases the diagnosis may be made by auscultation of the heart. Metallic blowing or churning sounds are heard if air has found its way into the vessels.

The introduction of small quantities of air is easily borne by the body; the greater the quantity of air, the more pronounced and graver are the symptoms; unrest, anxiety, dyspnea, cyanosis, fluttering pulse, unconsciousness, cramps, and death, which may supervene almost immediately, or after the elapse of a very stormy period. The symptoms in air-embolism are the result of interference with the pulmonary circulation, the associated cerebral anemia, and the supervening cardiac failure.

Prophylaxis is very important. Every incised vein should be carefully ligated. Should the wounded vein be a large one, the operative site should be lowered so that it is lower than the level of the heart. In my experience it is better to lower the head during the removal of large goitres and other vascular cervical tumors; while the pelvis should be lowered during operations in the vicinity of the large abdominal veins or on the liver. In certain instances where a sudden complication may occur, as for example the laceration of large veins or even lung tissue during the luxation of a very large retrosternal goitre, the patient should be prepared for the immediate administration of intratracheal anæsthesia with a positive pressure apparatus. In cases of this type, general anæsthesia is preferable to local anæsthesia, in that the gasping and straining coincident to the sucking of the thoracic wound is under better control. This is especially true in the nervous patient.

Should the previously mentioned swishing noise direct the attention of the surgeon to the advent of air-embolism, the suspected opening in the vein should be closed immediately with the finger or with a gauze tampon. If the closure is successful, then the following measures can be carried out in an orderly way while the finger or tampon continues to occlude the opening. If the closure is not successful then the greatest speed is necessary. The field of operation is lowered, the wound is filled with saline solution (Treves) and then pressure is applied to the wound. During expiration the pressure on the vein should be carefully released while the force of expiration may be reinforced by bilateral manual pressure on the thorax. The lumen of the vein, can then, as a rule, be recognized by the flow of blood from the laceration of the vessel. The opening is then grasped and closed either by ligation or in certain instances by suture.

The management of the resultant air-embolism consists of stimulation of the heart by the usual remedies and by lowering the head. In desperate cases one may try to remove a portion of the aspirated air. Magendies' suggestion to withdraw the air by pushing a catheter through the point of injury and thence to the right auricle is dangerous and of little avail. If removal is indicated it would seem simpler to withdraw the air by direct puncture of the heart. A long, thin hypodermic needle, to which is attached a syringe, is inserted vertically, deep into the third intercostal space, 1.5 cm. from the right margin of the sternum when aspiration is attempted. The prospect of these measures being successful is not good, since the blocking air bubbles are no longer confined to the right heart, but are found in the pulmonary artery as well. In desperate cases in which less radical procedures are of no avail, and in which auscultation and x-ray establish with certainty the presence of large quantities of air in the blood vessels, one should consider exposing the large vessels, as in the Trendelenburg operation, when the air can be removed by direct puncture.

Acidosis and Alkalosis. Within recent years clinicians have come to realize that a variety of pathologic conditions cause an alteration in the hydrogen-ion content of the blood. Under ordinary conditions the buffer substances in the blood serve to maintain a constant or nearly constant reaction. Imperfect combustion of fatty acids results in a depletion of the alkali reserve and the production of the state of acidosis, while the loss of chlorides from the blood in the vomiting of high intestinal obstruction results in the condition known as alkalosis. As long as the increased acidity or alkalinity can be taken care of by the buffer substances in the body, the acidosis or alkalosis is not symptomatically demonstrable. However as the reserve is exhausted the symptoms set in.

In acidosis these are headache, nausea, vomiting, shortness of breath, restlessness, insomnia and general exhaustion, and in severe cases, stupor, coma and death. An investigation made by Stegemann and Jaguttis in my clinic showed that two-thirds of all those operated on show acetone in the urine immediately after operation. They also showed that about 14 percent of the patients show acetone in the urine before operation. In women and in children, acetonuria is more frequent before and after operation than in men. The quantity of acetone excreted varies, but the quantity of acetone and of diacetic acid vary directly. The type and extent of the operation has evidently little influence on the postoperative excretion of acetone. I have observed its presence frequently in various types of hyperplastic thyroid disease, in acute appendicitis, and in other acute infections. It is often noticeable in psychically excited patients.

A definite association between acetonuria and clinical symptoms of acidosis is by no means constant. From observations in my clinic I can not accept the widespread view that the appearance of symptoms of acidosis will be hastened in every case through shock, hemorrhage, imperfect kidney function, purging, cold, eventration, tugging on the abdominal viscera, the length of the operation and anæsthesia. Even if acetonuria exists previous to the operation, one can not say that such a condition will continue or become exaggerated after operation, if the proper treatment is instituted. Therefore the assumption is not necessarily correct that acetonuria is a contra-indication to anæsthesia and operation, or that the prognosis is worse because of this. I do not believe that it is necessary to attempt to treat acetonuria if it is unassociated with symptoms other than to supply carbohydrates. I except of course the acetonuria of metabolic disease (for the treatment of the acidosis of diabetes see page 37).

2. Urinary Apparatus

The methods of examination, evaluation and management of the urinary system follow directly after the discussion of the cardiac, because of the intimate interrelation of the two systems. Disease of one can not exist for long without a resultant involvement of the other. In fact it is often difficult to determine which system is the seat of the primary disease, and which of the secondary. The methods for investigating the functional capacity of these systems are in many instances the same, and an evaluation of one system will frequently lead to evidences of the functional capacity of the other. Improvement in the function of one often improves the other.

The preoperative examination of a patient is incomplete unless the kidney function is determined. Likewise constant observation of urinary function is often of the greatest importance in the postoperative care. Routine examination of the urine should include the determination of the specific gravity, the presence or absence of albumin, sugar, bile pigment, acetone bodies, casts, cylindroids, epithelium, and red and white blood cells. In specific instances the twenty-four hour intake and output should be measured.

The twenty-four hour **intake and output record** is in many cases valuable. We obtain from this an indication of cardiac and renal function. The normal twenty-four hour output varies from 1000 to 1800 c.c. I have measured the daily urinary output of all seriously ill patients who have associated cardiac or renal disease, and of patients whose intake of nourishment is restricted, or who receive fluids other than by mouth. The intake and output are recorded on the temperature chart in the form of vertical, colored columns. This chart of intake and output is, to me, often more important than the temperature or pulse record.

In **acute nephritis** the operation is if possible postponed until improvement occurs. If this is not possible, ether or chloroform should be avoided, because they act as kidney irritants. **Chronic nephritis,** in the absence of definite clinical symptoms, is not a contra-indication to operation if the functional capacity is not too greatly impaired, but even here, local or spinal anæsthesia is preferable.

Infectious processes of the urinary apparatus should be treated if possible before operation. Large quantities of alkaline spring water or water to which alkalies have been added should be used. Urinary antiseptics, chiefly urotropin and pyridum, have been found useful. In cystitis lukewarm bladder irrigations of the milder antiseptics such as potassium permanganate may be used two or three times daily. In inflammation of the bladder or in urinary retention the use of an indwelling catheter and suction gives excellent results.

Numerous **tests** have been described, from which the degree of kidney impairment can be determined, and the effect of this on the capacity of the patient to withstand operation deduced. These tests assist in estimating the improvement under treatment, and the results should be used in deciding whether treatment has converted an inoperable patient into an operable one. Such investigations must be made routinely in patients with hypertrophy of the prostrate and with other diseases of the urinary apparatus, especially where nephrectomy is contemplated. In the latter instance a differential kidney function test is essential. These functional tests are of especial value in cardiovascular disease and give data of prognostic import.

The tests depend either upon examination of kidney function (direct examination), or upon examination of the blood for increased nitrogen content as a result of insufficient kidney activity (indirect examination). Because of the importance of the results of the investigation of kidney function I have adopted a chart for my records which has in it the normal curves, and on which can be placed the results from the case under investigation. One can, at a glance, see any deviation from the normal and can from day to day visualize changes in the functional capacity of the kidney.

(a) The most useful direct test is Volhard's **dilution and concentration test.** Healthy kidneys can eliminate rapidly large quantities of fluids which are taken by the individual. They furthermore have the power to concentrate the urine quickly after the excess of fluid introduced has been eliminated. The more incompetent the kidneys, the more sluggishly and incompletely do they respond. This test is in some respects similar to those of Albarran and Straus-Graunwald. I believe that they give valuable information and should be more widely used than they are at present.

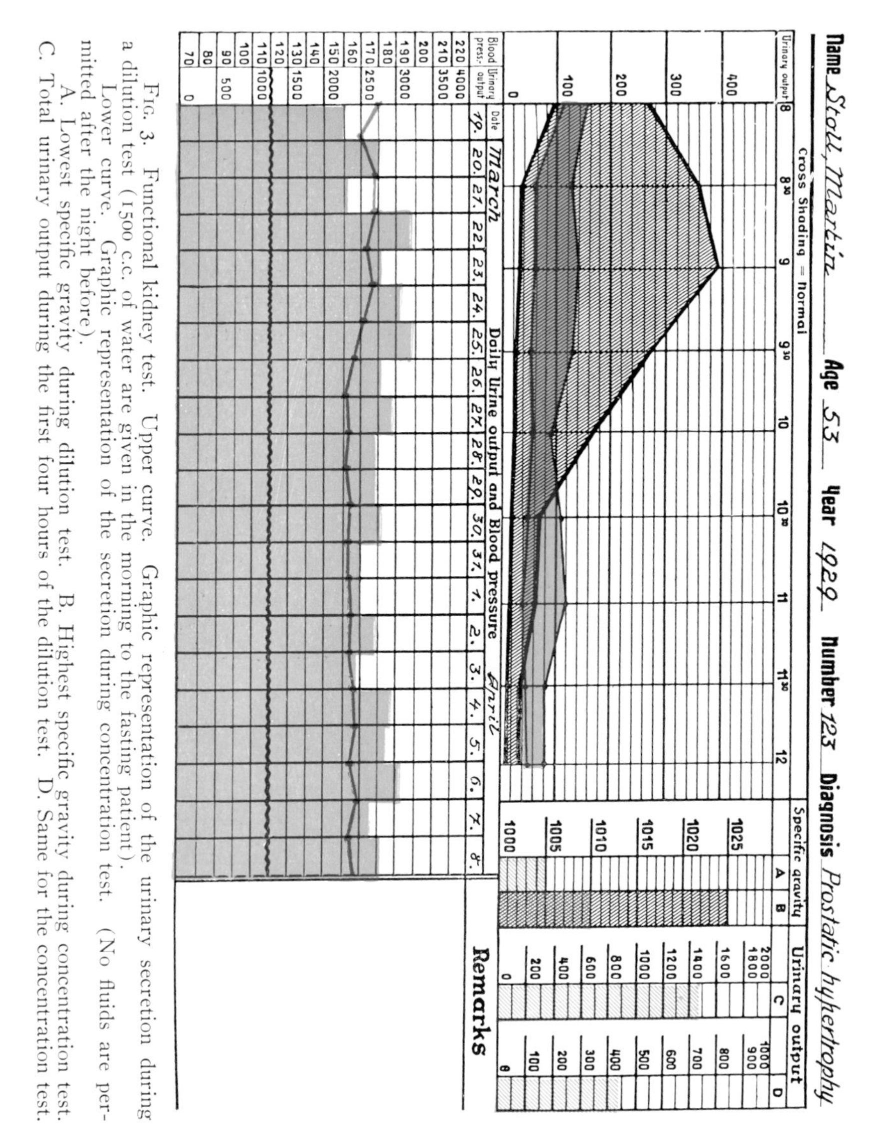

Fig. 3. Functional kidney test. Upper curve. Graphic representation of the urinary secretion during a dilution test (1500 c.c. of water are given in the morning to the fasting patient).
Lower curve. Graphic representation of the secretion during concentration test. (No fluids are permitted after the night before).
A. Lowest specific gravity during dilution test. B. Highest specific gravity during concentration test. C. Total urinary output during the first four hours of the dilution test. D. Same for the concentration test.

The Volhard test is carried out as follows: In the morning, after voiding, the fasting patient, at rest in bed, drinks one and a half liters of weak tea within a period of a half hour. The urine is collected every half hour and each specimen is kept separate. The quantity is measured and the specific gravity is determined. An individual with healthy kidneys eliminates the one and a half liters of fluid in four hours. The sooner the elimination begins (best in the first half hour intervals of a half liter at a time), and the more rapidly the specific gravity drops to about 1002, the more elastic are the kidneys. After the four-hour period, in an individual with healthy kidneys and on a dry diet, the specific gravity rapidly increases, and a specific gravity of 1030 will be reached the same evening. As the specific gravity increases the quantity of urine diminishes. The more inflexible the kidneys, the smaller is the half hour output of urine, the longer is the period of elimination, and the longer is the period before the specific gravity returns toward normal. Kidneys which are unable to concentrate the urine to a specific gravity of 1015 should be looked upon with suspicion. This figure is the lowest limit which the surgeon should accept from those presenting themselves for elective operations.

(b) **Water Restriction Test.** The fasting patient is given no fluid or nourishment after the evening preceding this test. The bladder is emptied at 7 o'clock in the morning. From 8 a.m. to 12 noon the urine is collected every half hour, the amounts are measured and the specific gravity estimated. Where kidney disease is not present the amount of urine excreted decreases steadily, so that at 8 o'clock not more than 100 c.c. are obtained, and this amount rapidly falls to 20 c.c., and finally to not more than 5 c.c. The specific gravity rises to 1025 or even higher. The more diseased the kidneys, the further the results deviate from the normal.

(c) Cryoscopy or **determination of the freezing point** of the blood is the simplest indirect test. It depends upon the following principle: The blood, that is the blood serum, is a solution of salts whose concentration in the healthy is nearly constant. The depression of the freezing point of a solution depends upon the quantity of salt present. The more concentrated a solution is, the more its freezing point falls below that of distilled water, which at atmospheric pressure is 0° C. One can thus determine the molecular concentration of this solution from the difference between the freezing point of it and that of distilled water and from this, determine the existence of a normal or abnormal balance between the blood and urine. The blood serum of an individual with healthy kidneys has a depression of the freezing point Δ of 0.56° C. The higher the kidney threshold for these salts, the greater Δ becomes and assumes a value of 0.65° C. or more. A normal value for Δ indicates nothing as to the condition of the individual kidney, but demonstrates merely that, as a whole, there is present enough functionally capable kidney tissue to maintain a normal nitrogen threshold. If one kidney is entirely destroyed and there is an increase in the value of Δ we know that the second kidney is diseased, because one normal kidney is capable of eliminating the waste products of metabolism and of maintaining a normal Δ value.

Experience has taught us that patients with nitrogen retention are not good risks for the more extensive operative procedures. Kümmel advises against operation on patients when Δ is greater than 0.60° C.

The freezing point of the blood may be determined with Beckmann's apparatus (Fig. 4). A very sensitive thermometer divided into 1/100 degrees projects well into a glass cylinder, in which the fluid to be examined is kept steadily in motion by means of a platinum stirrer. The glass cylinder is immersed in a freezing mixture and constantly stirred. The meniscus of the mercury column should be carefully watched. It continues to fall as the solution is stirred, then suddenly begins to rise. The instant the fluid freezes, the column of mercury rises to the freezing point and remains stationary for a time, later to fall slowly, from further cooling. The freezing point is the maximum height of the mercury at which it is stationary for some time, after its initial fall. The freezing point of distilled water should be determined first and then the freezing point of the defibrinated blood. The difference between the two figures gives the value of Δ.

(d) Analysis of the blood for **nitrogen retention** is a most useful method in hospital practice. The methods now used are simple enough to be conducted in any well organized laboratory, and yield information which is important both from the standpoint of diagnosis and prognosis. While it is possible to estimate urea nitrogen, uric acid nitrogen, the amino-acids, ammonia nitrogen, creatinine, and creatine, it is now generally accepted that the most useful information with regard to kidney function is obtained from an estimation of the blood urea and non-protein nitrogen.

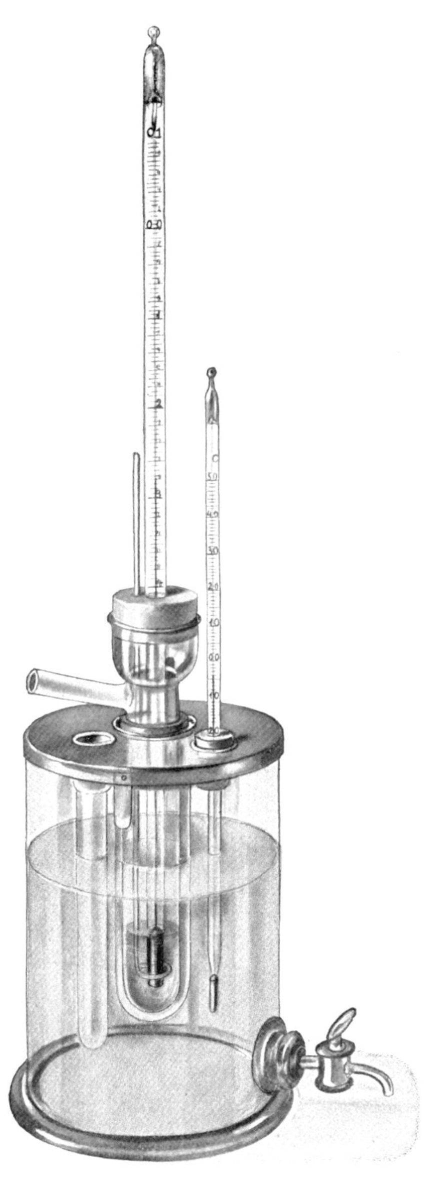

FIG. 4. Beckmann's apparatus for determination of the freezing point (cryoscopy).

Since the surgeon will not conduct these examinations himself, the technic is not included here. In certain forms of kidney damage, nitrogen products are held back by the kidney, so that these products tend to increase in the blood. The normal blood urea nitrogen value is from 12 to 20 mg. per 100 c.c. of blood, while that for non-protein nitrogen is 20 to 40 mg. per 100 c.c. It should be remembered that conditions other than nephritis may cause an increase of these substances in the blood. Thus prolonged vomiting, intestinal obstruction, and certain acute infections may cause nitrogen retention in the blood. If any of these conditions exist, or if there is any doubt as to which of two lesions is in a major part responsible for the nitrogen retention, the urinary urea should be estimated. If the nitrogen retention is due to renal disease the urinary urea will be lower than 2 per-cent, while in non-nephritic nitrogen retention the urea will be more than this.

It is well to remember that the nitrogen retention is not always proportional to the renal damage. Some authors hold that the estimation of the blood creatinine is of greater value, a content of over 1.5 mg. per 100 c.c. of blood supposedly being a definite sign of renal damage. Experience seems to indicate that the estimation of urea and non-protein nitrogen, which includes all the soluble nitrogenous products excepting protein, will as a rule give the information which the surgeon needs in making a decision for or against operation, on the basis of the retention of nitrogenous products in the blood.

(e) There remains one other commonly used method for the determination of kidney function. This method depends on the ability of the kidneys to eliminate certain dyes when injected into the blood stream. The use of indigocarmine and phenolsulphonphthalein as differential function tests will be discussed later, but the latter is used so extensively as a test of the function of both kidneys that it is included here.

The method was first described by Rowntree and Geraghty. The patient drinks 8 to 10 ounces of water and fifteen or twenty minutes later empties his bladder. One cubic centimeter of a specially prepared solution of the dye is injected either intramuscularly or intravenously. The urine is collected 65 minutes and two hours and five minutes after injection. The content of dye of each specimen is estimated separately, after making the specimens alkaline with 25 percent NaOH. and then making the volume of each up to 1000 c.c. with water. A sample is removed and read in a colorimeter against a known dilution of the dye. During the first hour a normal individual will excrete 50 percent or more of the dye, and during the second hour 20 percent of the dye. Any amount below a 65 to 70 percent total output of the dye can be regarded as an indication of functional deficiency of the kidneys.

Since, in many cases the kidney function can be improved by appropriate treatment, it is possible by repeated tests to estimate the improvement and to operate in elective cases when conditions are more favorable. An improvement of the pathologic changes of the diseased kidney, especially when fibrosis has occurred, can not be brought about by therapeusis. However, the renal function increases in many cases and with this improvement in function an improvement takes place in the general condition of the patient. The medical management in these cases should be entrusted to the internist and consists in improving the hygiene, in a frugal, non-irritating diet, low in proteins and salt as indicated, in regulation of the intake of fluids, in regulation of the intestinal action, and in improvement of the circulation.

I have adopted an exceptionally effective régime for handling those cases in which the urinary disturbance is due to an obstruction to the outflow of urine (hypertrophy of the prostate, urethral stricture). When the urinary retention is the result of prostatic obstruction slow decompression followed by some type of repeated drainage is essential. The establishment of an unobstructed urinary flow is an important feature in the care of these cases. This can, after slow decompression, be brought about through the drainage of the bladder by means of a permanent catheter equipped with suction, whether the urine is withdrawn through the urethra or through a suprapubic fistula. As a rule the kidneys respond to this procedure by increasing the output of urine, and by a gradual return to a more normal urine both in quantity and quality. It is well to await stabilization, since during the early period of increased urine output the general resistance of the patient is not good. It is often amazing how markedly impaired kidneys will again assume nearly normal function under such management, if the treatment is continued long enough. Thus the prognosis of the patient is improved.

We have discussed up to this time the methods used for the investigation of both kidneys. The information thus gained is sufficient when it is not planned to operate on the kidneys themselves. If such is the case one must know the **differential kidney function.** It is not permissible to operate on one kidney without knowing exactly the functional capacity of the other. Unless this rule is strictly adhered to, the surgeon will at times find himself in a very precarious position. The surgeon must ascertain whether the supposed or demonstrated kidney lesion affects one or both kidneys, and if only one, which one. If one kidney shows the major lesion will the kidney which is to remain be able to carry on the function of the two so as not to jeopardize life?

Some knowledge of the function of each kidney may be obtained by direct observation of the condition of the ureteral orifice and by observing the type of excretion from it, but preferably by collecting the urine from each kidney separately after ureteral catheterization and the subsequent examination of these specimens by procedures previously described for the total urine.

The inspection of the ureteral orifices is as a rule done by cystoscopy, exceptionally after suprapubic cystotomy. Rigidity of the orifice of the ureter or pathological changes around it indicate disease of the corresponding kidney. If in spite of prolonged observation of a ureteral orifice no fluid is seen to escape from it, while from the other side there is a normal flow, one can assume that one kidney is not functioning or that there is some obstruction to its outflow. If there is a discharge of pus from a ureteral orifice, or a concretion is observed, or if blood appears in the urine before the introduction of a ureteral catheter, there is clear indication of kidney disease. Chromo-ureteroscopy permits one by mere cystoscopic observation of the ureteral orifice to obtain valuable information as to the condition of the corresponding kidney.

The ease with which urine can be obtained by ureteral catheterization warrants this being done. The simultaneous catheterization of both ureters is desirable.

Urine obtained from each kidney in this manner, can be examined by the usual urine tests, which have been discussed previously, and by comparing the findings of the two specimens important deductions can be drawn. Besides the routine chemical examination these specimens should be examined for pus cells, cylinders, casts, epithelium, and bacteria. Cultures may be made and if tuberculosis is suspected a guinea pig should be inoculated with some of the urine. It must be emphasized that the finding of certain constituents, especially tubercle bacilli, in both specimens, although suggestive, does not prove positively a disease of both kidneys, because bacteria or other material in the bladder may be carried to the healthy ureter during the introduction of the catheter, and appear in the urine from the healthy kidney. Since the introduction of a catheter may traumatize a healthy ureter so that bleeding results, the presence of blood in the urine subsequent to ureteral catheterization is of little significance. The specific gravity of the urine from both sides, its urea and chloride content, can be determined and compared. It is possible to compare the quantity of urine eliminated by each kidney during a given time with the quantity of water ingested; to compare the percentage of dye elimination from each kidney, as well as the individual concentrating capacity of these organs. The absence of fluid or a reduction in its quantity from a catheter can only be accepted as evidence of a diminution or absence of kidney action, when it can be demonstrated, preferably after the administration of a dye, that no fluid is reaching the bladder by passing around the catheter. If a fluid of a low specific gravity flows continually from the catheter, instead of concentrated urine coming in regular spurts, there probably exists a dilatation of the kidney pelvis, or a hydronephrosis.

In studying differential kidney function, the use of dyes, which may be given intramuscularly or intravenously, is of the utmost importance. By this method one can determine first, the time elapsing between the intramuscular or intravenous injection of such a substance and the beginning of its elimination by the kidneys; second, the concentration at different periods, and third, the duration of its elimination. The more rapidly the dye appears, the more concentrated it is, and the shorter the period for complete elimination, the better is the kidney function. The comparison of the results obtained from each kidney permits one to estimate fully the differential function.

Indigocarmine is used for this work more generally than any other substance. In this test we place one tablet of carmine coerul, 0.08 gm., and sodium chloride, 0.1 gm., in a sterile flask, to which are added 20 c.c. of distilled water. The salts are dissolved by gentle heat. A 0.4 percent solution of the dye is thus obtained. After cooling the solution to body temperature, the entire amount is injected into the gluteal muscles, or better, 4 to 5 c.c. (in children 2 to 3 c.c.) of the solution are injected into an arm vein.

After the intramuscular injection, the healthy kidney begins to eliminate the dye in from 5 to 10 minutes, the dye reaches the maximum concentration in about 20 minutes, and elimination ceases after 12 hours at the latest. After intravenous injection the dye should appear in from 2 to 3 minutes, reach its maximum concentration a short time later, and be completely eliminated in one and a half hours. Delay in appearance, prolongation of the duration of elimination, and inability to concentrate the dye are evidences of impairment of kidney function.

There are other substances also used in elimination tests, such as phenolsulphonphthalein and phloridzin, as well as the urea and chloride content of the urine from each side. However, the results obtained by the use of indigocarmine and phenolsulphonphthalein have been so satisfactory that, except in exceptional cases, other elimination tests are unnecessary.

In the phenolsulphonphthalein test 1 c.c. of the dye (0.006 gm.) is injected intramuscularly or intravenously. In each collecting receptacle are placed a few drops of a weak sodium hydroxide solution. The appearance of the dye causes the solution to turn red. The healthy kidney begins to eliminate it in from 3 to 5 minutes after injection.

The urea determinations can be made by any one of a number of standard methods. Determination of the freezing point is carried out in the same manner as was described for the blood, except that 20 c.c. of urine are used instead of blood. If the urine from one kidney has a higher freezing point than the urine from the other kidney, it is evident that the former kidney is not functioning normally, and the closer the freezing point approaches that for water the more damage has taken place.

It is not necessary to make all the tests in each case. In most instances the function can be determined by a few examinations. If a kidney secretes the proper quantity of a light golden urine of normal specific gravity, within the proper interval of time, in which urine there are no pus cells, bacteria nor albumin, it is fairly certain that it is healthy and competent to assume the entire kidney activity. The longer one kidney has had to assume the entire burden, and still has been able to maintain adequate secretory function, the more definite is the possibility of unilateral nephrectomy without disturbance of the nitrogen balance. Any doubt still remaining may be satisfied by the indigocarmine test.

The x-ray examination of the kidneys and the ureters is valuable and in many cases indispensable. The healthy kidney is not always visualized in the roentgenogram. In the majority of instances it is necessary to determine its position, the position and form of the kidney pelvis, and of the ureters by the use of shadow casting substances, or the use of an opaque ureteral catheter. In the United States a sodium iodide solution is most frequently used. Much information can be gained from the ease with which the catheter can be introduced and the amount of fluid necessary to fill the kidney pelvis. The solution is introduced by gravity. In this manner we derive information as to the form, location, size and anatomical arrangement of the kidney and ureter. The horseshoe kidney and double ureter are frequently diagnosed by this method. It is also possible at times to demonstrate the presence of stones. Most stones give a distinct shadow; but here again it is advisable practice to use pyelography so that calcified glands or phleboliths may be eliminated. Lateral, or better, stereoscopic plates are often essential. These findings can be supplemented by the production of pneumoperitoneum, when if the patient is placed in a suitable position the air will reach the kidney to be x-rayed. According to Rosenstein, air inflation in the neighborhood of the kidney has not been given the attention which it deserves.

Since the introduction of **Uroselectan** by von Lichtenberg, the surgeon and urologist have added another method for pelvic, ureteral, and bladder visualization. The intravenous injection of 40 grams of this dye, which contains iodine, will permit of the visualization of the calyces, the pelvis, and the ureter without ureteral catheterization.

The last method of determining the extent and type of the kidney lesion is by operative exposure, where if necessary the kidney may be incised down to the kidney pelvis. Exploratory incision may be used to determine the extent and degree of the renal damage, or it may be used in order to determine the presence of a kidney which visually is not diseased and which apparently can undertake the function of the kidney to be removed.

It is impossible for some patients to urinate while lying down, and at times even while sitting. One may try to train them before operation. Should the patient be unable to void after operation and after every possible means has been used to stimulate voluntary urination, catheterization should be resorted to.

In some cases of **postoperative urine retention** one may obtain voluntary evacuation by the intravenous injection of 5 c.c. of a 40 percent uro-

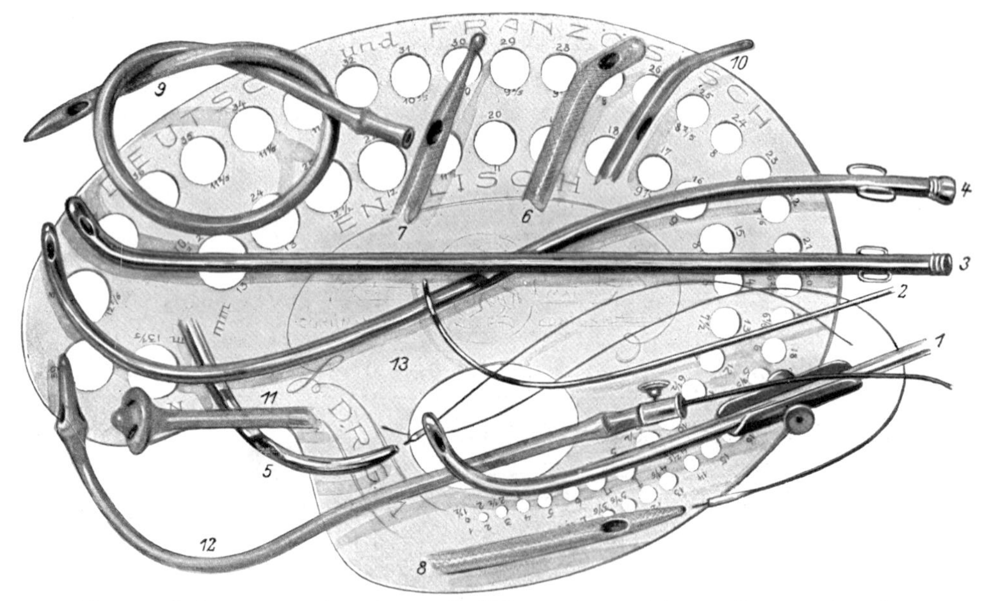

FIG. 5. Catheters of various forms, flexibility and materials. 1. Bent metal catheter of medium weight with sliding shuttle for lubricant. 2. Small metal curved catheter. 3. Metal catheter with Mercier's curve. 4. Double curved metal catheter. 5. Metal catheter with filiform bougie. 6. Silk catheter with Mercier's curve. 7. Straight silk catheter. 8. Silk catheter with filiform bougie. 9. Nelaton catheter. 10. Thiemann catheter. 11. Pezzer catheter. 12. Pezzer catheter on curved metal stylet. 13. Catheter gauge.

tropin solution (Vogt). If unsuccessful this may be repeated in 2 hours. This drug has often given satisfactory results when used orally in 1 gm. doses given every hour for 3 or 4 doses. I am of the opinion however, that catheterization is simpler, less dangerous, and more positive. After one catheterization the patient will frequently be able to void spontaneously. In other cases the disability persists for days. Then, according to necessity, the patient should be catheterized at least twice daily, or an indwelling catheter should be inserted.

Catheterization. Catheterization requires the same careful attention to asepsis as a major operation. The maintenance of proper asepsis is best accomplished, when the field of operation and the catheters are not touched by the operator's hands. This technic can be easily attained. The correct

third phase, which deviation the operator should carefully follow. The rigid catheter is removed by reversing the phases of its introduction.

The catheterization of man with semi-soft catheters is carried out in the same way as catheterization with a rigid catheter. The changes of direction in the various phases are not so sharply pronounced because of the flexibility of the catheter.

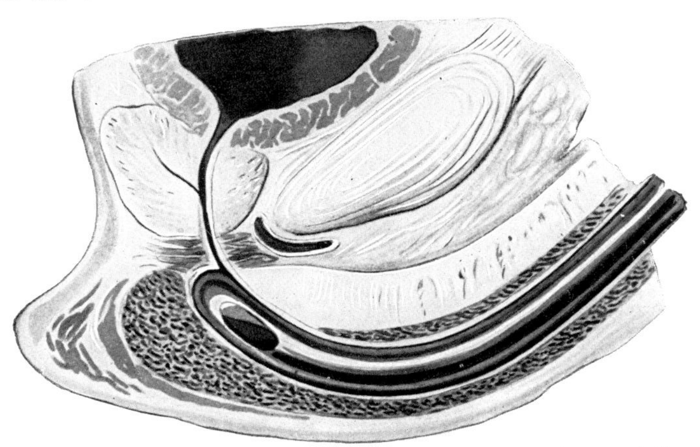

FIG. 13. The tip of the catheter is caught in a fold of mucous membrane of the posterior wall of the urethra.

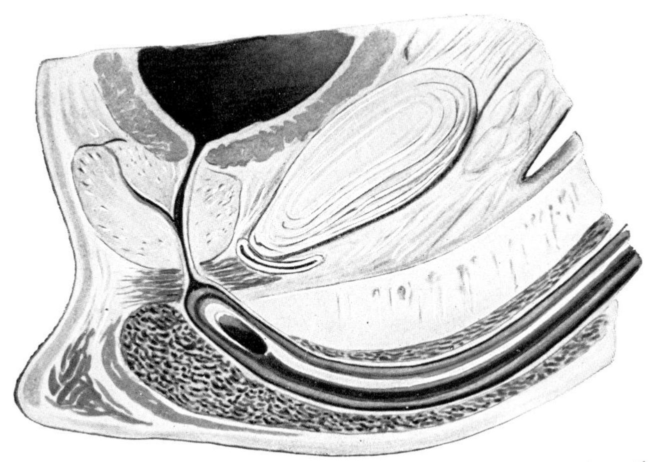

FIG. 14. By leverage the tip of the catheter is raised and pressed against the anterior wall. It is thus freed and can then slide into the bladder.

Catheterization in the female is simple with any kind of catheter. The catheter is introduced into the urethral orifice after properly retracting the labia.

Difficulties in Catheterization. If a phimosis blocks the entrance of the urethra, it should be split on the dorsal side, after injecting local anæsthesia. If the external urethral orifice is too narrow for the catheter, it should be either stretched, or split with the scissors in the direction of the frenum, under local anæsthesia. During introduction the catheter sometimes gets caught in a pocket of the mucous membrane on the posterior wall (Fig. 13).

The catheter should then be withdrawn and reintroduced making light pressure on the anterior urethral wall (Fig. 14). If this does not suffice one can facilitate matters by inserting the left index finger into the rectum and guiding the catheter forward (Fig. 15).

In the absence of an organic stricture of the urethra, there may also occur another point of resistance at the internal orifice as the result of a spasm of the sphincter. Making constant light pressure one waits, for several minutes, until the catheter, after the relaxation of the spasm, enters the bladder. Oftentimes the resistance of the sphincter can be gradually overcome by the

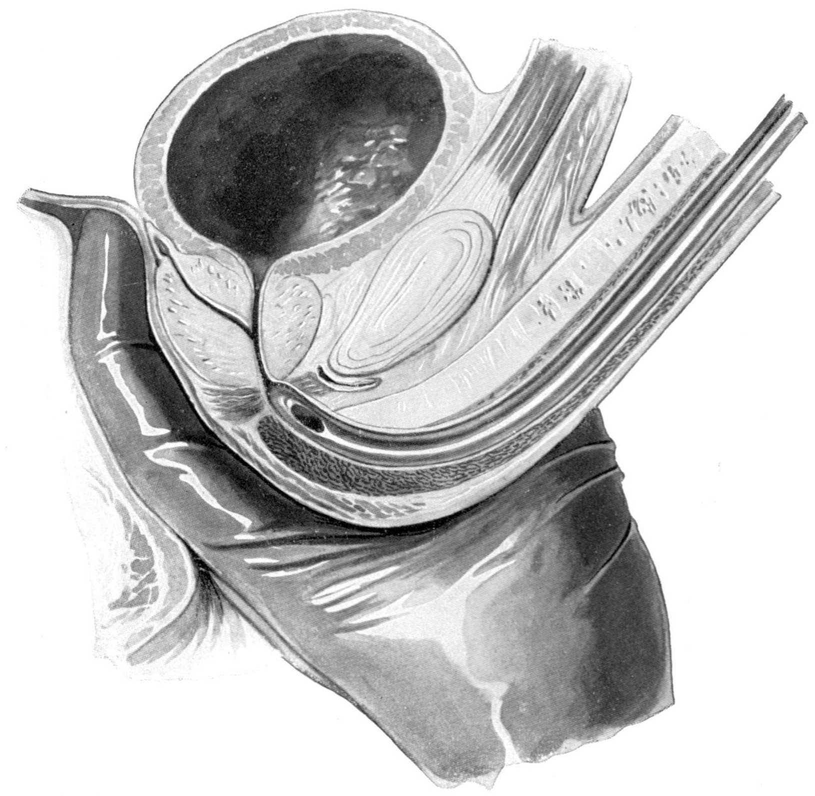

FIG. 15. The index finger introduced into the rectum, supports the rigid catheter as it is inserted.

water pressure of a closed irrigator, at a height of ½ to 1 meter. In the presence of a stricture of the urethra the stenosis can occasionally, though sometimes only after considerable trouble, be passed with a filiform attachment which is attached to a fine catheter, the latter following the filiform into the bladder. The passing of a filiform bougie succeeds more frequently however when one introduces a whole bundle of the filiforms into the locally anæsthetized urethra and tries alternatively to push forward the individual bougies.

The Permanent Catheter. The only practical permanent catheter is the soft Nelaton catheter. Only when its introduction proves unsuccessful, is it permissible and then only under exceptional circumstances, to leave a semi-rigid catheter in the urethra for a short time. The retention of the permanent catheter creates difficulties and in spite of numerous proposals there is, as yet, no entirely successful method.

In cases where it has been very difficult to insert and where retention is essential for recovery I have fastened it, in addition to using one of the methods described below, in man, by a silk stitch through the frenum; in the female, by a silk stitch through the lower part of the clitoris. After a few days the stitch may be removed.

We can successfully attach a permanent catheter to the penis for a period of time by adhesive plaster strips, or by a mastic elastic cloth. The fastening of the catheter with adhesive plaster and elastic cloth can be done either through a rubber ring, or cuff, provided with two safety pins, or by two silk threads.

The rubber ring, or cuff, is pulled on the catheter, as described in Chapter III, on the drawing of rubber rings on rubber tubes. The ring is fastened on the catheter at its exit from the urethra. Transversely through the rubber ring are placed two safety pins, a small tampon being wrapped around the catheter between the safety pins and the end of the penis, to prevent pressure of the pins on the glans penis.

The catheter is fixed by adhesive plaster in the following manner. A strip of adhesive plaster, about 25 cm. long, provided in the center with a small hole through which the end of the catheter passes, is attached along both sides of the stretched penis so that it presses the safety pins against the tampon on the tip of the penis. The retention of the adhesive plaster strip is insured by a second plaster strip wrapped around the penis in a spiral form (Fig. 16).

If one employs the mastic elastic coat, the extended penis is covered with mastic and over this is rolled a knitted webbing of proportional width. The safety pins of the rubber ring are fixed through the end of the webbing jacket and the jacket is tied over the catheter with a silk thread (Fig. 17).

If it is desired to use silk threads for further retention of the catheter, in conjunction with a mastic jacket or adhesive plaster band, these should be passed around the catheter, near the urethral orifice, and tied tightly enough to assist in the retention of the catheter but not to constrict it. Each silk thread is passed through either the webbing or the adhesive plaster (Fig. 17) and then tied.

The soft Pezzer catheter is self-retaining because of its mushroom-like tip (Fig. 5). Before introduction it is stretched over a stylet, and by this means the tip is elongated and offers very little resistance when introduced. If used in this way the stylet should be curved so that the catheter is introduced in the same manner as a rigid catheter. This may present certain difficulties in the male, but none in the female. For an indwelling catheter in the latter I prefer this type. The Pezzer catheter can be removed through the urethra with gentle traction.

Diabetes is a complication which effects adversely the prognosis in every surgical operation. The surgeon, however, is better able to take care of the surgical diseases of the diabetic since the introduction of insulin. The complications most feared in the diabetic after surgical intervention are acidosis and coma. In the diabetic there is a greater tendency to wound infection from a diminution of the resistance of the tissues, which is associated with the hyperglycemia that attends faulty carbohydrate metabolism. In many of these cases there exists also varying degrees of arteriosclerosis.

Insulin provides an effective means for controlling the hyperglycemia and assists in the prevention and treatment of acidosis and coma. By its use

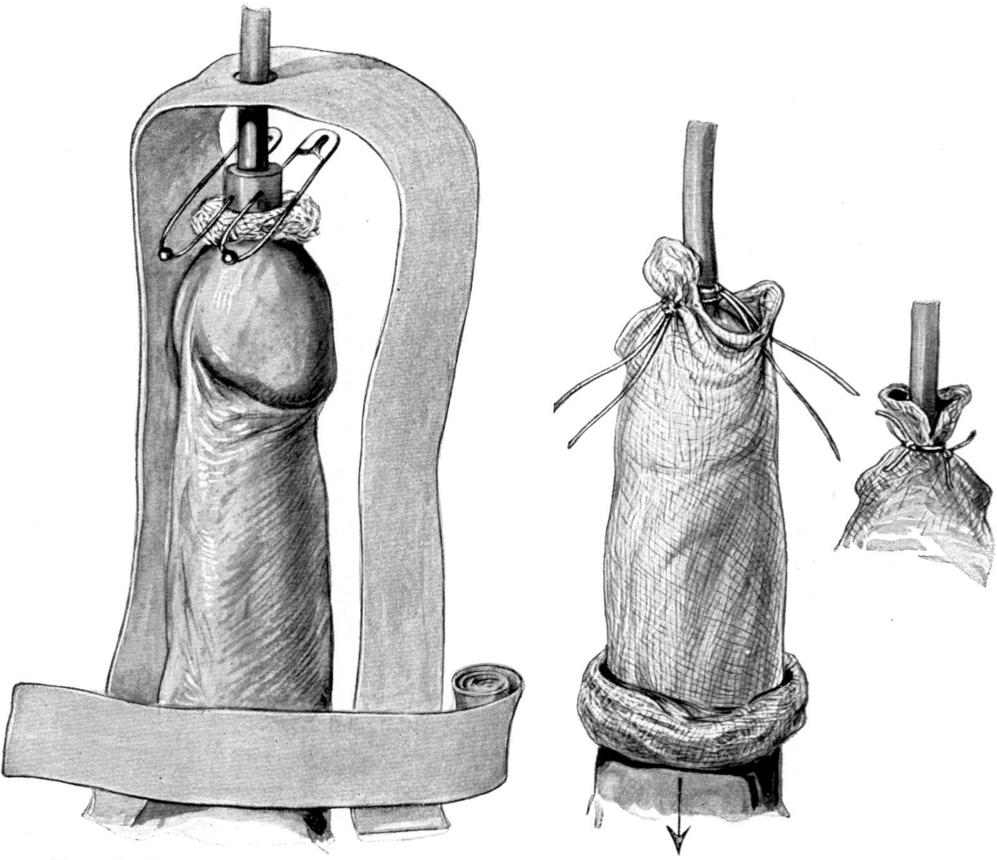

FIG. 16. Retention of a permanent catheter with adhesive plaster. A strip of adhesive to be fastened to the length of the penis is perforated for the passage of the catheter. When in place it immobilizes two safety pins fastened to the catheter by means of a rubber ring. The strip of adhesive is held securely in place by a second adhesive strip wrapped in a spiral turn.

FIG. 17. Fastening of a permanent catheter with a mastic covered gauze tube. Through the end of a gauze tube fastened to the penis with mastic, two silk threads tied around the catheter are stitched and tied.

the function of the organism is increased as is the resistance against infection. The possibility of successful operation can therefore be considerably increased with this aid.

Uninfected wounds in diabetics, whose diabetes has been controlled with insulin, unite as do those of the non-diabetic, nearly always by first intention. In the surgical treatment of carbuncle the postoperative course of the diabetic treated with insulin is often similar to that of the non-diabetic. In diabetic gangrene with a mild secondary infection I have observed that under insulin administration and proper surgical treatment the inflammation frequently subsides rapidly. In suitable cases one may confine himself to a mere minor amputation such as the removal of gangrenous toes or feet. This is especially true when there does not exist extensive arterial changes. On the contrary widely spread infections, in spite of intensive insulin therapy do not exhibit the same tendency toward recovery. (The individual with diabetes and severe infection presents a difficult surgical problem since the two conditions act in a vicious circle. I. S. R.)

I have found local anæsthesia most satisfactory in this disease. Adrenalin should not be used with the local anæsthesia since it counteracts the action of insulin by causing a hyperglycemia. Spinal anæsthesia is frequently well tolerated. If a general anæsthetic can not be avoided, nitrous oxide and oxygen are preferable to other agents. Chloroform and ether should not be used.

The operation itself should be carried out rapidly, with a minimum of trauma to the patient. The type of wound should be as simple as possible. Even if insulin therapy succeeds best when controlled by the internist, the surgeon should acquaint himself with its use so as to be able to use it in an emergency. Insulin can be given subcutaneously or intravenously, but it does not act when given by mouth. Its maximum effect when given subcutaneously occurs 2 to 3 hours after injection, and the frequency of the administration must depend upon the severity of the symptoms. It should be given from one to two hours before a meal. One unit of insulin takes care of from 1.5 to 2 gm. of sugar. In emergencies it is sufficient for the surgeon to know the amount of sugar in the urine, and the qualitative test for ketone bodies. However if time exists the blood sugar should also be ascertained, as well as the plasma carbon dioxide.

The patient must be carefully followed before and after operation, and constant use should be made of the laboratory. Unless this is done the dosage of insulin and the diet can not be carefully controlled. An overdose of insulin may cause varying degrees of hypoglycemia, the symptom complex at times going so far as to present the picture known as hypoglycemic shock. Hypoglycemia is recognized by unrest, irritation, tremor, palpitation, sweating, vasomotor disturbances, cramps, and finally by a loss of consciousness. As a rule hypoglycemia will not result as long as glycosuria is present. At the first indication of hypoglycemia, one should administer sugar by mouth or glucose intravenously with or without insulin, depending upon the amount of glucose injected.

It is exceedingly difficult to outline any exact method for the preparation of the diabetic patient for operation or for the postoperative care. The dosage of insulin, the method of its administration, and the question of glucose injection coincident with the insulin will vary in every patient. It should be further emphasized that unless the insulin dosage is very carefully controlled by blood and urine analyses disaster may result. The help of an internist interested in problems of this type should not be underestimated.

In instances where immediate operation was imperative and the patient was in coma, I have injected immediately 50 units of insulin subcutaneously and 50 units intravenously. After 2 to 3 hours more insulin can be administered, depending on the indications. In severe coma 200 to 300 units may be necessary in the first 24 hours, but I must again stress the fact that no exact rules can be laid down, for the measures to be taken depend on the blood analysis.

If operation is necessary in a moderately severe diabetic who is not in coma, insulin is best given before operation, or immediately after operation. In these cases I find that glucose and insulin give the most satisfactory results.

In operations where a short delay is possible, it is preferable to study the blood and urine before administering insulin. It may be possible by careful control of the diet to so reduce the hyperglycemia that insulin is not necessary. If after operation the diabetes is aggravated, insulin can then be given as indicated. If even though the patient is on a carefully controlled diet, hyperglycemia and glycosuria still persist, then the excess of carbohydrate in the blood can be reduced by the use of insulin. These patients require adequate nourishment, 30 to 35 calories per kilo of body weight. The exact ratio of protein, carbohydrate, and fat must be varied in different patients. One gram of protein should be given for each kilo of body weight. The carbohydrate is best given in the form of 5 and 10 percent vegetables.

The use of a basal requirement diet plus the use of insulin in gradually increasing doses until the hyperglycemia is brought under control marks a distinct advance in the preparation of the diabetic patient requiring surgical treatment. In some instances the blood sugar can be reduced to normal limits. In others the blood sugar may still be elevated, but there results only a slight glycosuria, and acetonuria disappears.

The diet should be of known caloric value, and the blood sugar should be estimated daily as well as a 24 hour estimation of the urinary sugar and the presence of ketone bodies. An intimate knowledge of the food-stuffs is essential in ordering a diet for the diabetic patient. One must know the amount of carbohydrate, fat, and protein in each article of the diet. From this the caloric value of each article of the diet can be calculated, since 1 gram of protein and carbohydrate is equivalent to 4 calories, and 1 gram of fat to 9 calories.

An increase in the diet will depend on how well the patient tolerates the basal diet. It is well to remember that in the early stages a rapid increase in diet is not always essential. The necessity for insulin and the dosage of this will depend on the capacity of the patient for taking care of the diet given. Insulin should not be used in the milder cases unless the patient can not take an adequate diet without support. The basal diet must of course vary with the age and weight of the patient. The adult requires 30 to 35 calories for every kilo of body weight, so that a patient weighing approximately 50 kilos requires about 1695 calories, while one weighing 75 kilos requires about 2520 calories. Women are supposed to require slightly less calories than men, while children require more.

It should be remembered that these are basal requirements, so that the surgeon should attempt as soon as possible to get his patient on a diet approximately 20 percent above the basal requirement.

Diets 1 to 4 are so constructed as to allow an increase of carbohydrate from 40 grams to 125 grams, with suitable increase of fat for a person of 60 kg. weight who is free of ketonuria. At the bottom of each diet there is given the total amount of fat that might be given to have a ketogenic anti-ketogenic ratio of 1 to 1.5, assuming that the urine is free of sugar. The amount of protein allowed should be that amount which will allow 1 gram for each kilogram of weight. The protein content can be varied by increasing or decreasing the amount of meat or eggs, and correcting for the fat of the eggs.

Diet 6, which is higher in carbohydrate and lower in fat is indicated when diacetic acid is found in the urine. (These diets were prepared by Dr. Leon Jonas of the Hospital of the University of Pennsylvania. I. S. R.)

The administration of insulin must be carefully controlled during the convalescence by examining the 24 hour urine output for its sugar content and ketone bodies, and by repeated blood sugar estimations. In the pyogenic infections it will be found that the dosage of insulin must be reduced as the infection is brought under control.

In ketonuria, glucose and insulin should be administered immediately, and the proteins and fats should be reduced. The amount of glucose, or glucose and insulin, necessary to cause a disappearance of the ketone bodies varies considerably. It is ofttimes proper to neglect the appearance of sugar in the urine on the day of operation, and to give glucose (50-60 gm. of a 5 percent solution) intravenously with insulin just before the anæsthetization.

The degree of ketosis or acidosis can be estimated roughly, but simply, from examination of the urine. The appearance of acetone bodies in the urine indicates an imbalance in the physiology of neutrality regulation. This acid-base equilibrium is a very complex one, and unless the surgeon fully understands the modern conception of this subject he should consult with some one who does. The term acidosis means a reduction or depletion of the alkali reserve. It is important to keep one thing in mind, a patient may be in a state of acidosis while the hydrogen ion concentration of the blood is normal. The reduction of the alkali reserve precedes the rise in the hydrogen ion concentration, so that the former is a valuable means for estimating when treatment is necessary.

When severe acidosis is present the carbohydrates should not be reduced since coma may result. Under such circumstances the diet must be carefully watched. The fats are first reduced, then the proteins, and lastly the carbohydrates. The use of insulin and glucose in the presence of coma should not be underestimated. One or two grams of glucose per unit of insulin should be given. The glucose had best be given intravenously if the acidosis is threatening.

The use of sodium bicarbonate in these cases is not agreed upon by all workers in this field. I have frequently used it, giving often as much as 10 grams per day either by mouth or by rectal drip in a 5 percent solution.

(A word of caution in regard to the use of glucose solutions by the rectal drip method may not be amiss. Evidence is accumulating that glucose is absorbed very slowly, if at all, by this route, so that it should not be depended upon in an emergency. I. S. R.)

Diet #1	P. 60	F. 76	C. 40
Grapefruit 75			5
Oatmeal 50	1		6
Cream 50	1	11	1
Egg 1	6	6	
Lister Bread 20	4	2	
Butter 5		3	
Tea or Coffee 10 c.c. Cream		2	
Meat 90	20	26	
Broth 200	4		
Vegetable—5%			5
Vegetable—10%			10
Lister Bread 20	4	2	
Butter 5		3	
Tea or Coffee 10 c.c. Cream		2	
Lister Bread 20	4	2	
Eggs 2	12	12	
Vegetable—5%			5
Orange 50			6
Butter 5		3	
Lettuce 50			1
Broth 200	4		
Tea or Coffee 10 c.c. Cream		2	
	60	76	39

Total fat allowed to have $\frac{K}{AK} = 1.5 = 110$ grams.

Total Calories = 1084.

Diet #2	P. 60	F. 117	C. 60
Grapefruit 75			5
Eggs 2	12	12	
Oatmeal 100	2		12
Butter 15		12	
Cream 100	3	22	3
Lister Bread 10	2	1	
Tea or Coffee 10 c.c. Cream		2	
Broth 200	4		
Meat 90	20	26	
Vegetable—10%			15
Vegetable—5%			5
Butter 15		12	
Lister Bread 10	2	1	
Tea or Coffee 10 c.c. Cream		2	
Eggs 2	12	12	
Vegetable—5%			5
Lister Bread 10	2	1	
Butter 15		12	
Orange 125			15
Tea or Coffee 10 c.c. Cream		2	
	59	117	60

Total fat allowed to have $\frac{K}{AK} = 1.5 = 150$ grams.

Total Calories = 1533.

DIET #3	P. 60	F. 135	C. 80
Grapefruit 75			5
Bacon 15		9	
Oatmeal 100	2		12
Egg 1	6	6	
Butter 15		12	
Cream 100	3	22	3
Lister Bread 20	4	2	
Tea or Coffee 10 c.c. Cream		2	
Potato 50	1		10
Meat 90	20	26	
Vegetable—10%			10
Vegetable—5%			5
Butter 20		18	
Lister Bread 20	4	2	
Tea or Coffee 10 c.c. Cream		2	
Eggs 2	12	12	
Vegetable—5%			5
Lister Bread 20	4	2	
Butter 20		18	
Orange 100			12
Potato 90	2		18
Tea or Coffee 10 c.c. Cream		2	
	58	135	80

Total fat allowed to have $\frac{K}{AK} = 1.5 = 190$ grams.

Total Calories = 1748.

DIET #4	P. 60	F. 156	C. 100
Grapefruit 150			11
Eggs 2	12	12	
Oatmeal 125	3		15
Butter 20		18	
Cream 100	3	22	3
Bacon 30		18	
White Bread 25	2		13
Tea or Coffee 10 c.c. Cream		2	
Meat 90	20	26	
Butter 25		21	
Vegetable—5%			5
Vegetable—10%			10
White Bread 25	2		13
Tea or Coffee 10 c.c. Cream		2	
Butter 25		21	
Broth 200	4		
Eggs 2	12	12	
Vegetable—5%			5
Orange 100			12
White Bread 25	2		13
Tea or Coffee 10 c.c. Cream		2	
	60	156	100

Total fat allowed to have $\frac{K}{AK} = 1.5 = 230$ grams.

Total Calories = 2044.

DIET #5	P. 60	F. 181	C. 126
Grapefruit 150			11
Eggs 2	12	12	
Oatmeal 125	3		15
Butter 20		18	
Cream 100	3	22	3
Bacon 30		18	
White Bread 25	2		13
Tea or Coffee 10 c.c. Cream		2	
Meat 90	20	26	
Butter 25		21	
Vegetable—5%			5
Vegetable—10%			10
Potato 100	2		20
White Bread 25	2		13
Tea or Coffee 10 c.c. Cream		2	
Butter 25		21	
Broth 100	2		
Eggs 2	12	12	
Vegetable—5%			5
Orange 150			18
Oil 25		25	
White Bread 25	2		13
Tea or Coffee 10 c.c. Cream		2	
	60	181	126

Total fat allowed to have $\frac{K}{AK} = 1.5 = 280$ grams.

Total Calories = 2369.

DIET #6	P. 60	F. 54	C. 125
Grapefruit 150			11
Oatmeal 150	3		18
Milk 100	3	4	5
Egg 1	6	6	
Tea or Coffee 10 c.c. Cream		2	
Meat 90	20	26	
Broth 200	4		
Vegetable—5%			5
Vegetable—10%			10
Potato 90	2		18
White Bread 25 gms.	2		13
Tea or Coffee 10 c.c. Cream		2	
Eggs 2	12	12	
Potato 75	2		15
Vegetable—5%			5
Orange 100			12
Broth 200	4		
White Bread 25 gms.	2		13
Tea or Coffee 10 c.c. Cream		2	
	60	54	125

50 grams of rice may be substituted for 60 gms. of potato or 100 gms. of orange.
Total Calories = 1199.
This diet is to be used when a low fat-high carbohydrate diet is indicated, *i.e.*, mild acidosis.

While simple postoperative acetonuria in the non-diabetic requires no special treatment, if clinical symptoms of acidosis occur, such as: dryness of the mouth, vomiting, rising pulse rate, restlessness, sighing respiration, and stupor, they are indications for immediate treatment. These symptoms are similar to those seen in the acidosis of diabetes, but they are rarely observed in so aggravated a form. The treatment consists in the administration of glucose, with or without insulin, so that the excess fatty acids can be oxidized and thereby not deplete the alkali reserve. Sodium bicarbonate may also be used. The ingestion of carbohydrates counteracts acidosis. If the patient is unable to take food by mouth, a 5 percent solution of glucose should be given intravenously. Such infusions not only counteract the acidosis but have a definite alterative effect on the patient.

While glucose may be given alone in many cases, occasionally it is necessary to give small doses of insulin with it in order to obtain the desired effect. In these cases 5 to 10 units of insulin are injected subcutaneously five minutes after the glucose has been administered. In cases of collapse with evident acidosis striking results have been obtained by the use of 50 percent solutions of glucose. If large amounts of fluid are also desired it is well to give the glucose in weaker concentrations, 10 to 15 percent. Insulin is often of value in these cases, but the amount can not be definitely stated since it must be determined for each individual patient. However, it should not exceed one unit for every two grams of glucose administered.

3. Lungs

The danger of postoperative pulmonary complications in the form of bronchitis, broncho-pneumonia, lobar pneumonia, atelectasis or embolism is great, especially after operations in the upper abdomen and the upper respiratory passages. About 27 percent of our postoperative deaths are associated with pulmonary complications. Patients suffering from respiratory disease should be operated on only when an emergency demands it. In other instances the surgeon should wait until the patient has been adequately treated and has been put in the best possible condition.

During an epidemic of respiratory infection in the community it is well to operate only on those patients where the operation is one of necessity, and to delay elective operations. Many of the postoperative pulmonary complications which occur during such a period are the result of lowering the resistance of the patient to the infecting organism. In a certain group of patients, especially the heavy cigarette smokers, a morning cough will persist indefinitely. However if there are no physical signs in the lungs operation may be resorted to with reasonable assurance that all will go well as far as the respiratory system is concerned.

Plenty of fresh dust-free air and sunshine are the best available means of preparing patients with chronic bronchitis for operation. Rest in bed is not essential in the majority of instances. If prolonged rest in bed, due to the basic cause, can not be avoided, I try to relieve the exhausting cough by putting the patient in the sitting position. I realize that some authors favor a head down position so as to favor ciliary action, but in my experience the sitting position has proved more satisfactory. I minimize hypostatic congestion by frequent change of position, systematic breathing exercises and by free movements ("Promenade in bed!"). The overhead suspension renders a distinct service in these cases, providing an easy means for the patient to lift himself and alter his position. (Fig. 2.) The breathing exercises, reinforced with periodic inhalations of carbon dioxide, stimulate pulmonary ventilation. After an acute respiratory infection one should postpone nonurgent operations for some time.

Careful oral prophylaxis should be practised before operation. Besides careful cleansing of the teeth previous to operation, all decayed teeth and tartar should, if possible, be removed before operating on elective cases. In all patients susceptible to repeated infections of the respiratory organs, local anæsthesia is to be preferred and ether is to be avoided. Many of these postoperative pulmonary complications are due to chilling as a result of exposure during transport of the patient from his room or ward to the operating room through poorly heated or draughty corridors; to waiting in an insufficiently heated anæsthetizing room; to needless exposure in the operating room; to the cold bed provided for receiving the patient after operation, and to poorly heated or draughty rooms used for the patient after operation. While a healthy individual may not be affected by such conditions, a sick person is extremely sensitive to them, especially while under an anæsthetic. During anæsthesia the heat regulating apparatus is disturbed and the patient's cutaneous area assumes the temperature of the surrounding media. As a result of this, preparation, anæsthesia, and operating rooms should have a carefully regulated temperature. Although a temperature of 25° C. is disagreeable for the operating staff it is best for the patient. The patient should be dressed in warm underwear even during the operation, and only that part necessary for adequate exposure for the operation should be removed.

Heated operating tables have not proved satisfactory. In special instances patients in need of heat are placed on an electrically heated pad and we also place around them warm water bottles. A fresh warm gown should be put on the patient at the completion of the operation. The bed, in which the patient is placed after operation, should be warm. The blankets and other covers can be kept in a warmer during the operation, and an electric pad used to reinforce these. We can not emphasize too strongly the care necessary to avoid burning anæsthetized patients with hot water bottles. It is therefore advisable, unless extreme care can be taken, not to use these as long as the patient is under the influence of the anæsthetic. During transportation through corridors the patient should be protected by woolen covers. **Embolic processes** play a rôle in postoperative pulmonary disturbances, and are discussed on page 14.

(Besides the factors already enumerated several others play an important rôle in the production of postoperative pulmonary complications. **Pulmonary hypoventilation,** resulting in a decreased vital capacity, occurs after many abdominal operations. This is due to the rise of the diaphragm which results in part from the entrance of air into the peritoneal cavity and in part from the splinting of the abdominal and lower thoracic musculature as a result of pain.

Various degrees of **pulmonary atelectasis** may result from the occlusion of a bronchus by a mucus plug. When this occurs the signs are frequently those of pulmonary consolidation. In atelectasis the heart is always shifted toward the affected side. This fact alone, plus the physical signs of lung consolidation, is sufficient to make the diagnosis. The roentgenogram will disclose the exact extent of the lesion. I. S. R.)

Even greater care is necessary during the early postoperative period than during the preoperative period in the prevention of respiratory complications. If a cough develops the patient should be placed in the sitting posture (Fig. 18) (although in some instances the flat or head down position which facilitates bronchial drainage gives more relief. I. S. R). A correct posture is essential in these patients whose resistance is already lowered. In order properly to regulate the patient's position a bed should be used in which adjustable inclinations can be obtained which support the body from but-

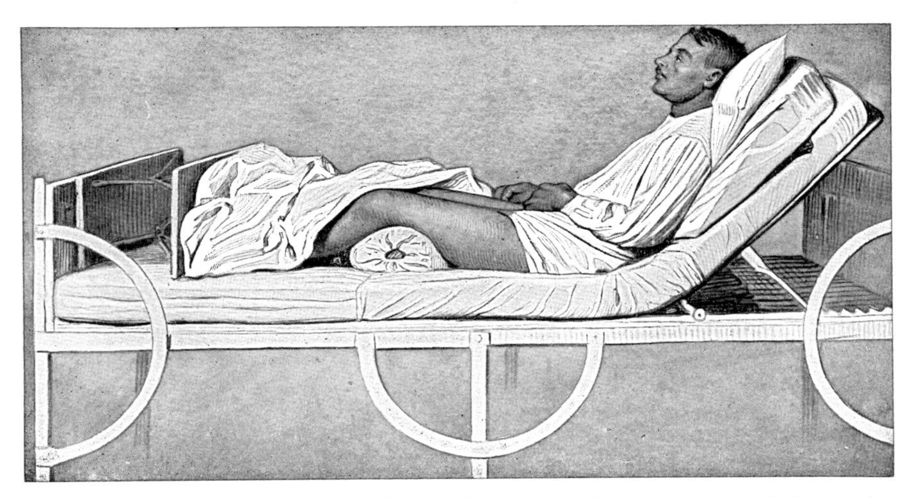

FIG. 18. Semi-sitting posture for the relief of cough. The upper part of the trunk rests upon an adjustable frame which has been raised to an angle of about 45 degrees. The feet have a firm buttress against an adjustable foot-board. The knees are slightly flexed by a pillow placed under them.

tocks to head. The use of pillows or wooden triangles is unsatisfactory because they are not adjustable to length or height, and because they are difficult to retain in position. When they are placed under the buttocks, the patient's head hangs backward like a weight. The inclined support should be of sufficient length to support the head. To prevent the patient from slipping down in bed there should be an adjustable foot-board against which the feet can rest, or the knees should be bent over a fixed roll or a double inclined plane. Regardless of which method is used the wood should be carefully covered so as to avoid pressure. Beds with adjustable frames which provide various inclinations for the head and knees are in common use and are very satisfactory as a rule.

Even the most comfortable position is not tolerated well for a long period of time by the sick patient. His position should be changed often. In the aged where hypostasis is feared the patient should be moved frequently and as soon as possible allowed to be out of bed.

Excessive coughing, especially after abdominal operations, can be relieved by the use of morphine or codeine. The dose can be so controlled as to relieve pain but not prevent expectoration. After laparotomies the pain which accompanies coughing and the danger of the breaking down of the suture line, which occasionally results from excessive coughing, can be prevented by applying a mastic abdominal supporter, by the skilful application of adhesive plaster strips, by a many tailed bandage, or by a laced abdominal binder. Abdominal wounds, which do not require dressing for seven or more days are preferably covered with a mastisol binder (Fig. 19). A muslin strip extending from the ensiform process to the symphysis is attached to the skin which has been covered with the mastic compound. The strip begins at the spinous processes and is carried around the front of the abdomen and tightly fastened on itself either with mastic or by suture. If the ab-

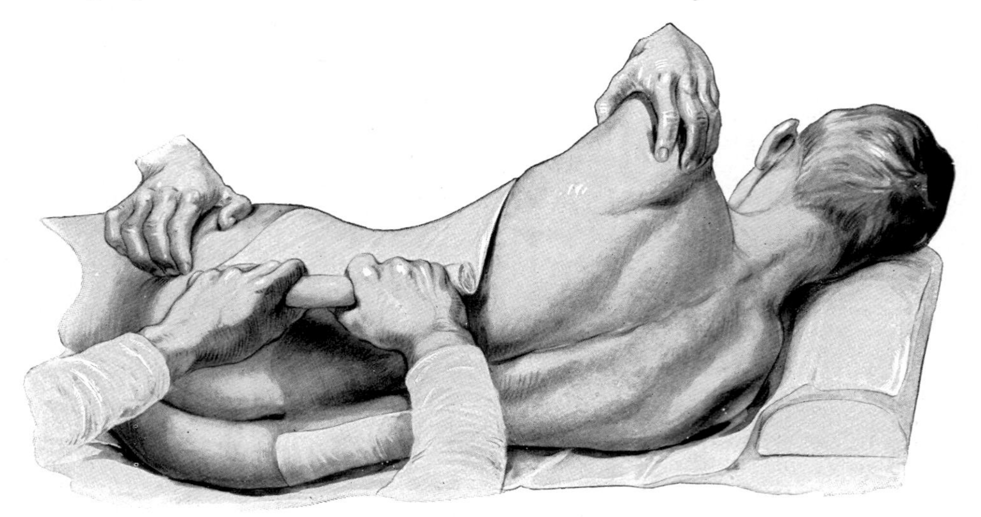

Fig. 19. Mastisol-abdominal binder. The mastisol is spread over the skin and a wide strip of muslin is stretched tightly over the abdomen in a girdle-like fashion. The ends of the strips overlap at the back.

dominal wound must be dressed often, I use the adhesive strips (Fig. 20) which can be laced together, or a many tailed binder (Fig. 21).

(In pulmonary atelectasis it is necessary that the patient be relieved of the bronchial obstruction. This may be released by cough, by gravity, by alteration of position, or it may have to be removed by bronchoscopic aspiration. The latter method removes the major plug and thus provides an airway for reinflation of the lung. The obstruction causing the atelectasis should be removed as soon as possible after the diagnosis has been made, or pneumonia may result. I. S. R.)

The value of carbon dioxide inhalations for preventing respiratory complications may be open to some question, but in my experience they have proved very helpful. The inhalation of carbon dioxide stimulates deep breathing and thus provides a method for overcoming the reduction of the vital capacity. It can be given through a nitrous oxide and oxygen machine so that the patient breathes into a mask, or a rubber catheter can be placed

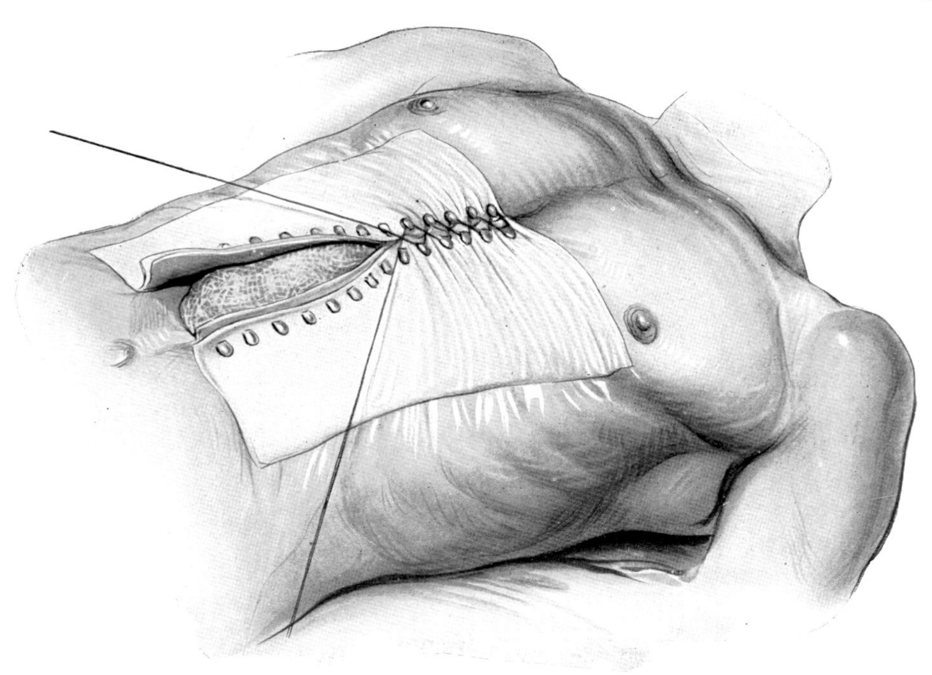

FIG. 20. Laced adhesive strips. Strips of adhesive, provided with hooks, are applied to either side of the wound and then laced together.

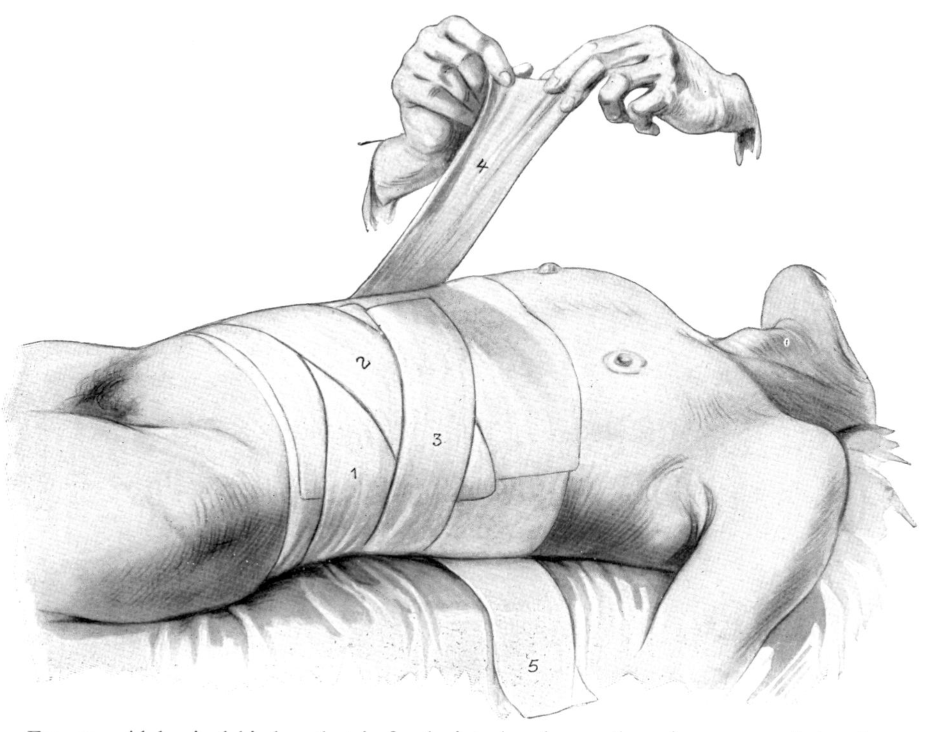

FIG. 21. Abdominal binder, that is firmly interlaced over the primary wound dressing.

in the patient's nose. It should not be given continuously but is best given for five or ten minutes every three hours.

Postoperative Hiccup (Singultus). Occasionally on the day of, or the day after an abdominal operation, less frequently after operations on the urinary apparatus, and rarely following other procedures, obstinate hiccup makes its appearance and may last for a week or more. Usually older men are affected and especially those who have lived well (Küttner). The remedies previously mentioned for the relief of pain have no influence upon this condition. The etiology is unknown. The patients are tortured day and night by the constant hiccup and may die from exhaustion. The treatment is not always successful. Narcotics are as a rule without effect, except as they provide sleep to the sufferers. The administration of cocaine or chloroform water is likewise as a rule ineffectual. The best result is obtained through blocking the phrenic nerve in the neck by an injection of a 1 percent solution of novocain between the sternocleidomastoid and the scalenus anterior muscles. The needle is inserted along the inner edge of the sternocleidomastoid muscle, the width of a finger above the jugular notch. The fluid is continuously injected as the needle is directed externally under the width of the muscle. In extreme cases, the nerve can be exposed and injected with alcohol or frozen with ethyl chloride.

4. Abdominal Organs

Possible tumors, an enlargement of the liver or spleen, or the presence of ascites, must always be looked for. Disease of the large parenchymatous abdominal organs, in particular the liver, pancreas and kidneys, lower the resistance to operative interference and to anæsthetization. The presence of such disease creates a relative contra-indication to operation. If, in spite of their existence, surgical procedures are necessary, then local anæsthesia is to be preferred. Nitrous oxide and oxygen is preferable to ether, and the latter is preferable to chloroform.

Especial foresight should be exercised in patients with **icterus.** These cases are apt to ooze considerably during and after operation. The majority of surgeons are agreed that the jaundiced patient should be specially prepared for operation and that the prophylactic measures instituted preoperatively should be continued for a definite time after operation. These will be described completely in the chapter on the arrest of hemorrhage. The use of calcium chloride and glucose is particularly recommended. The surgeon should exercise the most minute care in checking hemorrhage during the operation.

Patients should not be brought to the operating room with an overfilled gastro-intestinal tract. This is just as true when they are not to be subjected to laparotomy. **Vomiting** during the operation may result in interruptions and in aspiration. The subsequent rest in bed for many days after the operation, often causes intestinal stasis. Also food in the stomach and intestine raises the diaphragm and thus hinders pulmonary ventilation, which in turn predisposes the patient to pulmonary complications. In emergency operations gastric lavage may have to be resorted to, which in the case of continuous vomiting is often life saving. In non-urgent cases, I routinely give, and find useful, early on the day before the operation, a mild purgative so that the night's rest may not be disturbed.

According to the clinical researches made in my department (Frey, Surgical Congress, 1926) the preoperative emptying of the intestine does not influence the activity of the gut or its response to postoperative catharsis. The cathartic should depend largely upon what the patient is accustomed to taking. On the morning of operation the patients, especially children, should be asked to empty their bowels. If this is impossible spontaneously, a glycerine enema (50 parts of glycerine to 100 parts of water) should be given. If the bowel has not been thoroughly emptied it is possible that the patient may have an involuntary movement under anæsthesia. This is especially true in the aged, so that three times on the day previous to the operation I frequently give them 15 to 20 minims of tinct. opii.

In order to have the intestinal tract sufficiently empty the food intake must be restricted on the day before operation. Only small amounts of easily digested food of high caloric value are given. Finely chopped meat, fat in any form (butter), and white bread are suitable. If food is withheld the day before operation the patient feels weak, and there is nothing to be gained if the gastro-intestinal tract is not to be opened. Likewise, I believe it purposeless to withhold all food or drink from patients on the day of operation. To be sure, the stomach should be empty at the beginning of general anæsthesia or even during local anæsthesia, for it may be necessary to change to general anæsthesia. Since under normal conditions a meal has completely left the stomach in from three to six hours, patients who are to be operated upon during the latter part of the morning or in the afternoon should enjoy the quieting morning benefit of a cup of tea or coffee, with a piece of toast, the omission of which would distress even a healthy individual.

As a rule, following the operation there is a shorter or longer period of time during which food or liquids can not be taken by mouth. The length of time during which even liquids can not be given by mouth will vary according to the type of operation and the extent of nausea which exists. In certain instances nausea and vomiting are the only contra-indications to feeding. On the other hand in diffuse peritoneal infections and after operations on the stomach abstinence for a variable period of time is an essential part of the treatment. During this period fluids can be given by proctoclysis, by hypodermoclysis, or intravenously. Patients who have had several operations with subsequent excessive gastric irritability refuse all remedies since they believe they can shorten the postanæsthetic nausea by abstinence more quickly than by any other means.

For the most part the fears entertained in regard to abstinence from foods and fluids are exaggerated. Robust individuals are able to do without food for several days without any harm, even without great hardship. Debilitated patients, on the other hand, suffer from the loss of food and fluids and may be seriously injured by this. In them a restricted fluid intake with complete withdrawal of food may cause death in a relatively short time. Dehydration from water restriction is far more injurious than is the lack of food. Our main concern in such cases is to administer fluids. A rough estimate of the state of water balance is shown by the daily output of urine. It is as important to measure and chart the intake and output of fluid as it is to measure and chart the temperature. The 24 hour quantity of urine is normally a little less than 1500 c.c. Should the quantity of urine exceed this amount, we may conclude that we are giving the patient enough or even too much fluid; if it is less, we probably are giving him too little, assuming normal kidney elimination.

The introduction of fluid, if administration by mouth is impossible, is best done through continuous proctoclysis of warm physiologic salt solution, or warm tap water. This should be begun as soon as the patient returns from the operating room. If sufficient water can not be given in this way, salt solution is given intravenously. In serious cases the continuous intravenous drip is often life saving. Hypodermoclysis is painful and even though novocaine is used with it, I have never seen it given without discomfort to the patient. It is sometimes necessary in a patient who is markedly debilitated, and who can not take food by mouth, to administer glucose intravenously. As soon as the patient can safely be fed by mouth, he should not be subjected to the widely used "liquid diet", which often retards convalescence and fails to satisfy the patient's desire for food. The best guide, as a rule, is the patient's desire, which should be considered. Although in general, after major operations, particularly in bed-ridden patients, we prescribe a light diet, we must not deny, on principle, a patient's desire for some special food. Often the desire of the patient for a special article of food or drink can be gratified without any deleterious result, in fact, the gratification of such desires may work wonders in altering the mental attitude of the patient and so turn the tide in favor of recovery. In cream we have an easily digested, palatable, concentrated food. For those who do not like milk or cream it can be altered by the addition of a little salt, brandy, or flavoring, and so made more palatable; or it may be given as ice-cream. Children can add to their caloric intake by eating chocolate, whipped cream, and candies. And when the adult is attached to his cigarette, cigar or pipe, I fail to see any ground for denying him their use, in the absence of complications.

For the regulation of the bowels in bed-ridden patients, we must give particular attention to the addition of stewed fruits, and vegetables having a residue, to the diet. Reflex intestinal stimulation may also be brought about by the application of heat to the abdominal wall. In certain circumstances it is necessary to give the patient an enema or a mild purgative every second or third day.

Postoperative Acute Dilatation of the Stomach. After abdominal operations, especially those involving the stomach or biliary system, gastric dilatation is not a rare occurrence. This condition may occur any time after operation, but usually occurs between the third and fifth day. It is characterized by the vomiting of large quantities of dark or bile colored fluid, rapid, soft pulse and rapid, shallow respiration. Nausea, thirst, and hyperirritability torture the patient constantly. The vomiting of excessive amounts of fluid causes a reduction in the output of urine. Gastric peristalsis is visible. The body temperature is not increased. The constant vomiting causes a loss of chloride and base from the blood and **alkalosis** may result.

One of the causes given for this condition is a sudden reflex paralysis of the muscular apparatus of the stomach wall. Various degrees of atony may occur, so that the surgeon may observe various gradations of gastric dilatation. The relaxed stomach is not able to empty its contents through the pylorus. Some observers believe that the forward progression of gastric contents is inhibited by gastromesenteric ileus. The stomach wall secretes enormous quantities of fluids, so that the stomach is markedly dilated. The distended stomach may contain four or even more liters of fluid. The over-distended stomach sags, often causing an acute angulation at the pylorus, thereby preventing even simple drainage. The diagnosis is usually made from the persistent vomiting of excessive amounts of fluid.

If the condition does not improve spontaneously or under treatment, death ensues within a few days. The death is similar to that from high intestinal obstruction. Dehydration, toxemia, the loss of chlorides and the frequent presence of alkalosis, together with the mechanical disturbance of the heart, are the chief causes of death.

Treatment consists of early and regular gastric lavage. The patient may assume the knee-chest position for short periods of time, or may be turned on his right side. Draining the stomach with a permanent indwelling tube, such as the Jutte tube, gives excellent results. Supporting remedies, such as physostigmine, pituitrin, strychnine, have been recommended but are of doubtful value. Neither food nor fluids should be given by mouth, but saline should be given either by rectum or by intravenous infusion. If these measures are applied in time, they cause restoration of the gastric tonus and lead to cure.

Operative procedures, such as gastrostomy or gastro-enterostomy, have been found to be of very little value. We would expect this, since patients often develop acute gastric dilatation after gastro-enterostomy. Furthermore, since the stomach wall is stretched and atonic, the technical difficulties of this operation are considerably increased and one has no assurance that the suture line will be secure or the stoma will function. As a last resort jejunostomy offers a means of administering food, and gastrostomy a means of permanent drainage.

Again a warning note must be sounded against prolonged fasting and drastic purging before and after operation. Only after gastric operations is it necessary to withhold food by mouth for any considerable period of time.

Menstruation is not a contra-indication to operation. Since most women, at this time, feel psychically and physically debilitated, it is better not to undertake major abdominal operations at this time. It is better to postpone all major operations of election for at least one week after the cessation of menstruation. A few days after major abdominal operations many women begin to menstruate. This should be no cause for anxiety.

During **pregnancy** operations of election should not be done if they can be postponed until after delivery without danger to the patient. Any operation may precipitate an abortion or premature birth. The further the pregnancy is advanced and the greater the scope of the operation, the greater is the necessity for refusing to do operations of choice. Diseases which often cause trouble during the latter part of pregnancy, as for example, appendicitis and herniæ, are best taken care of early in the pregnancy. Of course in acute surgical diseases immediate operation is often imperative. If one is compelled to operate during pregnancy, purgatives and enemata should be used cautiously in both the precperative preparation and in the postoperative treatment. Local anæsthesia is to be preferred to general anæsthesia. After the operation, in order to prevent the onset of labor, morphine should be used to keep the patient as quiet as possible.

It is necessary to determine the possible existence of pregnancy by both a history of the menstrual cycle and by a physical examination, even though the contemplated operation does not involve the organs of generation.

5. Nervous System

A general idea of the mental characteristics of the patient is readily formed from the observation of the patient's appearance, his conduct, and his attitude. A complete physical examination should include testing of the facial nerves, of the eye movements, the pupillary reactions, the patellar and Achilles reflexes, the motility and sensibility of scars. Such an examination will prevent one from overlooking more serious maladies or a hyperexcitability of the nervous system.

Diseases of the nervous system of a trophoneurotic character, such as tabes and syringomyelia, do not seem to affect the ability of a wound to heal. Nevertheless, one should be extremely cautious in advising operations of an elective character in patients suffering from advanced mental or nervous disease. The trophoneurotic lesions of the feet are difficult to heal, but many of these are associated with vascular disease.

The hypersensibility and instability of irritable, nervous and hysterical patients, as well as those addicted to the use of alcohol or morphine, or those who have suffered pain over a considerable interval, require careful preoperative preparation and consideration. For the patient in whom nervous irritability is not a factor, it is well to remember that every operation, attended as it is with a sudden change of the surroundings, a lack of certain conditions which were thought essential to life, and with the numberless strange and fleeting impressions attending the operation, involves psychic trauma of considerable extent. The surgeon must do all in his power to attenuate the psychic shock connected with the operation and must consider each case individually. The following suggestions are not to be kept exclusively for the nervously or psychically disturbed patient, but are to be put into practice sensibly and according to indication in the mentally "normal" patient as well.

If during the physical examination the patient is found to be normal with the exception of his surgical lesion, he should not be rushed to operation, especially if this is a major procedure, until he has had the opportunity of accommodating himself to his new surroundings. Cases of a non-emergency character should be in the hospital for at least one day before the operation is done.

Particular attention should be given to this preoperative period so that the patient is not in contact with emotional patients. He should be kept from observing patients with painful or unsightly diseases; from listening to the noises which often emanate from the anæsthetizing room, or from the sight of patients recently operated upon or of those recovering from an anæsthetic; from observing the dressing of painful wounds or viewing desperately ill or dying patients. The nursing force must be quiet and orderly and must attempt to instil confidence. Many individuals rapidly prepared for operation, after such experiences, give up hope even before the battle is begun. It is much better to strengthen the faith of the one who has decided on an operation; to impress them with the fact that its progress will be a happy one, that the pain can be controlled, and that the operating and nursing personnel can be trusted. Faith in the surgeon and his staff is of the utmost importance in every serious surgical procedure.

The same precautions should be thrown around both the preoperative and postoperative cases. Small quiet rooms, with few beds, are more suitable for this than are large wards which are never quiet, and which owe their existence to a more economical management. In hospitals with large wards the fresh postoperative cases, and the very sick or unruly ones should not be brought into the ward but should be kept in adjoining small rooms. It is absolutely necessary to provide in the wards abundant and regular quiet especially at night. Patients admitted at night should not be placed in the general ward. The custom of early cleaning of the wards should be abolished, since it disturbs the patients. Nor should it be necessary to disturb the entire ward early in the morning so that a number of unnecessary temperatures can be taken. I say this even though I begin to operate before 7 o'clock in the morning.

During the day all sorts of distractions, which take the patient's mind away from his suffering, are valuable. They aid in the recovery of the patient and are to be regarded as remedial measures. These include certain games, reading of light literature, humorous magazines, the phonograph or radio, and simple hand-work such as is provided by occupational therapy workers. Visitors are to be received by the patient within the limits permitted by the surgeon. The patient should be protected regardless of his friends! In severe illness, but one visitor at a time should be permitted in the room, and only at infrequent intervals.

The treatment of an emotional, high-strung patient should begin several days before the operation. It consists, besides the proper environment, of rest in bed and sedatives, among which the most important I have found to be the bromides. Luminal, veronal, and various other barbiturates may be used, as well as morphine or Pantopan, if they are necessary. I give even the psychically normal patient a sedative the night before operation, so that, his anxiety for the events to take place the next day may not prevent a restful night.

After operation all patients with an excitable nervous system should be given narcotics until they are under perfect control. I have found that alcoholic drinks accomplish valuable results, and I administer them in reasonable quantities to patients who have been accustomed to using them. Likewise I hold in high esteem the soothing action of tobacco for those addicted to its use. Should it not be possible to control the psychic irritability with these remedies, and a true postoperative psychosis develops, I administer, in addition to large doses of the above mentioned drugs, chloral hydrate and scopolamine.

Patients with toxic goitre require careful preoperative and postoperative treatment. The prognosis depends very largely on the care with which this preparation is carried out. For this reason every patient with toxic goitre must submit to at least a week of preparatory treatment, during which time all excitement is carefully avoided and the patient is placed in the best possible environment. There is present an abnormal psychic state. These patients frequently must be prepared for some time, before operation can be considered. They should be put to bed in a quiet room, receive a diet which is high in caloric value yet is easily assimilated, and they should be given sufficient sedatives in the form of bromides or the barbiturates to keep them quiet. The usefulness of digitalis in these cases is questionable unless fibrillation is present. I have, however, frequently used it when fibrillation was not present, merely as a cardiac stimulant, and I believe that it served a useful purpose. It is my custom to use general anæsthesia for all toxic goitre operations.

Basal Metabolism. The determination of the basal metabolic rate is important in studying patients with thyroid dysfunction. It is of value in differentiating various types of toxic goitre from effort syndromes; the degree of hyper or hypo function of the thyroid gland; and it assists in evaluating the part played by the thyroid in various polyglandular diseases. Metabolism has to do with the utilization of food substances by the tissues. The chief process in this utilization is that of oxidation, so that metabolism is in a sense food and tissue combustion. This combustion can be measured, either by determining the heat evolved, the oxygen consumed, or carbon dioxide produced. The present day concept of basal metabolism requires that the patients be starved for a number of hours and that during this period they remain in bed with complete mental and physical relaxation. The basal rate is therefore an expression of the energy interchange which is necessary for the minimal requirements at complete rest. It can be expressed in one of several ways. This rate is flexible depending upon sex, age, body weight, and body surface. The actual calculations used in its determination must take these factors into account. Harris and Benedict have established normal values by collecting a large amount of data and their work forms the basis for the clinical determinations, in that so-called normal values are used as the basis for expressing the increase or decrease of the metabolism of the patient studied.

In determining the energy expended under basal conditions it is only necessary to determine accurately the respiratory gaseous interchange during a definite period of time. In clinical practice one estimates either the amount of oxygen used or carbon dioxide expired.

The determination of the basal rate may be done in one of two ways. The **calorimetric method** determines the heat production. Although this method is without doubt the most accurate it is not used in clinical practice, because of the technical difficulties and the expense of the apparatus.

The **gasometric method** which determines the gaseous interchange may be subdivided into two groups: (1) the closed method, and (2) the open method. (The description which follows has been slightly altered. I. S. R.)

Examples of the closed method are the Benedict, Knipping, Krogh and

Sanborn apparatus. They are similar in principle in that the subject breathes from a spirometer filled with oxygen which is protected with a water seal. The spirometer is connected with a mouthpiece through which the resting patient breathes and the expired air passes through a container holding soda-lime which fixes the carbon dioxide. The spirometer in many of the apparatus is fitted with a mechanical arrangement for recording the oxygen consumption in cubic centimeters.

With the Krogh apparatus the patient is put on a carbohydrate diet for two days prior to the test. The respiratory quotient approximates 0.9 with a fair degree of accuracy. At this point each liter of oxygen consumed equals 4.9 calories. The possible error of 0.1 is of very little importance in clinical practice.

When the patient is quiet he begins to breath in the oxygen while the expired air containing oxygen and carbon dioxide passes through the soda-lime where the CO_2 is fixed and the oxygen is returned to the spirometer. Thus the volume of oxygen in the spirometer is gradually diminished. The decrease in volume is read for a definite time interval. Several readings should be made to reduce the effect of an error due to temporary irregular respiration. The volume of oxygen used is then corrected for temperature and pressure and the metabolic rate is calculated from standard tables.

The open methods require gas analysis after breathing into a bag or chamber. Although quite accurate, these methods are much more complicated.

The importance of estimating the basal metabolic rate is no longer a matter of conjecture. Magnus-Levy found the basal metabolic rate remarkably constant in the same individual, a fact which has been amply confirmed by the investigations of Harris and Benedict. Experience has shown that it is possible to have a plus or minus error of 15 percent, and that a B. M. R. of + 15 or -15 may be considered normal. However, rates above or below these figures should be looked upon as abnormal.

The major use of this test, as I have said, is in the group of thyroid diseases. Hyperthyroidism causes an elevation of the basal rate, while hypothyroidism causes it to decrease.

In latent hypothyroidism the basal rate is between -15 and -20, while below this clinical hypothyroidism is present. The clinical picture and the B. M. R. parallel each other. Hypothyroidism can be controlled with thyroid medication. The dose of thyroid extract necessary varies in the individual case and should be controlled by repeated estimations of the B. M. R.

The cases of cretinism have thyroid hypofunction, but they may also have a normal B. M. R., or slight deviations to either side of the normal.

The majority of the investigations have been made with hyperthyroidism. In these cases the B. M. R. is very important in differentiating disorders of the sympathetic nervous system and effort syndromes from true thyroid hyperfunction. Hyperthyroidism causes an elevation of the B. M. R., the rate increasing in proportion to the degree of hyperfunction. Froell has observed a rate of 140, although 90 to 100 is as high as one may ordinarily expect to find it even in very toxic cases.

Plummer in the United States and Neisser in Germany have advocated the use of iodine in the form of **Lugol's solution** in preparing these cases for operation. Iodine causes a retrogression in the process with a reduction of the B. M. R. and an improvement in the clinical symptoms. This lasts for a short period of time, after which the improvement recedes and the patients again slip back to their original state. The maximum improvement usually occurs in from 8 to 14 days after the beginning of the Lugol's solution. The patient should be operated on when the maximum effect is obtained. The question of whether a unilateral lobectomy or a subtotal thyroidectomy should be done is a matter which requires judgment. The decision should be based not only upon the patients' condition after iodine therapy, but upon their condition when first observed.

Iodine therapy is contra-indicated in those cases of hyperthyroidism which have been precipitated by iodine therapy. It is also supposedly contra-indicated in toxic adenoma, but the contra-indications are not so definite here.

Iodine therapy should be continued for several days after thyroidectomy. In fact the B. M. R., after operation, should be the deciding factor as to when it should be discontinued.

The **psychic make-up of the patient** must be taken into consideration in the choice of an anæsthetic. One must consider in making this choice the innate characteristics as well as the personal wishes of the patient. It has been our experience (F. König, German Surg. Cong. 1922) that the rise in blood pressure associated with the use of local anæsthesia is closely related to the extent of psychical excitation which takes place. It is not right that the nervous patient should have to lie awake while his leg is being amputated even though he suffers no physical pain. For this reason all nervous and abnormal patients are given a general anæsthetic for every major operation. In organic disease of the spinal cord and brain, spinal anæsthesia is never used.

Most patients have a rise in the blood pressure when they are transported to the anæsthetizing or operating room. This is the result of psychic stimuli. In order to avoid such stimulation every patient, excepting those which are to receive spinal anæsthesia, is given, half an hour before the beginning of the operation, 0.01 to 0.02 gm. of morphine sulphate. Scopolamine is not used as a pre-anæsthetic narcotic because it depresses respiration so markedly. To spare the patient as much as possible the anæsthesia should be induced in a room adjoining the operating room, and in very nervous patients I often have it started in their own room. Unusually nervous patients are asked to give their consent to operation in writing, and then are anæsthetized and operated on unbeknown to them after the method suggested by Crile. The day previous to operation they are given nitrous oxide and oxide as "treatment" for a short interval, while on the day of operation this is given for purposes of anæsthesia, and the patient is operated on when complete anæsthesia has been induced. I use this method very often in the severe cases of toxic goitre. It is in this type of case that intravenous and rectal anæsthesia may play an important rôle. The patient whose operation is to be done under local anæsthesia should have his face covered before being brought into the operating room. In many instances it is preferable to plug the ears with cotton.

The patient who receives local anæsthesia has constantly at his side a "psychic or vocal anæsthetist". This individual talks to the patient, quiets him, dispels fear, and, in general, represents his interests during the operation. Any narcotics which may be necessary during the operation should be at hand.

Exacting care is required for all patients immediately after operation, so as to control postoperative wound pain, which is not so severe in those operated upon under general anæsthesia as in those in whom local anæsthesia has been used. I administer to all patients in good condition at the conclusion of the operation a strong narcotic. This is given as a prophylactic. After general anæsthesia I give Pantopon or morphine (0.01-0.02 gm.) subcutaneously, while after local anæsthesia, where nausea is not a factor to be met, I frequently use only analgesics (Pyramidon 0.5 gm., aspirin 1.5-2.0 gm.). A quieting word from the surgeon as to the success of the operation, the excellent prospects for healing and recovery, are the best sedatives for a mind that is disturbed.

C. POSITION OF THE PATIENT DURING OPERATION

In order that the surgeon and his assistants may easily view the field of operation and be able to operate without undue fatigue, it is necessary to have the patient placed in a suitable position. An adjustable operating table is needed, of which there are many good models. One of these is illustrated (Fig. 22). This model I have designed and have found particularly useful. A good operating table should be easily adjustable to height, either by an oil-pump or screw. The table illustrated is easily moved, being supplied with rubber tired wheels and a handle with which it can be turned or easily transported to another position. The section supporting the thorax should be adjustable from the horizontal to the vertical position. It should also be possible to drop the lower section to a vertical position. The table should be so constructed as to rotate easily and be supplied with firm leg and shoulder supports which can assist in supporting the patient in any position. The head-piece should be freely movable in all directions. The table should be movable on its transverse axis (Trendelenburg's position, low pelvic inclination), as well as upon its long axis (inclination to the right or left). With it an almost vertical Trendelenburg position should be possible. It should permit the patient to lie comfortably on his back, on his side, or on his abdomen. Through the combination of the various positions of the table, the patient's body can assume any desired posture. Furthermore, there must be accessible contrivances to flex or extend the patient's body in certain locations, so that access to the deep organs can be more easily attained. For this, besides the adjustable sections of the table and the special blocks and plates which can be raised from the table surface, variously shaped inflatable pillows are helpful. The air cushions have the advantage that their thickness can be adjusted by the quantity of air introduced into them. The patient is placed on the empty cushion and after he is anæsthetized the cushion is inflated to the desired thickness. Air can be released or introduced as may be desired during the operation. For example, the air is released in an abdominal operation as soon as suture of the abdominal wall is begun. The advantages of the air cushions over the hard pillows are as a rule so great, that I use air cushions exclusively.

The metal top of the operating table is covered with a pad, preferably with a 4 cm. thick pad of rubber-sponge, which is covered with a washable

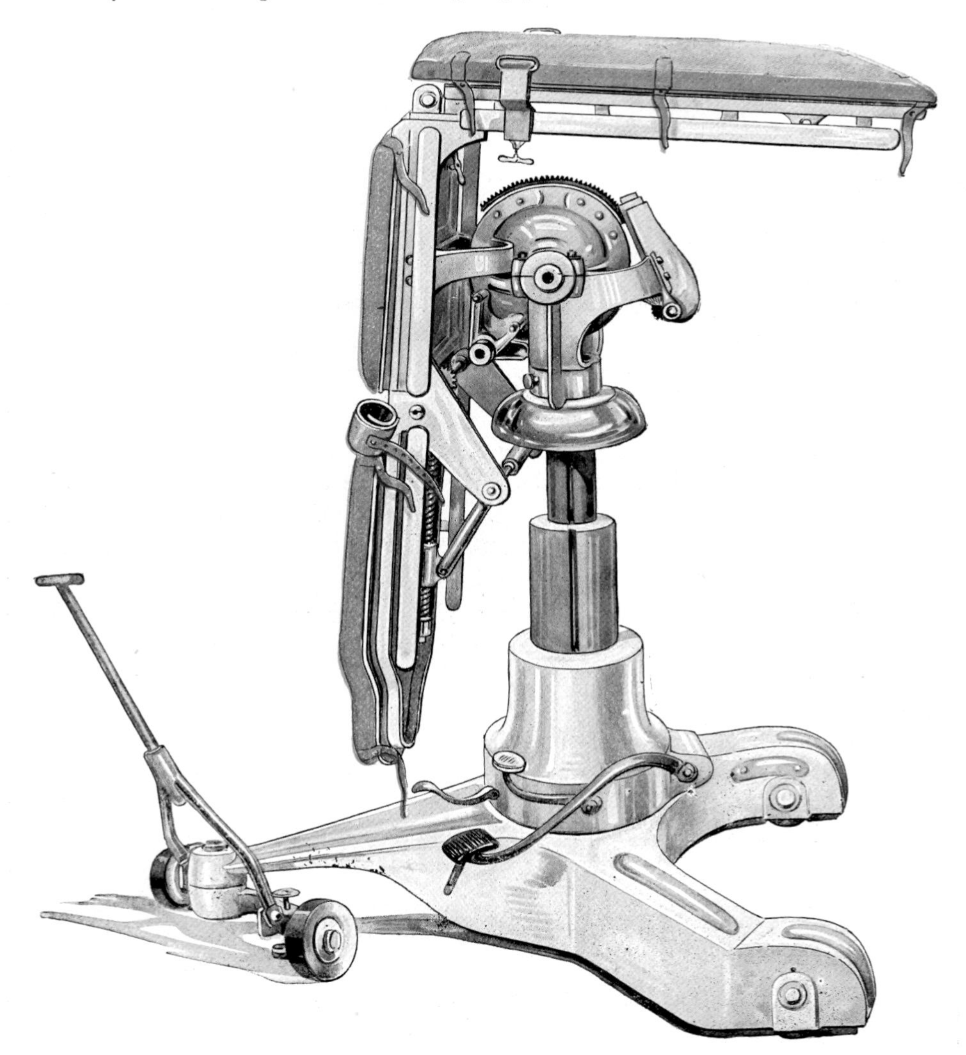

FIG. 22. Operating table (Kirschner-Windler). The patient may be placed in whatever position is desired and the table may be moved at will. A 90° elevation of the pelvis is possible. The large wheels and the handle make it easy to move.

rubber cover. A pillow is placed under the patient's head. The rubber-sponge pad can be sterilized by boiling. It is especially recommended for emaciated patients, particularly when one operates under a local anæsthetic, and for the support of bony prominences. A warning against the much used sandbag is not out of place. They are dusty, unless covered with rubber, and they must be sterilized every time they are used.

In the ordinary recumbent position the patient lies flat on his back on the horizontal operating table. The arms are arranged in a comfortable position at the sides, in such a manner as carefully to protect the radial (musculo-spiral) nerve from pressure. Failure to do this may result in radial (musculo-spiral) palsy. The arms may also be strapped to special arm-rests by placing the shoulder- and elbow-joints at a right angle. Just proximal to the knee, the legs are tightly strapped with a leather belt which is carried around the table. In an abdominal operation an air cushion is placed under the lumbar region (Fig. 23).

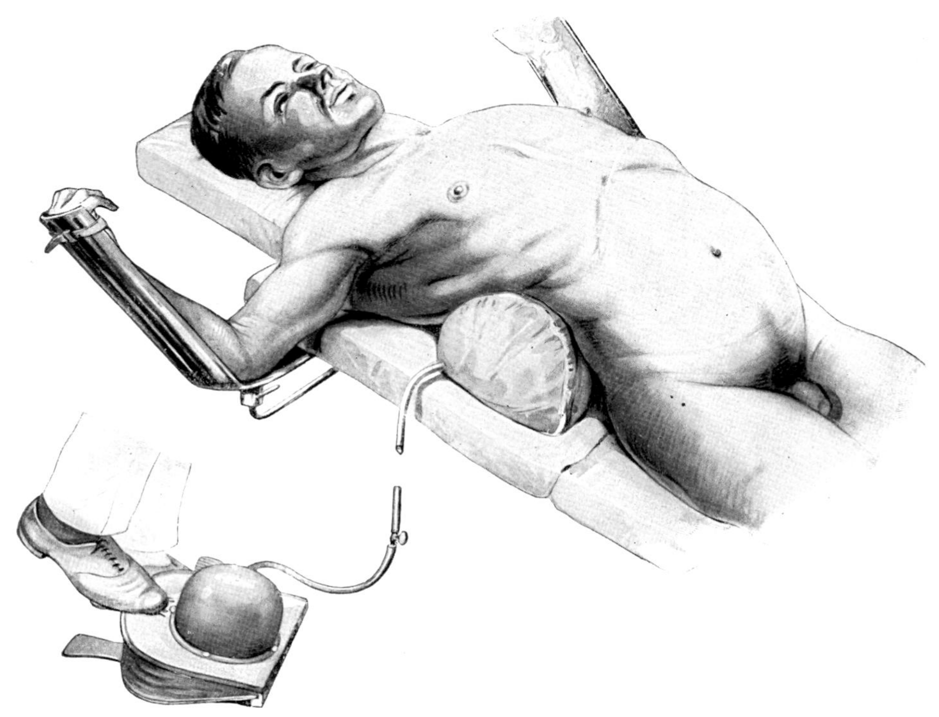

Fig. 23. Position for abdominal incision, especially for a mid-line incision above the umbilicus. By inflation of an air cushion placed under the small of the back the trunk is forced into the desired lordosis position. Before suture of the wound, the air is released so as to relax the abdominal wall. The arms are abducted to a right angle and supported by special arm holders. The operating table is padded with rubber-sponge cushions.

In Operations on the head and neck, the upper part of the trunk is elevated to reduce the blood pressure in the field of operation. It should not be raised too high, however, because of the possibility of air embolism. The position of the table can be immediately reversed if necessary. In certain operations, for example goitre operations, we do not raise the upper part of the body. When the trunk is placed in a vertical position, the feet are firmly placed against a transverse foot plate, and the strap over the knees maintains the legs in an extended position, so that the patient does not slide down. It is also possible to prevent the patient from sliding from the sitting position, by elevating the lower extremities so as to form a counterweight (Fig. 24).

Cranial operations require careful placing of the head, in fact, position is an important part of the operation. I have the head held by a special assistant, who uses a braided bandage sewed through the scalp or attached

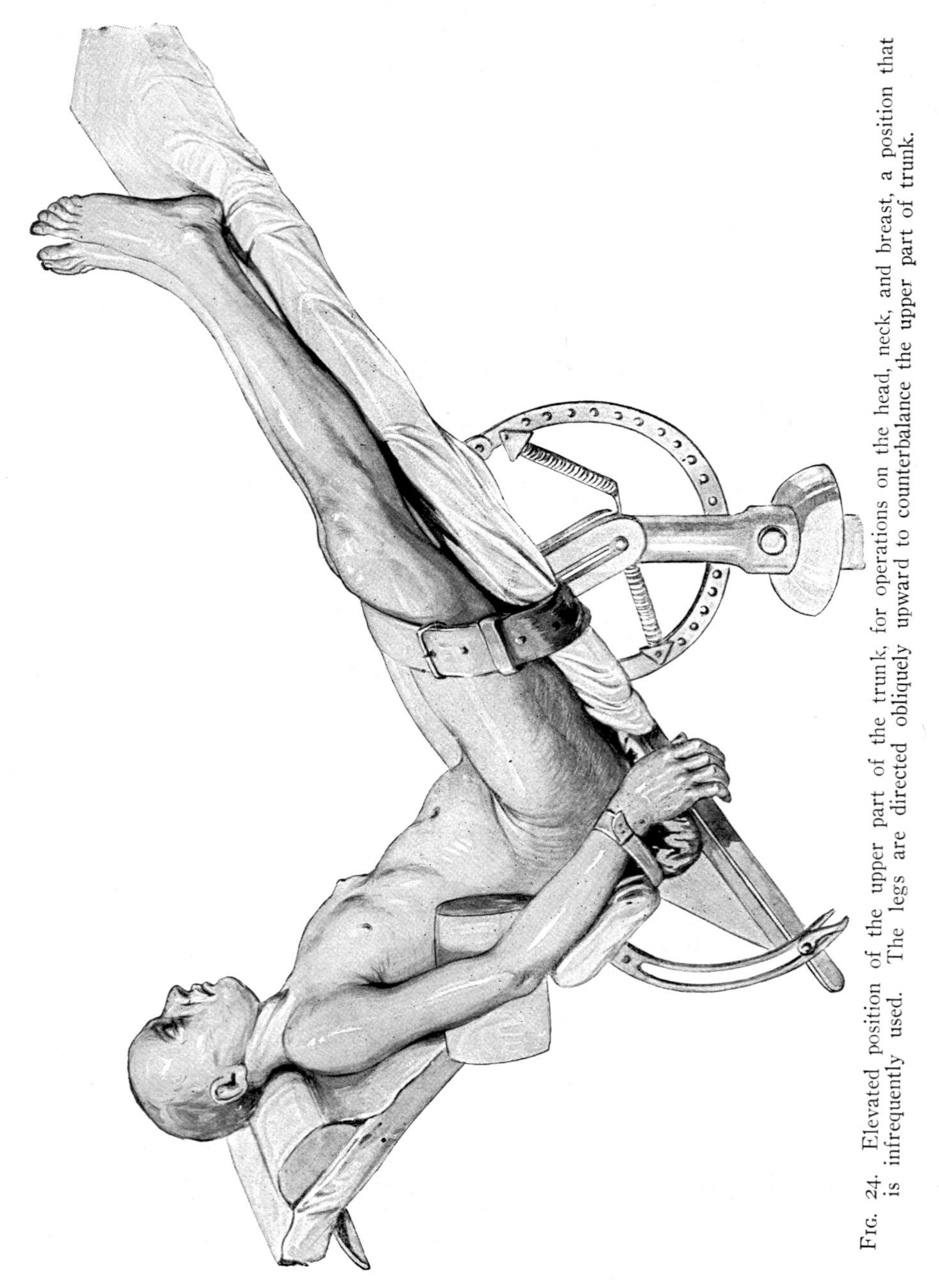

Fig. 24. Elevated position of the upper part of the trunk, for operations on the head, neck, and breast, a position that is infrequently used. The legs are directed obliquely upward to counterbalance the upper part of trunk.

with mastic, or after the position has been obtained, special attachments may be used so as to retain the head in the desired position.

While unilateral exposure of the cerebellum can be well carried out with

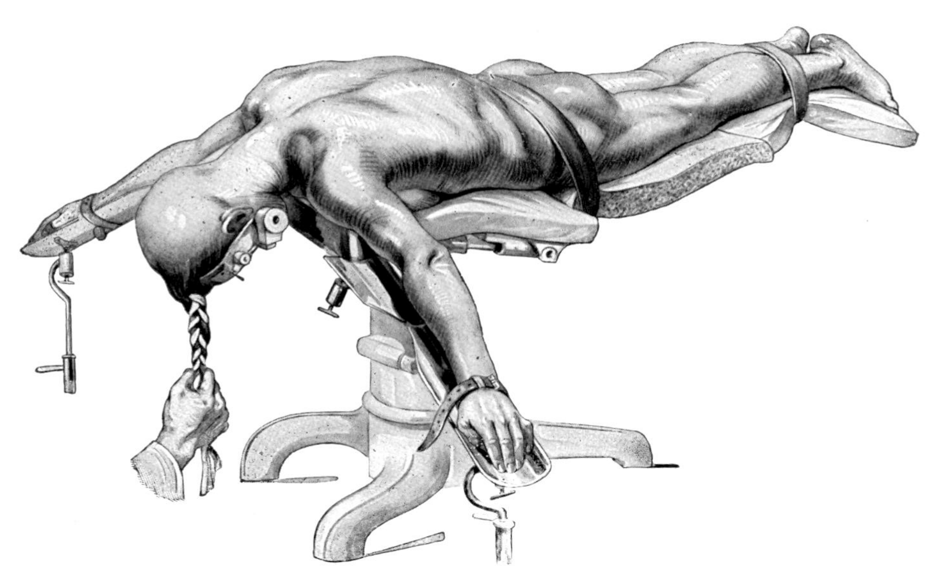

FIG. 25. Horizontal position for use in suboccipital craniectomy, or for operations on the spine or back. The face rests against a ringlike frame, through which the patient breathes and is anaesthetized. By tilting the table the head-end can be raised or lowered.

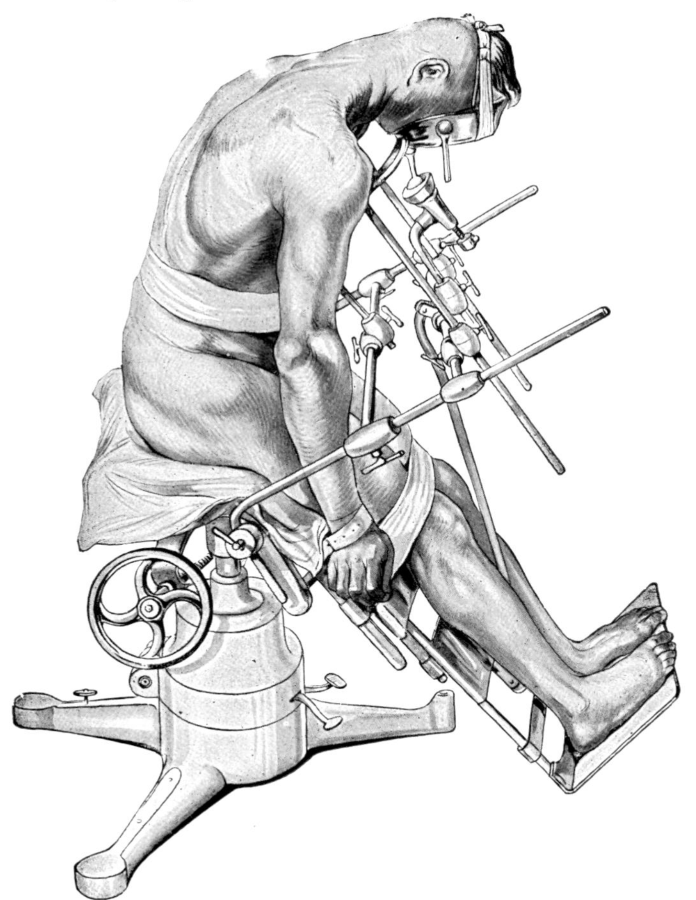

FIG. 26. Sitting position for suboccipital craniectomy.

the patient on the side and the head flexed on the chest, the exposure of both cerebellar hemispheres can not be done in this position (Figs. 25 and 26). For this it is best to put the patient in a sitting position, with the trunk and head inclined forward, and the head supported as illustrated, or in the position illustrated in figure 25 which also permits adequate access to the cerebellum. The sitting position permits of greater possibility of air embolism and is unsatisfactory when the blood pressure drops to shock levels.

In operations where the head must be extended, as in operations for cleft-palate, the head can be supported on a special table, or it can be placed

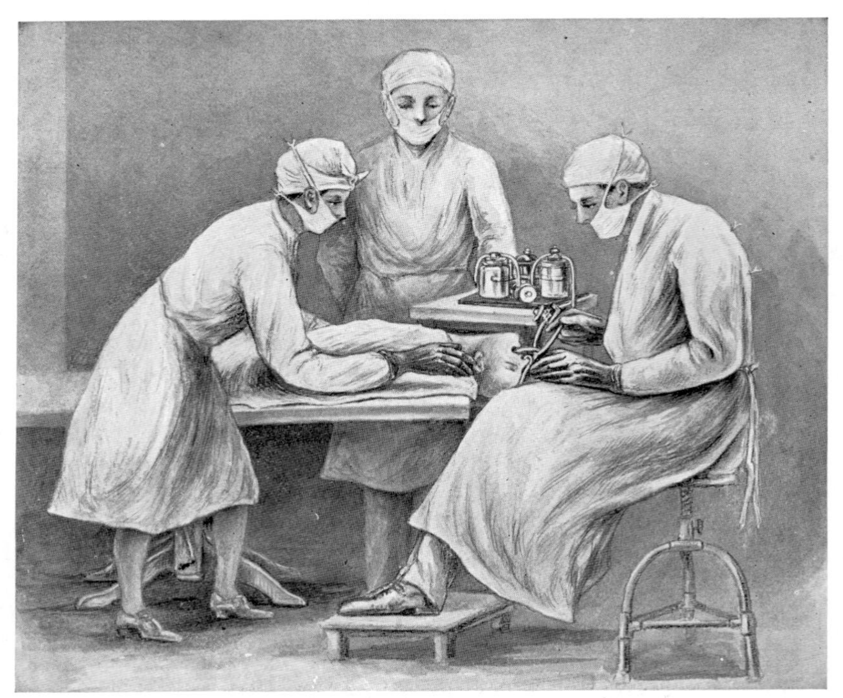

FIG. 27. Position of the head for operations on the palate or oro-pharynx. The head of the child rests on a frame held between the legs of the operator. The head is supported laterally at the ears by an assistant who also pulls the jaw forward. The anaesthesia is being administered by the intrapharyngeal method.

between the operator's knees (Fig. 27). The surgeon can easily change the position of the head by altering the position of his knees. This is of value if aspiration is threatened and is useful when the position must be altered during different steps of the operation. On the other hand, if the head is placed on a support the operator can shift his own position at will, working at times to the right or to the left, from above or from below. I therefore prefer the use of a support.

Small children, especially **infants,** can easily free themselves from the usual restraints and must be bound securely. I use a method which permits of perfect restraint of the four extremities and which is illustrated in figure 28. The child is first wrapped in a sheet and then bound as shown. This is very useful in facial operations in infants, such as operations for hare-lip.

After wrapping the infant in a sheet he is attached to a narrow tilting table which is adjustable on its transverse axis. In operations where the trunk must be exposed, the four extremities are firmly fixed by sheets so placed as to permit exposure of the operative field. One should avoid in binding them the danger of overheating.

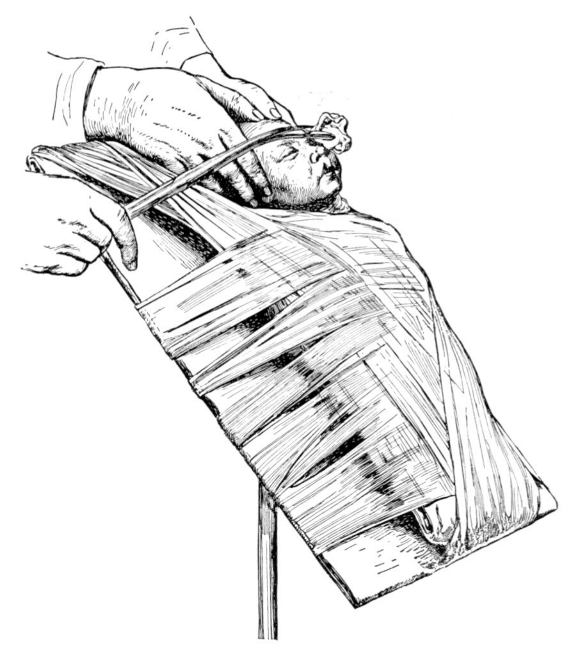

Fig. 28. Position of infant for operation on the face. The child is wrapped in a sheet and tied to a table that can be inclined.

In all **operations on the trunk** below the umbilicus, such as inguinal, or femoral herniæ, appendectomy, gynecological or rectal operations through abdominal incisions, the patient is so placed on the operating table that the Trendelenburg position can be immediately assumed (Fig. 29). The legs are bent at right angles at the knees and are fastened to leg supports or the drop leaf of the lower end of the table in such a manner that the weight of the patient is properly held. Further support can be obtained by the use of shoulder supports. If the legs are

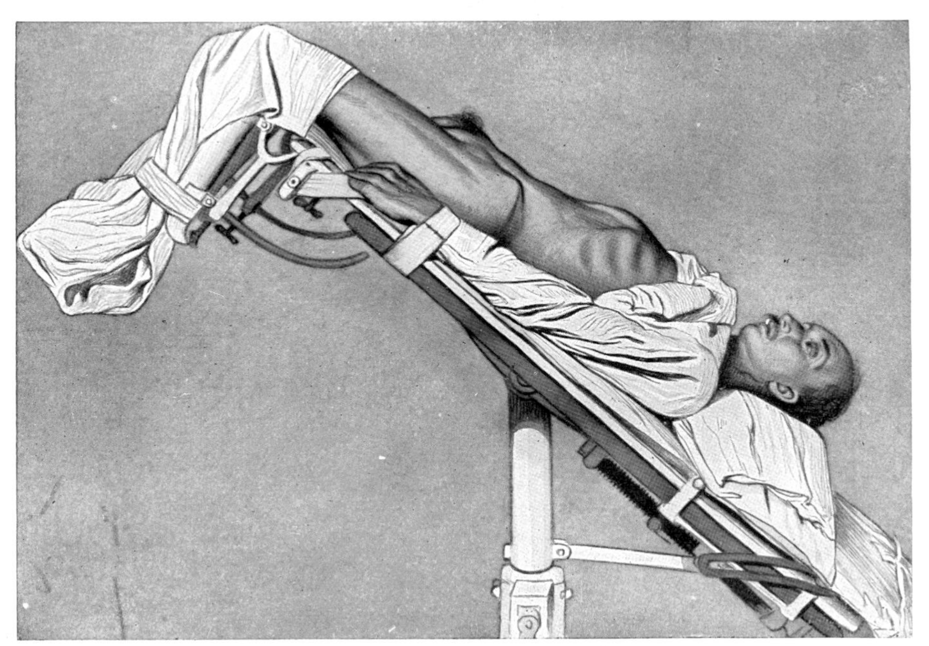

Fig. 29. Trendelenburg's position for operations in the true pelvis. The body is held by the legs which are bent at right angles at the knees. Shoulder supports can be used if desired.

separated in this position one assistant can stand between them. When using the Trendelenburg position the head of the patient should be directed toward the source of light. In the aged, inclined as they are to congestion, or in arteriosclerotic patients, care should be exercised as to the degree and the dura-

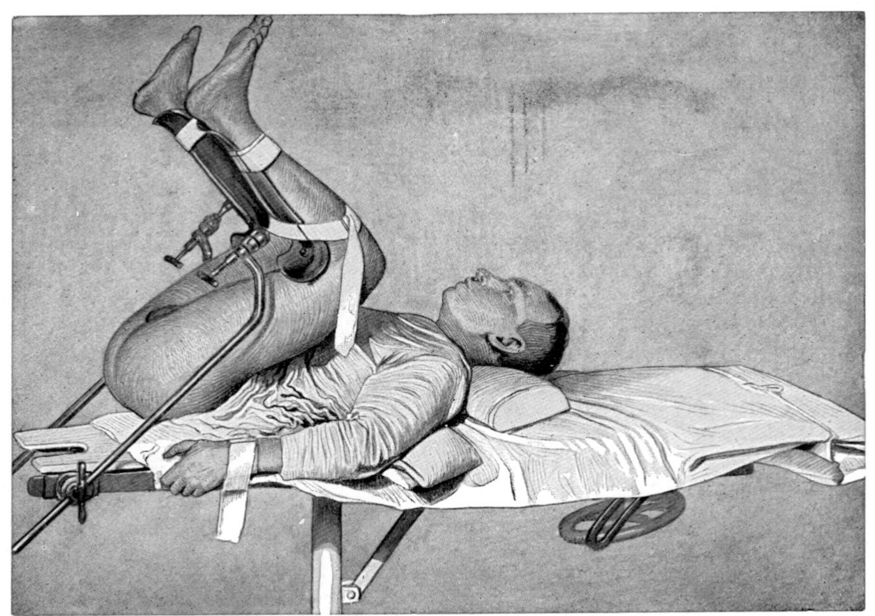

FIG. 30. Position for perineal operations (anus, prostate, urethra, vagina). Leg holders separate and elevate the lower extremities so that the soles of the feet are turned upwards. The scrotum, which cannot be shown in the illustration, is held up by a binder, which passes around the neck, or by fastening it with two towel clamps.

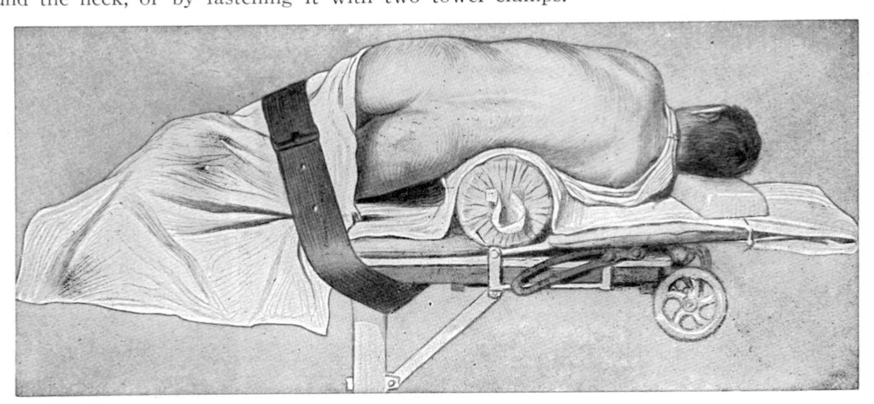

FIG. 31. Position for exposure of the retroperitoneal space (kidney) from the side. The patient lying on the side is arched by an inflatable roll placed under the opposite lumbar region.

tion of the Trendelenburg position. The fear that a collection of pus in the pelvis will tend to be carried toward the diaphragm in the Trendelenburg position is without foundation. Animal experimentation in my clinic demonstrated that this view is fallacious (Grube, German Surg. Cong. 1927).

In operations on the **anus**, the **perineum**, the **female genitalia**, and on the **buttock** and **posterior surface of the thigh**, the lithotomy position is ex-

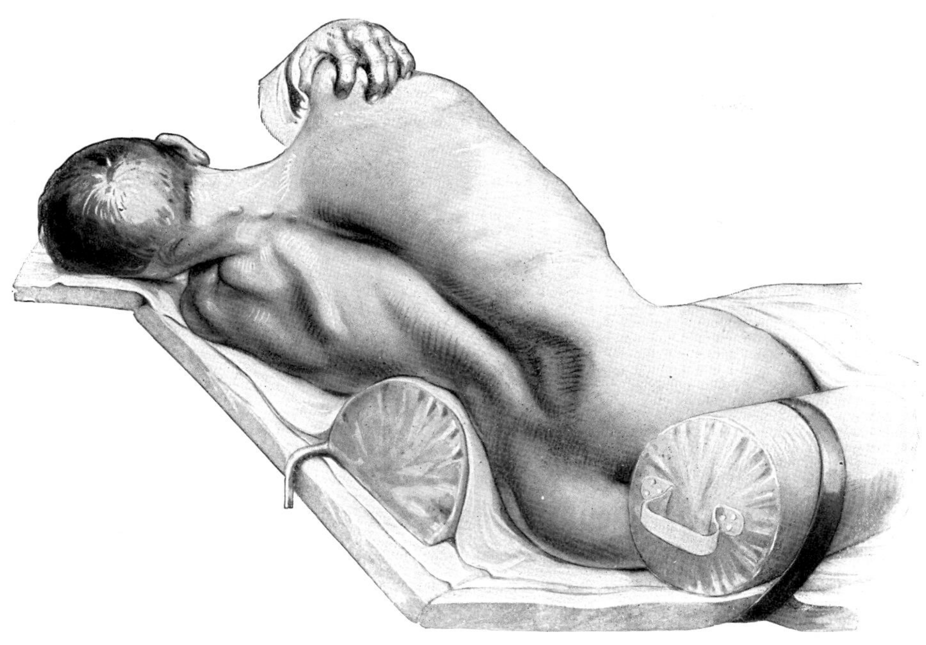

FIG. 32. Lateral position for operations on the thorax. The patient is in a semi-sitting posture. The side to be operated upon is thrown forward by an air cushion, the scapula is drawn forward and upward, to make the posterior portion of the upper ribs more accessible.

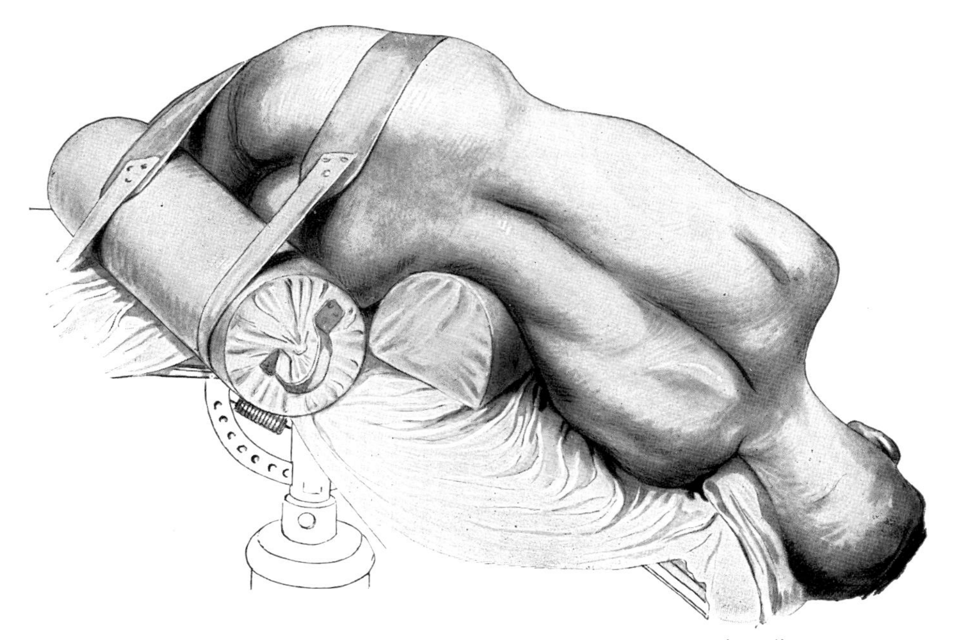

FIG. 33. Position for operations on the thorax in unilateral suppurative disease to prevent pus from entering the healthy lung during anaesthesia.

tremely useful (Fig. 30). The slightly spread legs are fastened to strong leg supports in such a way that they are acutely flexed at the hip-joint, while at the knee-joint they are bent so that the leg and thigh make an angle of about 135°. The soles of the feet are approximately parallel with the ceiling of the room. Technically, the best position is obtained when after fastening the leg to the holder, all screws are loosened while one assistant places the extremity in the desired position and a second assistant then tightens them. If the scrotum interferes with accessibility to the site of operation, it is tightly clipped to the right and left of the penis to the abdominal wall, or held up with a scrotal sling which can be passed around the neck of the patient.

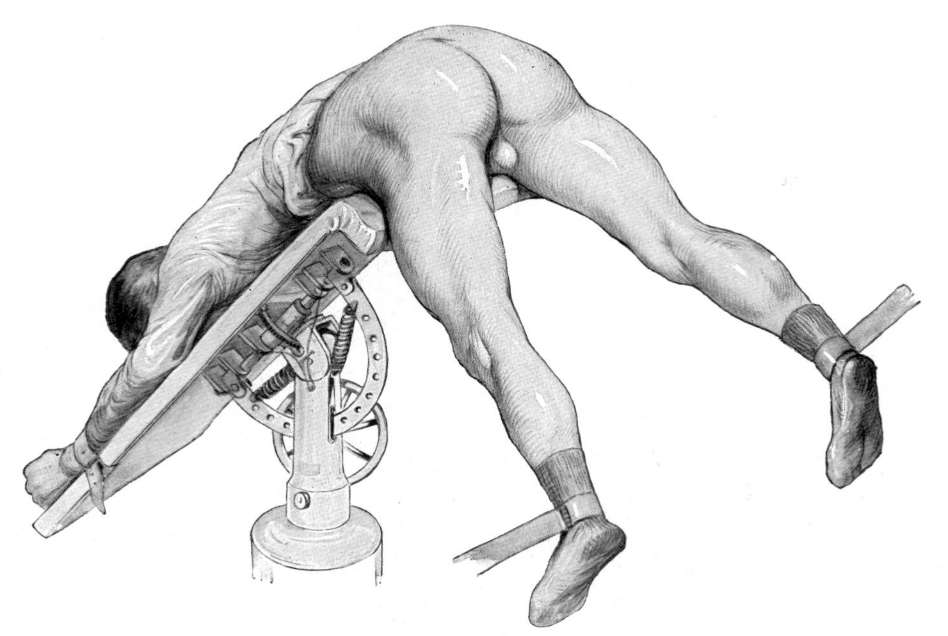

FIG. 34. Position for anal and sacral operations. The lower extremities are abducted.

Operations on the back, as for example laminectomy, can be done with the patient in the lateral position or on his abdomen. I favor the former because the blood flows away from the field of operation, and respiration and access to the mouth are not obstructed. The lateral position is best maintained by flexing the lower extremities to a right angle at the hip-joint, and placing a pillow against the patient's abdomen. The patient is then retained with straps passing around the table in such a way that the field of operation is not interfered with.

For the **exposure of the retroperitoneal space** through a lateral incision (kidney incision), a large air cushion is placed under the opposite lumbar region. This increases the distance between the iliac crest and the rib margin (Fig. 31). Before suturing the incision the air is released from the cushion. The air cushion is preferable to the kidney rack supplied on many operating tables.

Operations on the thorax are, as a rule, done with the patient in the lateral position. The upper part of the trunk is elevated and a soft air cushion is placed so as to throw the chest forward. The upper extremity on the side to be approached is carried upward and forward (Fig. 32).

If the trunk is elevated, as it frequently is, sliding can be prevented by flexing the thighs at the hip-joints and knees, and supporting the buttocks by a well strapped cushion.

In unilateral suppurative disease of the lung care must be taken that during the operation purulent material is not aspirated into the healthy lung. This can be accomplished by placing the patient in the head down position (Fig. 33). Respiratory movements of the healthy side should be restricted as little as possible. Occasionally it may be necessary to place the patient nearly over on his abdomen. If necessary the operator must inconvenience himself for the best interests of the patient. Special operating tables for pulmonary surgery seem to me unnecessary.

Whenever possible I avoid **the abdominal**

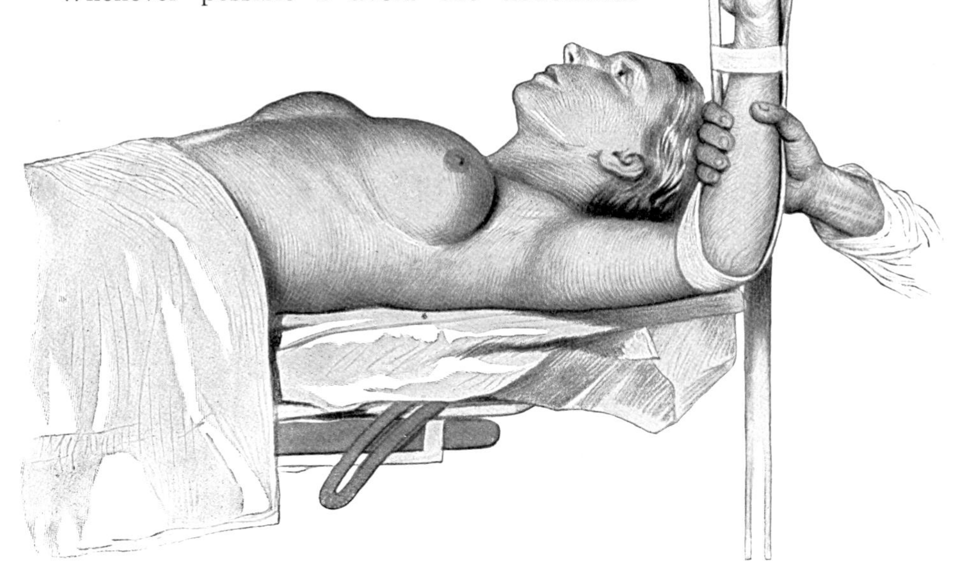

Fig. 35. Right-angle abduction of the arm in axillary exposures (breast amputation with axillary dissection). The forearm is fastened in the desired position to an upright in such a way that it can be easily adjusted.

position. It hinders respiration and prevents ready access to the mouth, disadvantages which can be partly met by placing a pillow under the chest. When the abdominal position is used the arms are best carried above the head.

The **abdominal-suspension position** provides an easy access to the anal and sacral regions (Fig. 34). The patient lies with the head down and the arms extended over the head, where they are attached to the sides of the operating table. The lower extremities are bent to a right angle at the hip-joint, and hang vertically over the table edge. They are spread by supports placed on the side of the table or by bridle-bandages which can be fastened

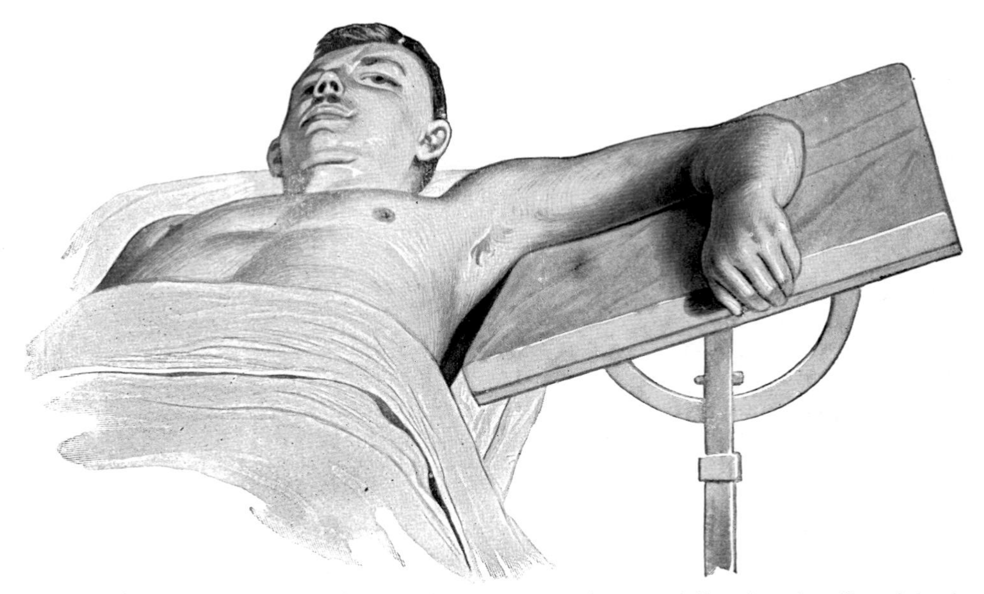

FIG. 36. Position for operations on the upper extremity, especially when the elbow joint is to be moved during the operation. The elevated extremity is placed on a table, adjustable to height and inclination; so as to reduce the amount of blood in the part. The table is covered with a rubber sponge cushion.

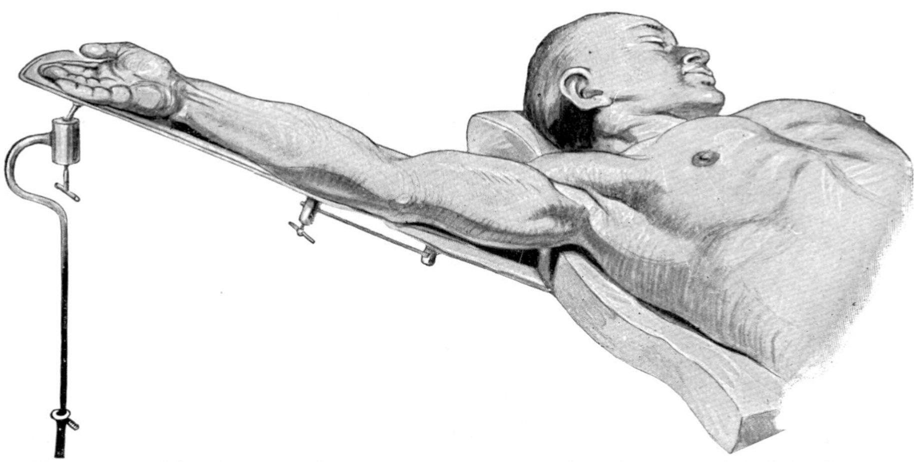

FIG. 37. Position for operations on the upper extremity when the elbow joint is not to be moved during the operation. In order to lessen plethora the extended limb is elevated upon a narrow support, adjustable to height and inclination, which is fastened to the operating table at one end and rests upon a leg at the other.

to the walls. The operator stations himself between the legs of the patient. This position is so uncomfortable for the patient that it should only be used during general anæsthesia.

In operations involving the axilla the arm is abducted at the shoulder-joint. Care should be taken when this position is maintained over long periods that there is no drag on, or injury to the brachial plexus. To hold the arm in the desired position it is suspended from an upright, and can be further supported by an orderly who need not be sterile (Fig. 35).

When performing operations on the extremities in which a tourniquet is not used, the position must be so arranged that there is a constant incline of the operated extremity towards the heart. For the arm, a small table is used, which can be screwed to the operating table and is supported by a special leg (Figs. 36, 37). For operations on the extensor surface of the elbow-joint the arm can be carried over the body.

One should never be misled into operating on a patient sitting on an ordinary chair, or perhaps even standing. If the patient collapses, the asepsis suffers. The patient should be placed on an operating table for every operation. He should be strapped whether local or general anæsthesia is used so that he will not interfere with the asepsis by any movement. Do not depend upon the assurance of the rationality of the patient himself. Naturally an explanation should be given to the conscious patient as to the necessity for the restriction.

D. GENERAL PRINCIPLES OF OPERATIVE TECHNIC

The aims of operative procedures vary according to the lesions which present themselves. They are attained, or striven for, by division, by suture, by displacement, by excision, by transplantation of tissues, or by the implantation of foreign bodies.

1. Division of Tissues

An exact knowledge and a constant consideration of topographical anatomy is indispensable for safe and careful surgery. A lack of consideration of anatomy and the use of one's intuition may occasionally bear fruit, but it is more often paid for by the patient. I am of the opinion that, with very few exceptions, all those structures which fall within the exposure of the operation should be systematically searched for and should be exposed by careful dissection. It is only with such care that accidental injuries can with certainty be avoided. The exposed anatomical structures offer, like the navigation points to the sailor, the only trustworthy sign-posts which permit the surgeon to continue with safety. **A perfect anatomical preparation is the foundation of every systematically planned operation.**

Of primary importance is the eyesight of the surgeon. All errors of refraction should be corrected. This is especially true of those suffering from presbyopia. For especially delicate dissections I utilize the Zeiss spectacles which have a two-fold magnification. They have the further advantage that they do not hinder the ordinary vision or the use of glasses for errors of refraction. The operator can stand at a distance of 20 cm. from the operative field when using the Zeiss spectacles.

For adequate exposure of the operative site it is necessary that the incision be of sufficient size. Unusually small skin scars should call forth no admiration. It is likewise true that an incision may be unnecessarily long or mutilating. The skin incision need be no longer than the incision necessary in the deeper parts. The wound should not be funnel-shaped, but should be rectangular in longitudinal section.

The greatest care and gentleness should be used in making the incision, in advancing through tissues, and in exposing deeper structures. Tearing, pulling, and boring through tissues have no place in surgery. Even in opening abscesses and phlegmons, care is necessary lest blind puncture damage surrounding or deeper structures. An incision made with a sharp scalpel inflicts the least possible damage and is therefore the least susceptible to infection. The knife is the most important instrument of the surgeon, the token of his

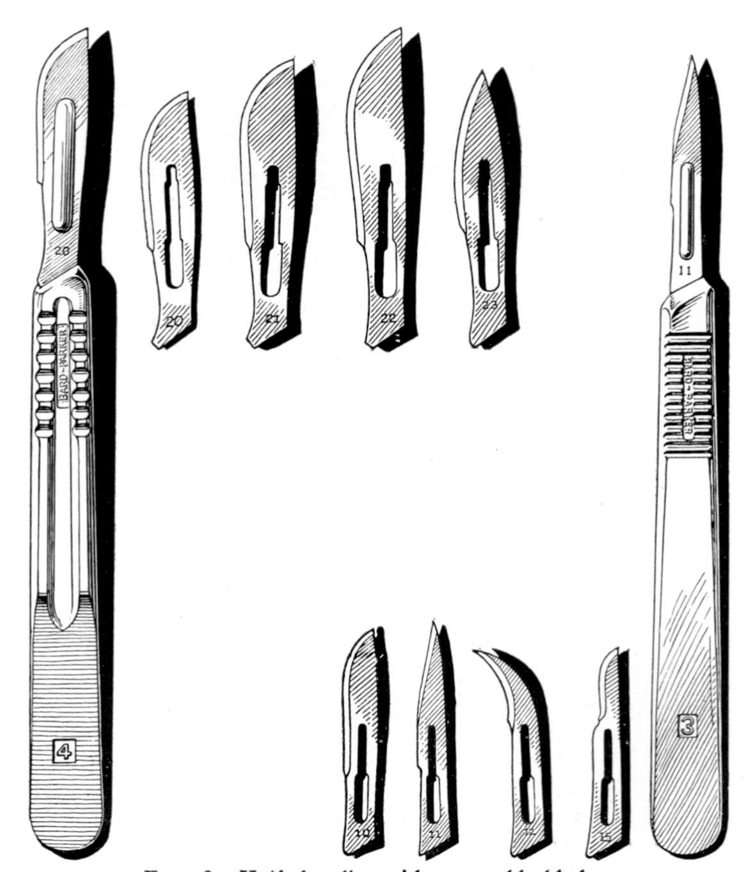

Fig. 38. Knife-handles with removable blades.

craft. It should always be sharp, for it is difficult to do good work with poor tools. One can often tell a poorly conducted clinic by the knives provided for the surgeon. Scalpels with changeable blades (Fig. 38) are excellent where the facilities for keeping the knives perfectly sharpened are not at hand. The keenness of the changeable blade is, I believe, considerably surpassed by a well sharpened solid knife. The changeable blades suffice for the ordinary incisions but do not satisfy me in dissection of dense tissues. I have not found the stainless steel knife as serviceable as those made from finer steels.

The **technic of holding the knife blade** at an acute angle against the skin is to be condemned, even though it is frequently recommended. The surgeon should have no fear in using a sharp scalpel. The handle of the scalpel is solely for holding, and it should not be used as a blunt dissector, for which unfortunately it is too frequently employed. The scalpel is held differently according to the thickness and density of the tissue to be divided. The writing-pen grasp (Fig. 40) is used for delicate dissections, the violin-bow grasp (Fig. 41) for skin incisions, the table-knife grasp (Fig. 42) for amputation incisions, and the stiletto grasp (Fig. 43) for transfixion. The choice of these lies in the sense of touch.

All attempts to control the hemorrhage which results from the use of the scalpel by crushing or pressure, by the use of the Paquelin, or electric cautery, seem unwise. The actual amount of tissue damage which results

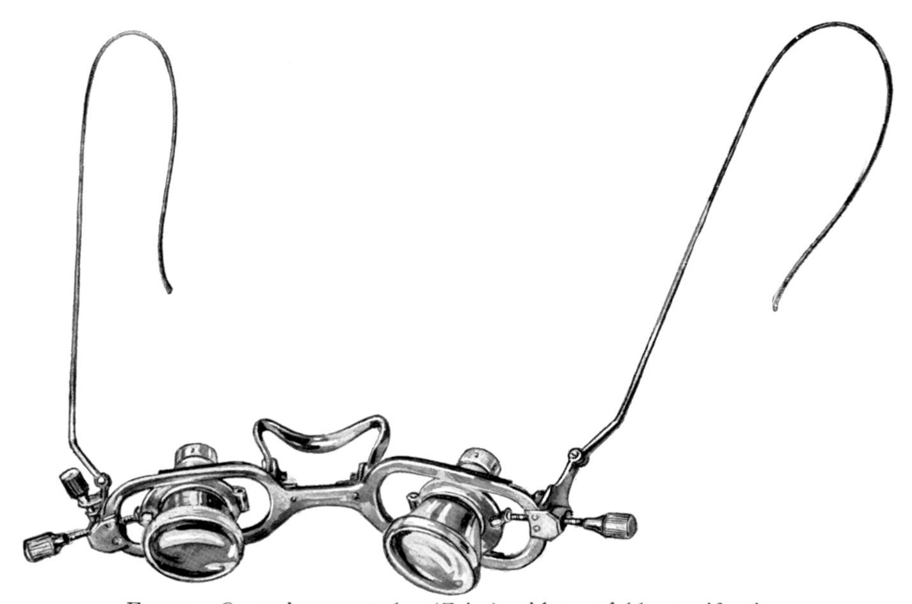

FIG. 39. Operating spectacles (Zeiss) with two-fold magnification.

from the use of these procedures cannot be estimated, and the type of injury which results from their use is not conducive to primary wound healing.

Electro- or Thermocoagulation. The current used for diathermy and electro-coagulation is a high frequency current with rapid alternation. It is a current of low potential, below 100 volts. The heating action is proportional to the square of the amperage and the resistance of the tissues. With a constant current strength of 0.2 to 0.3 amperes, one can increase the heating action to the thermal death point by union of the current paths. The blood in small vessels can be coagulated and the vessels can then be divided without hemorrhage. High frequency currents are utilized in surgery in four ways:

1. As a spark point, using the Forest needle or a needle of this type.
2. For coagulation of an entire area, as a tumor.

3. For control of hemorrhage.
4. For dissection.

An electrode is attached to the patient at a location removed from the site of operation. A pad saturated with saline solution is best placed between the skin and the electrode. The active electrode can be fitted with the desired device for a spark, for coagulation, or for cutting. (The Bovie apparatus

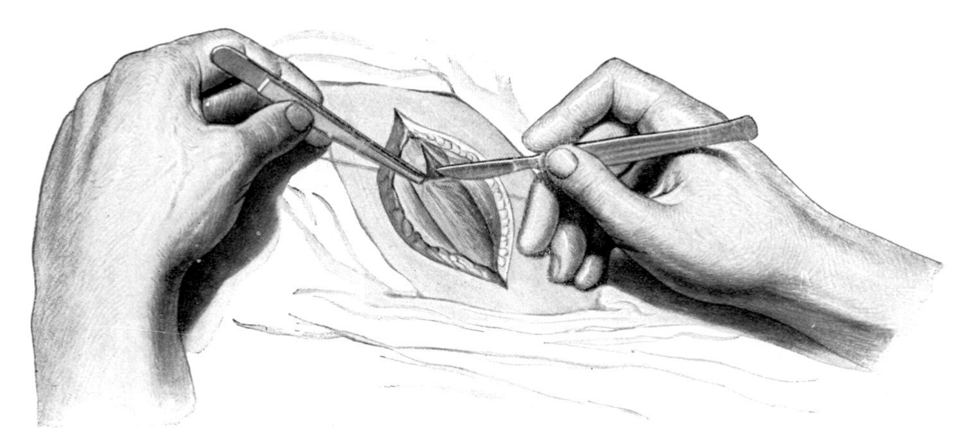

FIG. 40. Writing-pen grasp of knife. This is useful in the finer dissections.

embodies the best principles of this kind of apparatus now obtainable in the United States [Fig. 102]. The active electrode is applied to the surface to be treated. I. S. R.)

The point-electrode is used for the treatment of superficial skin lesions, angiomata, etc. The needle is applied at intervals of 2 to 4 mm. This procedure causes practically no pain.

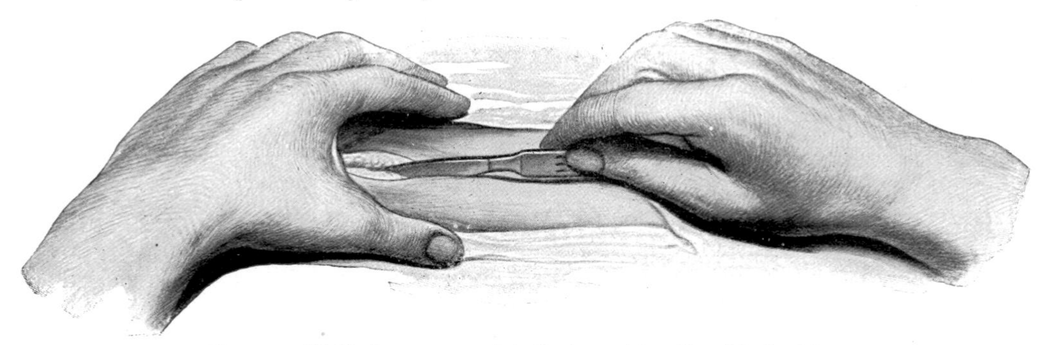

FIG. 41. Violin-bow grasp of knife in making the skin incision.

For coagulation an electrode about 0.25 to 0.5 mm. wide is placed on the tissue to be destroyed and the current is applied for about 30 seconds. This current should give no spark, nor should it crackle. Through continued action the tissue becomes discolored and takes on a cooked appearance, at which time it is necrotic. The action is greater if the blood supply to the part can be cut off while the electrode is in action.

With various types of electrodes tissue can be cut through with as sharp an edge as a knife can make. Coagulation and dissection may be carried on at the same time by using two active electrodes. The wound as a rule can be closed by primary suture. This method is also useful in opening abscesses and in removing malignant growths.

No exact rules can be given for this type of work since each type of apparatus varies and considerable knowledge of the instrument being used is necessary in order to obtain the best results.

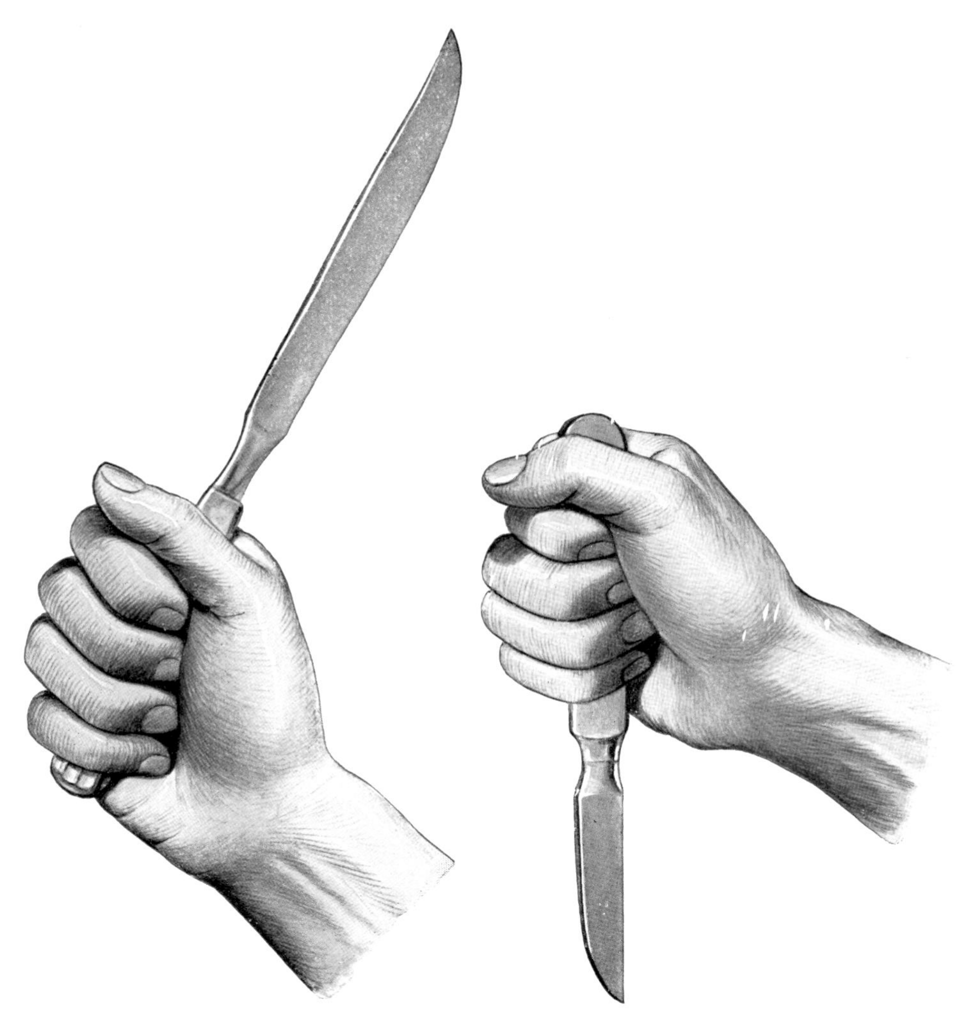

FIG. 42. Grasp of knife in amputations. FIG. 43. Grasp of knife for transfixion.

For grasping vessels and individual tissues one of the types of surgical forceps, with fine teeth, is very useful (Fig. 44). Anatomic forceps are not suited for grasping unless they are used very carefully for they injure the tissue grasped. They are however very useful for holding sponges, sutures, compresses and tampons. They are also useful in replacing the omentum, or removing it from the field of operation, for replacing protruding fat, during the suture of a wound, or for inversion of stumps, such as the stump of the appendix. In deep wounds long forceps are preferable.

Exposure of important structures, such as arteries, is accomplished by stretching the overlying connective tissues and dividing these layer by layer with a scalpel. In doing this the individual connective tissue layers are grasped and elevated with surgical forceps, a pair being held by the left hand of both the operator and his assistant. The raised fold is incised vertically. The forceps should be held like a writing pen with the fingers, not with the palm. Timidity, with resulting scratching, with a scalpel held at an angle, is to be attributed to lack of self-confidence or to lack of skill. The use of a groove director or anatomical forceps pushed bluntly under the overlying connective tissue, which is then divided, is not recommended, nor is the method of dividing the connective tissue by tearing to be tolerated even in the inexperienced.

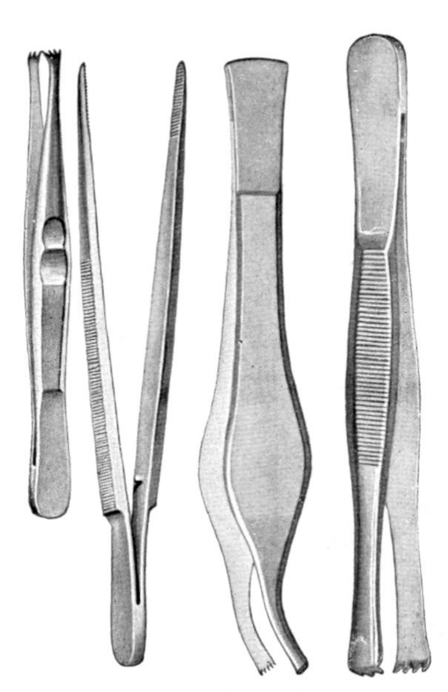

FIG. 44. a, c, d, various types of surgical forceps. b, anatomical forcep.

To free the exposed structures from any adherent connective tissue, and for pushing aside already divided tissue, I use the so-called tampon-holder, or dissecting forceps (Fig. 45). The dissecting forceps is handed to the surgeon equipped with a tampon, and after being used should be exchanged for a fresh one. The tampon must be firmly held by the end of the forceps so that it is not easily displaced. The use of a tampon in this way is much to be preferred to the use of the finger, the use of a tampon or piece of gauze in the hand, or the handle of a scalpel or other instrument. The use of the scalpel in this manner endangers one's assistants and is not in accord with careful surgical technic. Sharp dissection with a knife should alternate with blunt dissection with the tampon forceps until the area desired has been completely exposed.

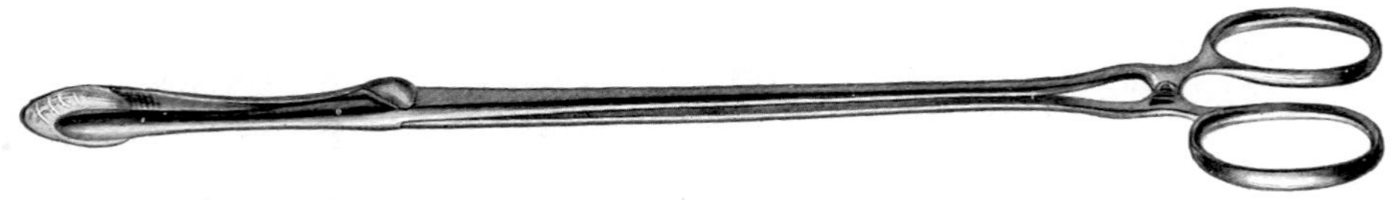

FIG. 45. Tampon-holder or dissecting forceps for the retraction of layers of loose tissue.

In separating thick layers of connective tissue, in which there are no important structures or large vessels, as for instance in the separation of the subcutaneous tissue after the skin has been incised, the skin is retracted and elevated with two sharp hooks, which puts tension on the fascia so that it can be divided easily with a few strokes of the scalpel (Fig. 46).

The divided skin and subcutaneous tissues are retracted with sharp or blunt hooked retractors of various forms and sizes, so as to expose the underlying structures. I find the most useful hooked retractors are those with from one to eight short sharp prongs (v. Volkmann) (Fig. 47); the blunt flat retractor of v. Langenbeck which is made in various widths and lengths; the long bladed sharp or blunt muscle retractors; the vein retractors, and the Roux retractors which resemble the last very closely (Fig. 48). The use for each is self evident.

Should the surgeon want to limit the number of assistants, or to make use of the added hands to better advantage, if there are not enough assistants at one's disposal, or if the wound margins must be retracted over a long period, self retaining retractors render excellent service. There are a number of different types of these, according to the type of wound to be retracted

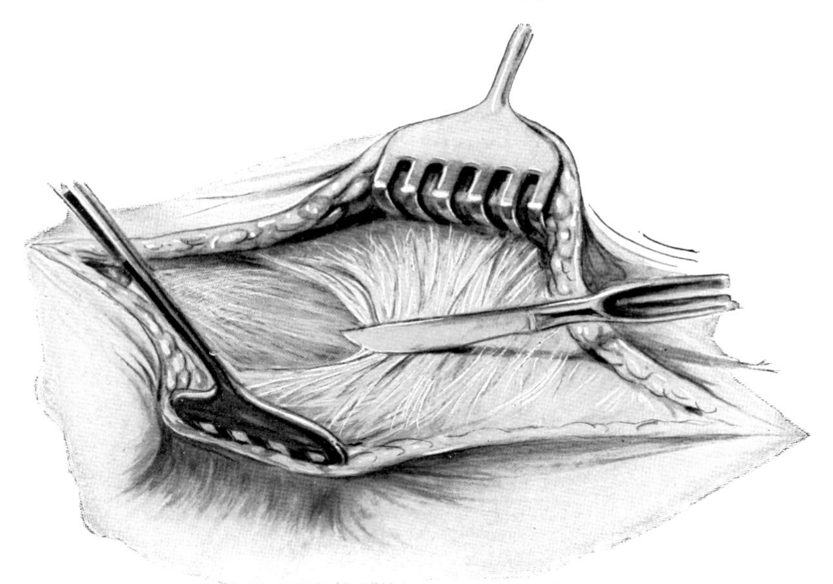

FIG. 46. Division of subcutaneous tissue with long strokes of the scalpel. The cutaneous tissues are retracted and raised by pronged retractors.

(Fig. 49). Some clinics use weighted hooks for self-retaining retractors, but these have the disadvantage of shifting their position and even falling to the floor. I have therefore devised a weighted hooked retractor with a double set of prongs, which is self retaining, which lies flat, and which will hold even thin tissue layers firmly (Fig. 50). Blunt retractors can be mounted on a frame and used as self retaining retractors (Fig. 51). Such a retractor replaces an assistant in an abdominal operation, and has the advantage of indefatigableness and uniformity.

If it is necessary to retract fascial margins, hernial sacs, the margins of the common duct or the dura mater, or small tumors, these can be grasped with Allis forceps or with various types of tenacula (Fig. 52). The larger types are particularly useful in grasping and manipulating large, dense structures. If these instruments hinder the view of, or access to the wound, one can use silk threads for retraction (Fig. 53). This type of traction is very

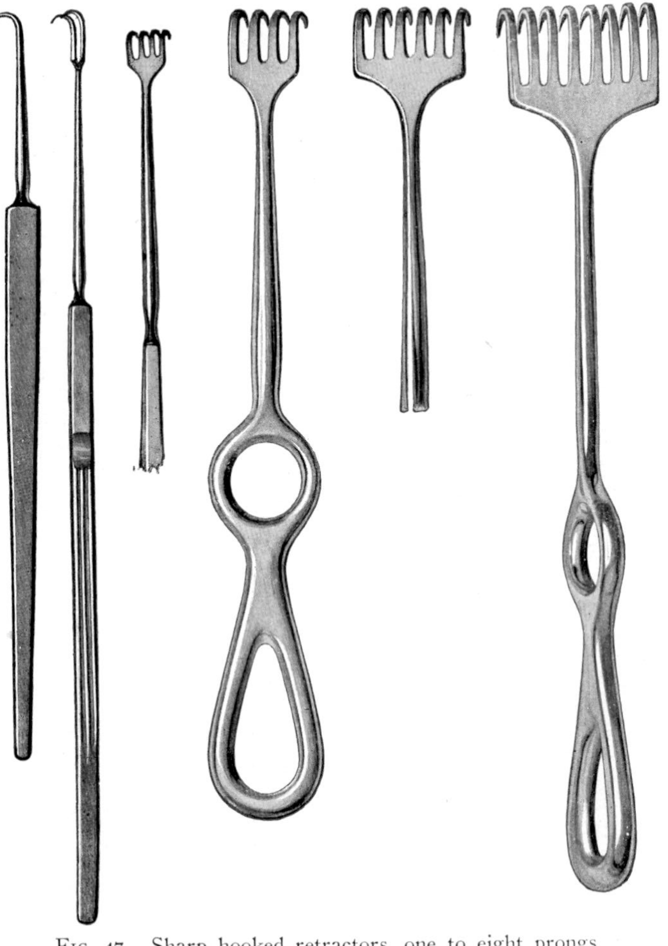

Fig. 47. Sharp hooked retractors, one to eight prongs.

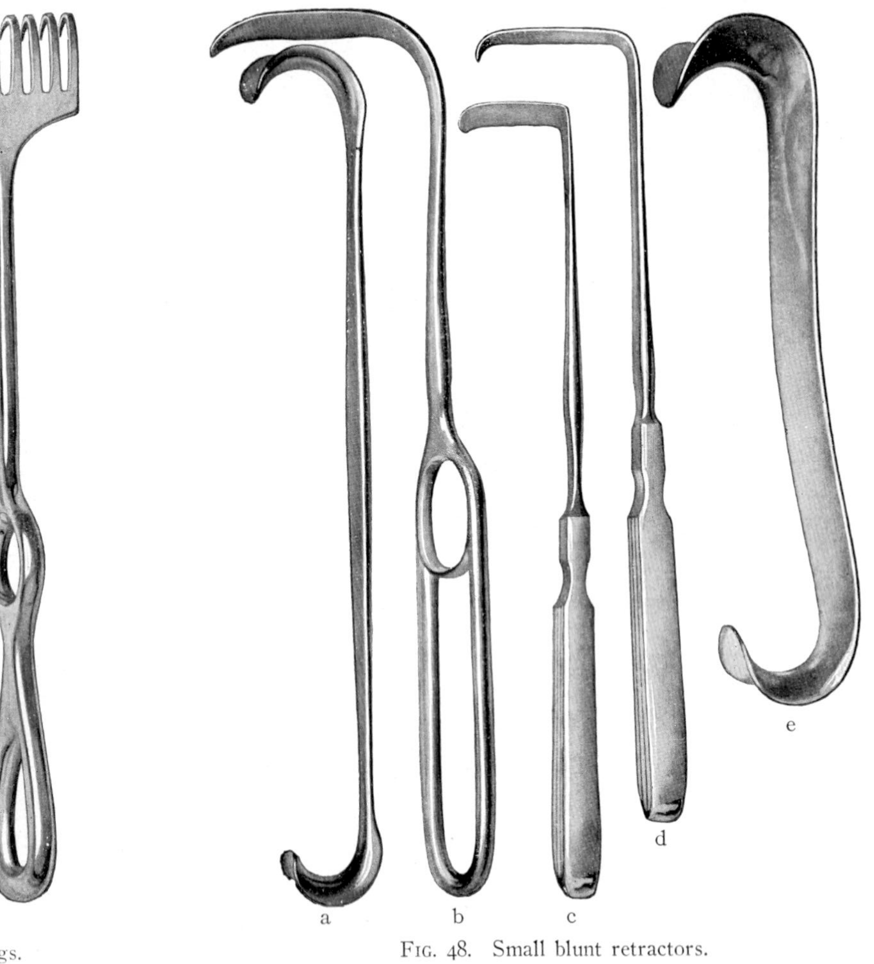

Fig. 48. Small blunt retractors.

The high hopes once placed in substances which supposedly dissolved cicatrices, such as fibrolysin, choline chloride, urea, and pregl-pepsin, have not been fulfilled. These remedies when used are injected either locally in the cicatrix and the surrounding area, or like fibrolysin may be injected at a distance. Likewise the results of the injection of human fat (humanol) have not been satisfactory. If the re-union of cord-like structures is to be pre-

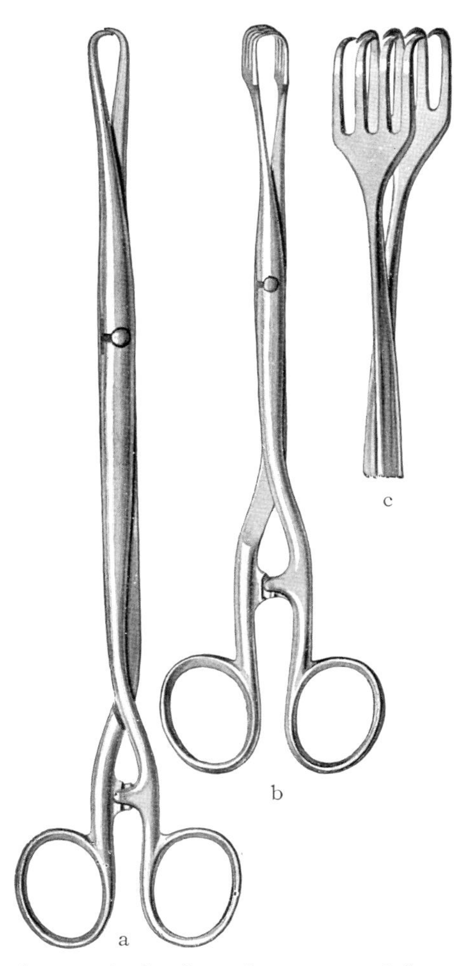

Fig. 52. a. Tenaculum forceps; b. Small; c. Large pronged forceps for grasping tissues.

vented, simple division does not as a rule suffice and it is best to excise a piece of the tissue. In this manner one can destroy permanently the function of tendons and nerves. In the division of blood vessels it would seem more advisable to resect a part of the vessel, rather than to ligate it in continuity or simply to divide it between ligatures. The separation, especially of tendons and nerves, is made more certain after division if the ends are turned back so as to make a sling, as was suggested by Nicoladoni in the treatment of flat feet after division of the tendon of Achilles (Fig. 55).

The Dilatation of Strictures. The dilatation of fistulous openings, strictures of the anus, of the esophagus, of the urethra, of the papilla of Vater, of the cervix, etc., can be accomplished in many instances by blunt dilatation. Conical shaped instruments of gradually increasing thickness are inserted through the stricture, beginning with the smaller sizes. Dilators are shaped according to the form and length of the channels to be dilated, so that many types exist: the short Hegar bougies (Fig. 56), the curved urethral bougies (Fig. 57), the long esophageal dilators, and many others. The instruments are either rigid and are made of metal, or they are elastic and made of rubber or silk covered with lacquer. The olivary tips either singly or in series are very useful in the treatment of esophageal strictures (Fig. 58).

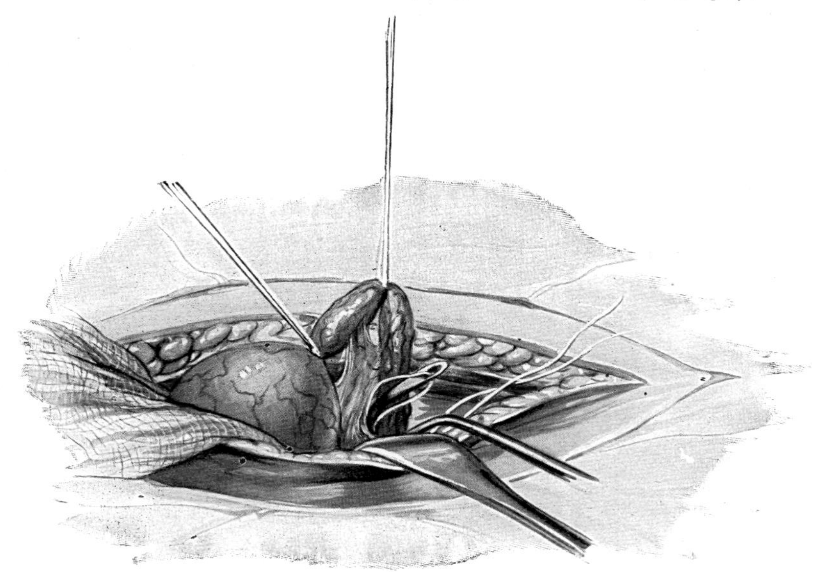

FIG. 53. Placing of ligatures at intervals with an aneurism needle. These ligatures can be used for retraction.

To push the instruments through the stricture requires a certain force. Since the operator cannot see the tip of the dilator, this force is not without danger. Sudden overcoming of the resistance may mean passage through the contracture or perforation of the wall. The utmost caution and care must be exercised whenever a bougie is used. The danger of perforation can be lessened by using a filiform bougie which is attached to the end of the larger dilator. The filiform is first passed through the stricture and this acts as a guide for the larger dilator (Fig. 57). This procedure is not entirely safe, since the thin filiform may break. The safest method, which, however, is not always possible, is to pull the dilator through the stenosis. If this is possible greater force can be used without danger of perforation. A thread is passed through the stricture and to the end of this the dilating instrument is attached. For the esophagus and for the intestine, a thread provided with a small shot (Fig. 59) is carried through the stenosis by peristaltic action. Through an opening in the stomach, the intestine, or urinary bladder the thread is recovered. The dilatation is accomplished by fastening to this

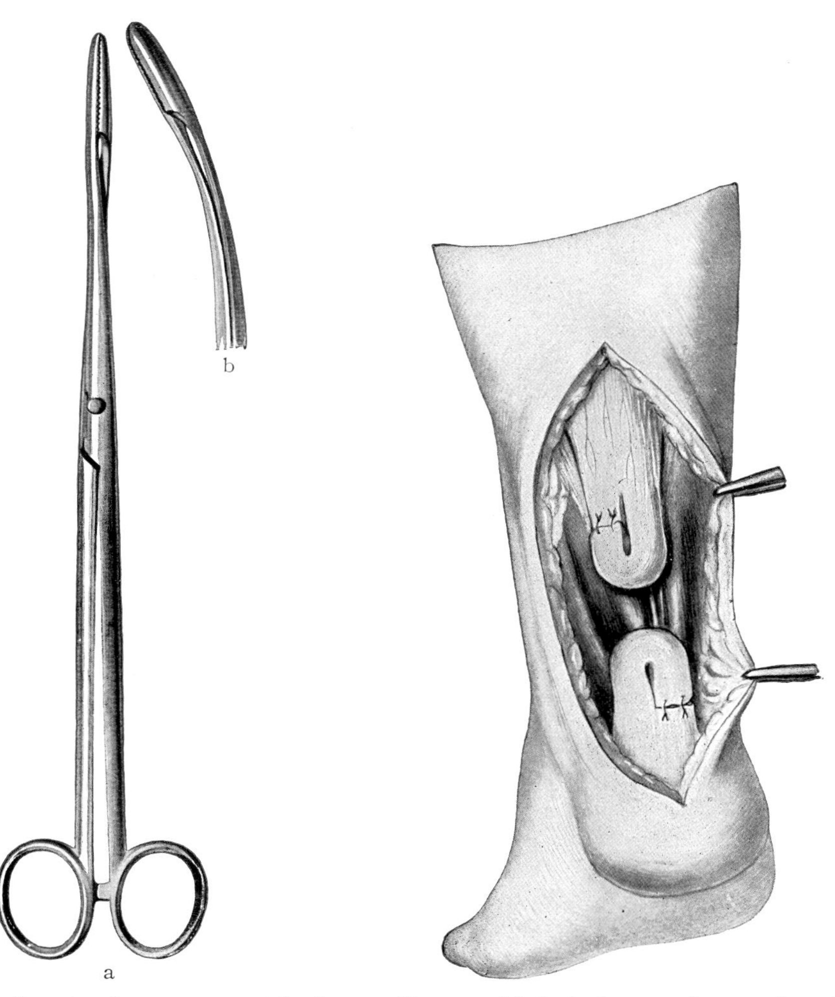

Fig. 54. Dressing forceps—a. straight, b. curved.

Fig. 55. Method of preventing reunion of tendons, *i.e.*, the tendo achilles.

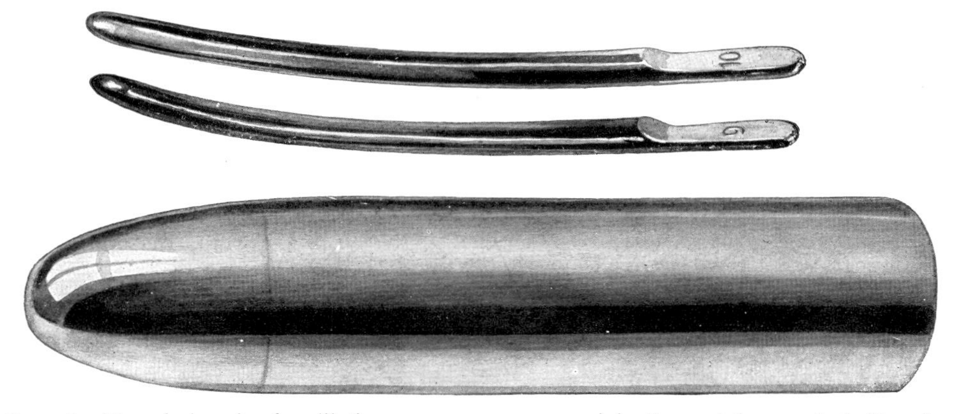

Fig. 56. Hegar's bougies for dilating narrow passages, originally used for cervical dilatation. The large forms are useful for anal dilatation.

thread either olives of gradually increasing size (Fig. 58) or flexible dilators (Fig. 60) which are then pulled retrogradely through the stricture.

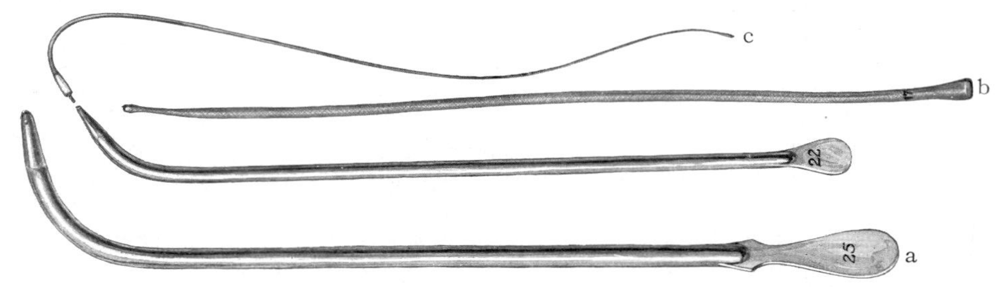

FIG. 57. Bougies for the dilatation of strictures, especially of the urethra. a. Metal, b. lacquered silk, c. filiform bougie.

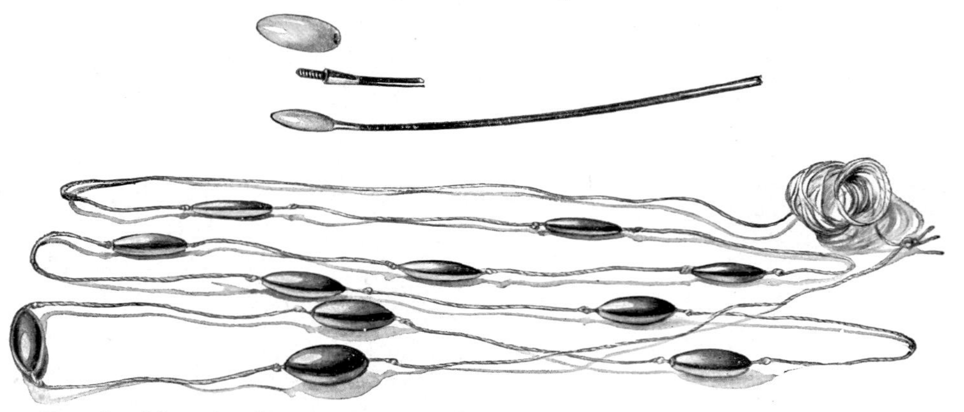

FIG. 58. Olives for dilatation of strictures, especially of the esophagus. The first type is introduced on a fishbone sound, while in the second type olives increasing in size are attached to a silk thread for "sounding without end."

An exceptionally useful instrument for blunt dilatation of short stenoses is the screwtop (Fig. 61), which is made in various sizes. With gentle screwing it dilates the stricture quickly and without danger.

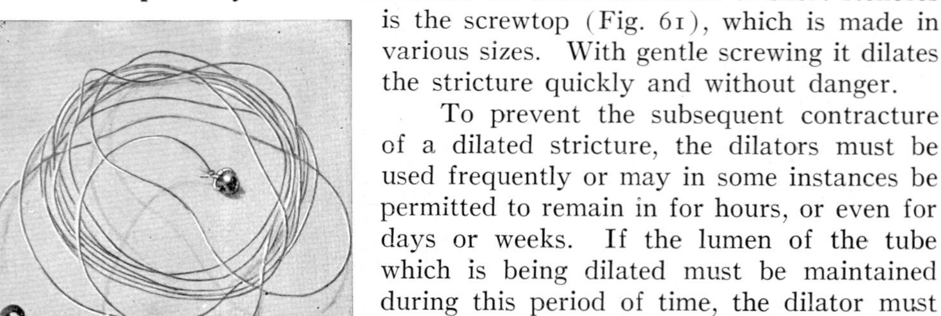

FIG. 59. Thread with shot, which is carried through the stricture by the peristalsis of the esophagus or intestine, so as to make possible repeated bouginage with the "thread without end."

To prevent the subsequent contracture of a dilated stricture, the dilators must be used frequently or may in some instances be permitted to remain in for hours, or even for days or weeks. If the lumen of the tube which is being dilated must be maintained during this period of time, the dilator must be hollow.

The dilatation of a narrowed lumen can also be accomplished at times by using materials which expand when introduced into the body. This is often a very useful method. For narrow stenoses catgut may be used; while for larger openings laminaria crayons (Fig. 62) are more effective. The crayons are inserted after they have been

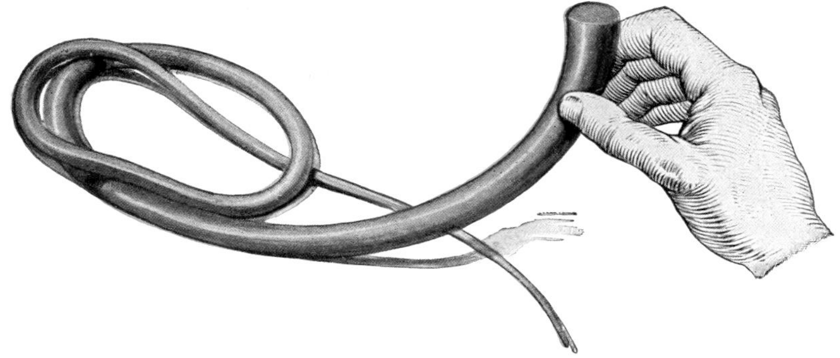

Fig. 60. Whip-like rubber bougie, for dilating strictures, especially of the esophagus.

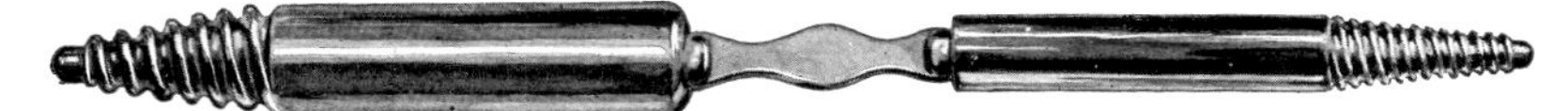

Fig. 61. Screw for dilating strictures.

immersed in boiling water for a few seconds and then squeezed dry. They remain in place for a variable period up to 24 hours. They have a thread attached at one end which prevents their being sucked in and permits of easy removal. V. Hacker has taught us to use, for a similar purpose, the elasticity of rubber tubes (Fig. 63). During stretching the rubber tube becomes thinner, but when the force is released it assumes its previous proportions. A rubber tube is stretched over a rigid sound and is thus introduced through the stenosis and the sound then withdrawn. The rubber tube contracts and thickens so that it makes pressure against the stricture. It is removed after a time and is replaced by a tube of larger diameter. The procedure is continued until the desired effect is obtained.

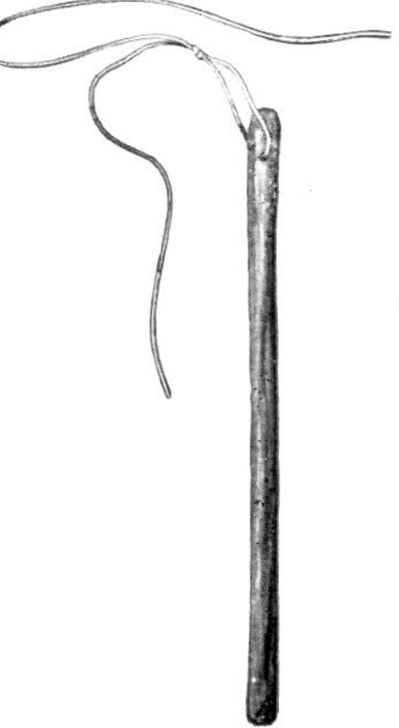

Fig. 62. Laminaria. Introduced dry, it expands by absorption of moisture and stretches the stricture.

If the desired effect cannot be obtained with the use of blunt dilatation, the cicatricial ring may be divided by radial incisions and the stenosis prevented from recurring by subsequent blunt dilatation. This method has not been very successful in the extensive strictures of the larger tubes. If the incision can not be made under the guidance of the eyes, then one should use

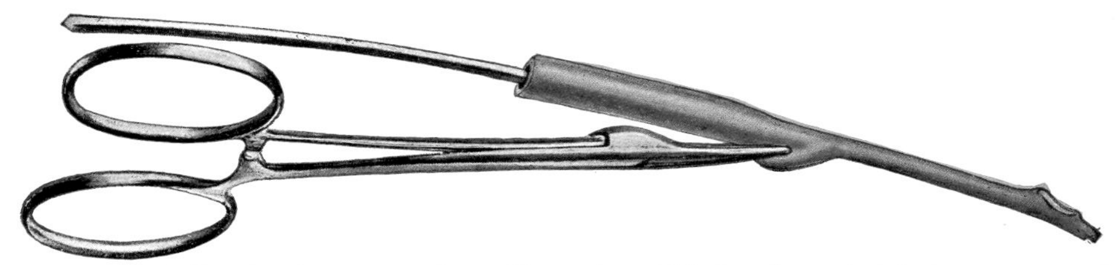

Fig. 63. Dilatation by means of a rubber tube which has been stretched over a sound. When the sound is withdrawn the diameter of the rubber tube increases and thus exerts pressure on the stricture.

one of the types of electrically lighted cannulæ or one of the knives enclosed in a sound, which knife is released after the tip of the dilator has passed the stricture (Fig. 64). The stricture is sectioned during the withdrawal of the instrument. This method has been very useful in the treatment of urethral stricture.

If measures such as those described fail to give the desired result, that portion of the tube which is stenosed should be excised and an end to end suture of healthy surfaces should be made, if possible. If end to end suture is not possible, some other type of plastic operation must be resorted to. Skin flaps whose outer surfaces are turned inward have been used. These may be pedunculated or may be free epidermis grafts. The epidermis grafts are fastened for this purpose on a suitable form made of rubber or dental compound. The grafts should be larger than the area to be covered. The details of this procedure are discussed in Chapter V, "Operations on the

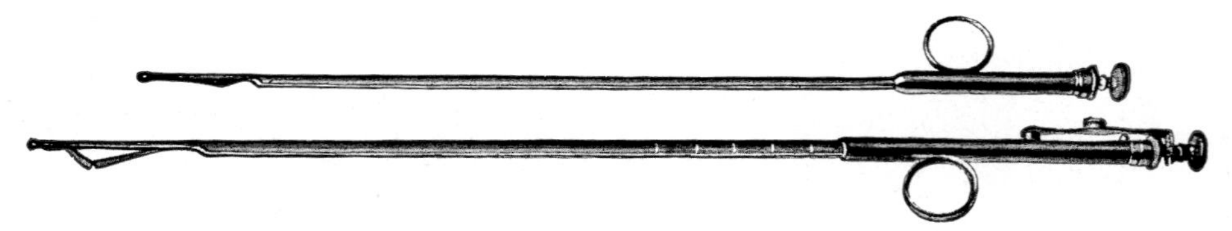

FIG. 64. Sounds with concealed knives (urethrotome). These are carried through the stricture with the blade concealed and are withdrawn with the blade exposed, thus dividing the stricture.

Skin." Although it may be doubted, I have found that for various defects the skin can be used satisfactorily to replace destroyed mucous membrane.

2. WOUND REPAIR

Union of wounds made at operation or resulting from injury is brought about, if possible, by direct suture of tissue planes, or, if necessary, by plastic operations, which may require lengthening, shortening, or the displacement of tissue, such as muscles and tendons. The purpose of repair is the establishment of permanent and firm union. It is obtained through the various forms of tissue suture.

In discussing the strength of tissue suture the factors of time and of the conditions of wound repair must be considered. The initial union depends solely upon the suture, and this we have become accustomed to designate as the **primary, or inorganic, union** of the wound. Gradually the coaptation becomes a permanent union through proliferation of fibroblasts between the two wound surfaces, and this we designate as **secondary, or organic, union.**

INORGANIC TISSUE UNION (COAPTATION)

Artificial union of tissues results from suture. In this manner close contact of the tissues can be obtained, and with the exception of certain plastic operations, the reconstruction of separated tissues leads to the restoration of normal anatomical relations.

In suturing tissues a threaded needle is passed first through one side of the wound and then to a point opposite this on the other side of the wound.

The ends of the suture are made taut to approximate the edges of the wound and the suture is tied, or if the suture is to be continuous the procedure is repeated without tying except at the beginning and the end of the suture line. It is possible to unite large wounds by multiple **interrupted** sutures, **or** by one **continuous suture.** The single sutures are more detailed, and consume more time, but they are safer than the continuous suture, since the entire suture line is jeopardized by the suture breaking at one point. The continuous suture on the other hand is more rapid and makes the suture line

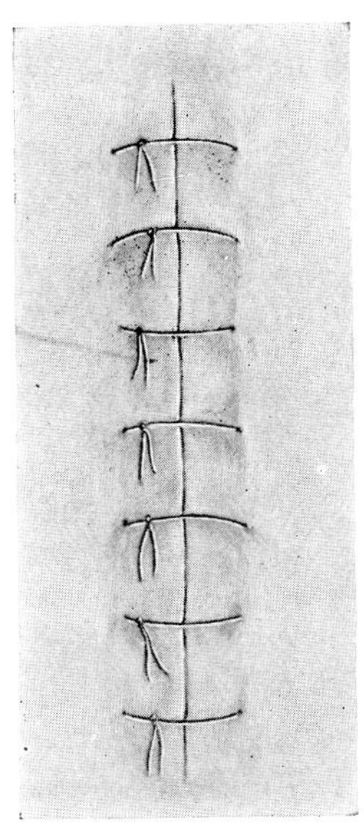

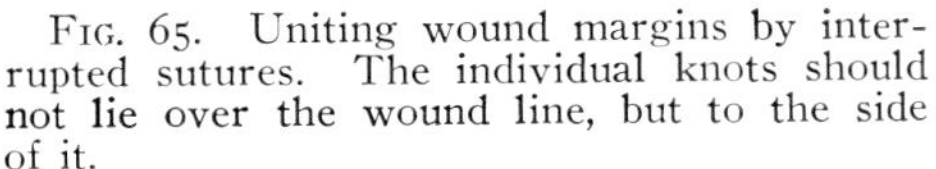

Fig. 65. Uniting wound margins by interrupted sutures. The individual knots should not lie over the wound line, but to the side of it.

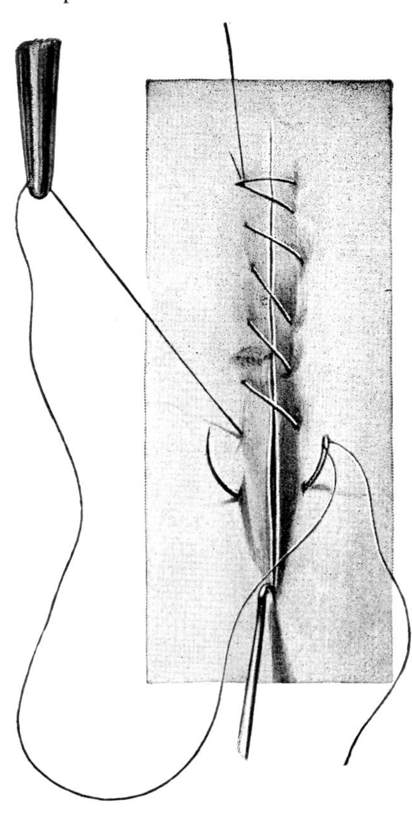

Fig. 66. Uniting wound margins by continuous suture. The suture is held taut with forceps by an assistant.

tighter than the interrupted suture with its intermediate spaces. It is, therefore, often preferred when the suture line is to be air and water-tight, or where the suture is being used for the arrest of hemorrhage. Either type of suture, if placed too close together and drawn too tight, may cause tissue strangulation, which eventually may lead to wound suppuration. The purpose of the suture is primary retention only, which must be made permanent by cicatrization.

When using the interrupted suture the thread is carried once through each side of the wound, and then tied securely in a knot (Fig. 65). The knot should be tied to either side of the wound, not over it. In continuous suture the thread, after it is carried through both wound margins, is knotted in the same manner, one end cut short and the suturing continued with the other end (Fig. 66). The approximation of the wound margins is obtained by tension on the suture which is held firmly by the assistant. He may use anatomic forceps or a special suture holder (Fig. 66).

The continuous suture is finally tied by drawing the thread only part way through one side, so that a loop is left, and then passing the end of the suture through the opposite side, thus providing ends for tying. If the suture is not long enough for this, a single stitch may be placed at the end of the wound and one end of this used to tie with the end of the continuous suture.

The complicated methods of suture formerly used have today at most only a historical value. Next to the simple interrupted or continuous suture, the **mattress suture** is of most importance (Fig. 67). This stitch may be of a continuous or interrupted type, the latter being preferable in most instances. The **recurrent stitch** is used chiefly for the arrest of hemorrhage (Figs. 69 and 70). The stitches overlap so as to completely surround the wound. The mattress stitch can be inserted so that the edges of the wound are inverted or everted. (Figs. 68, 71 a and b.) In the one instance the buried portion of the suture is at right angles to the wound, while in the other it is parallel to it. Either of these stitches may, however, cause interference with the circula-

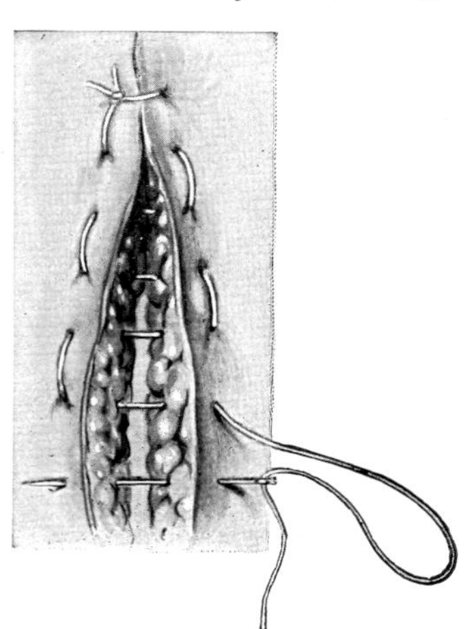

Fig. 67. Continuous mattress suture of the skin.

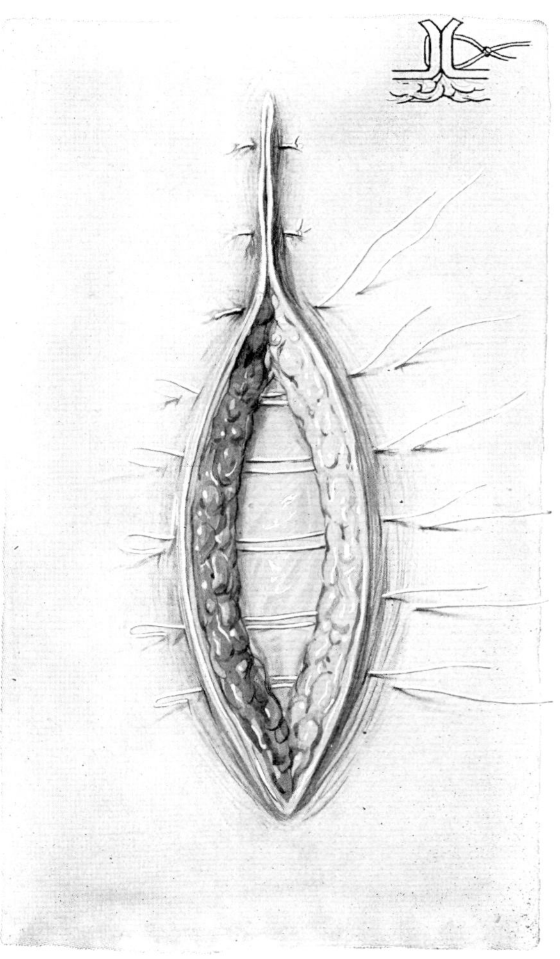

Fig. 68. Vertical mattress suture for eversion of wound edges.

tion of the wound edges. The interrupted **vertical mattress suture** (Fig. 68) does away with this difficulty. The suture passes through both sides of the wound at a considerable distance from the edges of the wound and then is passed back parallel to the first stitch but just catching the skin margins. This is a very useful suture. Many other stitches find favor in different countries, but as a whole they are modifications of the sutures already described. The various sero-muscular sutures are examples of this. It is for this reason that they are omitted from any separate description here.

For any type of suture a sharp needle is most important. While I prefer **needles** with a cutting edge or lancet shaped point (Fig. 72), some surgeons prefer the rounded points for certain types of suture. I prefer the sharper pointed needles because they penetrate tissues with greater ease and smoothness. The threading of the needle is made easier if the needle is provided with a split-eye. For intestinal surgery the needle may be integrally

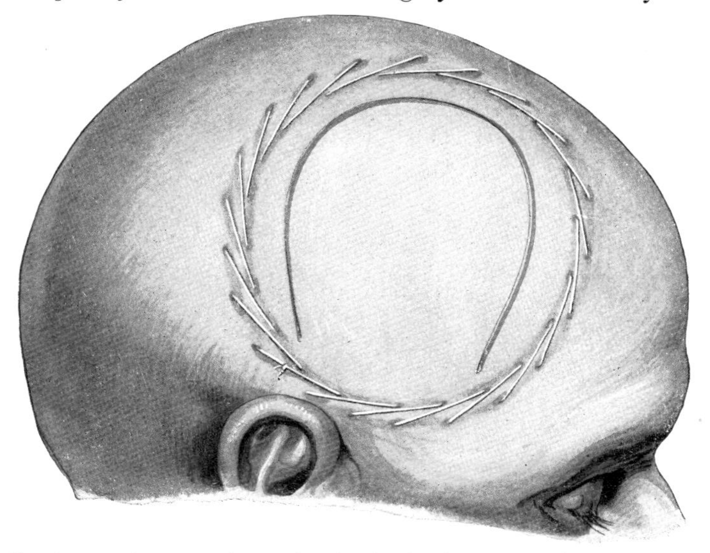

Fig. 69. Continuous (recurrent) overlapping back-stitch suture for control of hæmorrhage, in craniectomy. The stitches are so placed as to enclose completely the area outlined for the flap incision.

fixed to the catgut so as to be atraumatic. The size and shape of needles vary according to their use and the preference of the surgeon. The majority of needles are curved, the radius of curvature and the length of the circular arch varying. Curved needles should always be used with a needle-holder. Of these there are many types from which the surgeon may choose that one which suits him best.

I have personally used the Deus needle-holder for many years (Fig. 73). It has the advantage of holding the needle firmly without breaking it. Another very popular holder is the Mayo modification of the Hegar needle-holder (Fig. 74). For suturing in deep wounds the long, slender holders are to be preferred. For cleft-palate operations, the bayonet-like curved needle-holder is extremely useful (Fig. 75). For suturing the skin, the intestine, or in vascular suture straight needles are often used. For these no holder is necessary. For dense tissues the Reverdin needle is very satisfactory. (Fig.

76.) It is pushed through the tissues with the eye closed; the eye is then opened, the assistant inserts the suture and the needle is withdrawn.

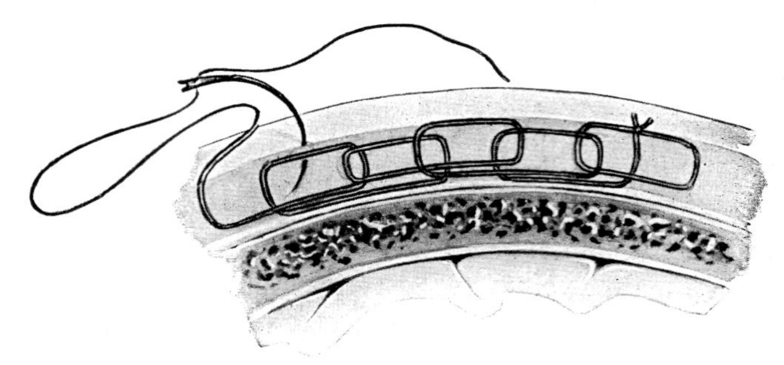

FIG. 70. Continuous (recurrent) overlapping back-stitch in cross-section (diagrammatic).

For **suture material** we use a variety of materials, linen, silk, catgut, wire, silkworm-gut, horsehair, kangaroo tendon, and living fascia. These suffice for every kind of work. If the materials are carefully selected one

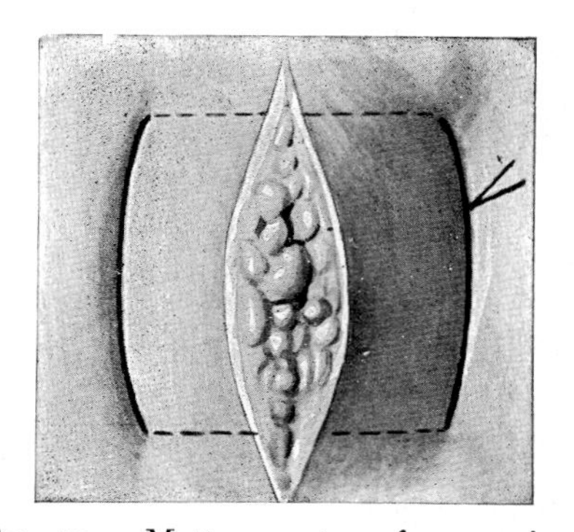

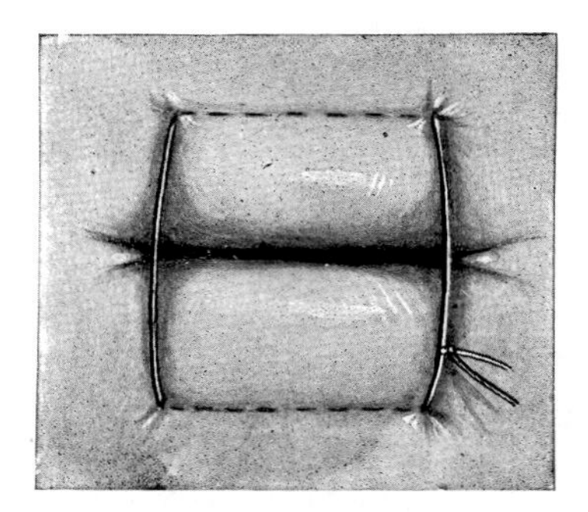

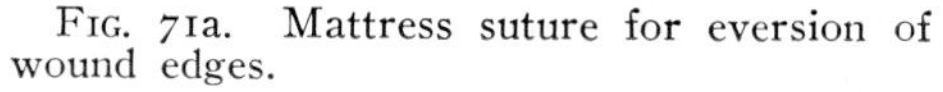

FIG. 71a. Mattress suture for eversion of wound edges.

FIG. 71b. Mattress suture for inversion of wound edges.

need not worry about their strength. Suture material does not, as a rule, break after the completion of the knot, but before or during the tying of the knot.

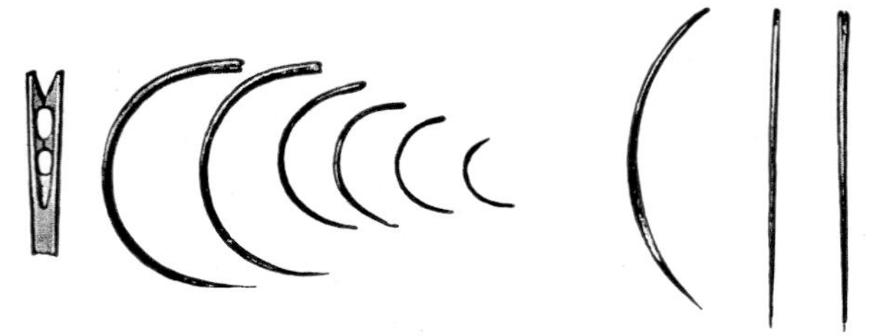

FIG. 72. Various types of straight and curved needles. Self-threading eye enlarged.

I usually use silk or catgut for the deeper sutures. For very delicate suturing of the skin horsehair is still my favorite. The various types of wire sutures, silver, bronze, rustless steel, or the braided Vienna, are used where very strong material is desired. Sutures, their preparation and applications, will be discussed more fully in Chapter III, "The Control of Infection." The surgeon should attempt to use as thin a suture material as is consistent with safety. In considering which type and size of material to use one should not depend on the strength of the material at the time of use, but upon the demands which may be made upon it later. Not only should the strength of the material be considered, but the reaction of the tissues to it. The greater the tension necessary to bring tissues together, and the thinner the tissues, the more difficult it is to select the material for suturing. Only in exceptional instances should doubled suture material be used.

In my clinic we use different sizes of silk. No. 36 is used in exceptional cases; #20 at times in herniorrhaphy or for suture of the rectus fascia; #4 for ligatures and for some cutaneous suture work; #1.5 for finer skin suturing and for gastro-intestinal surgery; while #00 is used for blood vessel suture.

My early experiences with the use of strips of fascia, especially fascia lata, for suture were not as satisfactory as I had hoped they would be from the enthusiastic reports of other surgeons.

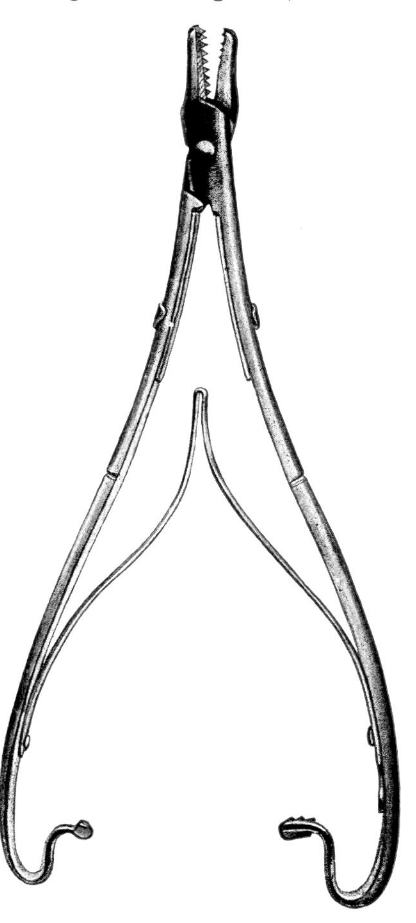

Fig. 73. Needle-holder. (Deus).

A number of sizes and types of catgut should always be available. As a rule I keep six sizes on hand. Unfortunately the sizes are not always uniform, even those from the same manufacturer. The same may be said of the strength of the gut. The smaller sizes are preferable if the desired strength can be obtained. Plain catgut should be used for the ordinary ligatures, while iodine or chromic gut should be used where rapid absorption is not desired. The smaller sizes #00 or #0 as a rule suffice for tying the ordinary vessels, while #1 or #2 should be used for the larger vessels. It is rarely necessary to use catgut in sizes larger than #2, but these are kept ready should the occasion arise.

The ordinary suture materials are tied in a knot. Wire is twisted or soldered together. The method of tying the knot is extremely important since upon this depends to a large extent the integrity of the wound closure. The knot should be firm and secure, since literally life may hang on a thread and the slipping of a knot may indeed be disastrous.

In many operations the tying of the many sutures and ligatures occupies the majority of the time. It is, therefore, of great importance that the knots be made automatically, uniformly, quickly and dependably. For this the method of double knotting is most satisfactory. It is essential for the security of the double knot that the end of the thread be passed to and from

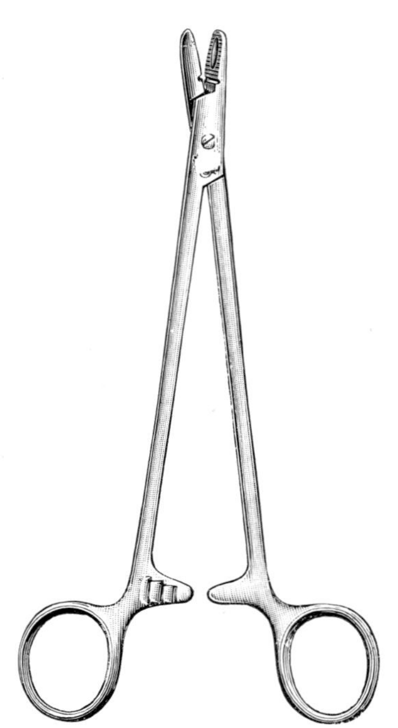

FIG. 74. Needle-holder. (Hegar-Mayo.)

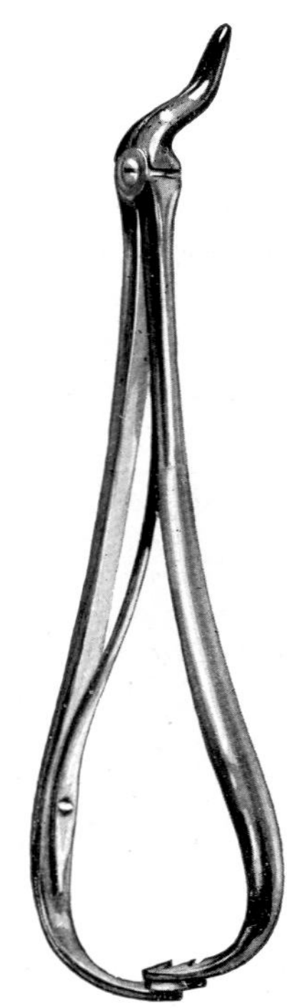

FIG. 75. Bayonet-shaped needle-holder, especially useful for suturing a cleft-palate.

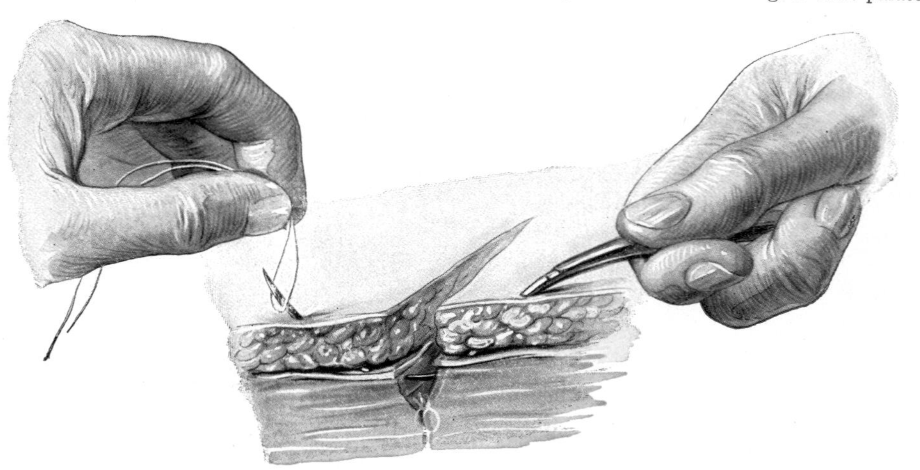

FIG. 76. Reverdin's needle. The needle is pushed through the wound margins with the eye closed, the eye is then opened, a suture is inserted by the assistant, the eye is closed and the needle withdrawn.

the surgeon as it is being tied. It is thus that the true, reef or sailor's, knot is tied (Fig. 77), the threads entering the knot on the same side of the loop. The sliding or granny knot (Fig. 78), in which the thread ends enter the knot on opposite sides of the loop, has no place in surgical practice. The surgeon and his assistants must acquire the ability to tie the true, square (Sailor's) knot with perfect ease and dexterity. The entire procedure should be done without the necessity of thinking of the individual movements.

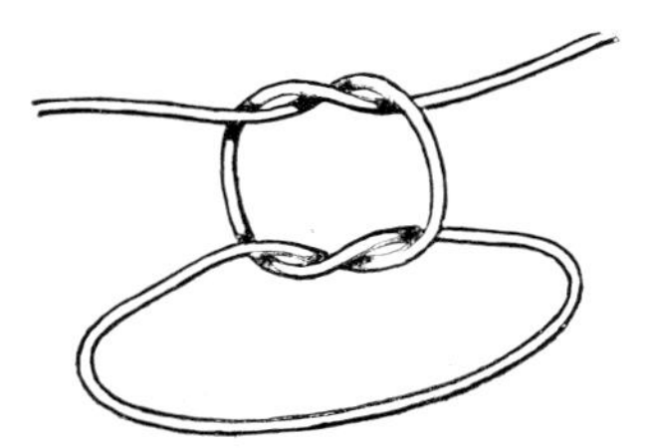

FIG. 77. True knot (Sailor's knot). At each side the thread ends enter the knot on the same side of the loop.

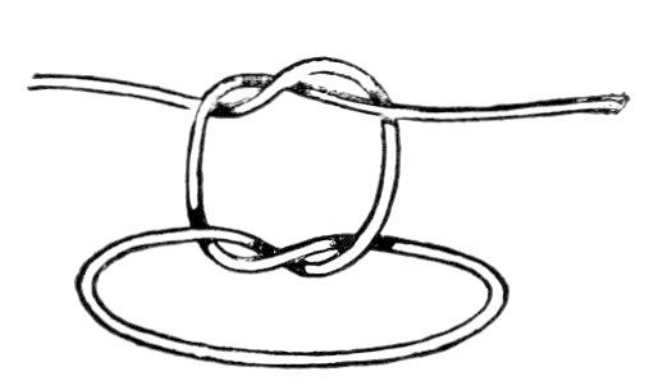

FIG. 78. False knot (Granny knot). At each side the thread ends enter the knot on opposite sides of the loop.

(To describe the individual movements of the hand would be superfluous. A study of the diagrams and constant practise can do more than any description of the finger manipulations. I. S. R.) A properly tied true (Sailor's) knot does not necessitate a third knot to make it secure.

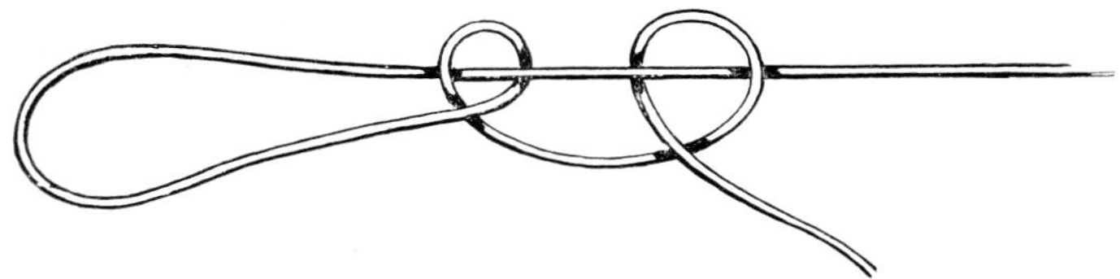

FIG. 79. Though the true (Sailor's) knot is correctly formed, if it is pulled unevenly during tying it will form a slip knot and will not hold.

It is possible at times to use only one knot. This, however, is only true when the force to be exerted against the knot is negligible. In general, however, one should use a knot which becomes tighter the more it is pulled upon, so that the place of the single knot is limited to the tying of very small vessels.

It often happens that the first knot slips while the second one is being tied. This results from a transitory relaxation of the suture. Thus the second knot is tied down on an insecurely tied first knot and the tie is not secure, in fact a slip knot is formed (Fig. 79). The surgeon's knot (Fig. 80), which is merely the first step of a single knot once repeated, prevents the first turn from slipping. It usually obviates the necessity of the assistant holding the first knot with a pair of anatomic forceps, since the friction of the two turns is sufficient to hold the knot secure until the second knot is tied. The second knot is tied without the double turn. If the first knot should tend to slip, the assistant should hold it until the second knot is applied (Fig. 81).

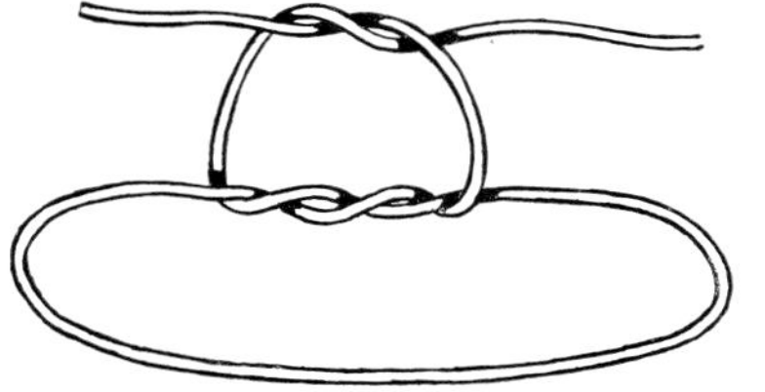

FIG. 80. Surgeon's knot, in which there are two turns in the first half and one turn in the second half of the knot. This prevents slipping during completion of the knot.

The exact method which each surgeon should use for tying the knots can not be described. Constant practice is necessary, and if this is indulged in each surgeon will evolve his own method, which for him becomes the method of choice.

In general it is preferable to use absorbable sutures in most subcutaneous surgery. These are well tolerated and after a short period disappear, so that the tissues are exposed to a foreign body for a minimum period. The only difficulty with catgut is that it is often too easily absorbed, thereby menacing wound healing. It is for this reason that I still use silk. Furthermore, moisture causes swelling of the gut, which tends to loosen the knots.

This loosening of the catgut knot does not as a rule appear clinically, since it is concealed by the onset of the organic wound healing. It is, however, a weak point in the retention of a suture placed for maintaining tissue apposition. This drawback can only be partially obviated by cutting the catgut suture further from the knot than one cuts the silk sutures.

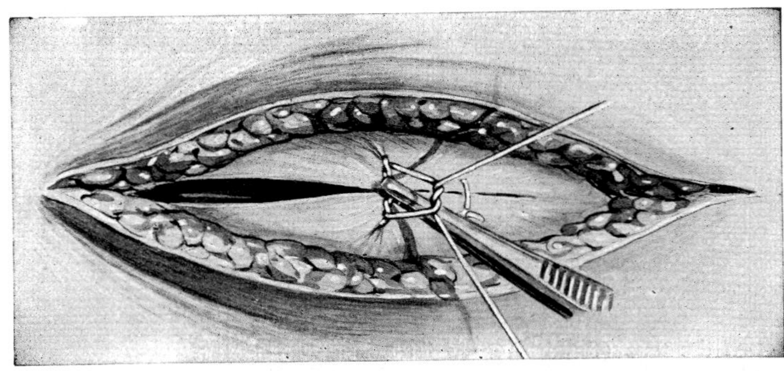

Fig. 81. Holding the first loop of a knot with an anatomic forceps, while the second loop is being tied.

Therefore, while I ordinarily prefer catgut for buried sutures, because of its absorbability, when particularly strong sutures are desired I resort to silk, as for example, in the ligation of large arteries, or for the closure of large hernial openings. In other cases, the catgut suture is often reinforced by the insertion of silk or wire tension sutures, as in the closure of a median incision of the abdominal wall. One may also suture the deep tissues with a non-absorbable suture material in order to obtain firm and permanent closure, but with the idea of later removing the suture so as not to leave a foreign body permanently in the tissues. As a rule, however, the non-absorbable sutures are used as interrupted tension sutures, while the remaining wound is closed by absorbable buried sutures. The figure of eight suture is excellent for the obliteration of dead spaces. It should be used as an interrupted suture. The suture can be placed in two ways, in that it may or may not pass through the skin of the side opposite to its entrance. The alternate sutures begin on opposite sides of the wound. They pierce the deep tissues on both sides and after crossing catch the more superficial layers.

When interrupted sutures are used the strength of the wound depends on a series of knots, so that the loosening of one knot may be of no special significance as far as good wound healing is concerned. In the continuous suture, on the other hand, the integrity of the suture depends on the beginning and the end knots. If the catgut does not break and if these knots remain intact the security of the wound is assured. In order to further secure the knots in a continuous suture I tie these with a silk ligature, as

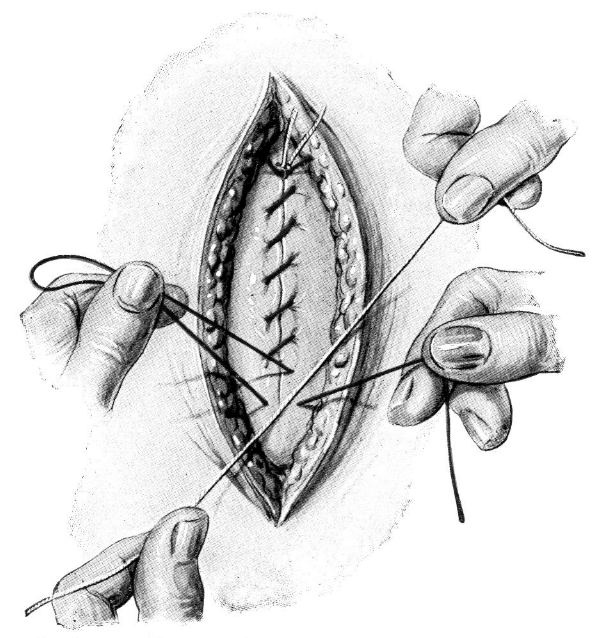

FIG. 82. Securing the knots of a continuous catgut suture by tying over a silk thread which is then tied on the catgut knot.

shown in figure 82. The silk thread is tied under the first catgut loop and is in turn tied over the completed knot so that it cannot slip or come loose.

In **wire suturing** the ends of the wire are either twisted or soldered together, or the wires may be retained by fastening lead plates and beads on their ends. Wire has the advantage over silk and catgut of being easily sterilized; it does not absorb any moisture, and it is not weakened by tissue juices. It has the disadvantage of being unwieldy and inflexible, so that its fixation is more difficult. It remains in the tissues permanently as a foreign body, so that it must often be removed at some later date. I use it chiefly for tension sutures, where it is easily removed, and for the fixation of bone in certain types of fracture.

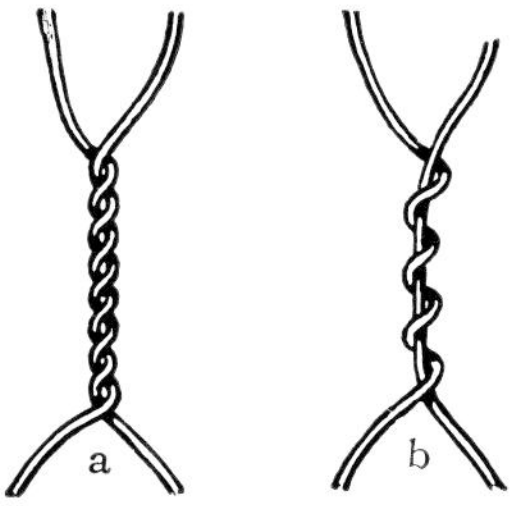

FIG. 83. Twisting the ends of two wires, (a) in a correct symmetrical form, (b) in an incorrect irregular form.

If the ends of the wire are twisted together for retention care must be taken to twist the wires one over the other. Figure 83 illustrates the correct and incorrect methods of doing this. If one end is merely twisted around the other, the retention is poor. A pair of smooth forceps or pliers should be used in twisting the ends and this demands some skill if one is to prevent breaking the wire.

Excellent retention of wire sutures is afforded by Braun's wire-plate method. I employ it mainly in reinforcing difficult closures of the abdominal wall (Fig. 84). For this Vienna braided wire is most suitable. It is sufficiently rough to prevent the slipping of the lead plates and beads. The lead beads which I have found most satisfactory are those used in various types of business for sealing a package or box to prevent tampering. These are better than the drilled lead shot. A small rubber pad is placed against the skin, a lead plate over this, and the retention beads, two on each side, against the lead plate. The wire so prepared on one end is pulled through both wound margins with a needle. The same plates are placed on the free end and the lead beads are pressed against the wire after considerable tension has been made to bring the wound margins together. The bead closest to the skin should be fastened first.

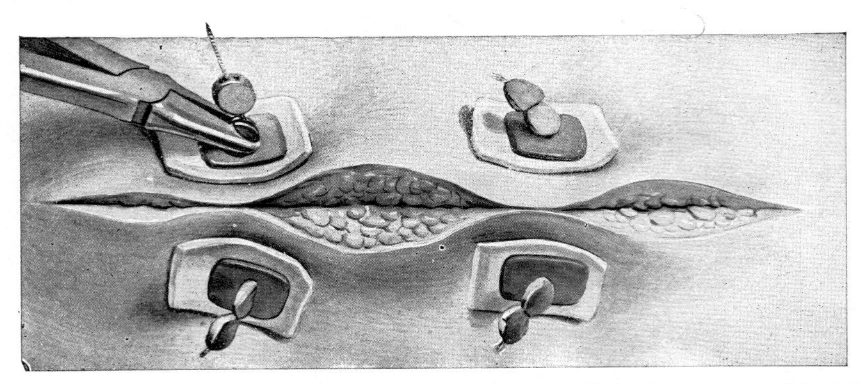

Fig. 84. Wire suture. A Vienna wire, provided on one side with two pressed lead beads, a lead platelet and a rubber pad, is carried through the wound margins and here passed through a rubber pad, a lead platelet and two lead beads. The beads then are tightly pressed while the wire is held under tension.

The compress tension suture depends on a similar principle (Fig. 85), but instead of wire, strong silk is used. In the middle of a long strong silk thread a gauze compress is tied. Both thread ends are threaded in a needle and are carried through both sides of the wound at a suitable distance from the wound edge. The needle is removed and the threads are tightly stretched thus drawing together the wound margins, and are then tied together over a second gauze roll.

The **firmness of a wound** after suture depends unconditionally on purely mechanical factors. If one assumes that the thread and knots are dependable, the strength of the suture depends on whether or not the wound edges can be brought together without causing the sutures to cut through the tissues. The various tissues respond differently to sutures, especially where tension is necessary for tissue approximation. The more yielding the tissue the less danger there is of the suture cutting through. Fat and muscle will withstand less tension than fascia and peritoneum. In suturing, therefore, an attempt should be made whenever possible to grasp the more resistant tissues or at least to include these in the suture. In suturing a muscle which has been divided across the direction of its fibers, the major emphasis in repair should be put on obtaining a good approximation of its fascial sheath.

As a rule the finer the suture the more easily it cuts through the tissues. A thread of 1/10 mm. diameter has half the resistance of a thread of 2/10 mm. Nevertheless, since it is not good surgical technic to use the heavier sutures when finer ones are possible, this consideration is not the deciding factor in the choice of the size of the suture. Finally, the less tension there is on the individual suture, the less danger there is of its cutting through. If two sewed wound surfaces are pulled apart with a force of 1 kilogram and this force is distributed over ten interrupted sutures, the load for each suture amounts to only 1/10 kilogram; if there are twenty sutures, then the load is 1/20 kilogram per suture, so that the load of each suture is decreased by half. The increased number of sutures used in the suture of a wound definitely increases the strength of the closure.

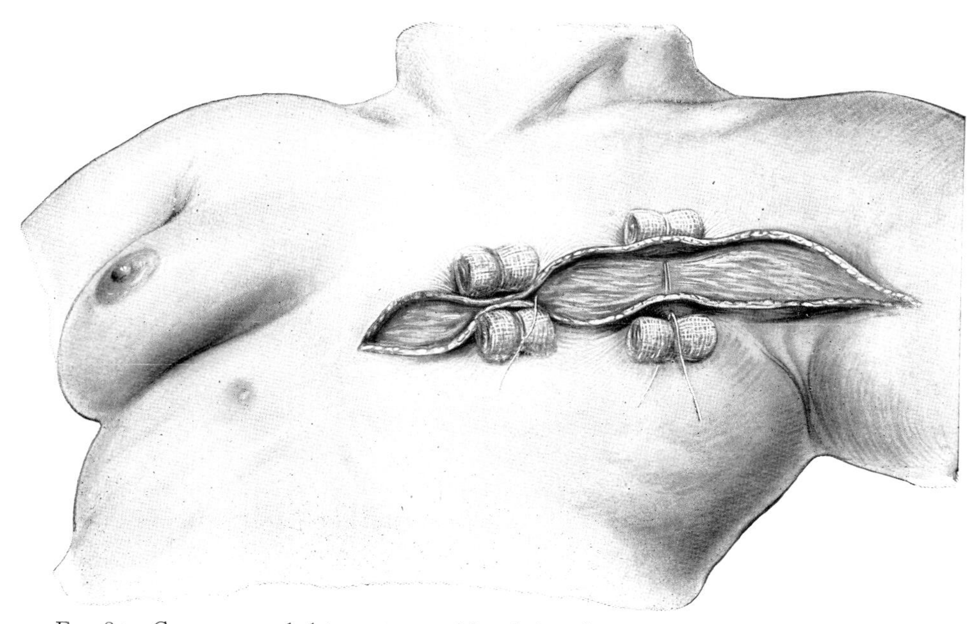

Fig. 85. Compress or bolster suture. After being tied around a small roll of gauze both ends of the suture are passed through the wound margins and tied under tension around a second roll of gauze.

The number of sutures used, however, must find its limit in the size of the wound. To insert too many is as harmful as to insert too few. If too many are used, the blood supply along the wound will suffer and thus wound repair be impaired. The number of sutures should only be increased if the presence of additional tissue layers necessitates this. It is often possible to resuture the fascia on either side of the wound over the main suture line thus reinforcing this; a pedicled flap can be used to cover the wound, or a free fascia lata transplant can be used (Fig. 86) to reinforce the suture line.

After the closure of wounds which are under considerable tension one must always keep in mind the fact that the sutures may tend to cut through slowly. This cutting is so limited at first, that it is not easily discernible. It is frequently only noticed when it is complete and the wound margins, suddenly deprived of support, separate. The more tissue incorporated in the individual suture, the longer will this serious complication be deferred. Hence, in placing sutures which will be subjected to considerable tension it is well to include a considerable amount of tissue between them. The tension suture has its place in this type of wound. Of these there are numerous types, of which the compress and wire suture are good examples. If it is desired to give the tension sutures the simple loop-form, the suture material should be fairly thick and it should be carried through the skin on both sides

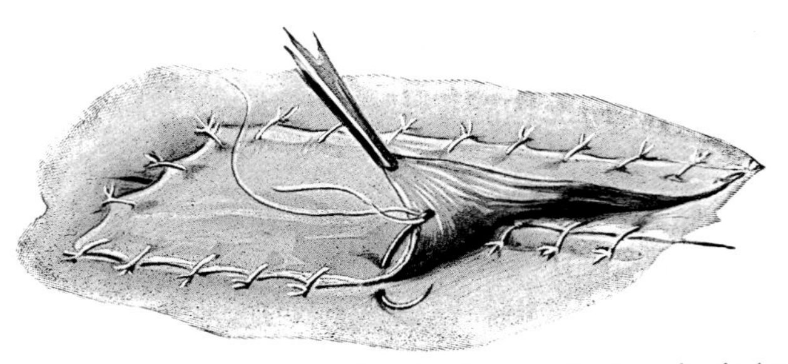

FIG. 86. Reinforcement of a suture line by the use of a free fascia lata graft.

of the wound, so that it can be removed later. Heavy silk, silkworm-gut, wire, or wire-plate sutures are used. The method of suturing can be such that the thread, before it tears out, must cut through thick tissue layers. The U-sutures, the "pulley-suture", and various other complicated sutures are used for this purpose. They also have a place in tendon suture. These sutures, however, materially impair the blood supply to the wound margins and in this way retard organic wound healing. The "pulley-suture" (Fig. 87) combines a tension suture with a coaptation suture. The needle is passed into the tissues well away from one side of the wound margin then out at a similar distance from the wound edge of the opposite side; it then passes into the tissues close to the edge of the first side and out of the opposite wound margin at a similar distance, where the ends are tied.

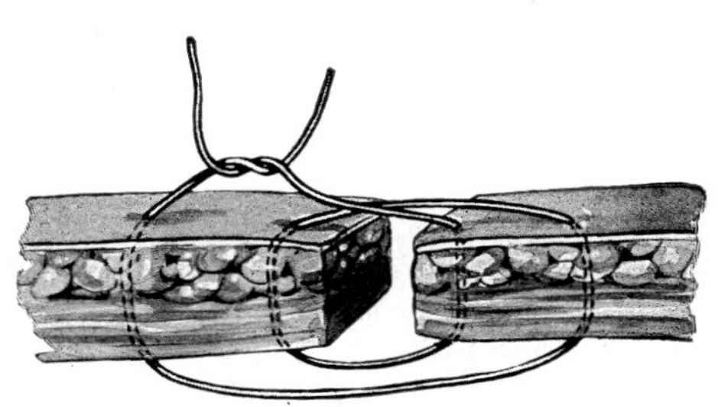

FIG. 87. Pulley-suture. This suture combines the tension suture with a coaptation suture.

There are a number of factors which tend to cause the separation of a wound after suture. The innate elasticity of tissues, constantly tending to retract after division, is a very definite factor. This is beautifully exemplified in the result of division of a muscle or its tendon. This defect can only be overcome by forceful tension. Distention, breathing, coughing constantly cause added stress and strain on an abdominal suture line. Disturbing forces should be reduced or controlled as much as possible to protect the integrity of the suture line. Too great tension on the sutures should be avoided by making use of the many procedures described in the various chapters where the problems of stress and strain are discussed, such as the proper position of an extremity after reduction of a fracture to relieve muscle pull, or the mobilization or displacement of structures to be united.

The burden on a wound should be reduced by properly applied bandages. From the standpoint of wound healing, it is unwise to permit a patient who has undergone an abdominal operation to get out of bed too soon. Bandages and adhesive straps should be so placed as to counteract forces tending to separate the wound. The use of abdominal binders (Figs. 19 and 21) after laparotomy can not be overestimated. The margins of superficial wounds which are only slightly separated can sometimes be brought together by adhesive plaster so that suture is not required, although experience has taught me that this is not always successful.

ORGANIC WOUND REPAIR

The organic union of a wound takes place in the course of approximately eight to ten days by the proliferation of fibroblasts. The new-formed connective tissue is at first frail and easily torn. It gradually becomes condensed and firm, but it takes some weeks before the repair gives rise to the completed scar. Scar tissue is never as strong as the original tissue. It is easily stretched under force, so that the surgeon attempts to obtain wounds with as small an area of scar as possible. Wound complications cause wider separation of the wound margins with a subsequently greater area to be filled with fibrous tissue.

The wider the gap between two wound margins, the more slowly it is filled in with cicatricial tissue, the wider is the cicatrix, and the later and more incomplete is the repair. The factors which cause a lack of firmness of the wound repair also retard the beginning of early organic wound healing, in fact widely separated wounds heal by granulation. Thus the wound is weak and herniation through it may easily occur. Hematoma of the wound may also cause a weak wound since this may serve as a nidus for suppuration, or it may be replaced by a wide band of connective tissue. Any wound which depends for healing on the process of granulation is a poor wound, although it is occasionally impossible to obtain repair by any other process. It is well known that age, strength, and the constitution of the patient play an important rôle in the rapidity and type of wound repair. As soon as fibroblasts have proliferated and organic wound repair has taken place the inorganic repair which resulted from suture is no longer of any significance.

The broader the wound surfaces, the more satisfactory the repair is apt to be. This is due to the stronger cicatrix which results in a firmer wound. This implies, however, not the distance between the healthy wound margins, but the depth of the scar. Ten square centimeters of cicatricial union in sagittal section is 10 times stronger than 1 square centimeter. I endeavor, therefore, wherever strength of the scar is essential to a good functional end-result to obtain broad contact of the surfaces. In order to obtain this the wounds may have to be specially prepared. Slanting, step-like, or feather-like union are simple methods of obtaining this in tendon suture. Other methods are those of fascia overlapping (Figs. 88, 89 and 90), the use of free fascial transplants (Fig. 86), and the use of pedunculated grafts. These all tend to increase the security of the repair and the subsequent strength of

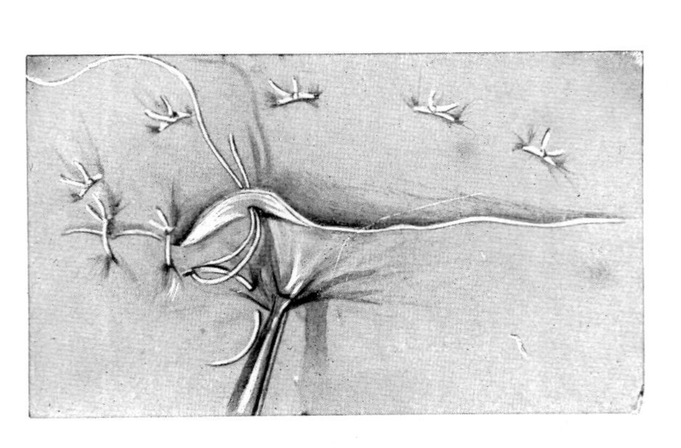

FIG. 88. Overlapping or imbrication of the fascia by a double row of sutures in order to increase the fascial contact and reinforce the wound suture.

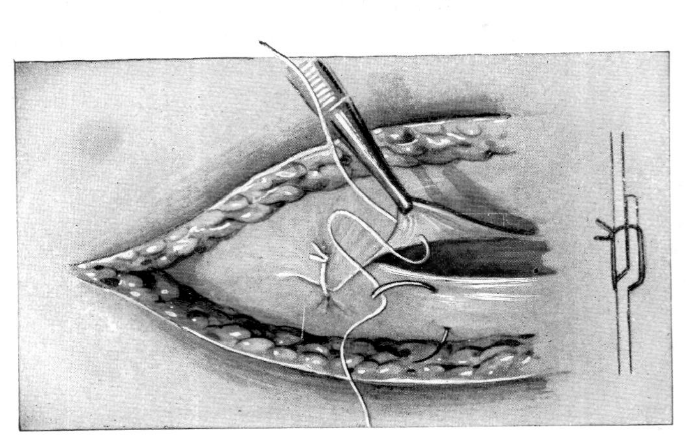

FIG. 89. Overlapping fascia with one line of sutures.

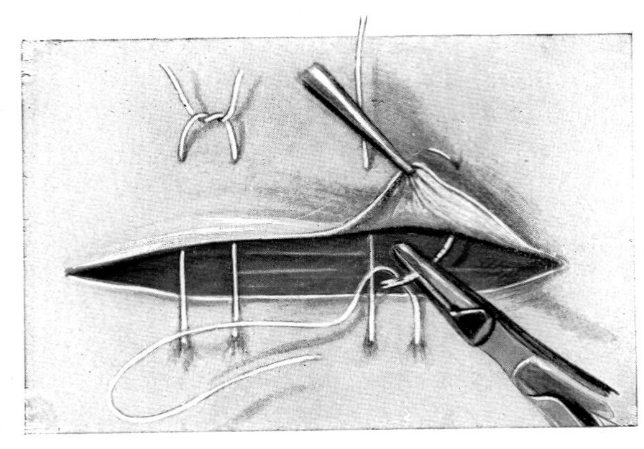

FIG. 90. Overlapping fascia with mattress sutures.

the wound. By their intelligent use an otherwise weak wound with its potentialities of later herniation may be made a permanently secure one.

3. Excision of Tissues and Removal of Foreign Bodies

EXCISION OF TISSUES

Accumulations of fluids inside the body in the form of cysts or abscesses can be emptied by aspiration. The technic which I find very useful for this is described on page 251. Aspiration serves two functions; it is partly diagnostic, in that it determines the presence of fluid as well as the nature of it, and partly therapeutic, in that it removes the fluid. Therapeutically the results of aspiration are only too often transitory, since the underlying cause is not affected by this procedure. For permanent cure of fluid accumulations the cyst must be obliterated by cicatrization, the fluid diverted into tissues capable of absorbing it, the entire cyst wall excised, or the causative factor producing the ascites removed.

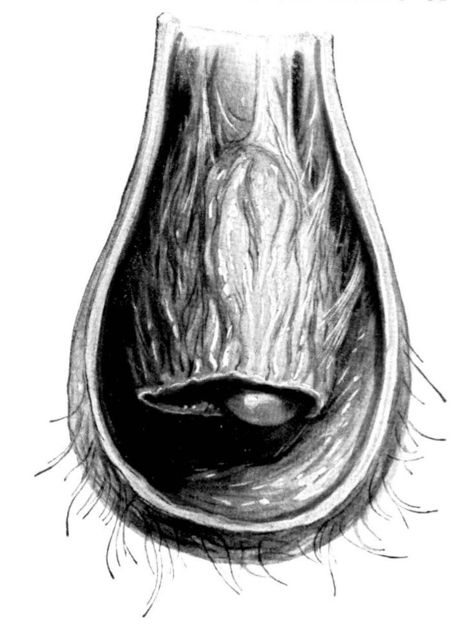

Fig. 91. Continuous drainage of a cyst into the surrounding connective tissue. The drainage of a testicular hydrocele into the subcutaneous cellular tissue, through removal of the tip of the sac, serves as an example.

The cicatrization and subsequent obliteration of the cyst wall only has a chance for success in those cysts whose inner lining is extremely susceptible to irritation. The cyst after being emptied of its contents has injected into it a few cubic centimeters of an irritating solution, such as tincture of iodine, weak phenol, alcohol, chloroform, 10 percent zinc chloride, 10 percent sodium chloride, 1 percent formalin, etc. Immediately after injection a rather severe local reaction occurs which subsides in a few days, and in favorable cases the subsidence of the inflammatory reaction is followed by fibroblastic proliferation which obliterates the sac.

For continuous drainage of the contents of a cyst into other tissues (Fig. 91) a hole as large as possible should be made in the cyst wall. Although this procedure may give good results, it is more likely not to, and if definite indications do not forbid it the cyst should be excised.

Should the drainage take place in an interstitial space like the peritoneal cavity, or in a hollow organ like the intestine, or onto the body surface, care should be taken to assure accurate apposition of the opposed surfaces so that a lip-fistula is established (Fig. 92). This will prevent closure of the opening and thus permit drainage over an indefinite period.

In spite of many precautions, the methods already described may fail to result in the alleviation of symptoms. The walls may not be obliterated, the opening for subcutaneous drainage may close, or the lip-fistula may

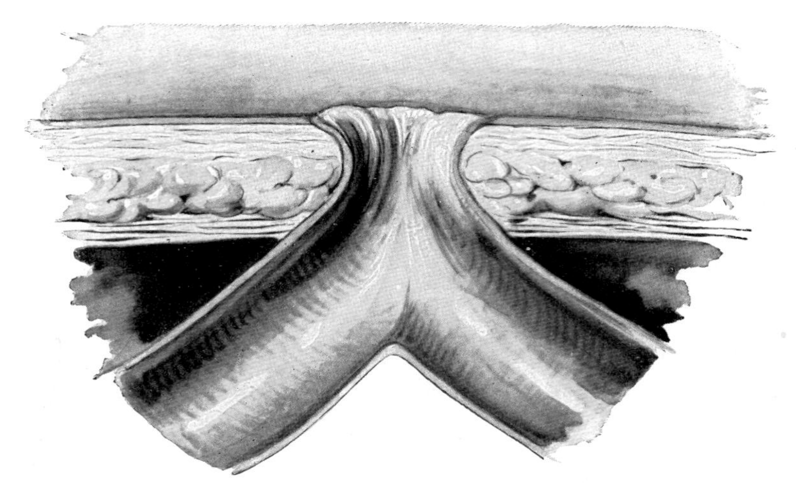

Fig. 92. A lip-fistula, in which epithelium meets epithelium, can only be cured, when the epithelial connection is completely interrupted. A lip-fistula between an intestinal loop and the surface of the skin is shown.

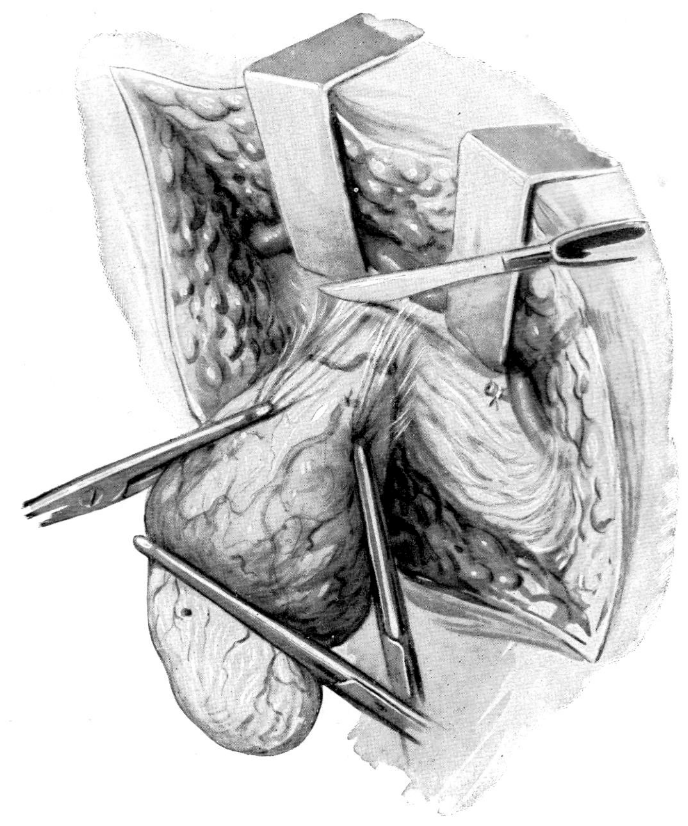

Fig. 93. Excision of a cyst. Because of the inaccessibility of the under side where lies a large artery, the cyst was first evacuated by puncture. The connective tissue bands between the cyst-wall and surrounding tissues were then stretched and divided. All divided vessels were doubly ligated.

not be entirely successful. The use of non-absorbable wicks for the drainage of fluids, such as the use of silk threads in hydrocephalus and elephantiasis, has been equally discouraging, although at times no more radical treatment can be attempted.

The **excision of a simple cyst** is carried in the same way as the excision of a non-malignant tumor. The exposure of the cyst is facilitated if the cyst is not drained, but remains tense. When access to the posterior side is difficult, the cyst can be emptied to facilitate this part of the exposure.

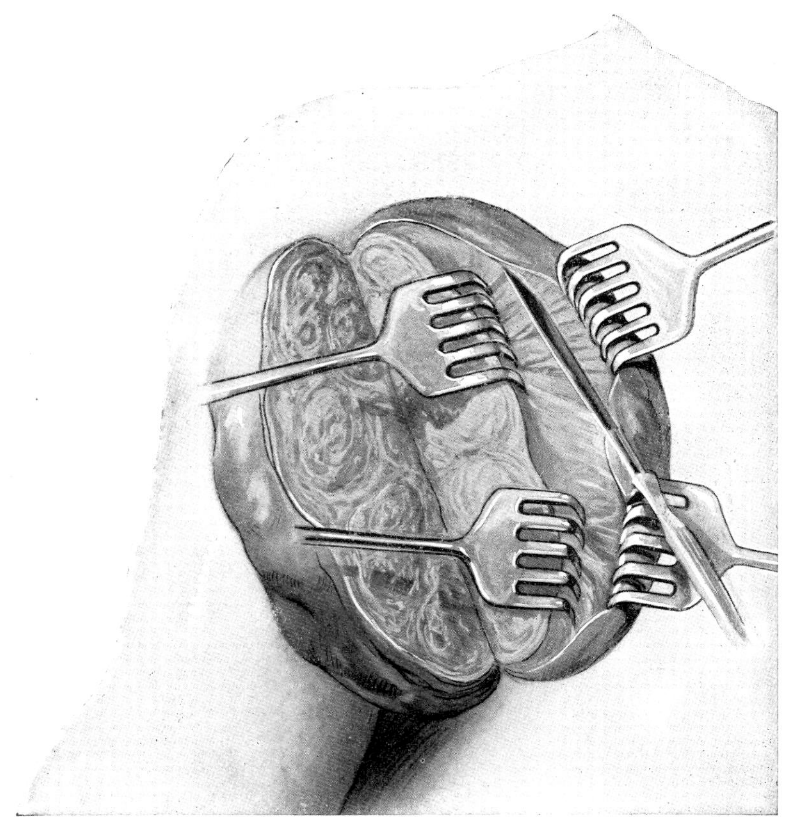

FIG. 94. Removal of a benign tumor. As an example a fatty-tumor is shown. The tumor is sectioned, so that the sharp border between tumor and healthy tissue may be clearly seen. The tumor may then be separated from the surrounding tissue, as a rule, without an extensive anatomical exposure.

It is only after excision that the surgeon can assure the patient of permanent relief (Fig. 93).

There is a fundamental difference in the technic for the **excision of benign and malignant tumors.** Failure to recognize this important difference frequently results in a poor end-result.

Benign tumors (Fig. 94) are removed by exposing fully the surface of the tumor and then by sharp dissection separating it from the surrounding tissues. Traction on the tumor increases the ease with which the dissection can be carried out, since it stretches the connecting bands between the tumor and the healthy tissues. The tumor can sometimes be separated by blunt dissection, and when this is possible bleeding is minimized. Any important structures around the tumor should be carefully exposed and then safeguarded during the remainder of the operation.

In the case of **malignant tumors** we start with the assumption that the disease has spread from the local lesion and that not only the area immediately surrounding the growth, but the surrounding fascia, the lymph

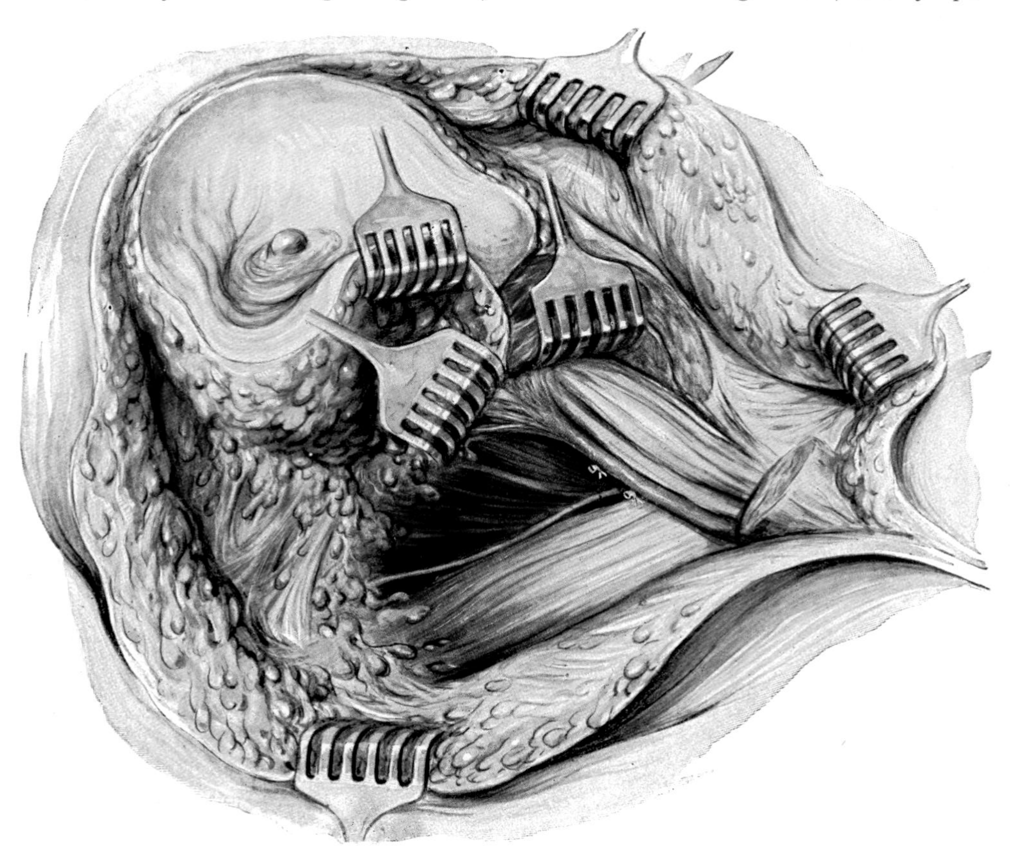

FIG. 95. When a malignant tumor is removed, as for example a breast cancer, the incision is made, on all sides, well into healthy tissue, so that as the dissection progresses the tumor is encased in healthy tissue and all possible lymphatic connections have been severed before the growth itself is disturbed.

vessels and the regional lymph glands contain malignant cells, even though there may be no macroscopic evidence of this. It is for these reasons that a malignant tumor should not be detached directly from the surrounding tissue, but that the entire area adjacent to it should be excised, together with large areas of the adjacent fascia and the regional lymph glands (Fig. 95). Whenever feasible, the entire area is dissected and removed en bloc in order to avoid implantation metastasis. In the field of operation only those tissues are left behind which can not be dispensed with without severe anatomic or physiologic injury. The incision is planned so that the dissection can begin at the periphery and be carried toward the tumor from all directions, thus enclosing the tumor in supposedly healthy tissue until the final part of the dissection permits the removal of the entire mass. There is left behind an anatomic exposure of indispensable structures, while the supposedly healthy tissue immediately surrounding the malignant tissue is removed. This procedure can not be carried out in every case, since the malignant tumor may have invaded adjacent parts and metastasized to regional glands so as to require sharp dissection from important structures which can not be sacrificed. This however does not change the principle of the plan of operation. In those instances where complete removal is not possible the prospects for permanent cure or even prolonged relief are greatly lessened. If it is impossible to do a complete dissection because it involves the sacrifice of vital structures, the lesion is not subject to radical operation and the sooner the operation is terminated the better, since it offers no hope for the patient.

Advanced lesions which are not radically operable, and which are being treated by x-ray or radium, frequently require some type of surgical treatment for the relief of unbearable pain.

X-ray and radium burns which do not respond to conservative treatment must also be treated by surgical procedures. The treatment is not unlike that used for the cure of malignant tumors. Excision of these lesions must be extensive since the tissue has become damaged as a result of the irradiation for a much wider area than is grossly visible. The damage consists essentially in an obliterative angeitis, involving not only the blood vessels but also the lymphatics. The resulting defect can be covered by skin grafts of one type or another.

It is for this reason that the wound even after excision may show little if any tendency to heal. The blood supply may be so impaired that a secondary ulcer results. The more radical the excision the better, since not infrequently malignancy is superimposed on the chronic ulcer. Bone involved in the lesion should also be excised up to the area of healthy tissue. The only thing which should permit one to forego as radical an operation as seems to be indicated would be the injury of major vessels, nerves, important joints, and the danger of opening certain of the body cavities.

It should be remembered that the skin surrounding the area of a radium or x-ray ulcer is devitalized, which makes it unsuitable for transplantation to the excised area. Even though telangiectases may not be present in the surrounding skin its usefulness for grafting too often is lost. Since the gap resulting from excision of an x-ray ulcer can be closed by direct suture only very infrequently, and since suitable skin can rarely be obtained in the vicinity of the area, the surgeon must use a pedunculated or free skin transplant to cover the excised area. The pedicle graft is to be preferred since it will be nourished while the graft is becoming accustomed to its new bed. Thus even though the blood supply of the area is impoverished, the graft is able to remain healthy while it becomes organized with the surrounding tissue. Free transplants of skin, however, often survive extremely well, contrary to expectation.

If, because of ulceration and the density of the surrounding tissues, it is impossible to recognize important structures, and if the lesion is severe enough to warrant it, amputation should be done. It is far better to do this than to temporize with so-called palliative procedures.

It is possible to remove parts of very highly developed organs, such as the liver, the thyroid gland, the thymus, the pancreas, or in some instances even whole organs, such as the spleen, one lung, or one kidney, without endangering the life of the patient. After adequate exposure of the field of operation, the real technical difficulty which confronts the surgeon is the control of hemorrhage. In each instance the management of hemorrhage must be met as the indications arise. In one instance the major vessels must be ligated, in another ligation of the smaller branches will suffice, while in still another it is necessary temporarily to interrupt the major blood supply to the organ while the operation is being done. The entire subject is discussed more fully in the chapter on "The Control of Hemorrhage". In complete excision (extirpation) of an organ, if it possesses no free surface, it should be detached from the surrounding tissues by double ligation of all bleeding points and by separation of the connecting tissue bands, as has been described earlier in this chapter. The pedicle containing the major vessels demands special consideration, and should, if possible, be taken care of early in the operation.

Biopsy. As a rule it is possible to determine in advance the extent of an operation, so that it may follow a definite plan. Occasionally, the diagnosis remains more or less uncertain, prior to operation, or during the operation it may prove to have been incorrect. Similar uncertainty and error occur particularly frequently in regard to the differential diagnosis between benign and malignant disease, and occasionally in regard to inflammatory disease. If the correct diagnosis becomes apparent during the operation, the operative procedure can be altered to meet the situation. Should, however, simple observation lead to no definite conclusion, then one must remove one, or more, characteristic portions of the lesion for microscopic examination (Fig. 96). The biopsy should be done at that part of the lesion which will show the actual character of the process, and not from tissue surrounding the lesion which may disclose only secondary changes. Sufficient tissue must be removed for careful microscopic, bacteriologic or chemical examination. This may be done at a preliminary operation, or better as the first step in a complete procedure. In the latter case the wound is kept open until the results of a frozen section are obtained from the pathologist. This consumes about ten minutes and it is done preferably in a laboratory adjoining the operating room (see 117A "The Set-Up of the Operating Room"). This short delay during the operation is counterbalanced by the advantage that, on the basis of the histologic diagnosis, the necessary operation can be carried out in one stage. Where doubt exists as to the diagnosis, the consent of the patient for radical operation, if necessary, must be obtained before anæsthetization. If this is done routinely it will avoid discussions at the operating table regarding consent, particularly when the operation has been begun under general anæsthesia. Emergencies may arise when it is necessary to obtain consent from patients who are anæsthetized, as for instance, when the exposure of a focus of infection discloses an unexpected gas bacillus infection, making it necessary to amputate a limb.

If one does not succeed during the preliminary stages of the operation in determining the nature of the tumor, I believe that the operation should be discontinued, or, in the simpler cases, the surgeon should proceed as if the lesion were benign. However this is rarely necessary, since a good pathologist can, in the majority of instances, state whether the lesion is benign or malignant from a frozen section. Should a more careful examination of the tissue change the diagnosis, then the radical operation must be undertaken as soon as possible. In such instances it is accomplished under less favorable conditions, since infection may have taken place after the primary operation, or is more apt to occur after the secondary one, and the spread of the tumor cells is more likely.

Immediate Examination of Specimens Obtained by Biopsy. A section about 3 mm. thick and 1 sq. cm. in area is boiled for 2 minutes in a formalin solution (1 part of 40 percent commercial formalin in 5 parts of water),

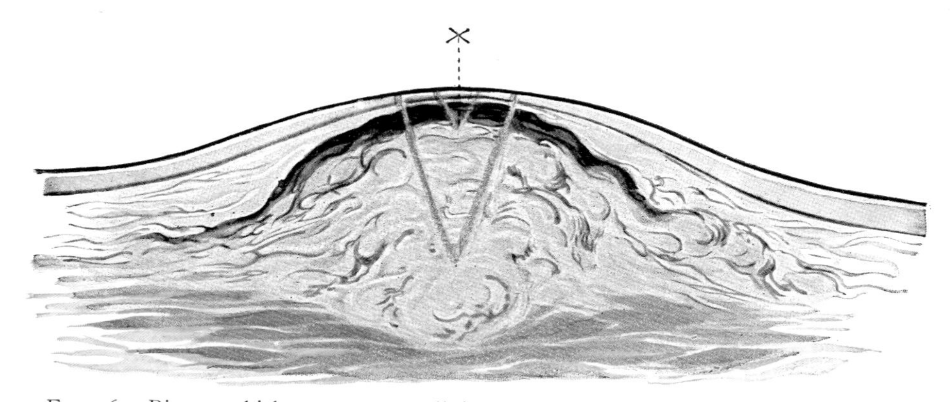

Fig. 96. Biopsy which penetrates well into the tissue to be examined. Removal of a small wedge (x) is incorrect, for the histologic picture at the margin of a tumor may lead to false conclusions.

frozen with carbon dioxide, and cut about 10 microns thick with a microtome. The section caught in water is drawn upon an object carrier or a cover-glass, pressed close with filter paper and stained with hematoxylin and eosin, after which it is ready to be examined microscopically. The entire procedure takes only about ten minutes. The time can be shortened by dispensing with the eosin counter-stain, or by using only one stain, for example, polychromatic methylene-blue. However the distinctness of the individual tissues and cells is not nearly so good, so that an exact diagnosis is more difficult or may even be impossible. It is for this reason that I favor the slightly longer method. In a case where the diagnosis is apparently doubtful the material obtained at operation should always be submitted to a careful histologic, bacteriologic, and chemical examination. Even though the diagnosis may be unquestioned, the laboratory examination should also be made. It is only then that complete statistical studies can be made.

Tissue Destruction with the Cautery. It is possible to destroy live tissue by the action of heat, such as the actual cautery. The necrotic tissue can then be removed by the surgeon or permitted to separate of its own accord. Since the line of separation can not be accurately predetermined, the use of the red hot iron is not advised where the line of separation must be exact or where subsequent suture must be resorted to, and tissue devitalization may prevent primary union. The use of the cautery for the control of hemorrhage is now rarely resorted to, for we can control bleeding much better by other means. When an exact anatomic exposure is not important; when one wishes to destroy the bed of a malignant tumor after its removal; when primary wound healing is not desired and the wound secretion can easily escape; when a large area of living tissue must be destroyed with a minimum of bleeding, or when, in the excision of tissues, it is desirable simultaneously to sterilize the wound surface and to control oozing, the cautery iron has occasionally certain advantages. If, however, during the cauterization of tissues large vessels are injured, the bleeding can not be controlled by heat, and the bleeding vessel must be ligated. The danger of the use of the cautery iron lies also in the damage which it may do to the vessel wall so that while hemorrhage may not occur primarily it may take place secondarily when the vessel wall undergoes necrosis. In such instances

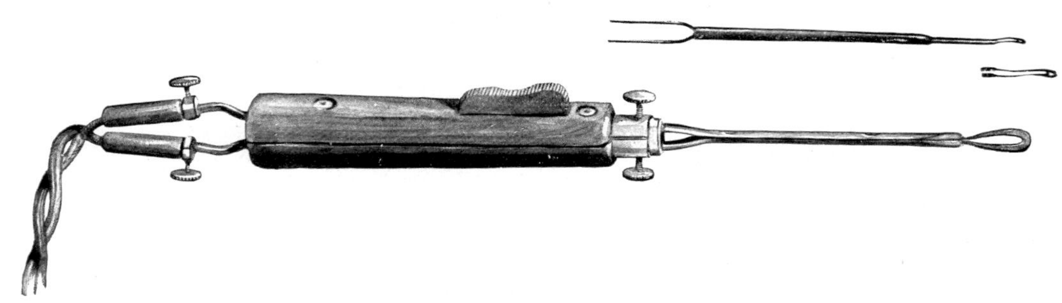

FIG. 97. Electric cautery with various attachments.

failure to supply emergency treatment may prove fatal. In order to prevent such a calamity the cautery iron should not be used in the immediate proximity of any large vessel.

For smaller procedures, such as division of the intestine, the cauterization of an appendiceal stump, and the cauterization of hemorrhoids, the electric cautery (Fig. 97), or the Paquelin cautery (Fig. 98) does very well. I believe however that even the use of these instruments, which are to an extent similar to the cautery iron, have no advantage over the scalpel. I use them, as Bier does, occasionally to destroy ulcerating fungating malignant tumors whose complete excision with the scalpel is impossible.

When in such instances it is necessary to destroy a large amount of tissue the smaller types of cauteries do not suffice. The special types of searing irons can be used for this purpose. I have had made a number of searing irons of special sizes and shapes which are provided with a metal handle (Fig. 99). These are sterilized with the other instruments. They are heated with a gas-oxygen blow-pipe burner. The burner consists of two metal pipes, the one fitting into the other (Figs. 100 and 101). The outer tube of the blow-pipe is connected with an illuminating gas pipe, as shown in the illustration, while the inner tube is connected to an oxygen tank. The gas is turned on and the escaping gas ignited. When an iron is to be heated, the oxygen is turned on. This mixes with the gas flame and changes it to a sharp pointed flame giving a heat of about 1600° F. The irons get red-hot within a fraction of a minute, and if permitted to remain in the flame they will melt. They should not be heated to more than a red glow. As soon as the burner is not needed the oxygen is turned off.

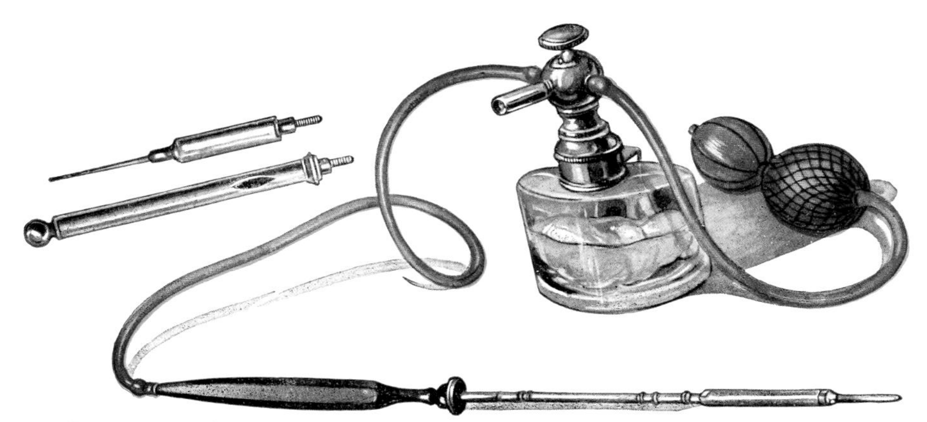

FIG. 98. Paquelin cautery. The platinum tip is heated by vaporized benzine.

The electric cautery iron (Fig. 102) can be used for similar purposes. It has the advantage of not needing a special flame to heat it. Furthermore it is provided with a number of variously shaped tips which are interchangeable, and the major portion of the heated surface is confined to a more easily controlled area. (I.S.R.)

The electric "surgical knives" have more recently come into wide use (Fig. 102). They can be used for dissection, do not cause damage to tissues

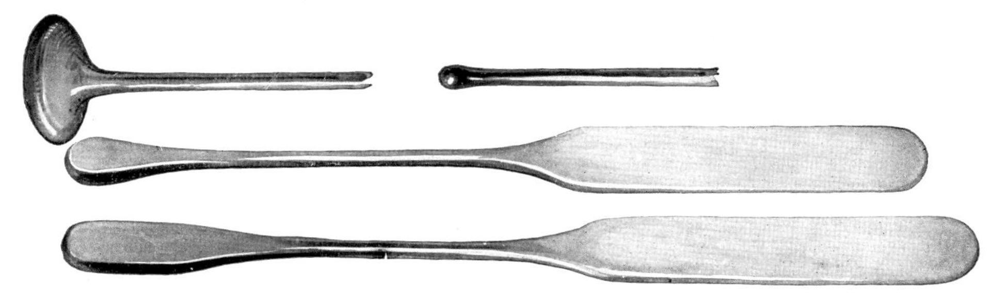

FIG. 99. Various shaped searing irons.

adjacent to the site of their use, and can also be used for the coagulation of blood. They will probably have a wide field of usefulness in the surgery of malignant tumors.

Recently I have used a large Paquelin cautery which has an electrically driven air pump, when a cautery larger than the small Paquelin was required. It is an exceedingly useful instrument (Fig. 103).

The Treatment of Tissue Defects. After the removal of tumors, after injuries, and after suppurative wounds there remain tissue defects which require closure. If possible the wound should be completely closed by suture. Unless this is done secondary infection may occur. In most instances it is

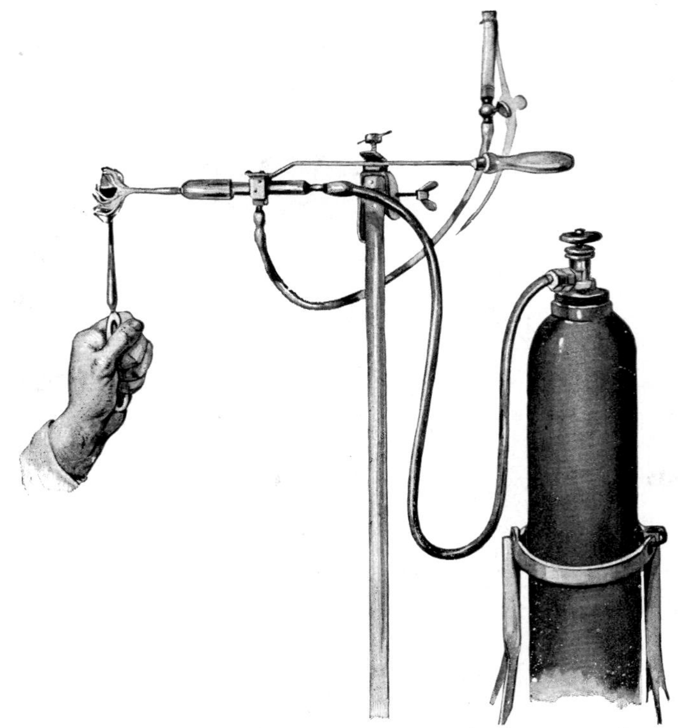

FIG. 100. Gas-oxygen blow pipe. The flame fed by illuminating gas and oxygen develops a heat of 1600° F., in which an iron can be rapidly heated.

possible to bring the tissues in apposition. Dead spaces should be carefully avoided, since nature, "abhoring a vacuum," will fill the space with blood and serum, which in turn invites infection. If it is impossible to obtain good

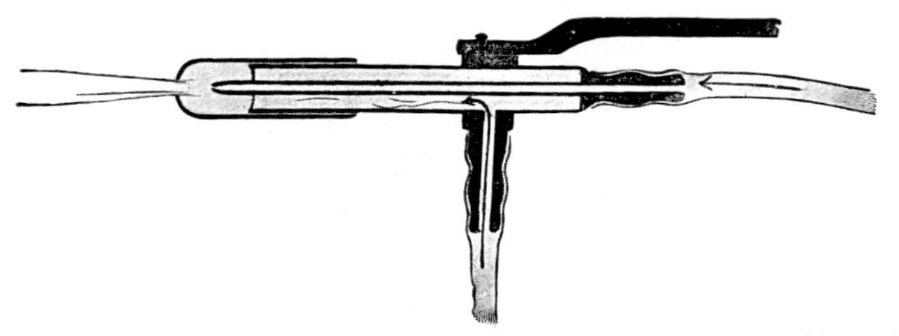

FIG. 101. A cross-section through the burner of the gas-oxygen blow pipe.

approximation of the wound edges, the wound should be drained. If the defect is large and if, even after mobilization of the wound edges, closure is not possible, the cavity should be filled with living tissue. This can be grafted from a neighboring muscle, or fat flaps may be used. If either of these is impossible, a free transplant can be attempted. For this purpose fat is suitable for the smaller defects, or where a denser material is desired fascia should be used. Inert materials such as wax or paraffin are not well tolerated

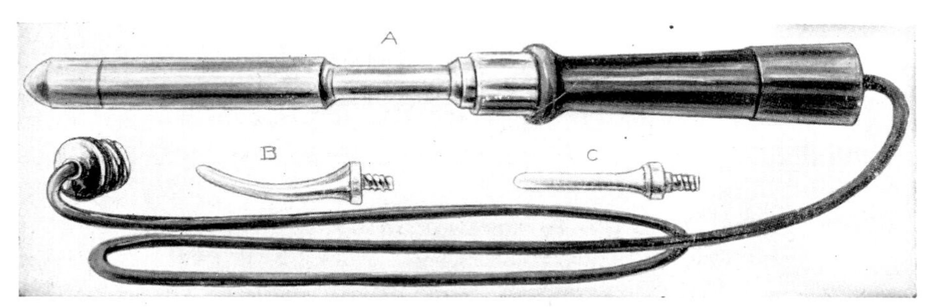

FIG. 102. A. Electric cautery with large rounded tip. B. and C., additional tips.

by the soft parts and their use is not recommended. The filling of bone cavities will be discussed in the chapter on "Operations on the Bones."

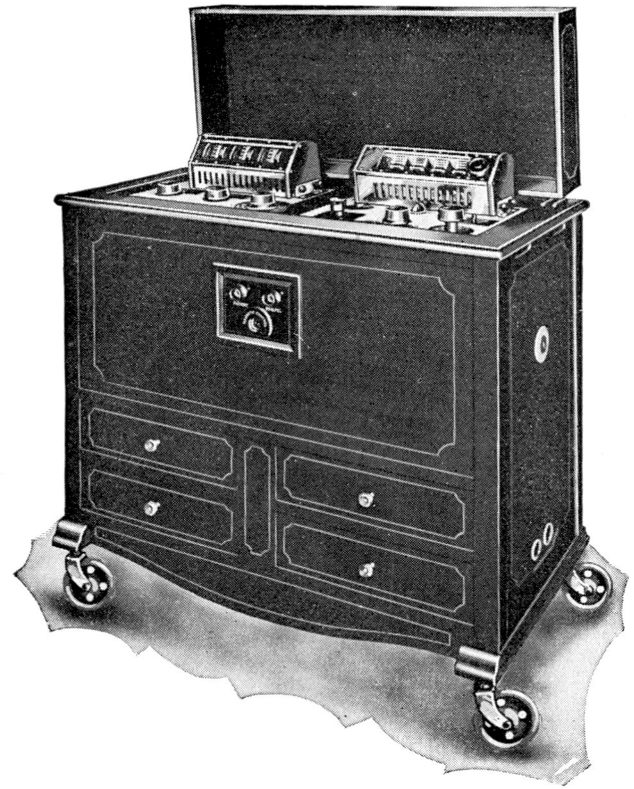

FIG. 102 a. The Bovie Apparatus.

When infection is present no attempt should be made to close the defect. The wound should be treated for the infection and when this is controlled the decision must be made either to permit the wound to heal by granulation, or to perform secondary wound suture. I still find iodoform gauze useful in stimulating the growth of granulation tissue.

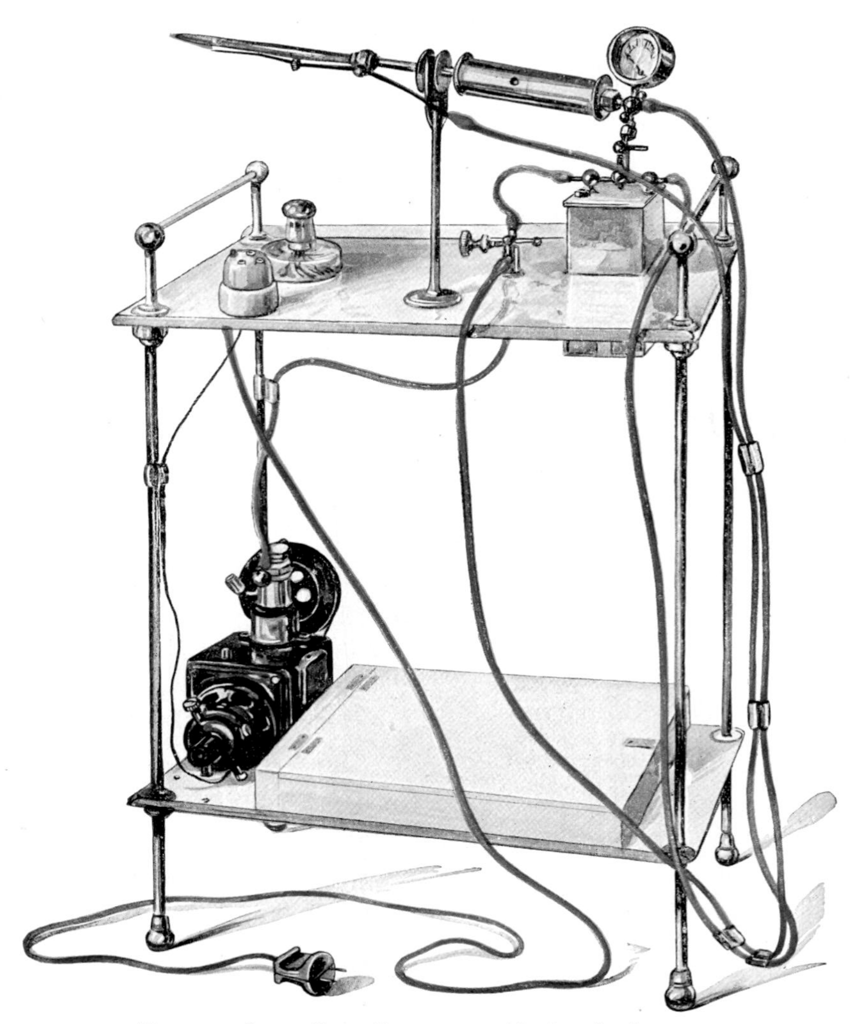

FIG. 103. Large Paquelin cautery with electric air pump.

REMOVAL OF FOREIGN BODIES

(a) Indications for the Removal of Foreign Bodies. Foreign bodies found in the body are, as a rule, either forced in during an accident, such as bullets, broken parts of pointed and cutting weapons, needles, chips of glass, wood-splinters, shreds of clothing, etc., or there may be imbedded in the body during operations such things as silk threads, metal plates, ivory pegs, dead bones, or foreign bodies may be left behind by mistake during operations. The latter include tampons, compresses, drains, instruments, etc. The mere presence of a foreign object in the body is not in itself cause for its removal. The indications for removal are definitely limited, and the surgeon who operates on every case is apt occasionally to find himself in difficulty. The indications depend upon the type of foreign body present, the damage that it is doing, or is apt to do, and the general condition of the patient. It is essential that the disturbance caused by its presence be sufficient to warrant its removal. The danger of removal, with its associated damage, must be weighed against the damage which its presence is causing. The more damage it is causing the more difficult it may be to remove the foreign body, and yet the indication for its removal exists. To cite an example, the damage and danger in the search for a foreign body lodged in the brain, has often no relation to the potential danger of its presence.

Since every case is different, the indications which I shall give are only relative, and the surgeon must consider the entire problem presented by each patient before he makes his decision. As is so often true, although the limits are fairly definite, the concrete indications must rest upon the good judgment of the operator.

The removal of a foreign body should be considered: 1. When a foreign body produces persistent pain. This is often the case when the foreign body is sharp and is constantly irritating the tissues in which it is imbedded. Even blunt objects may produce pain by pressure on large nerve trunks. The surgeon must be careful in attempting to explain all of the subjective complaints of the patient by the presence of the foreign body. Other lesions may coexist which actually may be the cause of the discomfort from which the patient is suffering. The results of the tissue injury associated with the penetration of a foreign body, such as scars, adhesions in the serous cavities, pleura and peritoneum, after chest or abdominal gun-shot or stab wounds, very often produce more pain than the foreign body itself. The attempted removal may increase the tissue alterations and intensify the patient's symptoms. One must take into account the patient's psychic make-up, since the idea that the foreign body will continue to cause tissue injury may become so fixed that nothing short of removal will help the patient.

2. When a foreign body is so superficial that the swelling it causes is perceptible to the eye or to the touch of the patient. In a superficial wound the removal of any visible object is one of the prerequisites of proper wound revision. When the foreign body is under the skin or mucous membrane its removal is so certain, simple, and without danger, that it should always be recommended. The mere fact that the patient knows of its presence in the superficial tissues is indication enough for its removal, and the patient will have little rest until he is sure that it has been removed.

3. When a foreign body offers a mechanical obstruction to function of a part. A needle may prevent the movement of a tendon or of a joint, or as a joint mouse, cause internal derangement of the joint. A foreign body may obstruct the passage of air through the trachea or bronchi; the swallowing of food through the esophagus, or prevent its moving through the stomach or intestine; while others may obstruct the flow of urine through the urethra.

4. When the foreign body causes constant irritation of the tissues in which it is lodged. Foreign bodies may produce an effusion into a joint and later lead to chronic joint inflammation; they may cause lung abscess or

pulmonary suppuration if lodged in a bronchus; or if lodged in the brain they may cause abscess or Jacksonian epilepsy, or both.

5. When the foreign body has a tendency to wander it is potentially dangerous. Bodies lying in the soft parts, which are pointed on one end and blunt on the other, such as stick-pins, sewing needles, glass-chips, and knife blades, are pushed forward, with the pointed extremity foremost by the movements of the surrounding tissues. They may cover long distances, some having been known to wander the entire length of the body. They may pass through the body cavities and the hollow organs, and in this way can cause considerable damage, even though the clinical symptoms may at the time not be very acute. Blunt objects, such as missiles, may also change their position. In very soft tissues, like the brain, they may tend to sink and in this way cause injury to very important structures. In denser tissue, such as muscle, they change their position after encapsulation only if an intercurrent infection takes place.

If the bodies lodge in the immediate proximity of structures such as the heart or the larger arteries, they may penetrate them and thus give rise to hemorrhage or, by weakening the wall, they may subsequently cause an aneurysm. Pieces of glass may break in the tissues and then by altering their position cause damage.

6. When a foreign body causes persistence of an infection early removal is indicated. In recent injuries, foreign bodies which are known to cause infection, such as shrapnel, and shell missiles, should be removed at once. To these may be added bomb fragments, wood splinters, and any object which may have carried even minute portions of clothing into the wound. On the other hand, smaller smooth objects, knife-blade points, rifle bullets, dagger points, etc., do not demand immediate removal, and if they are deep in the tissues may be left for subsequent removal if this becomes desirable.

In the presence of acute infection foreign bodies will tend to maintain and aggravate the infection. Their removal, therefore, generally speaking, is required in order to control the infection.

In many instances deep seated foreign bodies are responsible for the persistence of chronic suppuration. If a foreign body of some size is located in an infected area a fistula will often remain after the disappearance of the acute inflammatory symptoms. Inversely, if a fistula is present without visible cause and defies all efforts to cure it, the suspicion should arise that a foreign body is present in the depths of the wound. Besides foreign bodies entering the body through injury, like gun-shot wounds, one must consider substances intentionally left during operations, in the form of silk threads, wires, and metal plates, or foreign bodies such as tampons, sponges, instruments, drainage tubes, etc., which have been left accidentally during the operation or at a later dressing. Likewise necrotic unabsorbed tissues, such as bone sequestra, sloughs of fascia or tendons, or even urinary or gall-bladder calculi should be regarded as foreign bodies in this respect.

The immediate necessity for the removal of a foreign body is that, even though the wound may have healed primarily, latent infection may later become active and give rise to secondary suppuration.

7. When a foreign object may result in chemical injury to the body. The tissue fluids constantly bathing the foreign body may partially dissolve it and this in turn may injure adjoining tissues or result in constitutional injury. Such injurious irritation of the surrounding tissues has been known to occur in the eye. Lead poisoning has been known to occur from the presence of lead shot in the body.

It is not impossible that a foreign body composed of several metals, for example, copper wire soldered with zinc, could damage the tissue through the generation of an "electrical current." It would however be necessary for the metals to become separated, since an electrical current can only be produced when different metals are separated from one another by a salt solution, of which the lymph is an excellent example.

(b) The Localization of Foreign Bodies. Since the position of a foreign body may change from the time of its entry to the time of operation, its position should be redetermined just prior to operation for its removal. Besides the alteration of position observed in foreign bodies in the tissues, those which lie in abscesses, hollow viscera, joints, and other cavities may shift their position during alteration of the patient's position. It is important, therefore, to determine the position of the foreign body in the posture to be assumed during operation. Likewise during the operation through retraction or as a result of collapse of a viscus, such as the lung after pneumothorax, a foreign body is occasionally displaced. Such occurrences not infrequently alter the position of the foreign body.

The superficial cicatrix, which the entrance of the foreign body has left behind, offers little aid as to the exact position of the object at the time of its attempted removal. Disregarding secondary displacement, the penetrating object, especially if a bullet, may finally lodge at a site quite far removed from its site of entrance. I once saw a patient with a gun-shot entrance wound near the shoulder, and though no wound of exit could be found, we could not locate the bullet, until x-ray pictures subsequently showed the bullet to be in the gluteal region.

The simplest and surest method of determining the position of a foreign body is to feel it or the condensation of tissue around it. Unfortunately this is not possible in the more deeply lying foreign bodies. Further evidences of its position may be obtained by disorders of function to which its presence may give rise. The injury of individual centers and paths of the central nervous system, the paralysis of individual nerves, the absence of arterial pulsation, the limitation of motion of a joint or of certain muscles permit one to draw conclusions as to the position of the foreign body. However, these evidences are uncertain, since they may be the result of injury caused by the foreign body during its course. If the foreign body is in an infected area, it will usually be found in the depths of the fistulous tract.

The Localization of Foreign Bodies by the X-ray. A foreign body can best be localized when it is opaque to the Roentgen ray. Pieces of metal glass, rubber and iodoform gauze, which must often be searched for, belong to this category. Foreign bodies which cast no shadow, such as pieces of cloth or plain gauze sponges, may, when they are connected through a fistula with the periphery, be made to show contrast shadows by the injection of solutions which are opaque to the Roentgen ray, such as barium chloride, sodium iodide, etc. Examination will have shown that the end of the fistulous tract corresponded to the position of the foreign body, while subsequent to the injection of the solution the foreign body will be shown since it has become saturated with the salt. When a foreign body is located in a hollow organ, it can be easily located if it is opaque. Occasionally it is necessary to study its position by giving a barium meal. Stereoscopic plates are often very valuable. Even if an object in a fistulous tract casts a shadow I frequently fill the tract with a contrast solution, and after marking the skin exit of the tract with a lead marker, x-ray the patient so as to obtain additional information as to the exact course of the tract.

1. Fluoroscopy

A competent roentgenologist can accurately locate an x-ray body by studying its position when viewed from various positions through a fluoroscopic screen. Although this method is very valuable, it should be checked by x-ray pictures taken in various positions. The mere statement that a foreign body is present, without exact localization, does not add to the surgeon's knowledge. Superficial markers should be used in this work whether it is done by the fluoroscope or by the method of making plates. I fasten on the surface of the body either lead markers or wires, whose exact locations are marked with indelible colors. These markers should if possible correspond to definite anatomical points. Air, sounds, or catheters, etc., can be introduced into hollow organs (like the gastro-intestinal canal, kidney pelvis, urinary bladder, ureters, uterus, brain ventricles, or the subarachnoid space) to give contrast pictures.

When a foreign body moves with a movable organ (heart, liver, muscles, diaphragm), the foreign body is either in the structure or so close to it as to be affected by its movements.

The disadvantages of fluoroscopy are several. In the first place the roentgenologist must have had considerable experience with this method, in foreign body work, to be even relatively exact. Second, where the rays are not exactly vertical false images of the position of the body arise. Third, unless plates are also taken, the surgeon must depend on memory since he has no permanent records of the position of the object. On the other hand, the foreign body may be fairly well localized by fluoroscopy, its relative position marked, and then permanent plates made for the guidance of the surgeon.

2. The Two-Plate Procedure

A fairly good idea of the position of a foreign body can be obtained by taking two plates at right angles to one another after the object has been located by fluoroscopy. The use of various types of internal and external markers is just as important here as in fluoroscopy. The two-plate procedure combines the errors arising from false projection with the disadvantage that at the time of manipulation pictures made in only two directions are available. (Except for the head little is gained by taking pictures in three directions.) The procedure suffices very well for localizing large foreign bodies situated in a narrow bordered space, but is not entirely satisfactory for small foreign bodies located in the deeper tissues. Here again stereoscopic plates help considerably in the more difficult cases.

3. Determining the Depth of a Foreign Body

After preliminary Roentgen studies have been made the method of double exposure with displacement of the axis of the Roentgen rays will give

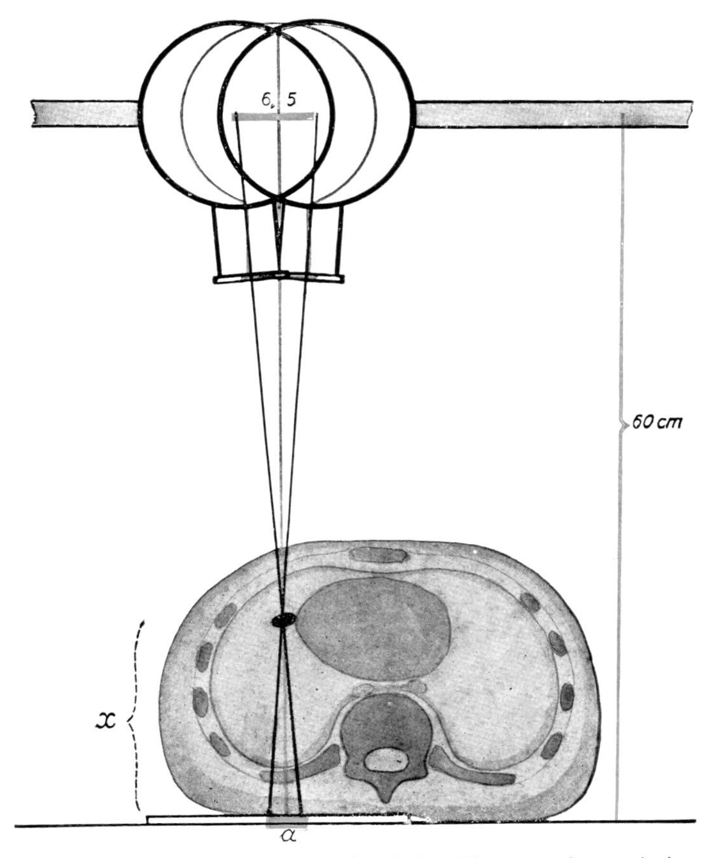

FIG. 104. Determining the depth of a foreign body. Two superimposed pictures are taken, the tube being moved a known distance between exposures. The red lines can be measured, so that x can be calculated and the position of the foreign body determined.

the final information that is desired. After placing the patient in the most favorable position as determined fluoroscopically, a plate is placed under the area to be examined, vertical to the direction of the rays. The central beam of the cathode is placed at a distance of exactly 60 cm. from the plate and focused on the foreign body. The cathode should be pushed for about 3.25 cm. to the right and to the left of zero and an exposure made in each position on the same plate. One sees then on the developed plate two foreign bodies, whose distance one from another is measured. One knows: (1) The distance of the shadows of the foreign body from one another, (2) The distance of the cathode from the plate = 60 cm., and (3) the distance of the cathode displacement for the second exposure = 6.5 cm. (Fig. 104.) From these the distance (x) of the foreign body from the plate can be calculated, using the formula $x = \frac{60a}{6.5 + a}$ where a is the measured distance between the two shadows of the foreign body on the plate. The distance can also be directly determined by using the table of Fürstenau. The result equals the distance of the foreign body from the plate and therefore, if the body lay flat on the plate, from the skin surface. If the body was not flat on the plate, as for instance in spinal deformity, then errors arise, for which a correction must be made.

4. Stereoscopic Localization

If the x-ray pictures are taken by stereoscopic technic, the films when placed in a stereoscope can be observed from one position so as to visualize the relative depth of all the shadows. It is the only procedure that affords a direct observation of the location of a foreign body. It is unnecessary to build space relations from the imagination when this method is used, since the pictures, properly visualized, give the exact position of the foreign body in relation to anatomical landmarks. A further advantage is, that by changing the plates in the exhibiting box one may see from the front as well as from the back. However, unless the stereoscopic adjustment is correct, errors may also arise with this method.

The stereo-technic consists in an exposure made on each of two plates at the same cathode distance (60 cm.), but with a movement of the cathode for a distance of about 3.25 cm. from zero to the right and left respectively during the exposures. The plates are placed in a special stereoscopic view-box and then studied. Hasselwander's apparatus has proved excellent as a viewing apparatus, and has the further advantage of permitting exact measurements during visualization.

5. The Spearing or Harpooning of Foreign Bodies

This method is frequently called Perthes' method. Harpooning is the simplest combination of x-ray technic with operative procedure. The foreign body is "speared" immediately before the operation, with the aid of the fluoroscope, by one or more specially made long needles. It can be carried out in at least two, and, at times, even more directions (Figs. 105 and 106). The needles are inserted so that the foreign body lies at their intersection. Purposely one needle is inserted in the plane corresponding to the direction of operative approach, so that it serves as a director during the operation. The needles must not be inserted in any direction in which important structures may be injured, and if it is impossible to avoid them this method should not be used.

If local anæsthesia is to be used it should be injected prior to the insertion of the needles, since its introduction subsequent to their fixation may cause them to shift their position. Perthes has devised several harpoons provided with barbed hooks, but these have no particular advantages. I use straight metal needles, which have mounted on their blunt end a metal ring with a cross-thread (Fig. 105). The needle is placed so that the shadow of

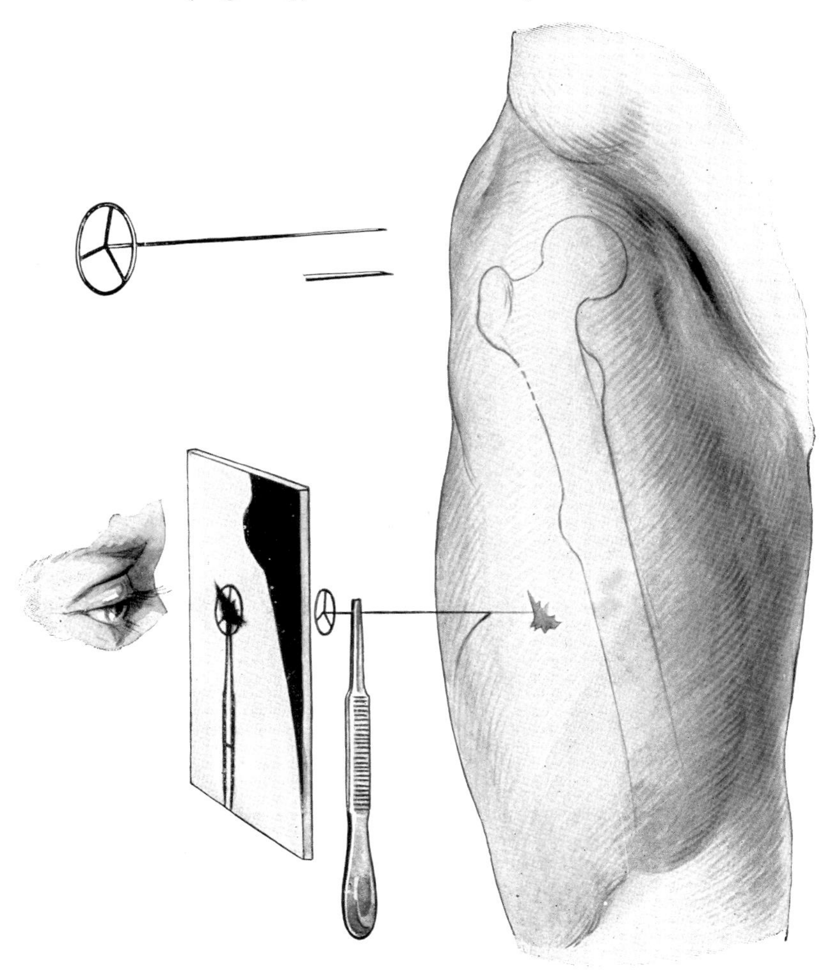

FIG. 105. Localization of a foreign body with the fluroscope. With the aid of the fluroscope the needle is inserted into the tissues until it comes in contact with the foreign body. It may be necessary to insert the needle in more than one direction. Left above: Needle with specially prepared circular end.

the foreign body falls on the point where the threads cross. In the simpler cases ordinary needles suffice. The method gives excellent results. It is especially useful when searching for very small foreign bodies. A foreign body which has evaded search can be "speared" through the open wound and then removed.

If the foreign body, due to its position, can be approached with a needle from only one side, or if one hesitates to leave the needle in the tissues, the line of the needle to the foreign body may be marked with color. Either methylene blue solution is injected into the tissue as a hollow needle is withdrawn (Foramitti), or some black china ink is dried on the needle before inserting and this deposits itself along the path of the needle. The incision then follows the line of pigmentation to the site of the foreign body.

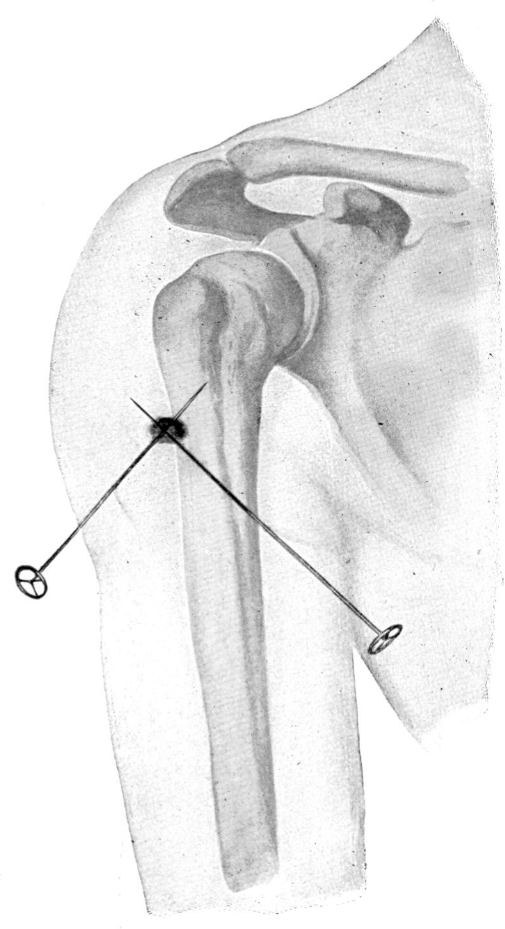

Fig. 106. The foreign body is approached from two directions with two needles. It lies at the intersection of the needles.

6. The Removal of Foreign Bodies with the aid of the Fluoroscopic Screen.

When this method is used it may be done in one of two ways. In the first place, the foreign body is localized fluoroscopically and the room is then lighted and the surgeon searches for the object. If he fails to find it, the fluoroscope is again used in order to ascertain how close the operator is to the foreign body. Sometimes the entire operation is done under fluoroscopic visualization. The latter procedure is not an anatomic operation, and it should be limited to those foreign bodies which are not in the proximity of important structures. A special fluoroscopic table (Fig. 107) is used for this, the tube carrier being freely movable. If the operation is started under direct illumination the fluoroscope is not utilized until the operator believes he is near the foreign body, when the room is darkened and an x-ray screen protected with sterile covers is held over the field of operation. A hemostat or forceps is inserted in the wound and if it is close to the object it is grasped and removed. If the object is close to important structures, direct illumination should again be used to remove the foreign body. Either of these methods has the disadvantage that it is often difficult to maintain asepsis, and that it is frequently time consuming.

The disadvantage of alternately using direct illumination and transillumination, with the loss of time necessary for accommodation of vision, may be overcome by using the Grashey monocle-cryptoscope so that one eye can be used for direct vision and one for fluoroscopy.

In my experience it is better to attempt to remove the foreign body after it has been localized by a good roentgenologist. If this fails then an attempt should be made to remove it fluoroscopically. In case a fluoroscope is not available, the operator should place a metal marker in the depths of the wound and then again x-ray the area for proper localization.

It is important to point out that the method for exploration and localization is not the all important item in foreign body removal, but that skillful surgery plays a very important rôle. A poor surgeon may fail with any method, while a good one may succeed with a relatively poor one. The more trauma the greater the danger of infection.

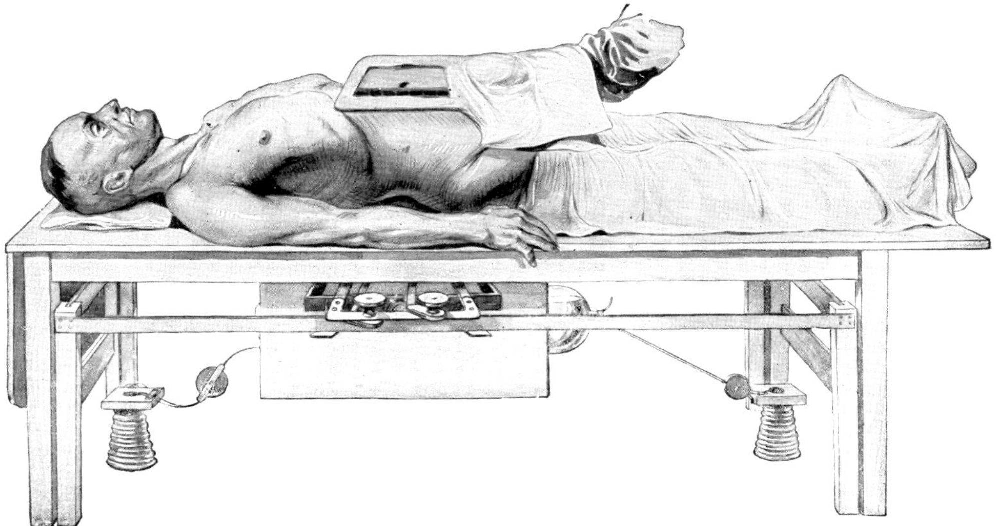

FIG. 107. Localization and removal of foreign bodies with the aid of a fluoroscopic table. This is especially useful in urology as well as in the localization of foreign bodies outside of the genito-urinary tract.

(c) The Technic for the Removal of Foreign Bodies. The removal of even non-irritating foreign bodies should be looked upon at most as only a conditionally aseptic operation. The skin is constantly contaminated, and frequently latent infection exists around the foreign body which is activated by the trauma of the operation. Therefore, the wound should be closed primarily only under the most favorable conditions. Since the removal of a foreign body present in the tissues for many years has been followed by tetanus, it is advisable to administer antitoxin before operation in any case where the foreign body may have carried such an infection into the wound. This is especially true if the foreign body has been in the tissues for some time and antitoxin was given at the time of the injury.

If a choice of approaches exists, that approach should be chosen which avoids important anatomical structures and at the same time permits adequate exposure without too much tissue trauma. If there are disadvantages to either approach, the shortest one should be chosen. The easiest cases, of course, are those in which the foreign body is palpable or when a short fistulous tract leads to it. When a tract is to be searched it should previously be injected with a dye to outline it. If the tract is deep and surrounded by considerable scar tissue it may be advisable to approach the foreign body through a clean, freshly made wound, so that the operation is accomplished under approximately aseptic conditions.

If search for a foreign body is to be made under local anæsthesia, it is best to mark the site for the incision on the skin surface, before the local anæsthetic is injected. The edema resulting from the injection may otherwise prevent proper orientation. In the extremities it is often advisable to use a tourniquet so as to do the operation bloodlessly.

The exposure should be made extremely carefully, lest rough handling of the tissues displace the object. It is not advisable repeatedly to explore the wound with a finger. One may frequently be led to the foreign body by scar tissue, or inflamed or suppurative areas. When the foreign body is located its removal is, for the most part, simple. It should be grasped with a forceps or hemostat and removed from its bed. If it can not be delivered in this manner the exposure should be enlarged and the foreign body removed with a small hook. If the body is embedded wholly, or in part, in bone it may be necessary to chisel it free. If it is situated close to large vessels or the heart, one must be prepared for hemorrhage. Small metal splinters can be easily removed by Susani's method. A hollow needle is pushed into the tissues with the aid of the fluoroscope and the splinter is caught in the needle where it remains while the needle is withdrawn. The electro-magnetic re-

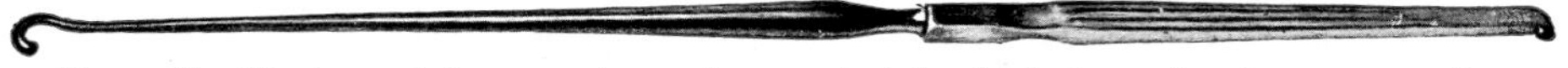

Fig. 108. Hook used in removing suture material which is prolonging suppuration.

moval of foreign bodies has not been as successful in general surgery as it has been in ophthalmology. However, when iron or steel is lodged in soft tissues, such as the brain, its removal by this method has been successful.

The Management of Suppuration Associated with Sutures. In operations where asepsis has been maintained sutures remain in the tissues without visible tissue reaction. Silk becomes surrounded and encapsulated by connective tissue if the wound remains clean, but even slight infection may cause oozing of cloudy serum from such a wound for weeks or months. Wire may become encapsulated in a like manner. Catgut is absorbed in a variable period of time, depending on its mode of preparation and its size. Infection may occur merely around the suture material with the formation of localized abscesses. These abscesses may rupture through the wound and form small fistulæ. Such fistulæ do not heal until the suture is extruded or removed. Non-absorbable sutures may become the site of infection years after their insertion into the tissues.

If the sutures in an infected wound do not extrude themselves, an attempt should be made to remove them. They may be "fished" for with forceps, or with a hook (Fig. 108). If these methods are unsuccessful, and suppuration is prolonged, the tract should be enlarged and the offending sutures removed under direct vision. If the sutures lie deep or in the vicinity of important structures, sensitive to infection (large vessels, abdominal cavity, etc.), the search may be difficult and dangerous. Such tracts should be injected with a dye before a search is attempted and the greatest caution should be exercised in the exposure.

When a suture has been found the search should not stop until the surgeon is satisfied that it is the sole cause of the trouble and that other fistulæ do not communicate with the one already explored. The wound should be permitted to close by granulation, or a secondary closure may be done when the infection has been controlled.

4. Transplantation of Tissues and the Implantation of Foreign Bodies

LIVING TISSUE

The displacement and transplantation of living tissues is known as plastic surgery. Several types of grafts are used: the pedicle graft, the free graft, and the migratory graft. Almost all tissues can be transplanted without any visible alteration of structure or function. The technic of transplantation of individual tissues will be discussed under the various kinds of tissue. Only the general rules governing grafting will be discussed here.

The most important rule in plastic surgery is to afford proper nutrition for the transplanted tissues. If the graft undergoes extensive necrosis, the entire transplant will as a rule be lost. The nutritional conditions of the free graft especially are considerably impaired by infection or by sanguineous effusions, so that the strictest asepsis and hemostasis are essential for good results. However, free transplants often do unite in spite of suppuration. The pedicled transplant has the advantage over the free transplant, in that nutrition can be maintained through the pedicle, while the free transplant is dependent on the tissue juices for nutrition until the capillaries from the surrounding tissue invade the graft. In order that the pedicle function satisfactorily for nourishing the flap, it must be large enough and it must not be twisted or stretched unduly. In skin grafting the pedicle should not be smaller than half the width of the broadest part of the flap. It is an advantage when the graft contains large vessels, and the pedicle should be planned so as to include a good sized artery.

The migratory graft is employed only in skin grafting. A pedicle graft is made and the flap transplanted to a new site. When this has established a lymph and blood vessel communication at its new site the pedicle is transplanted. The process can be repeated. Further details are given in the discussion of skin grafting.

The free graft is as a rule only successful when the patient's own tissues are used for the grafting (auto-plastic grafts). Tissues from the same species (homeoplastic) or from other species (heteroplastic) are at times successful, but this is not the rule. Only the tissues taken from one's own body persist anatomically and functionally. The homeo- and heteroplastic grafts, if they are not expelled, are replaced by connective tissues.

The grafts must be carefully protected for the first few days from mechanical, chemical or thermal injury. In skin grafting I therefore avoid skin disinfection, prior to operation, of the part from which the graft is to be taken. Nor do we scrub this area unduly, being satisfied with a careful cleansing with sterile normal saline solution. Deep tissues taken for transplantation should not be permitted to come in contact with the chemically disinfected skin or with any chemical solution. Normal saline solutions, as well as Ringer's solution, are included in this embargo. They are not only superfluous, but at times may be even injurious. Tissue should be transplanted as rapidly as possible after it is removed, so that the graft should not be removed until its bed is prepared.

It should be handled with the utmost gentleness, both during removal and transplantation. Mouse toothed forceps should not be used in handling it. The bed to which it is to be grafted should be dry. If after transplantation infection supervenes, the prospects for survival of the graft diminish with the severity of the infection. Primary wound closure should be done over buried transplants. Packing or draining invites infection. If infection results and suppuration develops, the graft is seriously endangered, but the end-result is not absolutely hopeless. The immediate relief of any existing tension, the improvement of the circulation, and the avoidance of any pressure on the grafted area are of importance.

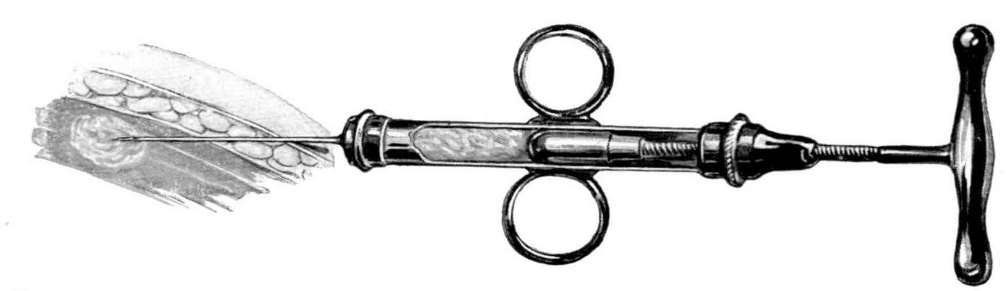

FIG. 109. Transplantation of tissue pulp with a metal syringe. The pulp is placed in the cylinder of the syringe. The high pressure necessary to force the pulp through a needle can be obtained by the screw piston.

Since the area which has been grafted will ooze lymph for the first few days, the thinner the graft the better are the prospects of its surviving. It is because of their thinness that fascial and Thiersch grafts are so successful. For this reason highly developed tissues (testicle, thyroid, ovary) should if possible be transplanted in thin slices.

The grafting of glandular organs (testicles, ovaries, thyroid, suprarenals) in order permanently to obtain their natural secretion has not been successful. No doubt grafts of this type persist and function for a period, but subsequently they degenerate and are replaced by fibrous tissue. However, if grafting is attempted, the grafts should be placed in a site which is well vascularized. Such sites as the rectus muscle or the bone marrow are to be preferred. Since in the transplantation of parenchymatous tissues, and also to a degree the skin, one does not care about form, but only about the cells and their secretions, it is possible to inject the tissues as suggested by Kurtzhahn. The tissues are pulped and aspirated into a special type of metal syringe (Fig. 109). The contents of the syringe are then forced into the desired location by screwing the piston. Although this procedure is extremely simple and can be repeated as often as desired, I have grave doubts whether the pulped transplant ever functions.

The transplantation of entire organs by means of vessel suture has not as yet been sucessfully done in man. The success of such procedures is frustrated by a lack of suitable material for grafting. The transfusion of blood is described in a later chapter.

INERT MATERIAL

Inert material for subcutaneous implantation should be differentiated as to whether it is partly soluble or absorbable in the tissue juices or whether it remains permanently as a foreign body. The soluble or absorbable materials are for the most part of organic origin, being derived from the human or from an animal. As a rule these materials are especially prepared before use in order to assure sterility and durability. Cargile membrane, artery walls, bone, serous membranes, fascia, kangaroo tendon, sheep-gut are some of the materials used. Sterility, above everything else, must be assured if they are used.

Of the inorganic metals, magnesium alone is removed by the body. It is disintegrated into magnesium oxide and hydrogen, and the former is absorbed, while the hydrogen gas is released and is supposed to stimulate the growth of connective tissue. It is for this supposed action that magnesium has been used in cavities whose obliteration is being attempted.

While absorbable materials vary in the time necessary for their complete disappearance, the non-absorbable bodies remain permanently unless they are removed by the surgeon or extruded by suppuration. If well tolerated they become surrounded by a connective tissue capsule. If suppuration occurs the foreign body should be removed as soon as possible. Even if the foreign body becomes encapsulated, it may, sometimes years later, become the site of suppuration. Since movement favors the expulsion of a foreign body, the use of non-absorbable materials in muscles is not recommended, while in rigid structures such as bone they are well tolerated.

As a rule the more precious a substance, the less it will be attacked by the body. Platinum, gold, chromium, even rustless steel, remain practically unchanged for years, and copper, bronze, and celluloid are also quite resistant. Silver, steel, iron, and ivory, on the other hand, are rapidly attacked. Silver is decomposed forming silver sulphide, while iron and steel form an iron oxide.

Silk and linen thread, silkworm gut, and rubber are also non-absorbable. Connective tissue slowly penetrates between the fibers of thread, and into the pores of rubber, so that after considerable time these materials gradually become intimately bound to the surrounding tissues.

CHAPTER II

THE CONTROL OF PAIN

The division of tissues is associated with pain, except in individuals with morbid disturbances of the consciousness or certain diseases of the central nervous system where pain is not perceived.

The ability to bear pain varies considerably. Women, as a rule, are more patient than men; the new-born, and old men are less sensitive than children or young adults. Racial groups, also, vary in their ability to withstand pain. Certain areas of the body are more sensitive than others. Thus the prepuce, nail beds, and cornea are extremely sensitive, while the intestine and stomach are relatively insensible.

It is possible to perform certain major operations without anæsthesia if one disregards pain. Until nearly the middle of the last century this was a matter of necessity. With anæsthesia at our command pain can now be controlled. The surgeon who wilfully subjects his patients to painful procedures without anæsthesia is guilty of a very serious offense.

Although history abounds with records of stoicism in the face of what undoubtedly was great pain, modern investigations have demonstrated that pain is a factor in the production of shock and postoperative psychoses. The surgeon is bound ethically and morally to use every available means to control pain, and failure to use these is evidence of incompetence and moral turpitude.

The control of pain in modern surgery dates from the work of Long, Jackson and Morton in the latter part of the first half of the 19th century. Long first used ether for anæsthesia in a surgical operation, while Morton first demonstrated its use before a group of surgeons. A few years after this, Simpson used chloroform. Since that time we have witnessed the synthesis of a large number of substances which can be used for the alleviation of pain, and every year brings forth new ones. The ability to perform any operation painlessly is, next to asepsis, the most important acquisition of modern surgery. Under anæsthesia the surgeon can perform major operations thoroughly and speedily, and he is not harassed by the torturing consciousness of martyrdom on the part of the patient.

Every operation can be performed under general anæsthesia, and most of them under local anæsthesia. The decision as to which type of anæsthesia should be used and the actual anæsthetic agent to be selected must be made after consideration of a number of factors, some of which have been discussed in Chapter I. Other factors will be discussed under the various types of anæsthesia and the various operations. The extent to which local anæsthesia can be used depends partly upon the temperament of the operator, and partly upon the skill which he develops in its use. That its use is often abused is as sure as the fact that many operators, from habit or indolence, persist in using general anæsthesia in all cases. Braun estimates that about half of all operations can be done under local anæsthesia, while the other half necessitates general anæsthesia, an estimate with which I agree.

Unless the emergency is very great, every patient should be prepared for anæsthesia. This has been discussed in Chapter I. The smoothness of the anæsthesia depends to a large extent on the thoroughness of this preparation.

Ether, ethyl chloride, and ethylene are inflammable, and should not be used during an operation in the presence of an open light, or exposed electrical apparatus, such as the cautery.

It seems hardly necessary to say that every patient who is to be operated on should have an operating sheet attached to his record. The practise is now nearly universal, but the majority of these sheets are practically worthless. The sheet should be begun before the patient goes to the operating room and should contain the following information: 1. Name of the patient; 2. Date of operation; 3. Location of the patient in the hospital; 4. Age; 5. Weight; 6. Diagnosis; 7. Diseases of especial significance to the anæsthetist (heart, lungs, kidneys, general debility, shock, stercoraceous vomiting, etc.); 8. The type of anæsthesia to be used; 9. Preliminary medication, dosage and time of administration. The anæsthetist during the operation records the pulse and blood pressure, and after the operation fills in the following data: 1. The operation and its number as recorded in the operating room book; 2. The operator and assistants; 3. The type of anæsthesia and the kind of anæsthetic; 4. The quantity of the anæsthetic used; 5. Duration of the operation; 6. The condition of the patient at the conclusion of the operation; 7. The sponge count. This sheet is then made a permanent part of the patient's record.

Every operating room should keep an operating room book which should contain the following information: 1. Number of operation; 2. Date; 3. Name of patient; 4. Age; 5. Disease; 6. Operation; 7. Location in hospital; 8. Operator; 9. Assistants; 10. Anæsthetist; 11. Anæsthesia; 12. Duration of operation; 13. Quantity of anæsthetic used; 14. Progress of anæsthesia.

A. GENERAL ANÆSTHESIA

General anæsthesia consists in the administration of a sleep producing anæsthetic substance, whose primary effect is on the central nervous system, principally the brain. The anæsthetic is carried to the brain by the blood stream. It may be administered by inhalation (inhalation anæsthesia), by bowel (rectal anæsthesia), or intravenously (intravenous anæsthesia).

Of fundamental importance in the safety of inducing anæsthesia is the ability of the anæsthetist to regulate the depth of anæsthesia, the proper length of time for its maintenance, and to be able to observe and correctly interpret the reactions of the patient. The administration of an anæsthetic which requires a single dose calculated before operation by weight does not take into consideration any of the idiosyncrasies of the patient. Inhalation anæsthesia thus fulfills the requirements more accurately than do the various types of intravenous or rectal anæsthesia. The major advantage of methods other than inhalation anæsthesia is that the psychic effect of anæsthetization is largely done away with and the patient goes to sleep without the attending nervous excitation.

Recently, I have overcome some of the objections to parapulmonic anæsthesia by introducing avertin as an intravenous anæsthetic. It combines safety and reliability, on the one hand, with protection against excitation, on the other. It is a highly satisfactory anæsthetic. It removes the major fear from the patient, the fear of anæsthesia. It lessens the mental shock. It is especially useful in operations for exophthalmic goitre because the day of the operation need not be disclosed. If this type of anæsthesia is used in small doses, just sufficient to cause light sleep, it can be reinforced with nitrous oxide and oxygen to obtain complete anæsthesia. Its use results in quieter patients whose relaxation is more profound than if it had not been used. (Sodium amytal [sodium iso-amyl-ethyl-barbiturate] is being used in the United States in a similar way. I. S. R.)

The anæsthetic substances used in general anæsthesia are eliminated by the lungs, intestine, kidneys or skin. In their course through the body they come in contact with all the body cells, and some of the anæsthetics have a deleterious effect on the cells of certain organs. The normal course and the various disturbances and dangers of the various methods of anæsthetization are similar. Since the drop method of inhalation anæsthesia is more widely used than any other method of anæsthesia, I will discuss it first, and then briefly describe certain of the other methods.

1. Drop-Anæsthesia

If one considers the use of inhalation anæsthetics throughout the world, ether and chloroform are the most widely used. For short periods of anæsthesia, ethyl chloride is preferred in many clinics. In the United States, nitrous oxide and oxygen, and ethylene are very widely used, while in Germany, narcylen (acetylene) anæsthesia has come into wide use.

For open drop anæsthesia ether has come to be accepted as the anæsthetic of choice. It is less dangerous and its margin of safety is very much greater than chloroform, so that in the absence of definite indications, ether should be used. In the United States chloroform is very rarely used in any of the larger surgical clinics. In Germany many surgeons still prefer it in inflammatory diseases of the respiratory organs, and as a preliminary anæsthetic for those resistant patients in whom induction with other anæsthetics is extremely difficult. Anæsthetists are now very generally agreed that the various mixtures of ether, chloroform and alcohol are not safe and offer no decided advantage. For this reason they are now rarely heard of. A well trained anæsthetist needs no such mixture for his work.

Chloroform, which has a boiling point of 61° C., is the quickest acting and most potent of the anæsthetic agents. It is because of this, however, that it is dangerous. The anæsthetic dose and the lethal dose are very close, so that the margin of safety is small. Furthermore, it causes degeneration of the cells of parenchymatous organs. It has a particularly deleterious effect on the heart, liver, and kidneys. In fact, if these organs are already diseased, the degeneration caused by its administration may prove fatal. It is only slowly eliminated from the body. For these many reasons it is rapidly being replaced by other substances as an anæsthetic agent.

Ether, which has a boiling point of 35° C., is not nearly so toxic. The anæsthetic dose and the lethal dose are more widely separated, so that the margin of safety is fairly great. Furthermore it is rapidly eliminated from the body. It irritates the respiratory system, leading to an increase of mucous secretion during anæsthesia, and no doubt predisposes the patient to post-operative pulmonary complications. It is to be avoided, therefore, in inflammatory affections of the respiratory organs. It causes some irritation of the kidneys, but has only a very slight effect on the liver or heart.

In the United States, anæsthesia is frequently induced with nitrous oxide and oxygen, and maintained with ether, or the ether is given with the gas. In Germany, the anæsthesia is often induced with chloroform and then continued with ether. The actual choice of anæsthetic depends on the surgeon, and he must decide this in each case. The decision should take into account the patient, the surgeon, and the individual administering the anæsthetic. Needless to say, a well trained anæsthetist is an essential part of every good operating team.

The anæsthetic agent should be chemically pure; it should have been made for anæsthesia, and it should not have decomposed. Deterioration of the volatile anæsthetics, ether, chloroform, and ethyl chloride does occur and their use after this has occurred may prove disastrous. To prevent deterioration they should be kept in dark bottles, in a dark, cool place, and should be used within a reasonable time, 12 hours, after opening the container. The larger manufacturers supplying ether and chloroform now test their product so carefully that it need not be tested before use if fresh material is used.

If one accepts the Meyer-Overton theory, inhalation anæsthetics exert their action by affecting the lipoids in the cells of the central nervous system. The intensity of the action of the anæsthetic supposedly depends upon the lipoidal solubility in the substance. Attempts have been made to explain the stage of excitement as one of stimulation, but this is not generally accepted. It is more generally thought to be the period when the normal inhibitions have been released. When the concentration of the anæsthetic in the blood reaches a certain point there follows a paralysis of certain portions of the brain. All portions of the brain are not affected equally or simultaneously. The cerebral cortex is first affected so that the perception of pain and voluntary movement are temporarily removed. The vital centers of the medulla oblongata which control the action of the heart, the tonus of the blood vessels, and respiration are not interfered with if the anæsthetic dose is not exceeded.

The depth of anæsthesia depends on the concentration of the substance in the blood and, therefore, in the brain and brain stem. If the concentration exceeds the optimum for anæsthesia, the action of the centers in the medulla are impaired and continuance of the anæsthetic at this point will lead to their paralysis and death. Thus the concentration of the anæsthetic must be under careful control at all stages of the anæsthesia, since a sudden increase in concentration during the stage of maintenance endangers the life of the patient. It is very important that the anæsthetist be able to inform the surgeon as to the exact stage of anæsthesia at any time. The concentration of the anæsthetic in the blood depends on the difference between its intake and its elimination and destruction. If in a prolonged operation the elimination of the anæsthetic is small in comparison with its intake, then gradually symptoms of overdosage appear. The anæsthetist must be able to recognize these and should always watch for them.

The total amount of anæsthetic which has been used throughout the operation is no criterion as to the stage of anæsthesia existing at any one time, nor to the condition of the various vital centers. On the other hand, the amount administered in a given unit of time has an important bearing on both of these. Death may result from the rapid administration of a few grams of chloroform, while ten times as much chloroform used sparingly over a long period will cause no harmful results. The anæsthetist must not permit herself to be persuaded to attempt too quick an induction of the anæsthesia. It is a dangerous undertaking and creates a hazard which the anæsthetist has no right to assume nor the surgeon any right to encourage.

The relation of surgeon and anæsthetist is not unlike that of the captain and navigator of a ship. Although the captain is, in general, responsible for what occurs, he must have faith in and rely upon his pilot. So too must the surgeon place faith and have confidence in the anæsthetist. He may offer suggestions, but the administration of the anæsthesia must be controlled by the anæsthetist, who should be specially prepared for this type of work.

The exact amount of anæsthetic necessary for anæsthesia varies in different individuals, as does also the time limit for its administration. These depend not only upon the patient, but also upon the type of operation and the skill of the anæsthetist. However, as a rule, the longer the operation the greater the danger of complications from the anæsthesia. In chloroform, ethyl chloride, and ether the great danger of prolonged anæsthesia is the damage which results in the large parenchymatous organs and which not infrequently causes death some time after the operation.

Classification of Anæsthesia. General anæsthesia is divided into two groups, complete and incomplete. The following discussion deals with complete anæsthesia. Anæsthesia is divided into four stages, which are not sharply delineated from each other.

1. The stage of conscious inhalation. } induction
2. The stage of excitement. }
3. The stage of deep anæsthesia. } maintenance
4. The stage of recovery.

To these could be added a fifth stage, the stage of paralysis of the medullary centers.

The stage of conscious inhalation begins with the administration of the anæsthetic. It and the succeeding stage are difficult and yet very important. Failure to realize their importance is the cause of many poor administrations of anæsthesia.

In the stage of conscious inhalation the pulse rate as a rule is increased. This is psychic and varies according to the temperament of the patient. The respiration is frequently irregular. The patient may temporarily stop breathing, or the respirations may become very shallow. Attempts may be made to pull off the mask. The patient may gag and expectorate. The reflexes as well as the sense of pain are at first increased. If an attempt is made to elicit the pupillary reactions the eye-lids close tightly.

The stage of excitement, or as many prefer to call it, the stage of the removal of normal inhibition, varies according to the habits and temperament of the patient and the skill of the anæsthetist. It is a stage which may cause considerable annoyance and delay the period of surgical anæsthesia. In

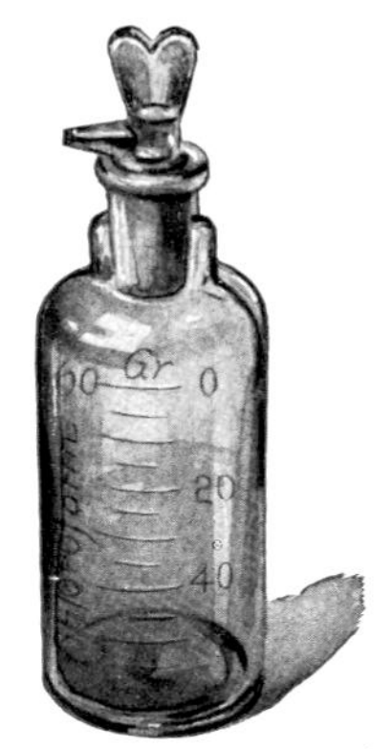

FIG. 110. Graduated drop-bottle of dark yellow glass for chloroform. The same type of bottle, but larger, may be used for ether.

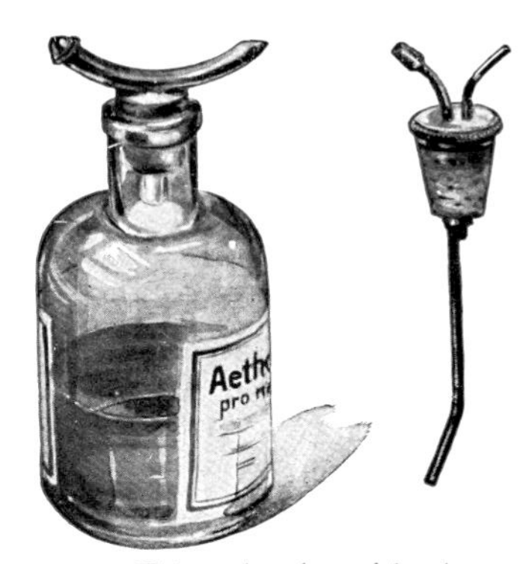

FIG. 111. Ether bottle with drop attachment; (b) another type of the drop attachment.

the stage of excitement the patient who may have been quiet, suddenly begins to struggle, sometimes violently, to shriek, curse or scream, and occasionally to have involuntary evacuations from the bladder or rectum. The pulse becomes considerably accelerated and the respiration jerky. The skin of the face is often suffused or cyanosed. The pupils are half dilated but react to light. The muscles are rigid. It is important to remember that this is not a necessary stage of anæsthesia in all patients. It can be eliminated or curtailed in most patients. The patient who has a tolerance for alcohol, however, reacts badly during this period.

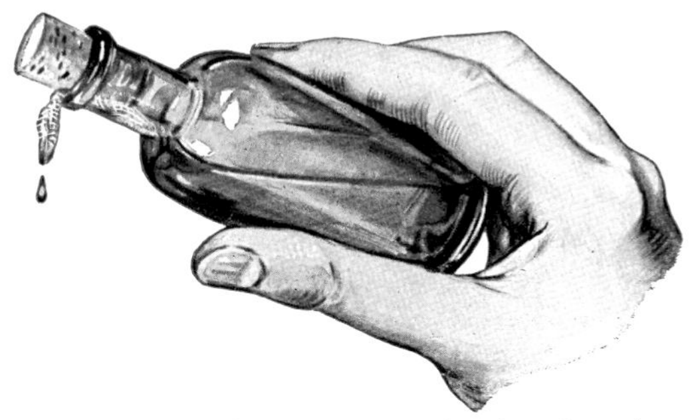

FIG. 112. Simple arrangement for dropping ether. It consists of a lengthwise groove cut into a cork, through which a small piece of gauze is inserted.

In the **stage of deep anæsthesia,** or maintenance, which is so often called the "quiet after the storm", the pulse is again slow, full and regular. Respiration is slow and regular. The pupils are contracted, but react to light. General relaxation exists and muscular reflexes are abolished. The cyanosis of the skin, which was present in the second stage disappears. The anæsthetist can vary the depth of anæsthesia during this period according to the sensitiveness of the tissues and the degree of relaxation desired. It is necessary for the anæsthetist to become acquainted with the surgeon with whom she works since some surgeons wish to restrict the amount of the anæsthetic, while others care nothing about this.

The stage of recovery begins when the anæsthetic is discontinued and ends when consciousness is re-established. During this period most patients exhibit nausea and vomiting. The pulse is again accelerated, and the respirations, which are at first slowed, may again become irregular. The face may

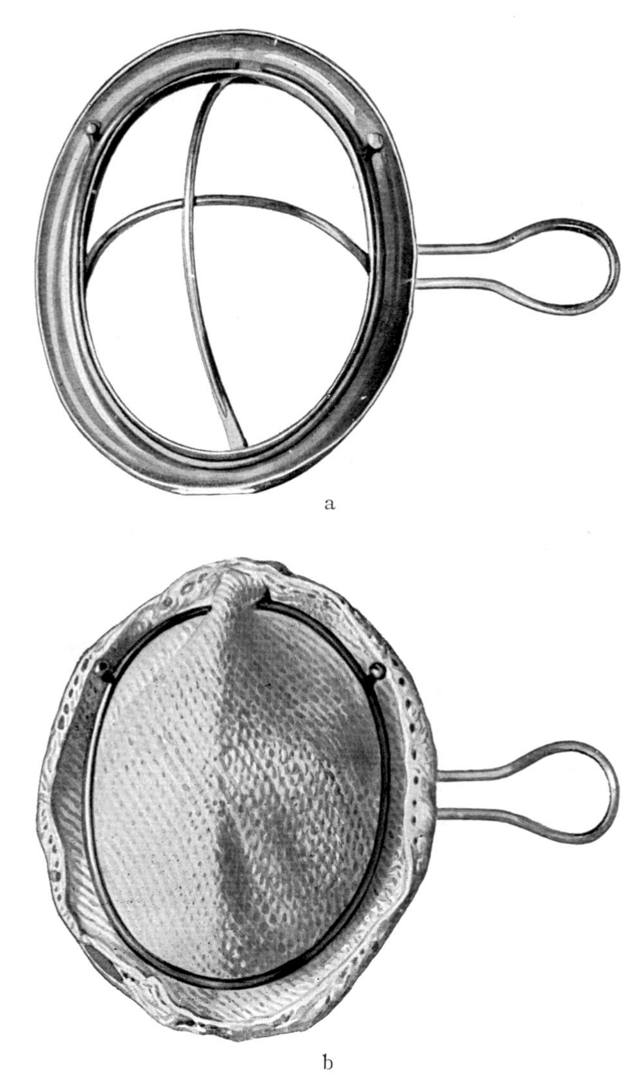

FIG. 113 a and b. Small chloroform mask (Schimmelbusch), without and with gauze cover.

again become suffused, and the pupils dilate slightly but react well to light. The corneal reflexes return. Muscular rigidity is again present. Care must be exercised during this period to prevent aspiration of vomitus.

In the **stage of beginning paralysis of the medullary centers** the pulse at first is slowed and then becomes more rapid, irregular, and weak. The blood pressure drops. The respiration at first slowed becomes irregular and jerky and cyanosis appears. The pupils are widely dilated and do not react to light. All other reflexes are abolished. Gradually respiration and cardiac activity cease, as the medullary centers suffer from a lack of oxygen.

The Technic of Inhalation Anæsthesia. The patients are given 0.01 to 0.02 gram of morphine sulphate and 0.0005 to 0.001 gram of atropine sulphate, hypodermically, 1/2 to 3/4 hour before anæsthesia is begun. The method most usually employed for inhalation anæsthesia is the drop method. While in Germany special bottles (Figs. 110 and 111) are used for this, in America ether is usually administered directly from the ether container. A simple drop bottle can be easily made by preparing a cork as shown in figure 112. If ether and chloroform are used in the clinic these should always be kept in different styled containers so that they will never be confused.

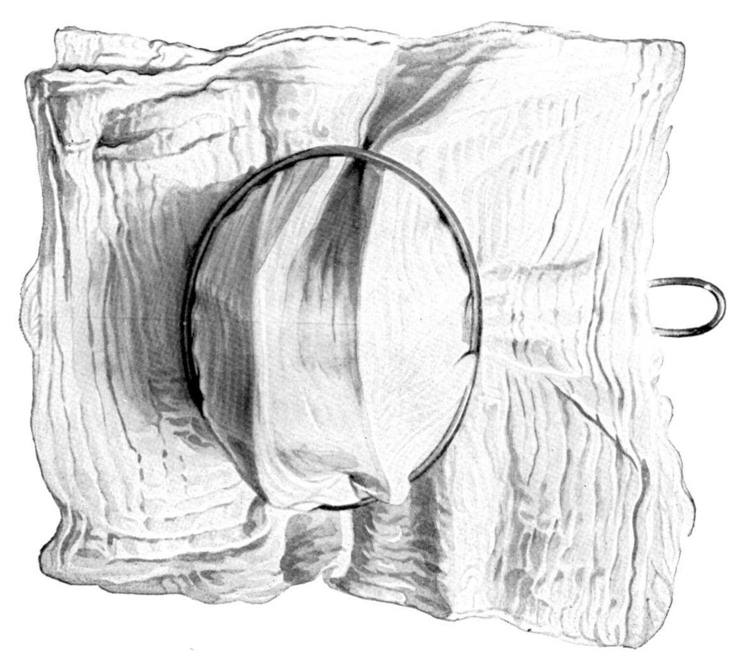

FIG. 114. Ether mask consisting of a wire frame with eight layers of gauze, which are fastened by a wire ring.

The anæsthetic vapor may be administered to the patient in a variety of ways when the anæsthetic is given by the drop method. The use of pieces of cloth or gauze without a mask is not efficient and is not economical. I use a simple wire frame (Fig. 114), which in size is between the small chloroform mask of Schimmelbusch (Fig. 113) and the large ether mask of Juillard-Dumond. The wire frame is boiled each time before it is used and is then covered with an eightfold layer of sterile gauze, which projects over the sides of the frame and is fastened to it by a wire ring which fits to the main part of the frame.

Interference with the supply of air by covering the mask with material which excludes air is no longer used. I no longer use carbon dioxide during the administration of the anæsthesia, although it is useful during the period of recovery. On the other hand, I frequently use oxygen while the anæsthetic is being given. When ether is given, the connection between the mask and the face can be made closer by placing a moistened cloth around the mask margin, and, by varying its size, the area through which air can be admitted through the mask may be limited (Fig. 115).

Before the mask is applied to the patient's face, the patient's eyes should be covered with a moistened compress or pad (Fig. 116) to prevent the anæsthetic agent from getting in the patient's eyes. Ether causes a very intense irritation of the conjunctiva and cornea, and if it should get under the pad the eyes should be irrigated with lukewarm physiologic salt solution. The face, which is to be covered by the mask, should be smeared with vaseline or cold cream to protect the skin from the irritating ether.

I permit no anæsthesia to be begun unless the anæsthetist has at hand a special table upon which are all of the necessary instruments and remedies for combating any possible contingency (Fig. 117). It should contain among other things a mouth-gag; a tongue forceps; a dressing forceps; some small sterile sponges; camphorated oil; adrenalin (1:1000); digalen; pituitrin; ampoules of alpha-lobelin; two sterile hypodermic syringes with suitable hypodermic needles.

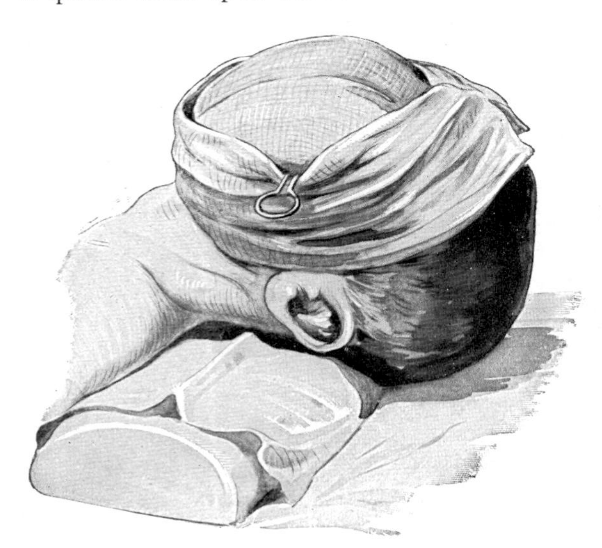

Fig. 115. Method for firmly enclosing the ether mask, by placing a moist towel around it.

It is the duty of the anæsthetist to interview the patient before attempting to induce anæsthesia and to reassure him. The anæsthetist should be familiar with the patient's peculiarities and with the results of the preoperative investigations. In my clinic the results of these investigations are incorporated on a special sheet which is prepared before the operation and accompanies the patient to the operating room. The anæsthetist must be sure that all loose articles are removed from the patient's mouth. He must also assure himself that the patient's bladder has been emptied. In stomach and intestinal operations the anæsthetist should be ready to insert a Jutte tube if vomiting occurs.

The amount of the anæsthetic varies during the different stages of anæsthesia and during the different periods of maintenance. No hard and fast rules can be given for the amount required, since this depends on the constitution, age, size, habits, and preoperative preparation of the patient. It further depends on the length of the operation, and the loss of blood and shock attending the operation. Just as every operation differs slightly, even though it may be for the same lesion, so every anæsthesia varies and demands the most careful control from the anæsthetist. The skill of the anæsthetist consists in being able to appraise the patient's condition throughout the period of anæsthesia and to administer the minimum amount of anæsthetic in every phase of anæsthesia.

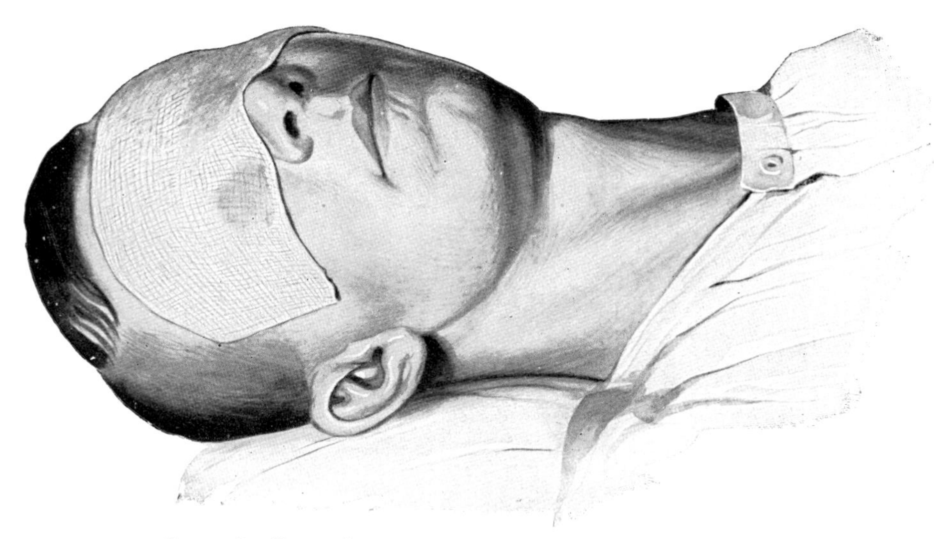

FIG. 116. Protection of the eyes during inhalation anæsthesia.

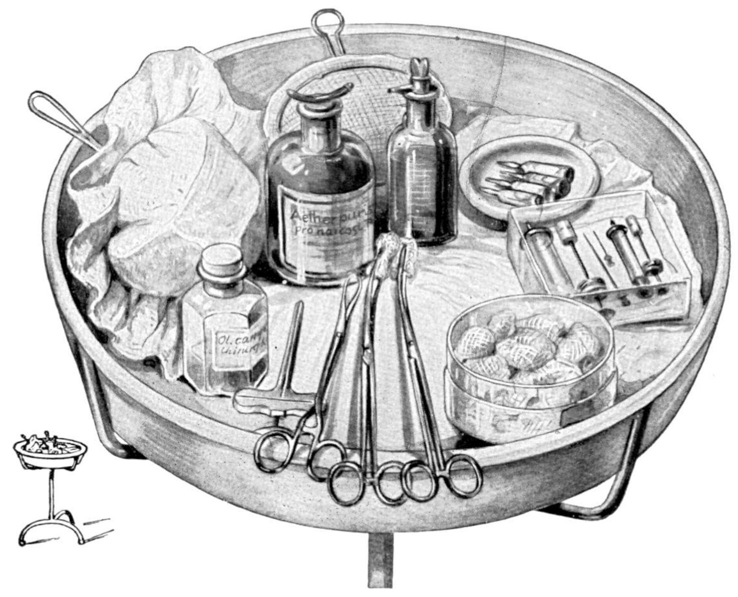

FIG. 117. Anæsthesia table, with the necessary instruments and drugs for general anæsthesia and for emergencies during anæsthesia.

Chloroform should never be poured on the mask, but should be dropped, always sparingly. The quantity of the anæsthetic administered can be regulated by varying the rapidity of the drops. A properly conducted general anæsthesia should be continuous; the mask should never be removed, but the anæsthetist should control the amount of the drug being used. The drops should be spread over the entire mask. The container should be held a few centimeters above the mask, for the non-vaporized anæsthetic may penetrate the gauze layers and thus burn the face, even though this has been protected with vaseline or cold cream.

The anæsthesia should be begun in a quiet room adjacent to the operating room. Very nervous patients should be anæsthetised in their beds. The atmosphere of the anæsthetising room should be as pleasant as possible. At least one capable individual should be ready to help restrain the patient if this becomes necessary. The patient's gown should be tied so as not to restrict breathing. During the period of anæsthesia the arms are held by restraining straps and a strap is placed just above the knees. In Chapter I, the avoidance of pressure palsy from faulty retention was discussed.

Although I have mentioned it previously, I repeat that the anæsthetist should examine the mouth of the patient before applying the mask, and if any foreign body is found it should be removed. He should attempt to gain

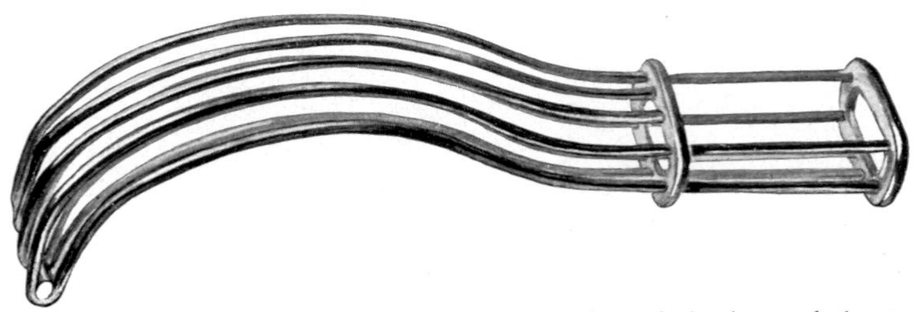

Fig. 118. Intubator (Mayo), which prevents retraction of the base of the tongue. The curved end is introduced into the pharynx, the other end is clamped firmly with its middle ring behind the incisors.

the patient's confidence with a few comforting words such as an assurance of a "good heart". He should quiet the patient and prepare him for the application of the mask and the odor of the anæsthetic. After this the dry mask is placed on the patient's face and he is asked to breathe quietly. The eternally repeated order, "Take a deep breath!" is senseless and irrelevant.

The anæsthetist may permit the patient to slowly count forward and backward, while he starts slowly dropping the anæsthetic, which may be preceded by a little cologne water or oil of orange. If the patient attempts to remove the mask, or holds his breath, the anæsthetist may temporarily remove or elevate the mask and then gently talk to the patient, gradually reassuming administration of the anæsthetic. Gradually the drops are accelerated until the patient is safely carried into the stage of deep anæsthesia, if this is desired. As the muscles relax, the lower jaw is brought forward, so as to prevent the tongue from falling backward and causing asphyxia. Should it be difficult to keep the tongue forward the Mayo intubator is introduced (Figs. 118 and 119). This is made of a wire frame which establishes an airway to the entrance of the larynx. It is a very useful instrument. The second ring of the intubator is fixed behind the incisor teeth so that it is firmly held. The pulse should be taken with the left hand, either from the carotid, the external maxillary (facial) close to the angle of the jaw, or from the temporal directly in front of the ear. The right hand is kept free for administering the anæsthetic and for testing the pupillary reflexes. Provision should be made for taking the blood pressure by attaching the blood pressure cuff before wheeling the patient into the operating room.

Surgical anæsthesia is recognized by muscular relaxation, complete absence of pain, and quiet and regular respiration. It should be borne in mind, that the morphine administered before the anæsthetization may so contract the pupils as to interfere with the pupillary responses. At the height of anæsthesia, the pulse is slow and full, the pupils are contracted, and the respiration is uniform and of medium depth. Gradual acceleration of the pulse, dilatation of the pupils, with sluggish reaction to light, irregularity of respiration, the return of muscular movements, and groaning indicate the advent of recovery. Excessive slowing of the pulse, sudden dilatation of the pupils which fail to react to light, irregular, shallow respiration, marked pallor or cyanosis of the face, darkening of the blood, and a drop in the blood pressure, with a corresponding lessening of hemorrhage from the tissues point to asphyxia and paralysis.

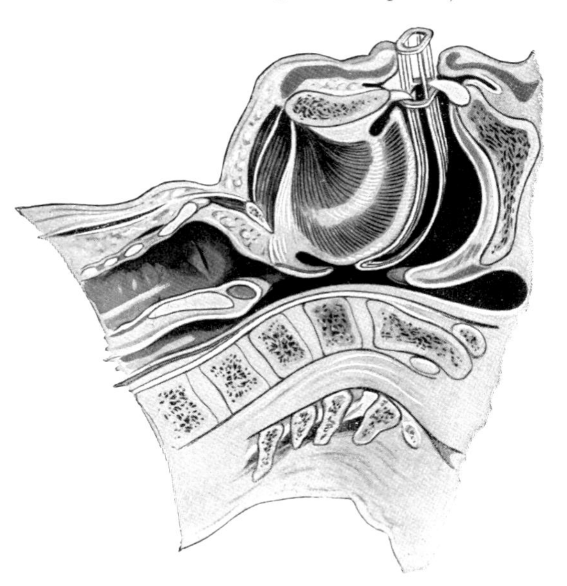

FIG. 119. Showing the Mayo intubator in position.

During deep anæsthesia the eye balls are fixed, the pupils contracted, the lid reflexes absent, and the corneal reflexes sluggish. The corneal reflexes should not be tested indiscriminately, in fact in my clinic no attempt is ever made to elicit them. It is very easy to damage and infect the cornea and the loss of more than one eye can be attributed to such an injury. Other ocular reflexes will give just as much information. If the pulse becomes weak, it may signify cardiac hypotonus or vaso-motor depression as a result of myocardial damage from the anæsthetic, of prolonged anæsthesia, of hemorrhage or shock. The pulse, respiration, pupils, and cutaneous color are constant, dependable indices of the degree of anæsthesia. They are the guides in anæsthesia.

When the general anæsthesia is deep and uniform, little ether is required to maintain the level of anæsthesia. In this stage, also, the depth is best controlled by a constant drop. Uneven administration of the anæsthetic results in uneven anæsthesia. Once deep surgical anæsthesia with relaxation results, the surgeon need not fear a return of rigidity if the anæsthetist gives the patient his undivided attention. Nor will vomiting or gagging occur until the patient shows signs of returning consciousness.

If it is desired that the stage of recovery begin, the mask is removed, and the patient may rebreathe a mixture of carbon dioxide (10 percent) and oxygen (90 percent). This stimulates respiration and induces a more rapid recovery. The operator should tell the anæsthetist that the conclusion of the operation is drawing near, so that the amount of the anæsthetic can be reduced. After the anæsthetic has been stopped the mask may be left on at first, and finally removed. The patient must be watched until the return of consciousness. If he vomits, the jaw is released and the head turned to the side, so as not to hinder the useful reflex movements of the tongue and pharyngeal muscles. The body is placed horizontally and no upright position should be assumed until the return of consciousness. As a rule, the attempt to wipe out the throat and pharynx of the struggling, vomiting, postanæsthetic patient is not only superfluous, but even dangerous.

2. Apparatus for Anæsthesia

The open or semi-closed drop-method of administering an anæsthetic is to be sure primitive, but it is quite safe for general use. The mixture of ether vapor and air cannot be controlled with any degree of accuracy. Also, the drop-method is not economical. The professional anæsthetist has therefore sought refinements in technic, and there has been developed a number of apparatus for the administration of volatile and gaseous anæsthetics. The drop-method is safer in the hands of a non-professional anæsthetist, it demands no special apparatus, and the necessary armamentarium can be obtained in any pharmacy. It is the method most suited to the general practitioner, and should be taught to every student of medicine. On the other hand, every trained anæsthetist must become familiar with several methods of administering anæsthetics and must be able to judge which of these methods is most suited to the case at hand.

It is impossible to describe all of the apparatus now at the disposal of the profession. They all depend upon the same principle, the vaporizing of liquid anæsthetics, and the delivery of the vapor or of a gas to the patient through a closed mask.

The masks, of different sizes, are made of metal, celluloid, or rubber, and are provided with an inflatable or kneaded rubber ring (Fig. 120). This makes an air-tight connection between the mask and the face of the patient. The face should be smeared with vaseline if the closure is to be absolutely tight. The masks can be adjusted to the patient's head with self-retaining elastic bands (Fig. 120). Every mask is made so that at some point it can be opened for the entrance of air, the size of this shutter is adjustable, and it can open and close during expiration and inspiration. The mask must be made air-tight: first, if positive pressure is desired; second, if the mixture of air and anæsthetic is not actively carried to the patient, but is given to him through respiration as occurs in rebreathing systems; and third, when surrounding air must be excluded, as in acetylene anæsthesia. The intake tube, as long as the anæsthetic does not flow in actively, should be protected by a recoil valve to prevent the entrance of the respiratory air. The pressure for carrying the anæsthetic mixture from the apparatus to the patient may be obtained with a hand operated bellows, an electrically driven air pump, or by the pressure obtained from an oxygen tank. It is not generally known that the valves and plugs of oxygen tanks, especially if they are oiled or greased, or protected with rubber washers, may cause ignition and explosion of the anæsthetic. This is especially true when acetylene or ethylene is used. For their use a specially constructed apparatus, which is carefully

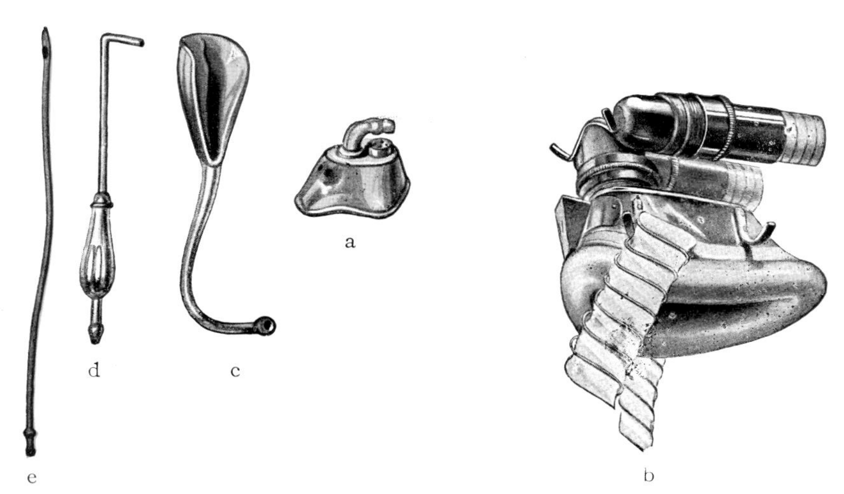

FIG. 120. Accessories for the administration of anæsthetics by a closed method. a. small metal or rubber gas mask; b. metal or celluloid mask with inflatable rubber ring, which insures an air-tight connection. c. anæsthesia "pipe". d. Salzer's cannula. c. Nelaton catheter for insertion into the nose.

grounded, should be provided. All apparatus coming in contact with nitrous oxide and oxygen, acetylene, or ethylene, should have perfectly clean pipes, joints, valves, etc., which should never have oils or greases in contact with them. Tools covered with oil should not be used around the apparatus, and fiber plates should be used for washers.

A special form of semi-closed mask is known as the anæsthetist's pipe (Fig. 120 c). It can be held in front of the nose, or nose and mouth, and is useful in operations for hare-lip.

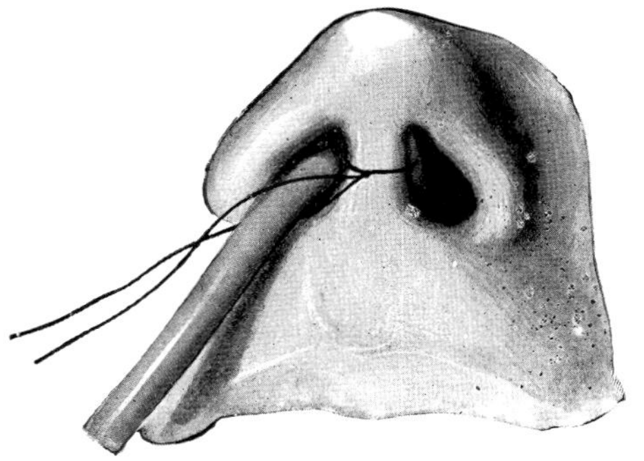

FIG. 121. Soft catheter introduced into the nose for the administration of volatile anæsthetics. It is held firmly in place by a suture which pierces the nasal septum.

For the direct introduction of vapor forming anæsthetics in the nose or mouth, or intrapharyngeally, the Salzer cannula (Fig. 120 d), or the Nelaton catheter (Fig. 120 e) is very useful. The metal cannula can be placed between the teeth, while the Nelaton catheter is inserted through the nasal orifice and then along the floor of the nose. It can be retained with adhesive strips or by suturing it in place (Fig. 121). These attachments are used only when a mask would obstruct the field of operation, as for instance in nasal, cleft-palate, and oropharyngeal surgery. They cannot be used unless some arrangement is at hand for forcing the anæsthetic to the patient from its container.

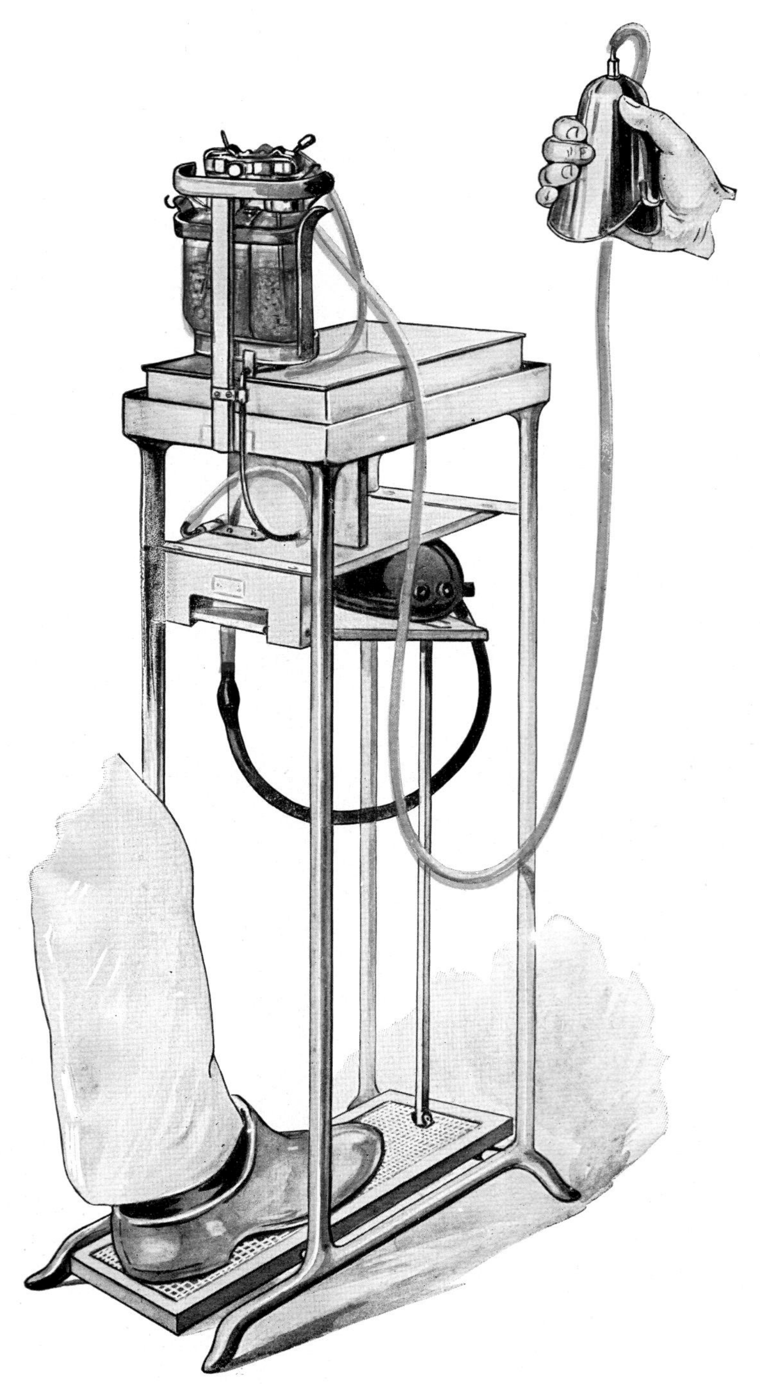

FIG. 122. Bellows worked by treadle for use with Braun's anæsthesia apparatus. This frees the hand of the anaesthetist.

Braun's apparatus (Fig. 122) is arranged for the administration of chloroform or ether, or both as a mixture. The air-current, developed by a bellows, is carried through the anæsthetic which is then vaporized. There are numerous modifications of this apparatus but it will serve as a type. The use of a hand bellows in this type of apparatus (Fig. 123) does not permit the anæsthetist to have his hands free for other purposes.

Ombrédanne's closed ether apparatus is very adaptable and convenient. It stands midway between the administration of ether through a mask and its administration through a gas machine. In principle it is somewhat similar to the Ben Morgan apparatus used in the United States, although it has no attachment for the simultaneous administration of oxygen. It is made in two types (Figs. 124a and 124b). It is in reality a closed method of anæsthesia, but it has a regulating valve which permits the anæsthetist to control the amount of air admitted to the apparatus. This valve is so constructed that only air will get to the patient, or a mixture of air and ether. Apparatus of this type are very economical, but require the services of a skilful anæsthetist. In his hands, however, the anæsthetization is, as a rule, all that can be desired, and if ether is used it can be administered by no better method.

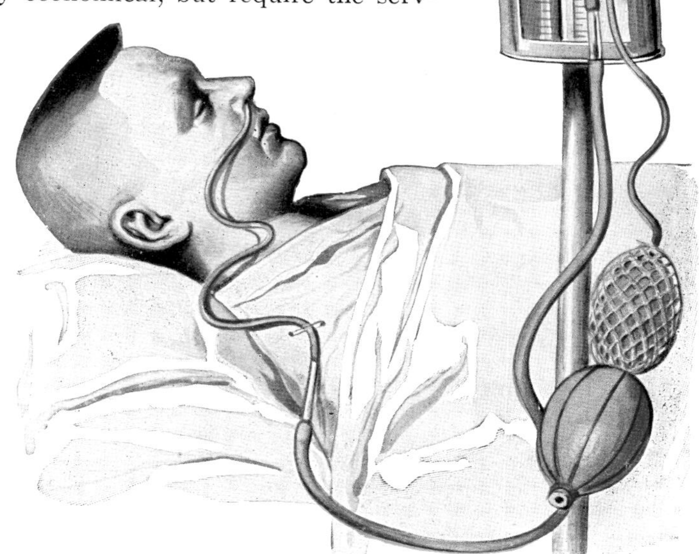

Fig. 123. Braun's apparatus for ether and chloroform anæsthesia. The air-current produced by the hand bellows is carried through ether or through chloroform or both, and the vapor is then conveyed to the patient through a Nelaton catheter inserted in the nose.

The McKesson apparatus (Figs. 125 and 126) is illustrated as one of a number of types of apparatus devised for the administration of nitrous oxide and oxygen with or without ether, or for the administration of ether with a gas. Carbon dioxide can also be administered through it. It permits the anæsthetist to regulate carefully the flow of the anæsthetic so as to control absolutely the amount to be administered. Furthermore it permits of an even mixture of anæsthetic substances, which was heretofore not obtainable.

Nitrous oxide and oxygen is a particularly safe anæsthetic in the hands of a professional anæsthetist. In the hands of a non-professional anæsthetist it is dangerous. It has little if any effect on the parenchymatous organs such as the liver and kidneys. The gas is rapidly eliminated from the body

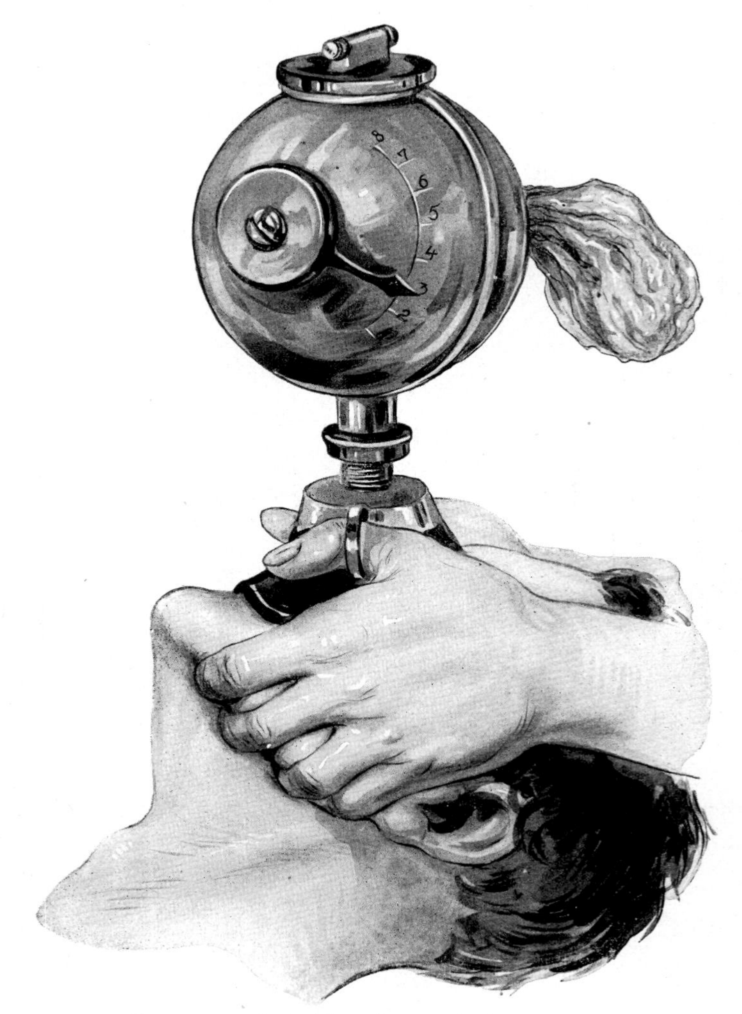

Fig. 124a. Ombrédanne's anæsthesia apparatus.

once the anæsthetic is discontinued. In these and many other particulars it is similar to ethylene anæsthesia. It differs from ethylene in not being explosive, in being nearly odorless, but in not relaxing the abdominal muscles to the same extent as does ethylene.

This type of anæsthesia is particularly useful in cachectic and anæmic patients where it is desirable to avoid visceral damage, and in hypotension, where an elevation of the blood pressure is desired during anæsthesia. It is particularly useful for prolonged anæsthesia. Muscular relaxation with ether anæsthesia is greater, but the dangers of complications with nitrous oxide and oxygen are less.

The efficiency of the anæsthetic depends on the preoperative preparation and medication, the purity of the gases, the flexibility of the apparatus, and the skill of the anæsthetist. Figure 125 illustrates the McKesson apparatus which has been used very successfully in the United States, although a variety of other makes have been equally successful. A mixing chamber is essential in every apparatus and the valves should be very carefully adjusted so as to deliver the gas evenly.

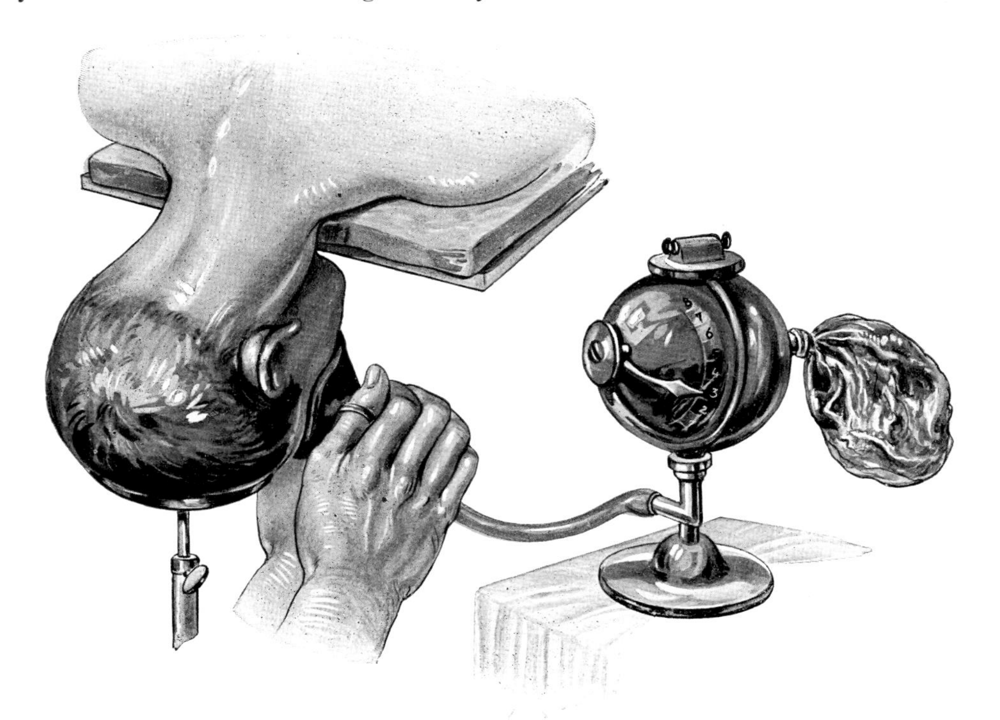

FIG. 124b. Ombrédanne's anæsthesia apparatus. The apparatus can be placed on a table and connected with the mask by a rubber tube.

A depletion of the blood oxygen and an increase of nitrous oxide above anæsthetic values are dangerous and unphysiological. Therefore the apparatus should indicate visibly the flow of each gas. Cyanosis is to be guarded against.

If the addition of 15-20 percent of oxygen in the mixture prevents deep anæsthesia it is better to reinforce the gas with ether than to decrease the oxygen concentration. The quantity of ether necessary is, as a rule, very small.

Patients who have been alcoholic or who have led outdoor lives are not easily anæsthetized with nitrous oxide and oxygen. Some selection of cases is necessary for uniformly good results.

Since this mixture causes a rise in blood pressure, patients with arteriosclerosis and hypertension, or advanced myocardial disease should, as a rule, not be given it. It is very useful in supplementing local, spinal, avertin or amytal anæsthesia, maintaining the patient in the stage of analgesia throughout the period of the operation.

On some apparatus attachments have been placed for removing carbon dioxide, thus permitting rebreathing of the nitrous oxide after the addition of oxygen. This may prove to be very economical. In the apparatus illustrated the quantity of each gas used per minute and the percentage of the mixture can be observed constantly. We have used paraffin oil in the mixing reservoir instead of water, and believe the results are much more satisfactory. At the conclusion of the operation a mixture of carbon dioxide (10 percent) and oxygen (90 percent) can be run through the same apparatus to promote more rapid recovery.

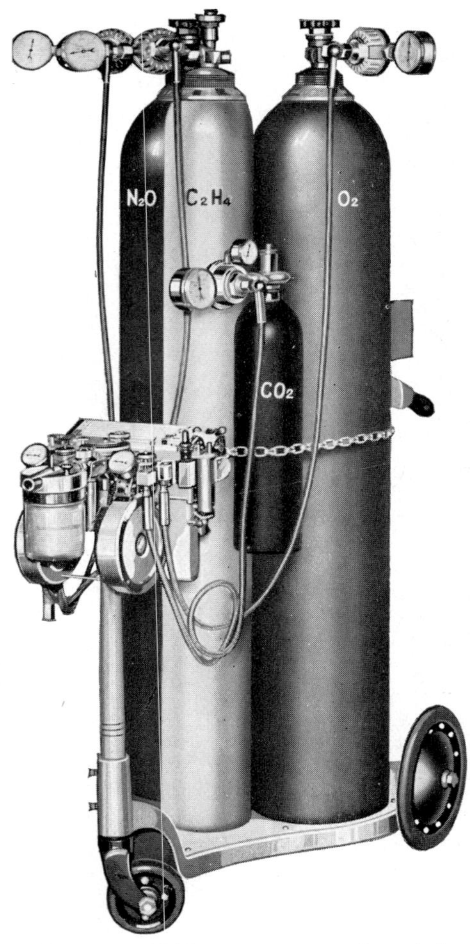

Fig. 125. McKesson apparatus for administering nitrous oxide and oxygen anæsthesia alone or with ether.

Technic. The patient should be given morphine or Pantopan about half an hour before anæsthesia is begun. In fact this may be given in divided doses, the first dose one hour and the second dose 15 minutes before operation. Atropine is not necessary because the gas does not cause any irritation of the respiratory tract. A mask which fits snugly to the face and which covers the nose and mouth should be used. If the gas is carefully administered the period of excitation is very short or even absent.

The surgeon should not be in too great a hurry to begin the operation. Ten minutes, at least, should elapse from the time of starting the anæsthetic to the time of operation. The main thing to observe is the color of the patient. If a pink color is maintained little fear need be held for the patient's condition. The breathing should be slow, regular and somewhat deeper than normal.

Recovery is rapid and postoperative vomiting not as frequent as after ether anæsthesia. Because of these many advantages nitrous oxide and oxygen occupies in the United States, and will occupy throughout the world, a permanent place in surgery. It is perhaps the safest anæsthetic for use by the skilled anæsthetist.

Acetylene (narcylen) **anæsthesia** (Wieland, Gauss) has found a field in anæsthesia in Germany in recent years. The anæsthetic is administered by a special apparatus. The compressed acetylene is mixed with oxygen and then compressed in another tank, from whence it flows, properly mixed, to the patient. The machine is constructed so that ether can be added to the mixture. The anæsthetic mixture is carried to the patient by means of an

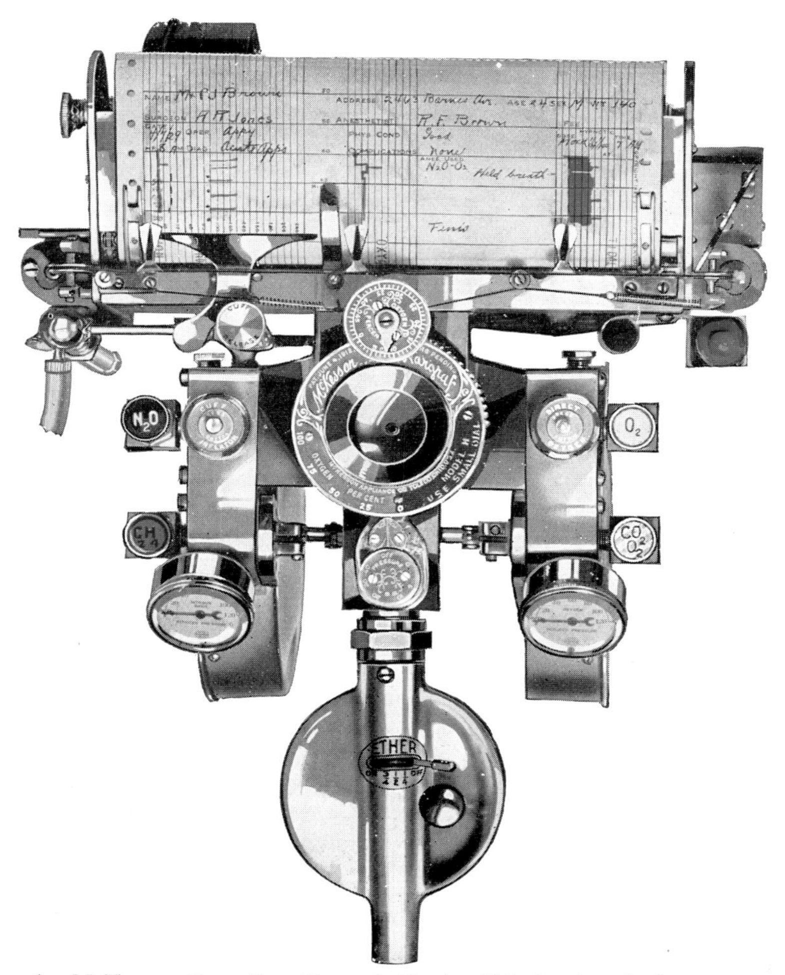

FIG. 126. McKesson Recording Nargraf Head. This head embodies every advantage known to the art of anæsthesia. It records time of anæsthesia, pressure of gases at inhaler, blood pressure (pulse pressure), percent of oxygen in mixture, volume of respiration, volume of rebreathing, character of respiration, and oxygen insufflation.

airtight mask. The expired air is carried through a potassium cartridge in which the carbon dioxide is removed and the purified acetylene is re-conveyed to the patient. An acetylene-oxygen mixture is highly explosive, just as is an ethylene-oxygen, or nitrous oxide-oxygen-ether mixture, so that extreme caution should be exercised when any of these is used. Open flames, electric cauteries, etc., should not be tolerated anywhere near the place where these anæsthetics are in use. Each apparatus should be grounded and the valves should be clean and free of oil or grease.

Acetylene (narcylen) anæsthesia properly controlled has in my experience been relatively safe. Administered by a skilled anæsthetist, overdosage has not been observed. It is well tolerated in shock and debilitated states in which the volatile anæsthetics are in general contraindicated. It causes a rise in systolic blood pressure. Deep anæsthesia is obtained in a few minutes, and recovery from deep anæsthesia to the return of full consciousness comes moderately quickly. The recovery is associated with little or no discomfort. The anæsthetic apparently does not cause any late visceral damage.

Complete muscular relaxation does not result in most cases, and in this it is more like nitrous oxide and oxygen anæsthesia. It is for this reason that I hesitate to use it routinely in abdominal operations, unless ether is used until the lesion is exposed. In all other operations, if position does not interfere with access to the mouth and nose, anæsthesia with acetylene (narcylen) can be carried out as well as with the other anæsthetics. As a result of the rise in blood-pressure, hemorrhage is freer than with the volatile anæsthetics.

3. Incomplete Anæsthesia

(a) **With Inhalation Anæsthetics.** If large quantities of these anæsthetics are administered to the patient in a short period of time it is possible in a few moments to induce a state of confusion or even unconsciousness, so that while the sense of pain is abolished, muscular relaxation is not obtained. This type of anæsthesia is most frequently obtained with ether, ethyl chloride and nitrous oxide. The patients may act as if they are in a delirium. This type of anæsthesia is not safe except for very short periods and is not recommended for any operation lasting more than a few minutes. Although the patients may act as if they felt pain, they have no knowledge of what was done when they awaken. Everything should be ready for the surgical procedure before the anæsthesia is begun.

When **ether** is used it should be poured over a dry mask. If the evaporation surface of the mask does not suffice to bring about the delirium, a second dry mask is placed over the saturated one. Ether is poured on this also and it is quickly placed under the first one. The procedure is continued until the desired effect is obtained. The delirium as a rule begins in ½ to 1½ minutes and is characterized by jerky respiration being succeeded by a more uniform type of breathing and the failure of the patient to answer intelligently. When the operation begins the administration of ether is interrupted, although the mask is permitted to stay in place.

Ethyl chloride is not as safe as ether even for incomplete anæsthesia. When used the ethyl chloride is dropped rapidly on a small fluffed piece of gauze which is held before the nasal orifices (Fig. 127). The ethyl chloride tube is grasped with the hand to warm it, and turned down so that the fluid can escape when the valve is opened. Two tubes may be used, but care should be exercised lest the patient receive an overdose even in the short period it is administered. The loss of consciousness is exceedingly rapid.

Nitrous oxide is widely used for this type of anæsthesia. It is not as safe as nitrous oxide and oxygen anæsthesia, but safer than ethyl chloride anæsthesia. It is very useful for the reduction of minor fractures, and the opening of abscesses, etc. The gas is given to the patient who elevates one arm. When this begins to drop and the patient fails to answer questions the operation can be begun. The anæsthetist should watch the patient so that he does not become too cyanosed.

(b) **Intravenous Avertin Anæsthesia (Kirschner).** In methods already described for anæsthetization forced inspiration is frequently necessary in order to obtain anæsthesia, and at least some effort is necessary on the part of the patient. It is this as much as anything else which causes the stage of excitation.

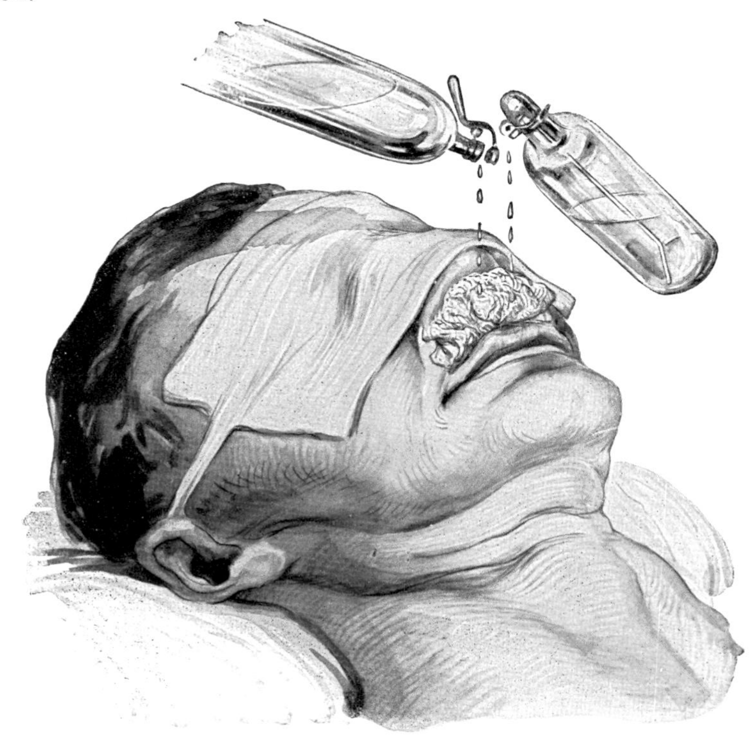

FIG. 127. Ethyl chloride anæsthesia. The ethyl chloride is dropped from one or two tubes on a small, loose pledget, which is held in front of the patient's nose or mouth.

I have recently been using Avertin intravenously and have been most favorably impressed with its possibilities. It can be given without causing the slightest suffering to the patient. The dose is regulated to the individual patient. While the effect of other substances now used for intravenous anæsthetization such as Somnifen, Pernocton, and sodium amytal may persist for hours or even several days, may lead to unpleasant periods of excitation during recovery, and may tax the vital cerebral centers, intravenous Avertin anæsthesia is rapidly recovered from and is accompanied by no unpleasant after effects. It may be supplemented by inhalation anæsthesia which may be used to maintain anæsthesia after the induction of sleep with Avertin.

It is very useful for short anæsthesia or as a preliminary anæsthetic to the use of any of the substances used for inhalation anæsthesia. The psychic factors are eliminated and the patient is quieter during the administration of the secondary anæsthetic. I have found the following apparatus very useful if Avertin is to be used and it may also have a field of usefulness in the administration of other anæsthetics which are given intravenously (Fig. 128). It is so made that it will deliver a known amount of the solution in a given time, delivering as much as 100 cc. in 40 seconds. A 3 percent solution of Avertin is used, which is prepared as follows: 145 cc. of physiologic saline solution at room temperature is placed in a cooled cylinder. With a Record syringe 5 cc. of a 100 percent solution of Avertin are placed in the saline solution. The Avertin should be kept in a dark, cool place, preferably, as I keep it, in an electric refrigerator. If a white precipitate of Avertin substance forms it should be removed before injection of the solution.

One should be sure that the solution of Avertin has not decomposed. It is unstable at temperatures over 40°C. The solution after being made ready for injection should not be warmed and all apparatus used while it is being made or injected should be cooled. The solution for injection should be kept at room temperature, since if it is cooled too much the Avertin precipitates out of the solution and thus the efficiency of the solution is seriously impaired.

The apparatus should be tested to be sure that it is in order. After filling the syringe all air must be excluded from the tubing. The lever of the apparatus is placed at the number on the cylinder corresponding to the weight of the patient in kilograms. The stop watch is set at zero. The intravenous puncture is made with the needle attached to a 2 cc. syringe and as soon as blood is freely aspirated the syringe is re-

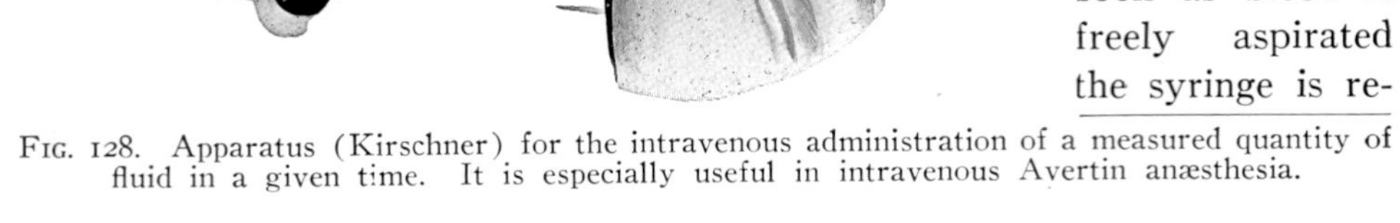

Fig. 128. Apparatus (Kirschner) for the intravenous administration of a measured quantity of fluid in a given time. It is especially useful in intravenous Avertin anæsthesia.

moved and the tubing is attached to the needle. Local anæsthesia can be used preliminary to the needle puncture. The rate of flow is regulated by a pinch-cock on the tubing. The calculated dose should be injected in approximately 45 seconds. The patient should be asked to count as soon as the injection is begun, and unconsciousness appears when about three-fourths of the dose has been injected.

If the patient is not asleep when the calculated dose has been given an additional amount is slowly and carefully introduced. Extreme care is essential. Consciousness returns in about 5 minutes after the injection has ceased.

4. Asphyxia or Syncope

A number of conditions which occasionally occur suddenly during anæsthesia and which threaten life have been grouped under the term, asphyxia, literally absence of the pulse, although in the accepted sense of the term, as it is now used, it denotes a deficiency of the blood oxygen. It would probably in most instances be better to use the term, now seldom employed, syncope.

When one considers the conditions arising during operation which affect the strength of the patient, such as hemorrhage, damage to the cerebrum, the section of nerves, damage to the myocardium, obstruction of the air-passages, air and fat emboli, and shock, then the serious conditions which inhalation anæsthesia in itself may precipitate are more clearly perceived.

In the **initial stage** of anæsthesia death rarely may occur as a reflex phenomenon, or it may occur as the result of over-dosage resulting in too high a concentration of the anæsthetic. The former is seen more frequently when chloroform is used than with any other anæsthetic.

In the **stage of excitement,** death may be the result of sudden cardiac reflex failure, or the result of aspiration during vomiting, or may occur from over-dosage.

In the **stage of maintenance** death may result from over-dosage precipitating the stage of paralysis of the medullary centers, or from obstruction of the respiratory tract.

In my opinion the majority of "table deaths" are associated with the anæsthesia. This is especially true when preliminary examination revealed no evidence of serious cardiac pathology. The deaths are the result of over-dosage of the anæsthetic or due to the untimely detection and faulty correction of an obstruction to free respiration by the anæsthetist. In the very rarest of cases, and then as a rule only in chloroform anæsthesia, does death occur after the first few inspirations of the anæsthetic. This type of death is due to reflex cardiac inhibition and can rarely be ascribed to fault of the anæsthetist.

Sudden death may occur when anæsthesia is administered to a patient who has status thymolymphaticus, which is discussed under "The Heart and Vascular System."

When death threatens during anæsthesia the all important thing is to be able to recognize its cause and as quickly as possible to remedy it. Prompt remedial measures are often life saving. A firm discipline must be maintained at all times. The anæsthetic should be stopped and the mask removed as soon as any untoward symptom appears.

If the cause of the untoward symptoms is not ascertainable immediately, the following procedure is recommended:

a. **Is the patient breathing?** The slightest degree of respiratory movement is seen best over the abdomen. Movements may be observed here when they can no longer be observed in the thorax. A small tab of cotton can be held before the nose or mouth in order to see whether it moves.

If the patient is not breathing, artificial respiration must be resorted to. First, the antero-lateral position of the thorax is compressed forcibly with

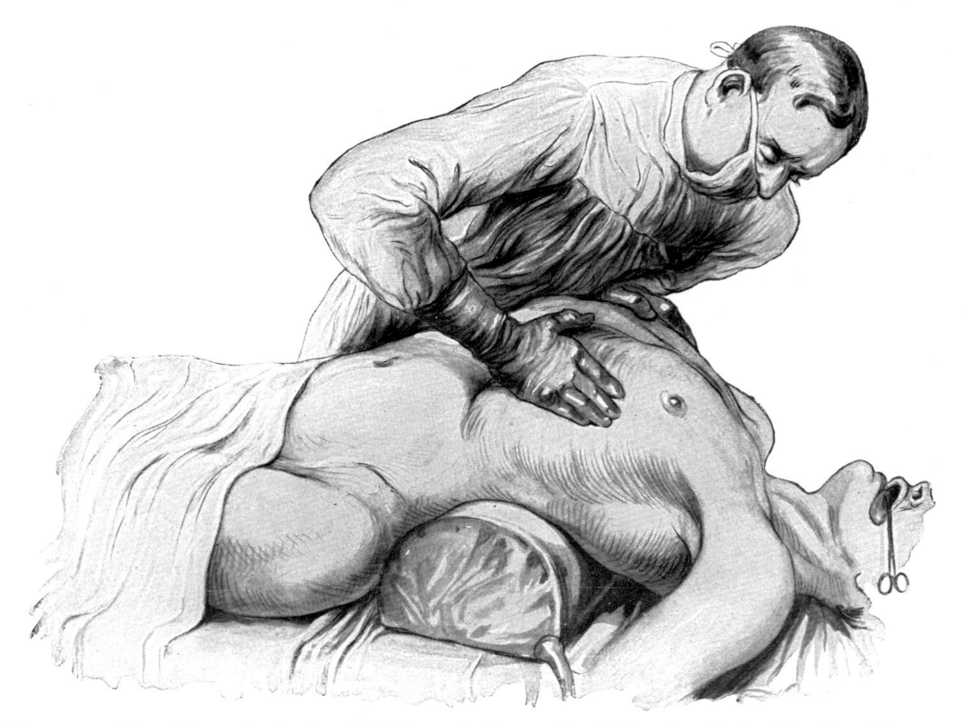

FIG. 129. Koenig's method of artificial respiration. Expiration is obtained by forcibly compressing the lower lateral thorax with the palms of the hands.

the hands laid flat on the lower ribs. The pressure is made and then released (Koenig) (Fig. 129). If respiration is not resumed in a short period of time, the arms are released, and a cushion is placed under the thorax, if that was not done previously, so that it arches the spine forcibly, and each of two assistants standing near the patient's head takes hold of an arm and carries it slowly and methodically, at first over the head (inspiration) (Fig. 130), and second down over the chest, where pressure is made on the thorax (expiration) (Sylvester) (Fig. 131). These rhythmical movements must not be carried out faster than about 16 times a minute. Artificial respiration should be continued until natural breathing is resumed or until death is definitely established. I doubt very much whether mere rhythmical traction of the tongue can stimulate breathing when it has stopped.

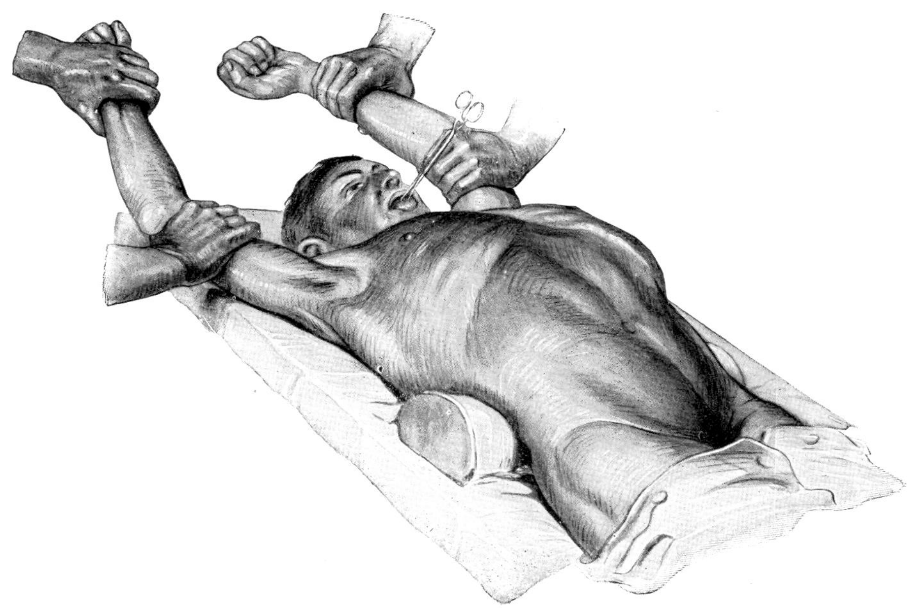

Fig. 130. Sylvester's method of artificial respiration. Inspiration is obtained by raising the arms well over the head of the patient. The thorax is arched by a pillow placed under the patient.

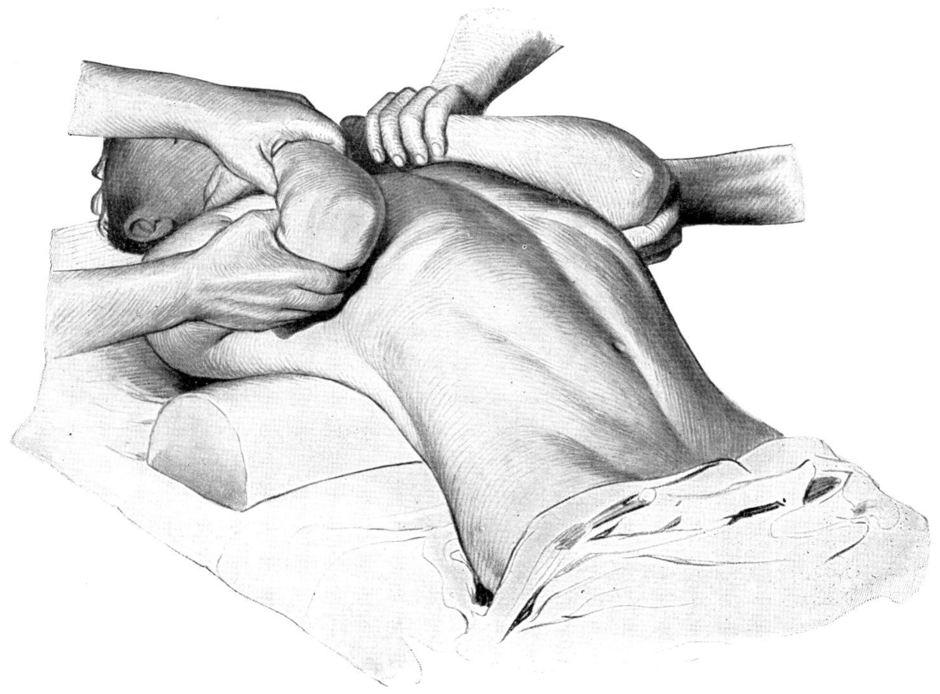

Fig. 131. Sylvester's method of artificial respiration. Expiration is obtained by pressing the arms of the patient against the thorax.

The use of positive pressure is often more successful. The positive pressure can be obtained from any of the good gas machines or from an intratracheal apparatus. The trachea can be intubated through a Jackson laryngoscope, a Kuhn tube may be used, or positive pressure can be obtained by fastening the mask firmly to the patient's face. The return of the patient's respiration is attempted by alternatingly expanding the lungs with positive pressure and then releasing this and pressing the thorax.

A mixture of 90 percent oxygen and 10 percent carbon dioxide is very efficacious as the gas for use. This can be given the patient through a

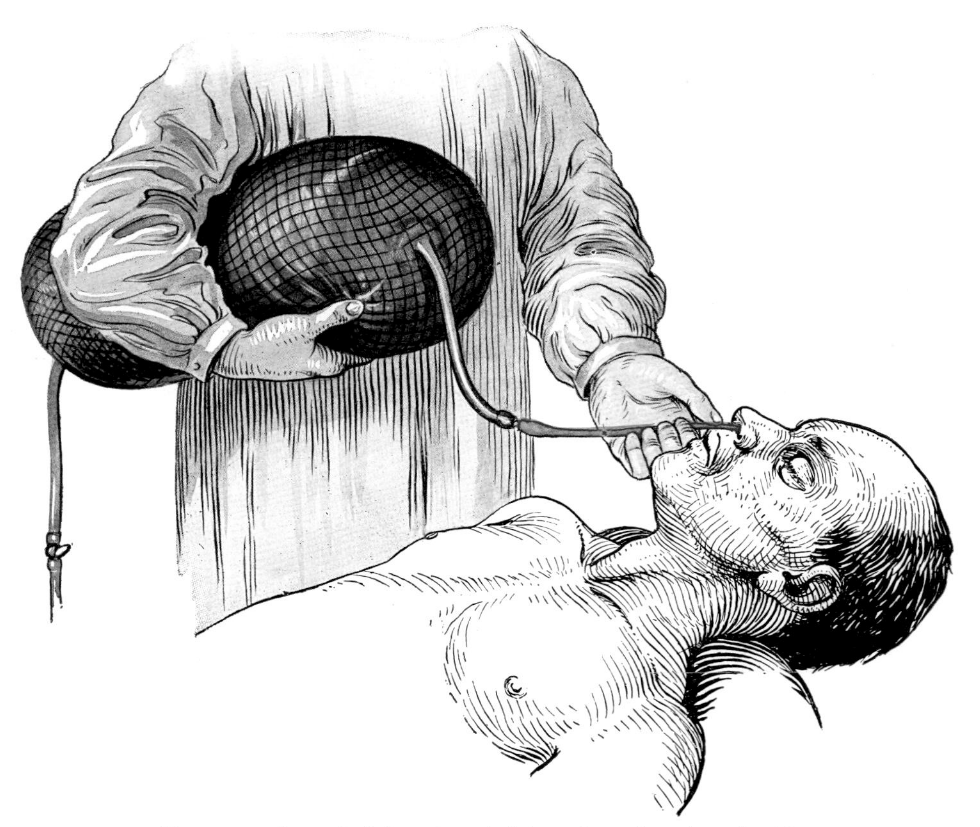

FIG. 132. A method for the administration of carbon dioxide.

nitrous-oxide and oxygen apparatus. This mixture serves as a powerful stimulant to the respiratory center. I keep rubber bags filled with carbon dioxide ready for instant use. It can be given through a Nelaton catheter inserted in a nostril.

(The apparatus recently described by Drinker and Shaw in which the principle of an alternating, external negative and positive pressure is utilized for forcing respiration, marks a distinct advance. At present its cost is considerable, but it will undoubtedly save many lives. I.S.R.)

If during asphyxia the patient makes active respiratory movements, or the respiratory movements are passively produced:

b. **Does** the **air,** during the respiratory movements **flow freely in and out the lungs?**

If an obstruction is present it must be removed.

The most frequent cause of respiratory tract obstruction is swallowing of the tongue. The best way to bring the tongue forward is by v. Esmarch-Heilberg's manipulation (Fig. 133). The anæsthetist places the palms of both hands flat over the patient's ears and the index fingers forward toward the symphysis of the mandible. The middle fingers are fixed under the angles of the mandible and with this grip pressure is made forward and upward so that the incisors of the mandible pass over those of the maxilla.

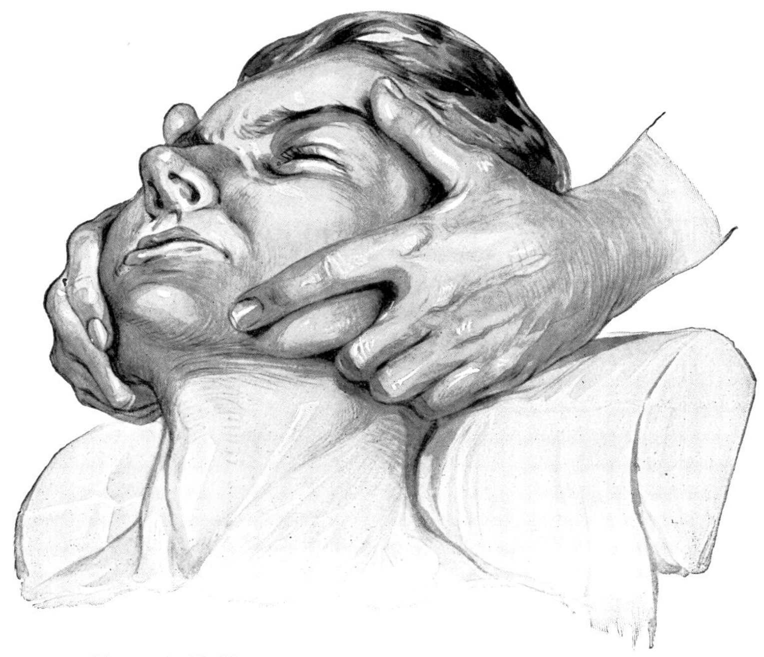

FIG. 133. v. Esmarch-Heilberg method of holding the lower jaw forward. The lower jaw is pushed forward and upward by pressure against both its ascending rami, so that the lower incisors are held in front of the upper incisors.

In this position the jaw can easily be held tight with the left hand. If it is impossible to bring the jaw forward by this procedure, the chin and the front teeth can be grasped with one hand and pulled forward. However, whenever there is difficulty in keeping the tongue forward so that the epiglottis is not hampered in its movements, the Mayo intubator (Fig. 118) should be inserted.

If in spite of these measures the tongue cannot be brought forward sufficiently, a mouth gag should be inserted, the tongue grasped, pulled forward, and then caught with a tongue forceps or a heavy silk thread in the region of the foramen cæcum (Fig. 134) and held forward. If all these measures do not help, the hyoid bone should be grasped with the index finger of the right hand in the pharynx over the epiglottis, and an attempt be made to pull the base of the tongue forward (v. Bergmann's manipulation), which has been modified by Gontermann (Fig. 135) who uses a straight handled tampon forceps.

The upper respiratory passages may also be obstructed by accumulated fluid, such as mucous, sputum, vomitus or blood, by foreign bodies, or pieces of tissue loosened at operation. This is recognized by the rattling respiration. Lowering the head and turning it to the side is not sufficient to relieve the

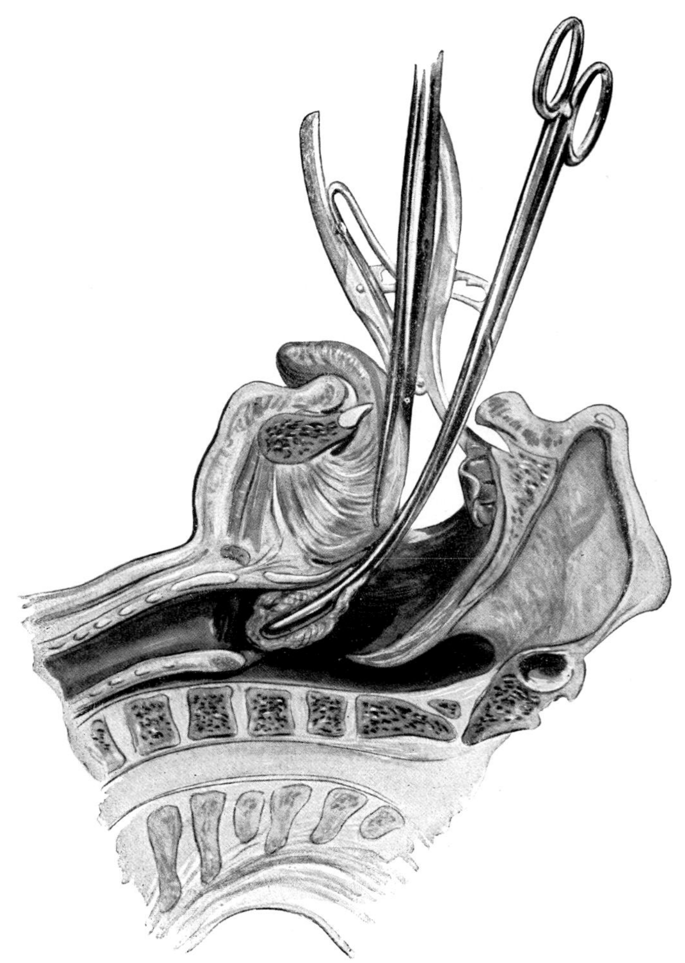

Fig. 134. Drawing tongue forward with sharp tongue forceps. The tongue is seized directly in front of the foramen caecum. The mouth is held open by means of a mouth-gag.

patient. The obstruction or fluid must be removed mechanically. First, the mouth should be opened widely with a mouth gag. The Roser-Koenig (Fig. 136), Heister (Fig. 137), or the O'Dwyer-Denhart (Fig. 138) are efficient types of mouth gags. They should be placed sidewise between the molars and opened slowly. If these are not available, a wrapped wooden spatula or a spoon handle may be used.

The tongue is then drawn forward as described above, and the mouth and pharynx and larynx aspirated. Any foreign body should be removed.

If the fluid is in the trachea or lungs the aspirating tube can be placed in the trachea through a laryngoscope and the fluid aspirated. The patient should be kept in the head down position.

If these directions are followed tracheotomy will rarely become necessary. After operations for large goitres tracheal collapse may occur, which may necessitate immediate tracheotomy, or this may be necessary when edema of the glottis prevents free respiration.

c. **Is the heart contracting** or not and what is the force of its contraction? It is the duty of the anæsthetist to observe the condition of the pulse and the blood pressure. It is his duty to recognize alterations in vascular tone and to acquaint the surgeon with these so that immediate steps may be taken to improve it. (Faulty respiration may be due to a depressed circulation. I.S.R.)

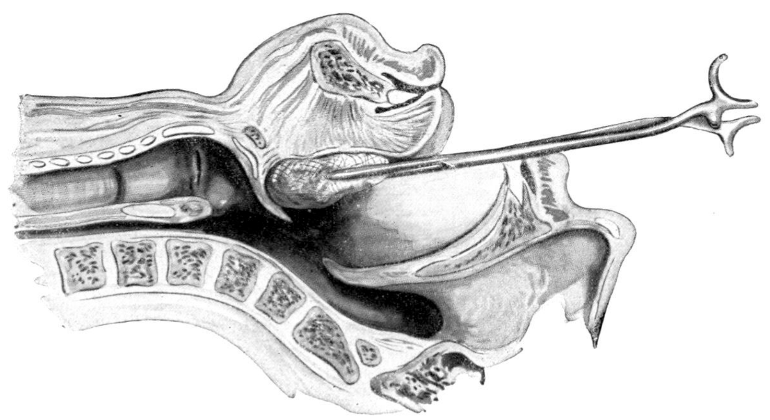

FIG. 135. Gontermann's manipulation. The base of the tongue is pressed forward with a sponge forceps, and thus the respiratory obstruction is removed.

If the heart beats become feeble, I administer subcutaneously according to the indications 10 cc. of camphorated oil or strophanthin (0.0005 gm.) intravenously. (Beware of the heart previously treated with digitalis!). In marked fall of the blood pressure I use 1 cc. of adrenalin (1:1000) intravenously or ephedrine (0.050 gm.). (See B. General Examination and Treatment, 1. The Heart and the Vascular System.)

If heart movements can no longer be demonstrated by inspection, palpation or auscultation, the only chance for resuscitation depends upon the direct introduction of drugs into the heart, and since this is probably futile, upon direct mechanical stimulation. All other efforts are purposeless gestures. Adrenalin is the only drug I use for injection into the cardiac muscle, and it is doubtful whether it really is worth while. It is injected into the walls of the left ventricle. For this purpose we introduce a long, thin needle 5.5 cm. to the left of the parasternal line, at the upper margin of the fourth intercostal space. The needle is passed perpendicularly until we feel the resistance of the heart muscle. The needle is passed a few millimeters deeper, and we assure ourselves, by aspiration, that we are not in the ventricle. The drug is then injected slowly. We consider it useless to attempt to cause resumption of cardiac activity by pressure on the chest wall alone. For effective heart massage the heart must be compressed directly. If the heart is not accessible because of the type of operation, the abdominal cavity should be opened by a midline incision below the ensiform process, so that the operator can insert his right hand. The heart is grasped by passing this hand up

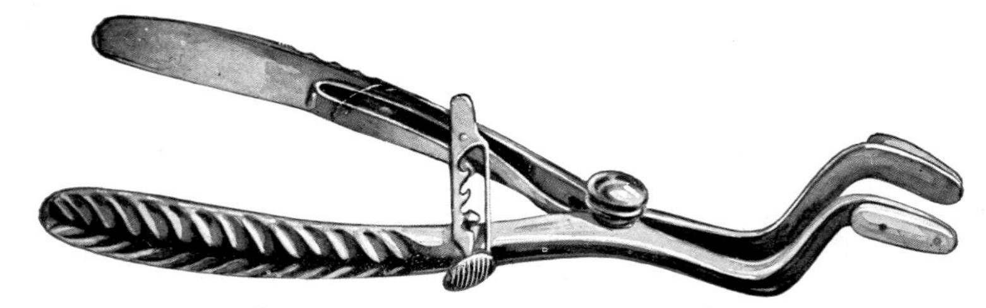

FIG. 136. Mouth-gag (Roser-Koenig).

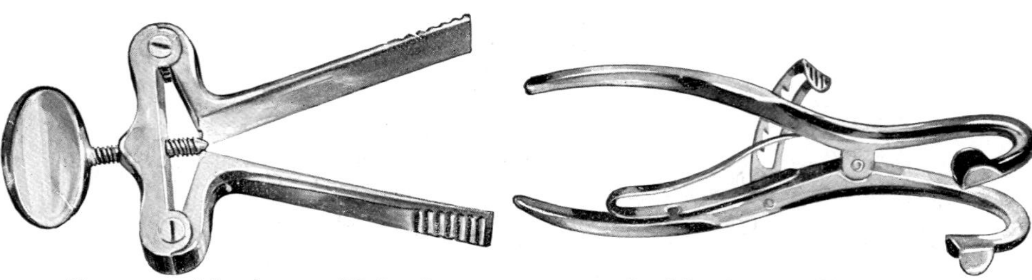

FIG. 137. Mouth-gag (Heister).

FIG. 138. Mouth-gag (O'Dwyer-Denhart).

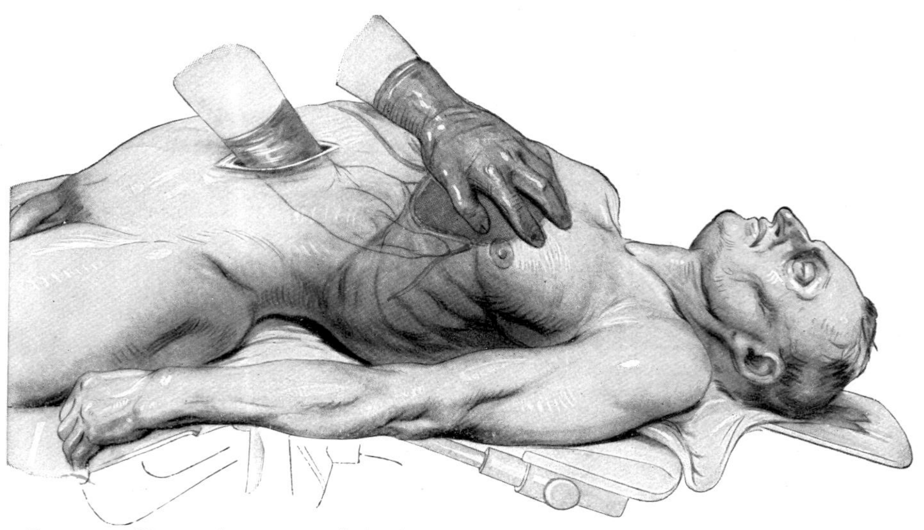

FIG. 139. Bimanual massage of the heart. Through a mid-line upper abdominal incision the operator places his right hand beneath and posterior to the heart by pushing up on the diaphragm. He then makes rhythmical pressure against the anterior chest wall which is reinforced by the left hand.

under the diaphragm to the left of the median line. The left hand is placed over the precardial area and the heart is massaged between the two hands, with a rhythm whose rapidity corresponds to the normal frequency of the heart (Fig. 139). The return of tonus and contractile power can be recognized by the surgeon in that the heart will be felt to relax and contract. The hand in the abdomen is not removed until the contractions continue after assistance has been withheld for some minutes. As soon as the danger appears to be over, the abdominal wound is sutured. It is necessary that careful asepsis be maintained throughout, or peritonitis may result.

Even though both respiration and heart action have ceased (apparent death), one should not give up all hope of resuscitation. While some of the procedures already described are being used a tube can be placed in the trachea and artificial respiration maintained by an intratracheal apparatus, or an apparatus such as that recently described by Drinker and Shaw, where respiration can be used if cardiac massage is not required. (It is useless to attempt to stimulate respiration with drugs when the circulation will no longer carry drugs to the respiratory center. A depressed respiratory center needs oxygenated blood and every effort should be made to supply this. I.S.R.)

The best gas to give intratracheally is perhaps pure oxygen, although the blood may not be able to take up more oxygen than is in the air.

The attempts to minimize the use of anæsthetics by reducing the circulation (Klapp), and thus to deprive a part of the blood of the influence of the anæsthetic so that an unaffected blood reserve may be maintained, have found few adherents. For this purpose both legs of the patient have tourniquets applied until all circulation is stopped (Fig. 140) before anæsthesia is begun. The tourniquets are loosened at the termination of anæsthesia or during it in case of danger. The procedure is annoying to the patient, puts an extra load on the heart, and may cause a wide fluctation of the blood pressure after release of the tourniquets. It is not a physiological procedure. Furthermore it increases the incidence of postoperative venous thrombosis. For these reasons it is not recommended.

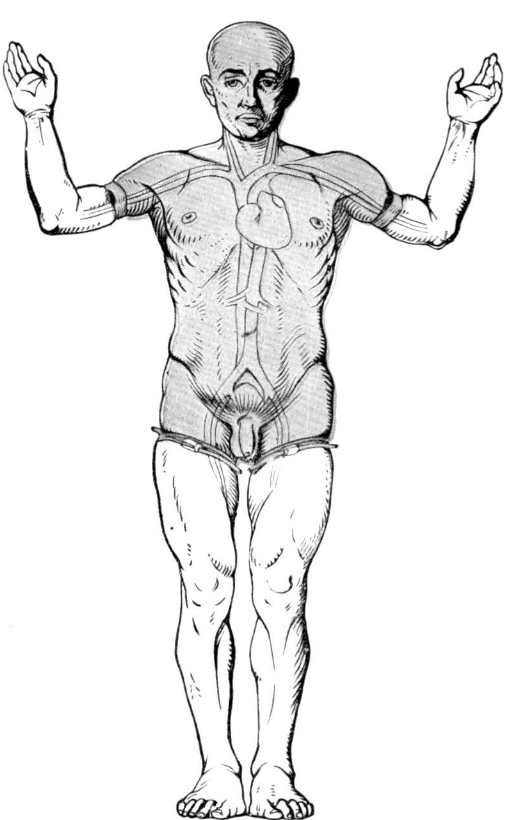

Fig. 140. Reduction of the circulatory system so that blood cannot get into the extremities, and arterial flow is maintained in the trunk and head.

5. Prevention of the Aspiration of Blood

In operations in the region of the upper respiratory passages (mouth, nose, pharynx, larynx) special precautions must be taken to prevent the aspiration of blood. Failure to protect the patient against aspiration may result in a postoperative pulmonary complication.

The preliminary unilateral or bilateral ligation of the arteries supplying the region to be operated upon, and the use of sponges in the field of operation do not as a rule suffice to prevent aspiration.

It is best to perform the operation under local anæsthesia, so that the cough reflex is not disturbed. If general anæsthesia is unavoidable, one may advantageously make use of Kuhn's tube (Fig. 141), or any other tube of this type. The Kuhn tube is a flexible metal tube which is passed through the mouth into the larynx where it remains throughout the anæsthesia. For this purpose, when deep anæsthesia is induced, the mouth is opened with a mouth gag, and the metal tube provided with a mandrin is passed along the index finger into the larynx (Fig. 141), where it remains while the mandrin

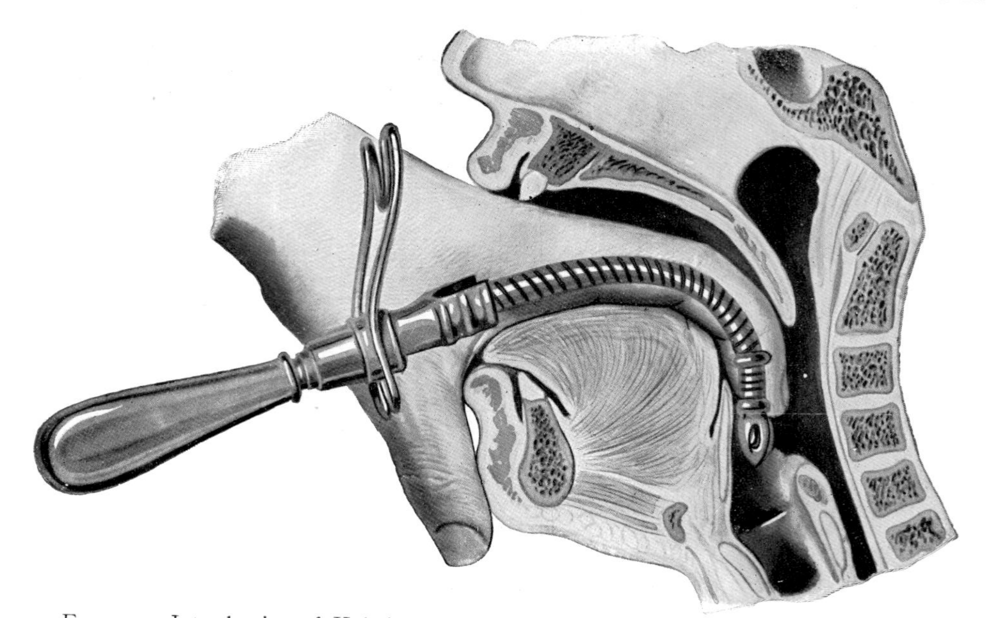

FIG. 141. Introduction of Kuhn's tube into the larynx. The left index finger draws the tongue and the epiglottis of the anæsthetized patient forward, while the aspirator, which has an attached mandrin, is introduced in the larynx, using the left index finger as a guide.

is removed. That portion of the metal tube projecting from the corner of the mouth can be held in place by fastening it around the neck with a rubber tube or a tape. To the metal tube is attached a funnel covered with gauze for continuing the administration of the anæsthetic. The funnel has a place for connecting a small side tube which is carried to the anæsthetist's ear, so that he can listen to the type of respiration (Fig. 142). When the field of operation permits it, after the tube is placed, the pharynx is packed with gauze strips, so as to prevent blood from gaining access to the larynx. Kuhn's apparatus is available in three sizes. It is worthy of recommendation.

If the operation warrants it, the inflow of blood in the air passages can be further avoided by a previous tracheotomy and the tamponing of the pharynx through the mouth or by obstructing the trachea with a special cannula that fits closely to its wall. When this is done access to the mouth and pharynx remains unobstructed. For an obstructing cannula one may use

I prefer a small glass tube. The shorter the distance between stop-cock and cannula, the less fluid this portion of the tube contains, and the more rapid the inflow once the stop-cock is opened.

If it is not kept sterilized, the apparatus should be sterilized before its use. In one of the cylinders physiologic salt solution is placed and kept continuously at 37°C., the other cylinder is filled with 1 liter of physiologic salt solution to which 50 cc. of pure ether has been added. This mixture is made by shaking the salt solution and ether at 28°C. The shaking should continue until the mixture takes on a milky color. The result is a 5 percent solution of ether. It should not be kept warmer than 28°C., nor should it ever contain more than 5 percent of ether. Stronger solutions may cause hemolysis. If the solution contains less than this amount of ether too much fluid must be given to the patient in order to obtain an adequate depth of anæsthesia.

The technical steps are as follows: Three-quarters of an hour before the operation, adults are given 0.0003 to 0.0005 gm. of scopolamine and 0.01 gm. of morphine, or instead of morphine, 0.02 gm. of Pantopon.

The solutions are poured into their respective cylinders and all air in the tubes is expelled. A vein in the anticubital fossa is exposed under local anæsthesia, and the intravenous cannula is inserted and tied in.

The rapidity of the flow of the solutions into the vein can be roughly adjusted by raising or lowering the stand. On the average, the solutions should be about 75 cm. above the vein. The finer regulation of the fluid flow is obtained by adjusting the screw-clamp just above the drop-bulb. For determining the rapidity of the flow, it is best to time the number of cubic centimeters leaving the cylinder. In accordance with Burckhardt's suggestion, the patient's face is covered during the anæsthesia with a mask made out of several layers of muslin, so as to permit rebreathing of the ether eliminated by the lungs.

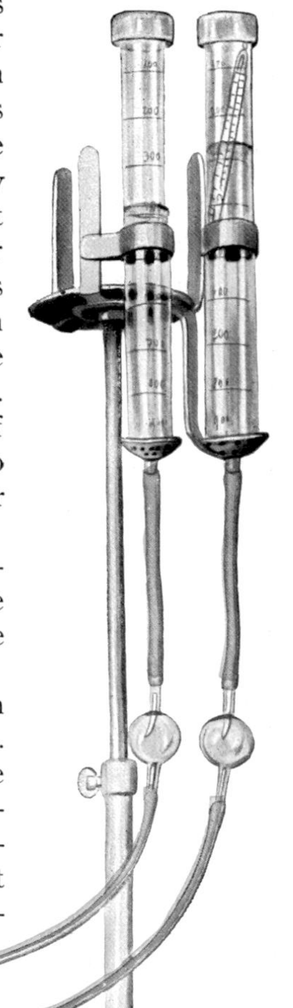

Fig. 145. Apparatus for intravenous ether anæsthesia. In one of the graduated glass cylinders is a solution of physiologic sodium chloride, in the other a 5 percent solution of ether. The flow of the ether into the vein is regulated by a three-way stopcock. Martin glass drop bulbs are inserted in the circuit. They are not absolutely necessary, but permit observation of the rate of flow.

The quantity of 5 percent ether-salt solution necessary to attain deep anæsthesia averages in men from 500 to 600 cc. and in women from 350 to 400 cc. The quantity required for induction and for maintenance throughout the operation depends on many of the considerations discussed under inhalation anæsthesia and upon the rapidity of the flow. To prevent asphyxia, it is advisable never to administer to an adult more than 75 cc. of the ether-

mixture per minute. At this rate of flow surgical anæsthesia is obtained in 5 to 10 minutes. As a rule one does not encounter sensations of suffocation or a real stage of excitement; there occur simply a few slight defensive movements. In the few cases in which deep anæsthesia is not obtained by this method, Burckhardt advises the inhalation of a few whiffs of chloroform. As soon as the patient goes to sleep the anæsthetic is continued carefully, observing the various signs, until deep anæsthesia is obtained, when the ether-solution is discontinued and the three-way stop-cock is opened to permit the slow flow of normal salt solution. From time to time, as required, the ether-mixture is administered. I have used over two liters of the mixture in a moderately strong man during a two hour anæsthesia, and 1200 cc. in a very strong man for a half hour operation. Other than watching the anæsthesia, the anæsthetist should permit a constant flow of saline so that blood does not clot in the cannula. In long anæsthesias several liters of fluid may be administered to the patient; and this can not be accepted as imposing a negligible burden on the heart.

When the anæsthesia is to be discontinued, the administration of the anæsthetic is stopped, the cannula removed and the vein ligated.

7. Rectal Anæsthesia

The administration of a general anæsthetic by rectum has the advantage that the entire procedure is consummated in one act, so that no anæsthetizing apparatus is necessary during the operation. It has the disadvantage, that the anæsthetic, in the event of threatening signs, can not be removed without considerable difficulty so that its immediate cessation is well nigh impossible. Nor can it be easily regulated. A further disadvantage is the inequality of absorption and the frequency with which irritation and even inflammation of the large bowel may occur.

Rectal Ether Anæsthesia. I am not a strong advocate of this type of ether anæsthesia, although I am aware of the fact that it is widely used by some surgeons. It does not seem to me to possess any advantage over other forms of general anæsthesia, and there is the added danger of severe rectal and large bowel inflammation. If it is to be used the patient should receive a cleansing enema 12 hours before the operation. A mixture of 50 cc. of olive oil and 50 cc. of ether is injected into the ampulla of the rectum 1½ hours and again 1 hour before the operation, and in case these quantities are not sufficient, a similar or a smaller amount is injected shortly before the operation. The patient should be kept in a quiet room and the face should be covered so as to promote rebreathing. At the conclusion of the operation the remaining fluid is syphoned off and the bowel is irrigated with normal saline solution.

I can not as yet give a favorable opinion in regard to the use of "E 107" which is made by the Farbwerke Leverkussen for general anæsthesia and which is given by rectum. Its use is apparently not free of all danger because of the very marked fall in blood pressure which may result.

Rectal Administration of Avertin. This method for the administration of Avertin has been widely used during the past few years. (It has the same advantages as sodium amytal anæsthesia and its administration is similar.

I. S. R.) The drug can be administered in such a way that the patient is unaware of it, sleep coming on gradually and quietly. However the many advantages which this method may have are offset by certain definite disadvantages.

There occurs, frequently, a marked drop in the blood pressure after its administration, and occasionally a perturbing period of excitation is observed during recovery. Furthermore, the depth of anæsthesia is not sufficient to carry out major abdominal operations with it alone, so that it must be reinforced with ether or nitrous oxide and oxygen.

Opinion is divided as to whether the advantages of this method are not outweighed by the disadvantages, since the advantages are obtainable by the intravenous method and the dosage is not as great. As with all new

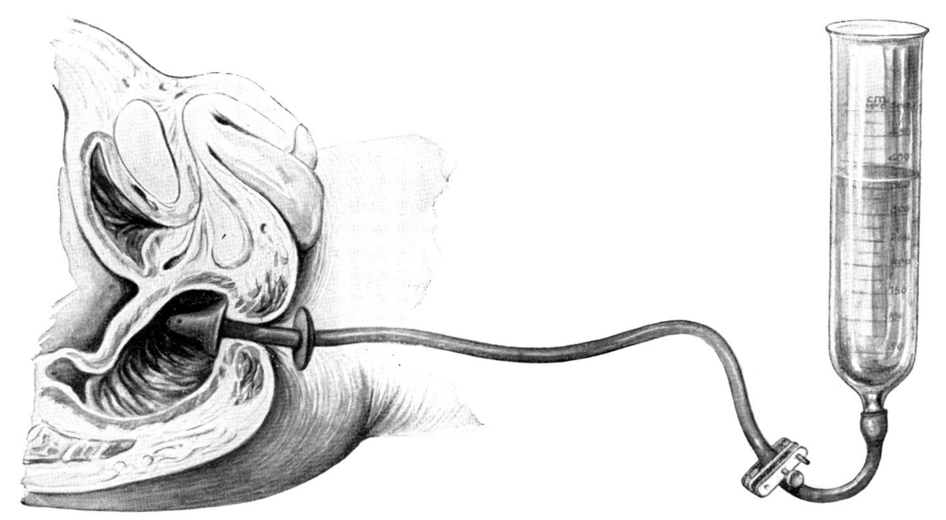

FIG. 146. Rectal anæsthesia using Butzengeiger's rectal tube. A graduated cylinder is attached to the tube. The tube is so constructed that the solution cannot be evacuated.

anæsthetic substances and methods of administration time alone will tell its real worth.

Butzengeiger's rectal tube can be used for administering all types of rectal anæsthesia (Fig. 146). In all of them a cleansing enema should be given before the anæsthetic is injected and a hypodermic injection of 0.01 gm. of morphine should precede the anæsthetic. The external anal ring of the tube is gently pressed close to the anus so as to prevent the escape of the anæsthetic solution. Sleep comes in a variable period, 10 minutes to one hour, depending on the substance used. The patient should be kept in a very quiet place. When the operation is completed the bowel should be irrigated thoroughly.

8. Scopolamine-Morphine Anæsthesia-Twilight Sleep

Scopolamine-morphine anæsthesia which has been widely used in obstetrics has not been used extensively in surgery. It has many disadvantages in that it depresses respiration, causes cyanosis, and frequently delirium. It cannot be removed from the system if danger signals appear. It is also difficult to determine hours before hand the exact time at which the operation is to be begun.

For twilight sleep the patient is kept in a quiet room, the eyes are covered and the ears are plugged. The usual dose is morphine sulphate, 0.01 to 0.02 gm., and scopolamine hydrobromide, 0.0005 to 0.001 gm. These are injected subcutaneously 1½ hours before the operation. Very large well built patients should receive 0.02 gm. of morphine, while unusually feeble ones should be given only 0.0003 gm. of scopolamine. If the anæsthesia is not successful inhalation anæsthesia must be resorted to. The solution of scopolamine should be freshly prepared, since it decomposes rapidly.

B. LOCAL ANÆSTHESIA

Local anæsthesia depends on breaking the connection of the peripheral sensory nerves at the site of operation with the center of pain perception. In most instances this is obtained by injecting into or around the nerves one of a variety of chemicals which can be used as local anæsthetics. Sometimes local anæsthesia is obtained by freezing (cold anæsthesia). Local anæsthesia is divided into: (1) cold anæsthesia, (2) superficial anæsthesia, (3) infiltration anæsthesia, (4) conduction anæsthesia, (5) venous anæsthesia, (6) spinal anæsthesia, (7) sacral anæsthesia.

1. Cold Anæsthesia

This type of anæsthesia, which depends on freezing the area of operation, can be used only on the surface and then for very simple procedures, such as incision of an abscess. Since the tissues which are frozen become rigid they can be penetrated only by force, and hence careful incision is not always possible. Since every operation done under this type of anæsthesia can be more successfully done under other types of local anæsthesia, I rarely, if ever, use freezing in my clinic, even in circumscribed acute inflammatory processes where, contrary to the generally accepted principles, I find no contra-indication to infiltration anæsthesia.

The evaporation of ethyl chloride is hastened by holding the ampoule well away from the skin (one-half meter or more). An electric fan can be played on the area so as to hasten evaporation, but blowing with the mouth should not be countenanced, because it endangers the asepsis. The surrounding skin may be touched with cold metal objects (Fig. 147). Freezing is accomplished more quickly when a tourniquet has been applied to the part, also, if cold water or carbon dioxide snow has been previously applied to the part to be frozen. Freezing, which occurs in from ½ to 3 minutes, is marked by a sudden whitening and hardening of the skin. The spray is continued for a few more seconds when the incision can be made.

2. General Considerations, Solutions and Instruments

The most extensive interruption of sensory pain stimuli is effected by the use of chemical substances, of which cocain is the oldest, though now rarely used, due to its toxicity. The substances are brought in contact with the nerves in various ways. Certain of them are absorbed from mucous membranes, and so reach the nerves (superficial anæsthesia). Others may be injected at the operative site (infiltration anæsthesia), or around the operative site (block anæsthesia), or in the large nerve trunks supplying the area of operation (conduction anæsthesia), into the cerebrospinal fluid after spinal puncture (spinal anæsthesia), and finally in the epidural space of the os sacrum (sacral anæsthesia).

Every anæsthetizing solution requires a time interval after contact with a nerve before pain stimuli are interrupted. After introducing the anæsthetic substance, one must wait 5 to 30 minutes before beginning the operation. I frequently inject the local anæsthetic and then complete the scrubbing of my hands and the disinfection of the patient's skin, so as to give the anæsthetic sufficient time for its action.

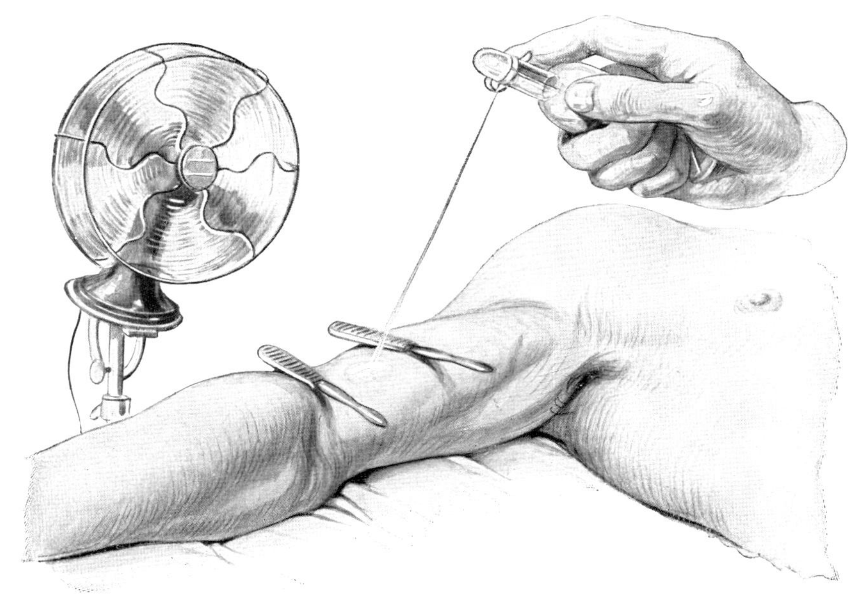

FIG. 147. Local anæsthesia with ethyl chloride. The stream from an ethyl chloride tube held at a distance, is directed on the site to be anæsthetized. Freezing is hastened by the air current from an electric fan and by placing cold metal instruments near the area.

The solutions used for local anæsthesia are slowly absorbed from the site of injection. As this occurs the perception of pain returns as nerve conduction is reestablished. Adrenalin prevents rapid absorption and anæsthesia can be prolonged if it is used with the local anæsthetic, except in the cerebrospinal fluid.

The more concentrated the solution, the more rapid and the more thorough is the anæsthesia. However, the strength of the solutions must be limited, since if large amounts are used they may cause the appearance of toxic symptoms. In general, therefore, the weaker solutions are preferable, since toxic symptoms depend on the amount of the anæsthetic substance absorbed in a unit of time. As long as cocain was used as the sole local anæsthetic and its absorption remained unchecked, local anæsthesia was definitely limited. But even here it found its master in Schleich.

The widening of this field of anæsthesia came only with the introduction of less toxic substances and with the elaboration of adrenalin. The most widely used local anæsthetic is novocain, which is used in strengths of from ½ to 4 percent. In Germany tutocain is a strong competitor, since the same effect can be obtained with solutions which are only one-fourth as strong. A 1 percent solution of novocain corresponds, for example, in its action to a 0.25 percent solution of tutocain. The synthesis of percain (Ciba) appears to have provided a valuable addition to the local anæsthetics. Its action persists for as long as 6 hours without the appearance of toxic symptoms. For certain local anæsthesias alypin, tropacocain, butyn, etc., should also be considered.

Adrenalin is added to the anæsthetizing solution, as a rule, in the proportion of 1 to 100,000. But here, too, the exact concentration varies in the hands of different surgeons.

It is extremely difficult to place a limit on the amount of local anæsthetic which can be safely used. The toxic effects depend, if we exclude those few individuals who have an idiosyncrasy to them, on the amount which is absorbed and carried to the brain in a given time. Absorption depends on a number of factors. The stronger the solution, the more rapid its absorption. Ten cubic centimeters of a 2 percent solution of novocain-adrenalin may be more toxic than 100 cc. of a 0.2 percent solution, although the same amount of novocain is injected in both instances. For this reason the weakest possible solutions are to be preferred. Furthermore, the absorption of the substance may be further retarded by obstructing the circulation to the part or by lowering the part injected. As a rule larger amounts can be more safely used at a distance from the heart than close to it, where the circulation is better. If during anæsthesia an Esmarch bandage is applied no general effects are observed.

In spite of large variations in the quantity of anæsthetic required, I have found that 300 cc. of a ½ percent solution, 125 cc. of a 1 percent solution, 50 cc. of a 2 percent solution of novocain are non-toxic to a strong healthy adult. Toxic symptoms may appear suddenly if during injection a vein or artery is entered and the solution is injected into the blood stream. The symptoms may be particularly alarming if the solution gains access to a vessel carrying blood to the brain. Large vessels should be carefully avoided and while the needle is being introduced fluid should be forced out so as to push aside the smaller vessels. If any doubt exists aspiration should be attempted before the injection is made. Nevertheless, accidents occasionally occur if this method is used in and around very vascular structures. This is particularly true in the introduction of anæsthetic solutions in the urethra and bladder, the walls of whose veins are so thin that they may perforate under relatively slight pressure. The majority of the cases of death from local anæsthesia have occurred during anæsthetization of the urethra.

It is not necessary to carry the toxic substance to the brain through the blood. In spinal anæsthesia, and accidentally in deep block (paravertebral) anæsthesia of the cervical nerves, the drug reaches the higher centers through the cerebrospinal fluid. Finally, threatening accessory effects can take place during local anæsthesia through interference with vital functions carried on by certain nerves, such as the vagus, phrenic, and sympathetics.

The symptoms of poisoning from cocain and its related substances are: nausea, vomiting, perspiration, dizziness, dyspnœa, pallor, cyanosis, palpitation, cramps, cardiac irregularity, and unconsciousness.

The Treatment of Poisoning. At the first sign of toxicity one should discontinue administering the anæsthetic. The injected region, if there is space for it, should be constricted with an Esmarch band and this should be slowly released as the symptoms of poisoning disappear. If the area has been incised it is well to promote bleeding. Alcohol, in the form of whiskey, is an excellent antidote for cocain poisoning, and recently toxic symptoms have been prevented by using the barbiturates previous to injection. If the symptoms disappear rapidly and are evidently the result of injecting the solution directly into a blood vessel, the anæsthetization may be continued. However, if any doubt exists it is best to discontinue its use and to change to some other type of anæsthesia.

Every fluid introduced into tissues which is not isotonic with the tissue fluids is a local cell poison, and may so injure the tissue as to destroy it. Isotonic solutions should therefore be used whenever possible. Since slight deviations in the isotonicity do not cause serious effects, one can neglect the small amount of local anæsthetic and adrenalin in the solutions, provided these are dissolved in physiologic salt solution.

Nevertheless, the anæsthetic solution, especially if it contains adrenalin, may injure the tissues so that necrosis results. It is therefore necessary to exercise caution in the use of local anæsthetics in arteriosclerotics and diabetics, when forming narrow skin-flaps, or in operations on the extremities where the blood supply is definitely impaired. Personally, I have never observed this type of injury.

As the action of the local anæsthetic disappears pain sets in. This is most marked 2 to 3 hours after the injection. It is more prominent after local anæsthesia than after general anæsthesia, since after the latter, the other post-anæsthetic complaints such as nausea and vomiting may distract the patient's attention from the wound pain. Furthermore, the pain is accentuated by the nerve irritation caused by a solution which may not be isotonic. The pain is more apt to be more acute when the tissue into which the solution is injected is not areolar tissue. The pain, as a rule, disappears within a few hours, but it may last for several days with considerable severity. It should be controlled with sedatives or narcotics, and the best results are obtained if these are given immediately after completion of the operation.

Method of Preparing Solutions for Local Anæsthesia. Since solutions containing adrenalin deteriorate rapidly and thus lose their effectiveness, they should, if possible, be freshly prepared on each operative day. Novocain solutions should be made from the best obtainable preparation. It should be either purchased in tablets of known weight or should be carefully weighed out and a chart kept. The salt should be water soluble. Good preparations can be boiled or sterilized in an autoclave without decomposing. Traces of sodium bicarbonate reduce the action of novocain, so that containers and syringes with which it comes in contact should be thoroughly boiled in distilled water and washed subsequently with physiologic salt solution. Many of the instances where novocain was apparently unsuccessful can be traced to this fault in technic. The solutions are more active when cold, than warm. I previously used as a solvent physiologic salt solution, and then, following Kochmann's and Hoffmann's suggestion, added potassium sulphate. The solution is prepared as follows: sodium chloride 7.0 gm., potassium sulphate 4.0 gm., distilled water to 1000 cc. Solutions are easily prepared for instant use if tablets or charts of known weight are kept on hand.

In preparing the solutions I use Braun's technic. The necessary number of tablets are placed in a heat resisting test tube, to which are added a few cubic centimeters of the solution and the mixture is heated until the novocain is dissolved (Fig. 148). The solution is then placed in a sterile

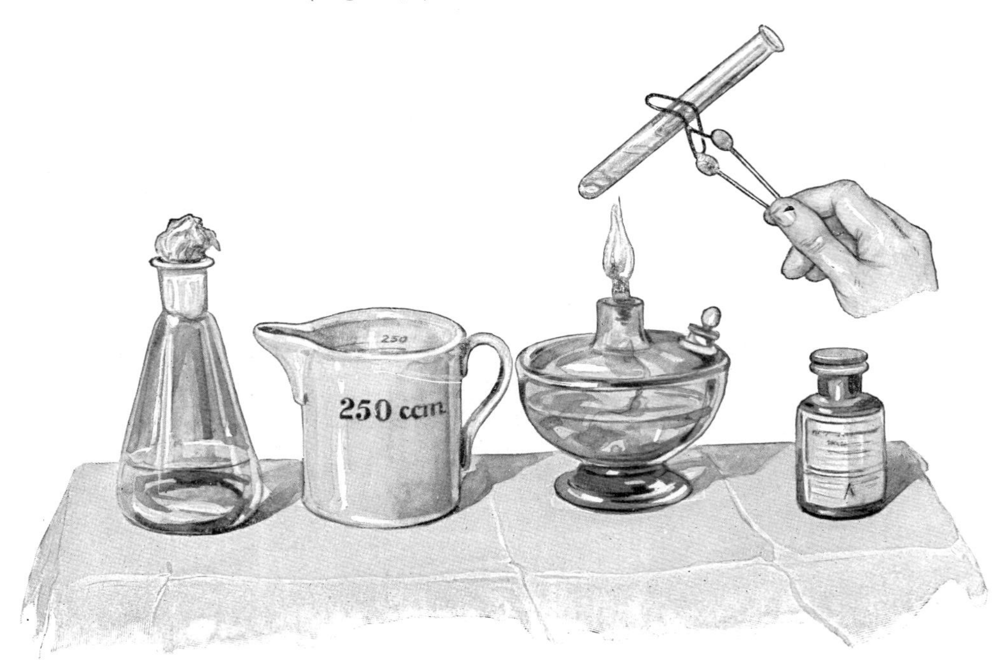

Fig. 148. Equipment for the preparation of solutions for local anæsthesia. The required number of tablets of novocain are taken from the supply bottle and placed in a test-tube with sterile salt solution and heated until dissolved. The solution is then poured into the sterile graduate and sterile salt solution is added from the flask to make the desired dilution.

graduate and sufficient cold salt solution is added to make the desired concentration. If all solutions and containers are sterile the solution is ready for use, or it may be placed in an Erlenmeyer flask and sterilized in the autoclave.

For urological operations we use a ½ to 1 percent alypin-adrenalin solution. This is made in a similar manner, but whenever adrenalin is used it should be added after the sterilization has been completed.

For anæsthesia of the nasal, pharyngeal and laryngeal mucous membrane we use a 5 percent solution of cocain, to which adrenalin is added. Stronger solutions are not necessary. Furthermore these solutions should be carefully labeled so that they are not mistaken for solutions of novocain.

A variety of special syringes have been devised for the injection of the local anæsthetic, but I prefer the simpler syringes. The Record syringe, made of a glass cylinder with metal ends and metal piston, seems to be the choice of the majority of surgeons. I use, as a rule, ordinary Record syringes of 5 and 10 cc. capacity, which are provided with rings for the thumb, index and middle fingers (Fig. 149). In order to prevent the glass cylinder from cracking during boiling, the syringe is taken apart and is not put together until the metal and glass have been cooled.

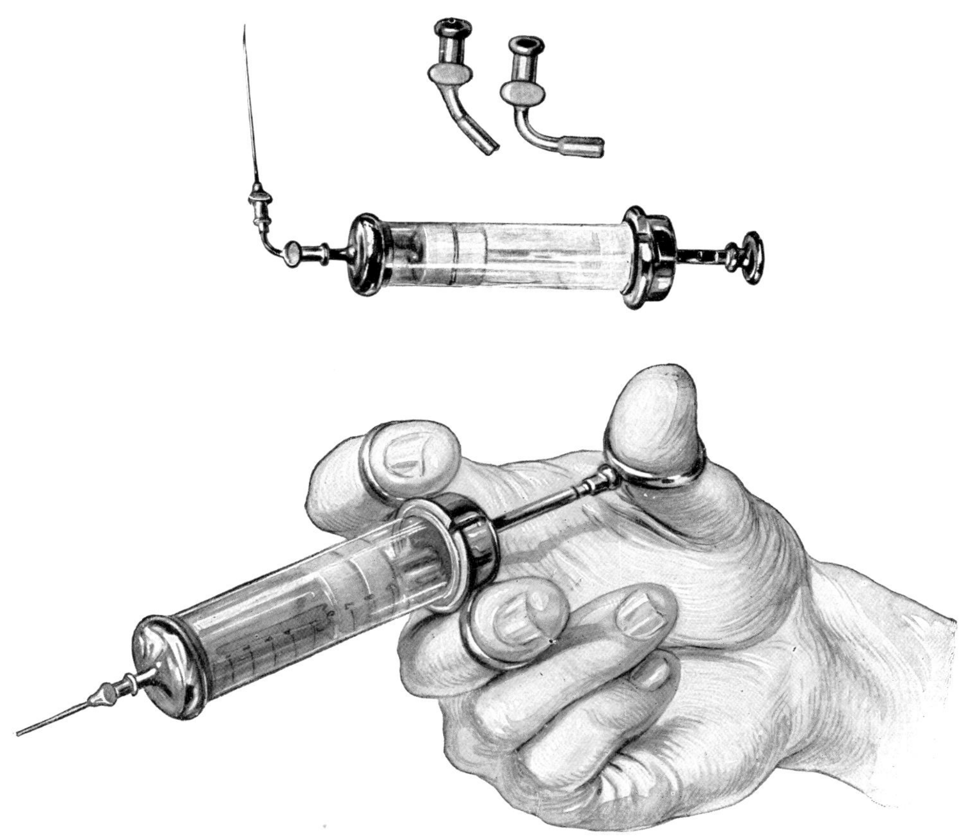

FIG. 149. 10 cc. Record syringe for local anæsthesia with and without thumb-ring and with angle tip.

A little sterile vaseline on the piston will permit easier action of the syringe. Exclusive of spinal and sacral anæsthesia, I use only three sizes of needles: a fine hypodermic needle 2.5 cm. long for anæsthetizing the skin; a #20 gauge needle, 5 cm. long, for subcutaneous injection; and one of similar size, 10 cm. long, for reaching the deeper areas. The needles should be made of rustless steel, and all needles and attachments must fit accurately. If the needles fit accurately and snugly, bayonet locks are not necessary. The needle should be pushed into the tissues only in a straight direction. Changes of direction after the needle has been inserted may cause it to break. If a long needle finds considerable resistance in dense tissues and threatens to bend, its exterior portion can be supported with a special needle-holder (See

Fig. 203). If the form of the body surface does not permit the use of a needle placed in the direction of the long axis of the springe, an angle-piece should be inserted between the syringe and the needle (Figs. 149 and 156).

3. Surface Anæsthesia

Mucous and serous membranes can be anæsthetized if cocain is brought in contact with these surfaces, and novocain may be used in wounds. The

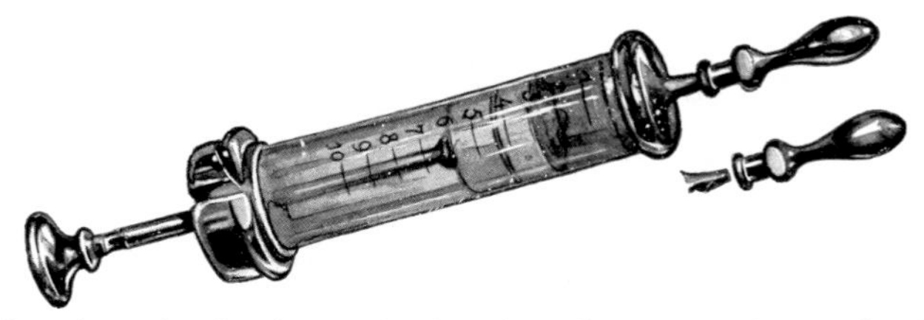

Fig. 150. Record syringe for local anæsthesia with olivary attachment for injection of the urethra and for fistulae.

mucous membrane of the nose, mouth, pharynx and larynx can be rendered insensible by application of a 5 percent cocain solution. However, only a superficial, rapidly disappearing anæsthesia is produced when this is done, so that I prefer submucous injection of novocain, or conduction anæsthesia for the more extensive operative procedures.

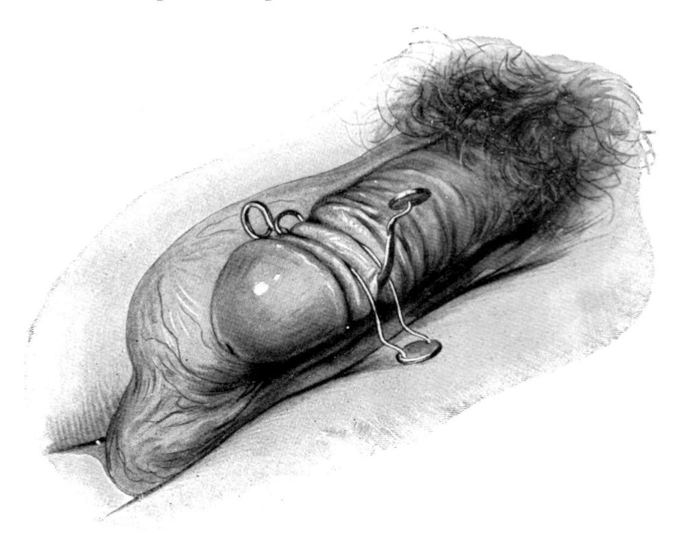

Fig. 151. Clamp for the retention of solutions injected into the urethra.

The mucous membrane of the male urethra, which is most sensitive in its posterior portion, can be effectively anæsthetized for catheterization and cystoscopy with a 1 percent solution of alypin. A Record syringe, provided with an olivary attachment (Fig. 150) should be used. After preliminary cleansing of the urethra, 10 cc. of the solution are injected through the external meatus and left in for 15 minutes by clamping the penis with a penis clamp (Fig. 151).

The female urethra can be rendered insensitive by using a cotton swab dipped in this solution, or for major procedures, 1 percent novocain may be injected around the urethra.

The urinary bladder can be anæsthetized by filling it through a catheter with a ½ percent alypin-adrenalin solution, after thoroughly washing it out. This is permitted to remain in for 30 minutes. If the bladder has only a small capacity, an irrigator placed 16 to 18 inches above the bladder and containing 100 cc. of the alypin solution is connected with the bladder by a soft rubber catheter. The bladder may at first expel the solution into the irrigator, but as the anæsthesia progresses it retains larger quantities of fluid.

It is important again to point out that the introduction of anæsthetizing solutions into the urinary passages may cause rupture of the thin walled veins and a rapid pouring of the solution into the circulation. Excessive pressure should never be used.

Joints are rendered insensitive in a few minutes after injection of a 1 percent novocain solution. Adrenalin should be used in these injections since absorption from serous surfaces is rapid.

4. Infiltration and Block Anæsthesia

By infiltration anæsthesia is meant that form of local anæsthesia in which the field of operation itself is infiltrated with the anæsthetizing solution.

The older method of infiltrating in stages the individual tissue layers as the operation progresses is now seldom used. In the rare instances in which we use infiltration anæsthesia we endeavor to infiltrate at one time all the layers of tissue which are to be incised. It is better to inject the deepest layers first and the more superficial layers later. I use, as a rule, a ½ percent novocain-adrenalin solution, but in exceptional cases I use a 1 or 2 percent solution. If one waits for 10 minutes from the time of completion of the injection before beginning the operation, the area will be completely insensitive. In fact, since the fluid tends to spread, the anæsthetic area is wider than the area injected. Beyond this zone sensitivity is acute and if the operative area must be enlarged certain difficulties may arise. A further disadvantage of infiltration anæsthesia is the edematous, glassy tissue which results after the injection and which makes accurate orientation somewhat difficult.

Since infiltration anæsthesia possesses no advantage over block anæsthesia, except that less solution is used, I use it only for small and simple procedures, such as for the anæsthetization of the point of insertion of a needle or for small puncture wounds. In all other cases I use block anæsthesia.

Infiltration anæsthesia finds its widest application in forming the intracutaneous skin-wheal (Fig. 152), which is necessary when a small area of skin is to be anæsthetized immediately, as for example, where a punctured wound is to be made, or a needle is to be inserted for exploration, or for the introduction of a local anæsthetic into the deeper tissues. In making the skin-wheal, a very fine hypodermic needle is inserted intradermally parallel to the skin surface just far enough so that the opening of the needle is covered. If the fluid is injected with a definite pressure, there appears at the site of injection a pale elevated area on which the skin pores are prominent. The skin at the site of the wheal becomes insensible at once.

Since the needle can be reinserted painlessly within and on the border of this first wheal, the adjacent tissue can be raised in a similar wheal and in this way long strips of skin can be anæsthetized either in a circle or

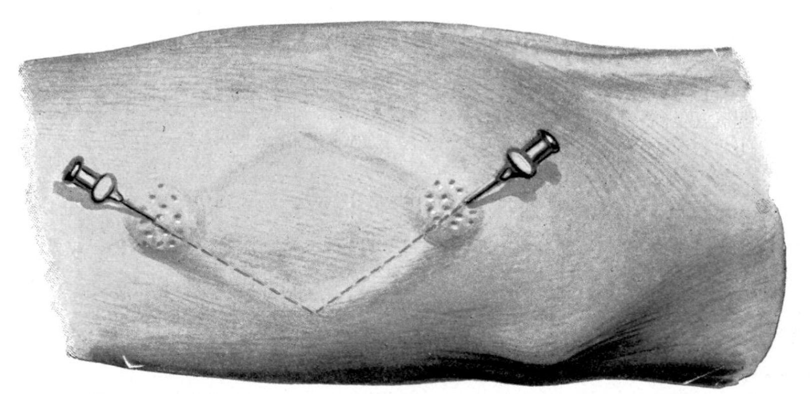

Fig. 152. Blocking a field through two intracutaneous wheals.

straight line without pain to the patient except for the initial skin prick. Since the skin wheal remains visible for only a short time, it is recommended when a series of wheals are being made to mark them with a colored solution which is applied to the skin.

Infiltration anæsthesia is today almost entirely displaced by block anæsthesia, which is local anæsthesia in the strictest sense of the word. It con-

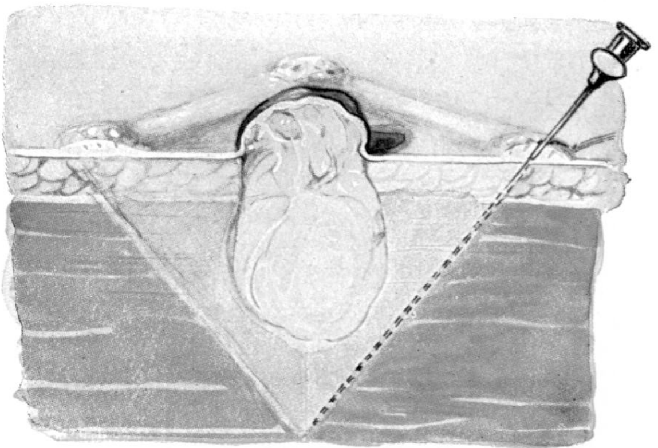

Fig. 153. The anæsthetic has been introduced through four intracutaneous wheals so as to outline an inverted pyramid. (Schematic.)

sists in blocking the area of operation by infiltrating the tissues around this area with a local anæsthetic so that all of the nerves supplying the area of operation are bathed in the solution and thus can not carry stimuli. The area of operation itself remains free from the anæsthetizing solution and therefore is unchanged in structure.

The simplest form of block anæsthesia is the outlining of a pyramid which encloses the operative area (Fig. 153). The infiltration is made through four or more puncture points in the following manner: If the area around a spherical tumor is to be injected, four points are marked out on

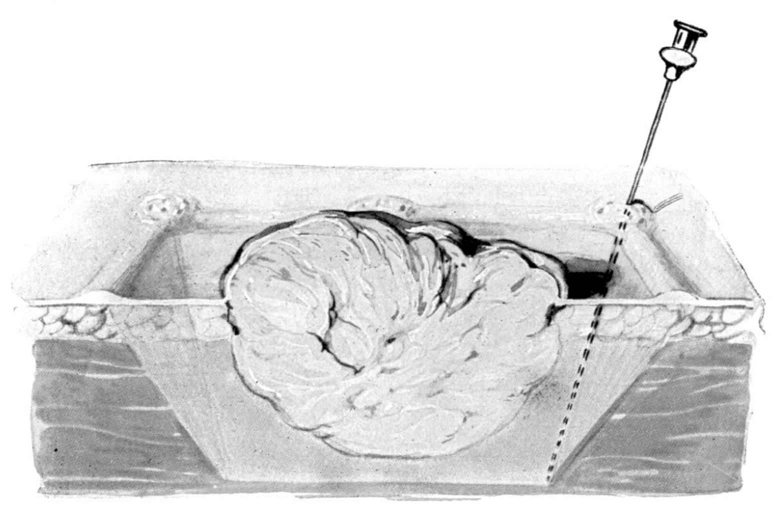

FIG. 154. Blocking of an operative area by cutaneous, subcutaneous, and deep injection of a local anæsthetic. (Diagrammatic.)

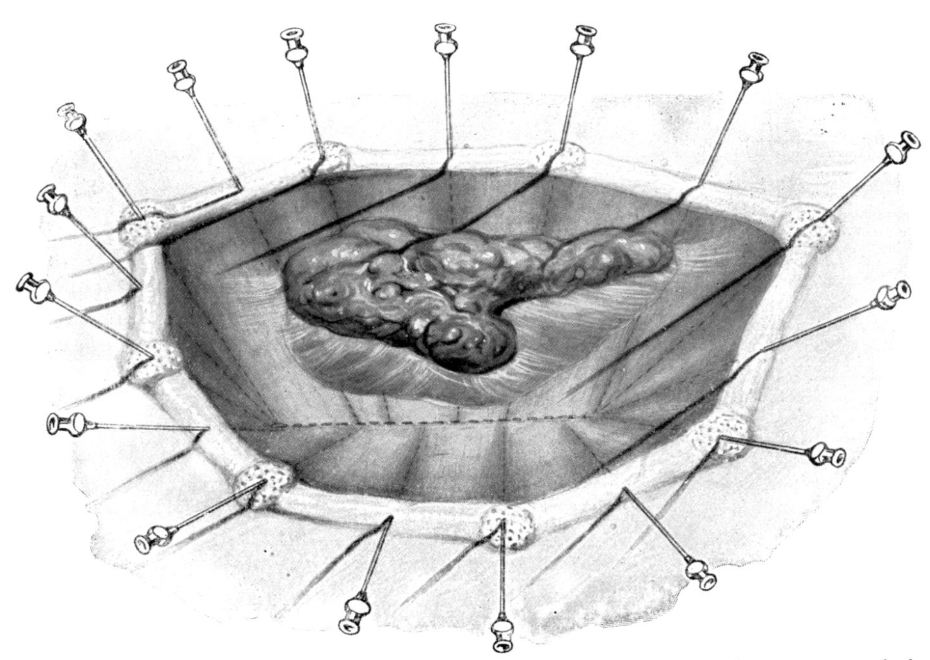

FIG. 155. Blocking an irregular shaped operative site by cutaneous, subcutaneous and deep infiltration of the anæsthetic solution through intracutaneous wheals.

the skin. The distance from one point to the other should be approximately 12 cm. These encircle the tumor and are joined by intracutaneous injections. The area of operation is then surrounded by a series of injections which tend to outline a pyramid. For the deep injections the four original wheals are used for inserting the needle. While the needle is being inserted through the tissues the solution should be forced out into them. The termination of the injection should be at a point under the growth to be removed. Additional skin wheals can be made for injection if this is desired. If this is done the infiltration can be more effectively accomplished (Fig.

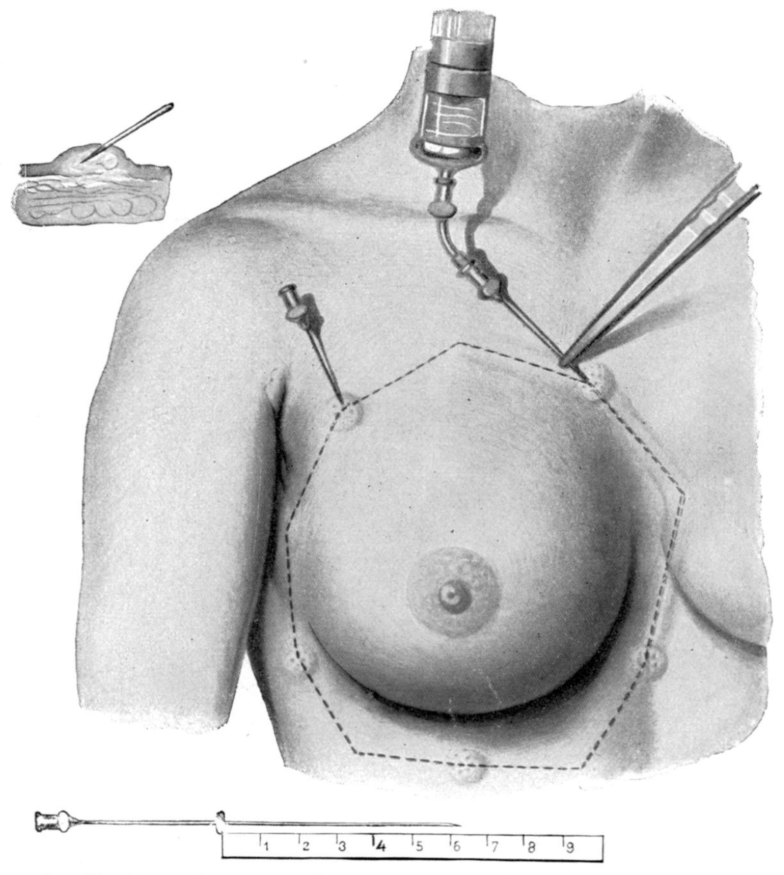

FIG. 156. Blocking of an operating area (female breast) by cutaneous, subcutaneous and deep infiltration. Above, to the left, intracutaneous infiltration wheal; below, a rubber marker is placed at the desired distance on a needle.

155). At the conclusion of the injection the entire operative area has been isolated by a wall of the local anæsthetic. Within 10 minutes the enclosed area should be insensitive. In accordance with the extent and shape of the field of operation one may deviate from this pyramidal form, in that the field of operation can be surrounded with any number of puncture points so as to outline various shapes and from which the block may be laid down. It is essential to enclose completely the operative field, the exact method by which this is done being unimportant (Figs. 152-156).

As a rule I use a ½ percent novocain-adrenalin solution for this type of injection although in certain areas, as in the region of the head or around inflammatory lesions, I use a 1 percent solution. During the introduction and withdrawal of a 6 cm. needle, 5 to 10 cc. of the anæsthetic are injected. During the injection the needle must be kept constantly in motion, so that if the needle accidentally enters a vessel only a very small amount of the solution will enter the circulating blood. The block should be completed at one time, preferably before the surgeon puts on his sterile gown or the operative field is finally draped, so that the solution may have time to take effect, and

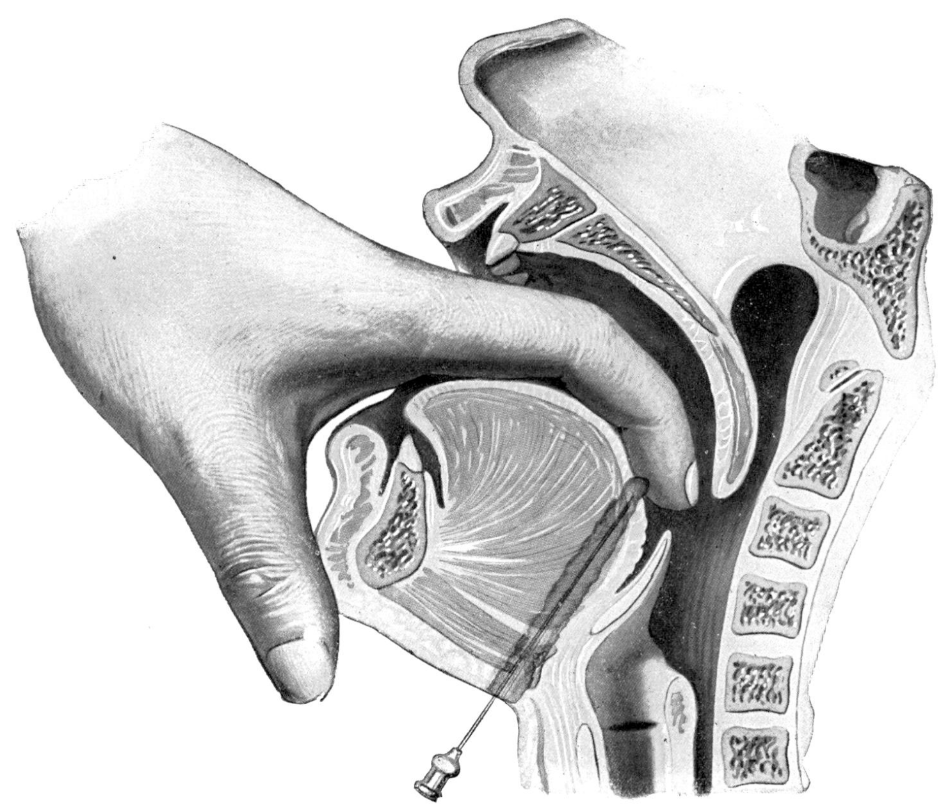

Fig. 157. Blocking a wide area which receives its nerves through its base. The tongue and submental area are anæsthetized by injecting the anæsthetic solution as shown in the illustration.

yet no time be lost in waiting for this. The injection has been unsuccessful if the operator is compelled, because of pain, to inject the field further during the operation. However, it is better to inject more solution, than to let the patient suffer. It is evident that block anæsthesia is only suitable where the extent of the operation is definitely known at the time of injection. Then, however, due to its unusual simplicity and because of the large number of available solutions, it is applicable to practically every region of the body.

Frequently block anæsthesia is more or less combined with conduction anæsthesia, in that while laying down the block individual nerves are injected, or in conjunction with block anæsthesia, individual nerves supplying the area of operation may be singled out for injection away from the site of operation.

Certain portions of the body can be rendered insensible to pain by infiltrating or blocking them at their base. If the part contains large nerves, a 1 percent solution of novocain should be used. In this way operations on the ear, the penis, the scrotum, the fingers and toes, the tongue (Fig. 157), or the arms and legs can be done painlessly, if the block has been laid down properly. For small parts such as the penis, fingers, or toes, two puncture points for the injection suffice; for larger parts, such as the arms or legs, four points are necessary. (Hackenbruch, Hohmeier, Sievers, Fritz Koenig.)

In the extremities a subcutaneous infiltration ring should be placed at least a hand's breadth proximal to the site of operation. From two, four, or even more points, a fan-like, cross-section infiltration of the soft parts should

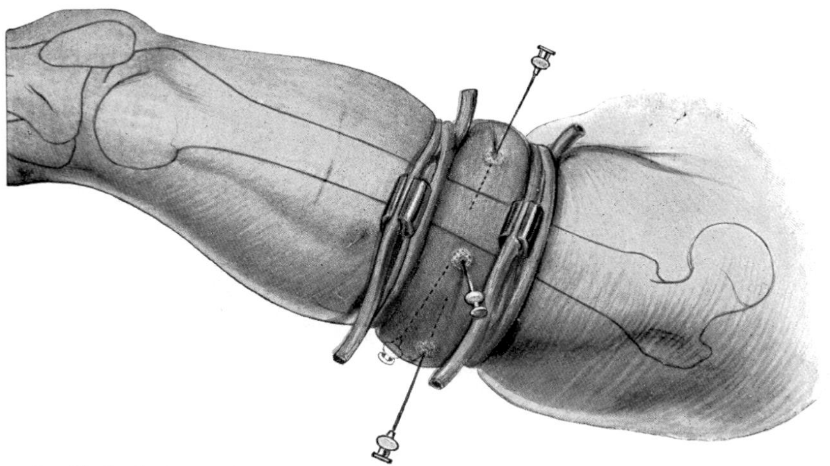

FIG. 158. Method of securing anæsthesia of the leg, by infiltrating an area approximal to the operative site. The anæsthetic is injected into the deeper tissues through a circular series of intracutaneous wheals.

be made down to the bone, after the cutaneous anæsthesia has been established (Fig. 158). When infiltrating in the location of the larger nerve trunks, 10 to 20 cc. of the solution should be injected. In these injections I also use a ½ percent solution of novocain, of which about 150 cc. is used for the arm, and from 200 to 250 cc. for the thigh. In the lower extremity I supplant this with 20 cc. of a 1 percent solution of novocain in the area of the sciatic and femoral nerves. Anæsthesia is more apt to be complete if an Esmarch bandage has been previously applied, and it occurs more quickly and more thoroughly when the infiltration is done between two tourniquets. It is not necessary to anæsthetize the bone, and the periosteum is rendered insensible if the infiltration has been properly done.

It is possible to reduce a fracture if a 2 percent solution of novocain is injected between the ends of the bone and into the hematoma surrounding the fracture.

Upon similar principles depends the efficiency of the elder Oberst's finger and toe anæsthesia. I no longer use a tourniquet for the fingers or toes having found that adrenalin suffices to restrict the circulation. A disadvantage of this method of anæsthesia is the very severe pain which frequently occurs after the operation. The pain is less the smaller the amount of anæsthetic used. It is also less if the block is carried out not in the region of the free fingers, but proximal to the webs, as will be later described.

The use of infiltration anæsthesia around inflamed tissues is not recommended generally, since it is believed that the bacteria are disseminated by the solution. I can not pass this by without further comment. I have used infiltration anæsthesia in the region of inflamed tissues (abscesses and furuncles), in hundreds of instances over many years, without having observed the most trifling disadvantage. It is true the injections are limited to the skin over the abscess, and to the skin around the furuncle. In diffuse, phlegmonous lesions I do not use this type of anæsthesia because of the pain which the injections would cause, and also because the extent of the lesion can not as a rule be determined before operation.

5. Conduction Anæsthesia

Conduction anæsthesia is that form of local anæsthesia in which one or more large nerve trunks supplying the area of operation, or the ganglia of these nerves are injected with an anæsthetizing solution so that they will not carry pain stimuli. The larger the nerve-trunk to be injected, the stronger should the solution be. A 1 percent solution is used principally, but for the large nerve-trunks of the extremities I use a 2 to 4 percent solution of novocain. The excellence of the anæsthesia and the rapidity with which this occurs depend on the accuracy with which the injection is made. Only in very rare instances should it be necessary to expose the nerves under infiltration anæsthesia before attempting to inject them under the guidance of the eye.

In the majority of instances the injection is made through a needle which traverses undamaged tissues. An excellent knowledge of regional anatomy is necessary to be successful with this method of anæsthesia.

The surgeon must be guided by the anatomical landmarks and must constantly keep in mind the relationship of other important structures to the nerves to be injected. The depth of the needle in the tissues is very important. The depth to which the needle has been inserted can be determined, if the entire length of the needle is known, by measuring the external portion, or better, a small cork or piece of rubber is placed on the needle before insertion at the estimated depth of the nerve to be injected (Fig. 156). In spite of the best efforts it is impossible to inject the nerve directly in every instance.

The surest sign that the needle is in the correct position is the occurrence of pain in the area supplied by the nerve, the needle point being shifted slightly from the supposedly correct position if pain in the distribution of the nerve does not result after introduction of the needle to the desired depth. In some cases, in which there are not sufficient landmarks present to indicate the position of the nerve, one may inject the anæsthetic by infiltration, laying down a line of solution perpendicular to the course of the nerve in a plane that must be traversed by it.

Often conduction anæsthesia is combined with infiltration anæsthesia. An exact knowledge of the nerves which supply the area in which the operation is planned is necessary, as well as the anatomical position of these, if the surgeon wishes to use successfully this method of anæsthesia to supplant in certain cases general anæsthesia. I shall describe certain of the

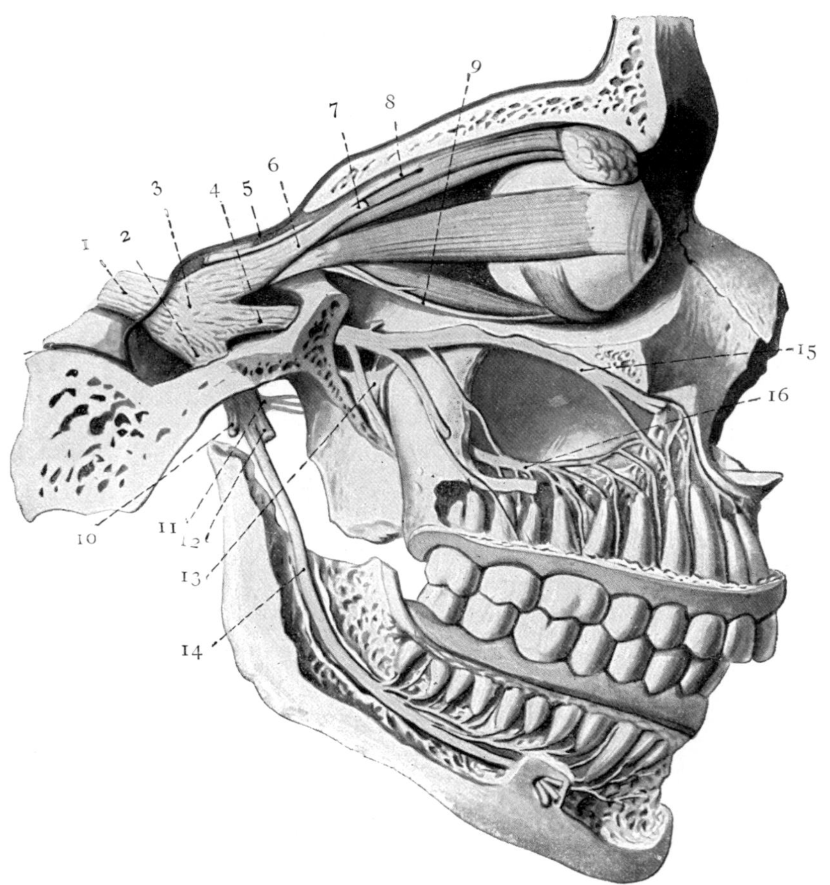

Fig. 159. Anatomy of the trigeminal (fifth) nerve (schematic). 1. sensory root, 2. third division, 3. Gasserian (semilunar) ganglion, 4. second division, 5. dura mater, 6. first division, 7. naso-ciliary nerve, 8. supra-orbital nerve, 9. zygomatic nerve, 10. auriculo-temporal nerve, 11. masticator nerve, 12. lingual nerve, 13. spheno-palatine nerve, 14. mandibular nerve, 15. anterior-superior alveolar nerve, 16. posterior-superior alveolar nerve.

important injections used for conduction anæsthesia and for whose elucidation we are indebted to Braun.

(A) BLOCKING OF THE TRIGEMINAL NERVE (FIGS. 160 AND 161)

The trigeminal nerve is the sensory nerve of the scalp, face and under half of the chin, the interior of the nose, that portion of the buccal cavity in front of the soft palate, and the orbit. It has a small motor branch. It has three major sensory branches (Fig. 159), ophthalmic, maxillary, and mandibular, which supply the areas of the face which their names indicate, but which overlap to a degree, so that it may be necessary to inject more than one branch in order to obtain complete anæsthesia in a given area.

The injection of the branches of this nerve or its Gasserian (semilunar) ganglion is of significance not only for anæsthesia during operative pro-

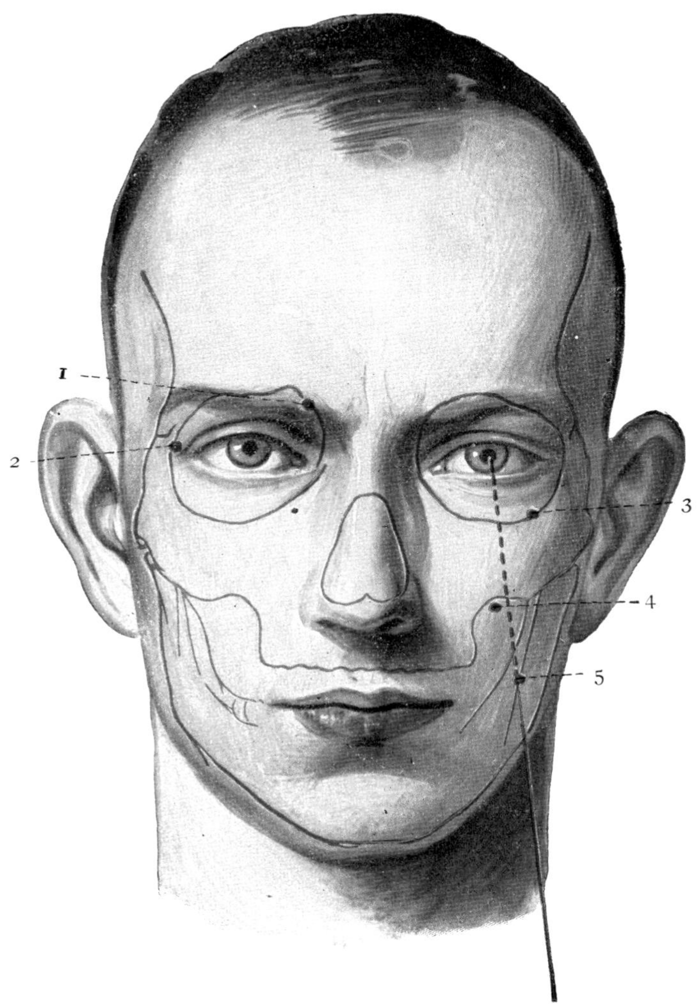

FIG. 160. Points of injection for blocking the various branches of the trigeminal (fifth) nerve (anterior view). For the explanation of the figures see the following drawing.

cedures, but is of importance in the treatment of trigeminal neuralgia (tic douloureux). For the latter, however, 1 to 3 cc. of absolute alcohol are used.

(1) Injection of the Gasserian (semilunar) Ganglion (Härtel).

By injecting an anæsthetic solution into the Gasserian ganglion, all three branches of the nerve are anæsthetized. The method of Härtel, who injects the Gasserian ganglion through the foramen ovale, is the one most widely used and I follow this in minute detail. The strictest asepsis is imperative, for the injection is to an extent an intracranial operation, especially since the sub-dural space may frequently be opened. The escape of cerebrospinal fluid through the needle indicates that this has occurred. Hence the needle should not be pushed through the mouth, nor through infected soft parts. The puncture is usually done in a semi-sitting position. The operator must be able to observe the patient from the front as well as from the side.

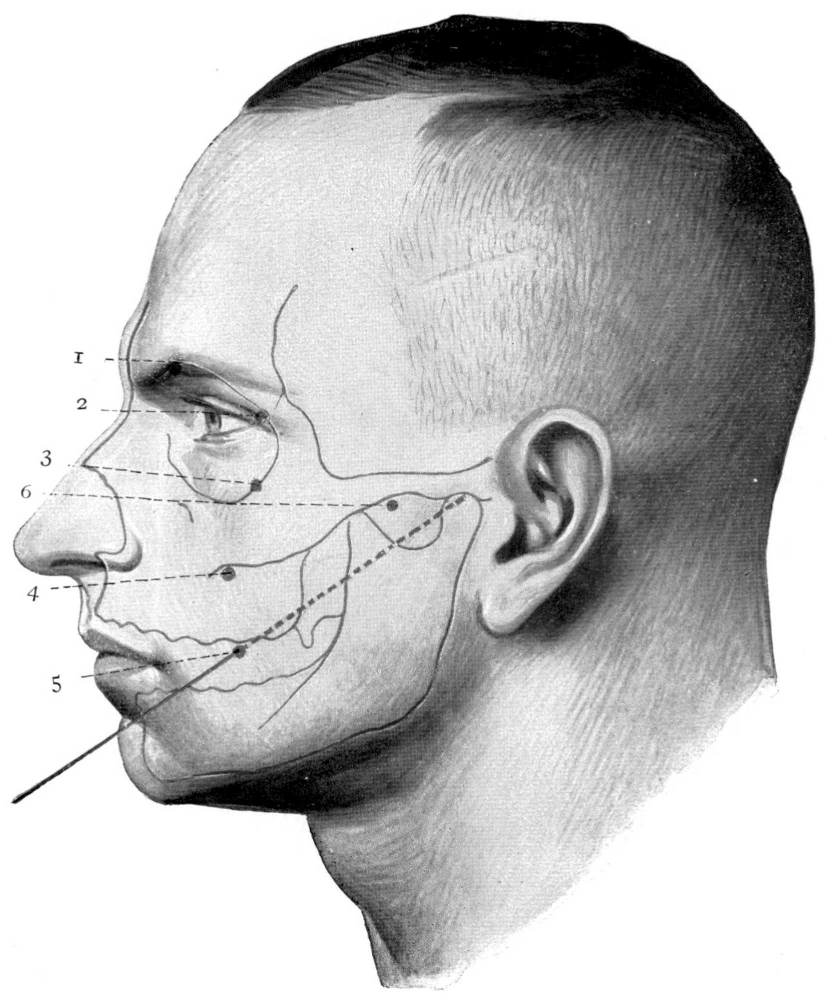

FIG. 161. Points of injection for blocking the various branches of the trigeminal (fifth) nerve (lateral view). 1. supra-orbital; 2. lateral orbital; 3. pterygo-palatine fossa through the orbit; 4. pterygo-palatine fossa from the side; 5. Gasserian (semilunar) ganglion; 6. otic ganglion.

A mark is made on the skin of the face with a colored solution 3 cm. to the side of and a similar distance above the angle of the mouth. The patient is at first carefully observed from the front (Fig. 162) and a line is drawn from the point of proposed entrance of the needle to the approximate location of the pupil with the patient looking forward. The patient is then observed from the side (Fig. 163) and a second line is drawn from the point of origin of the first to the articular tubercle of the same side. A wheal is made at the point where the needle is to be inserted. A needle at least 12 cm. long is used for the deep injection and a marker is placed 8 cm. from its tip. The needle is directed so that when viewing it from the front it parallels line #1, while in viewing it from the side it lies at a more acute angle to line #1 than line #2. It is directed toward the center of the zygomatic arch. The direction of the needle is maintained, without inserting a finger in the mouth of the patient, as the needle is pushed through the tissues. As a rough guide for direction, the continuation of the line of the needle lying in the foramen ovale should meet the scalp at a point 4 cm. in front of the lambdoid suture and 2 cm. to the opposite side of the midline. If considerable pain is felt while the needle is being inserted a few cc. of novocain should be injected. Aspiration with a syringe should be attempted in order to ascertain whether or not the needle is in a blood vessel. If the needle has been directed properly it should strike the bony resistance of the infratemporal plane at a depth of about 6 cm. From the side one observes whether or not the needle is in the direction of line #2, then viewing the patient from the front changes the direction of the needle by gently withdrawing it a short distance and then reinserting it, so that it is inserted more in the direction of line #2 and away from line #1. As the needle becomes parallel with line #2 it slides along the bony surface of the infratemporal fossa toward the foramen ovale, until it finally slides through this opening. Successful entrance of the foramen can be determined in two ways: objectively, by a sudden cessation of resistance against the needle; and subjectively, in non-anæsthetized patients, by radiating pains along the mandibular distribution of the nerve. The needle, as a rule, is 6 cm. deep, and this distance curiously is nearly always the same regardless of the size or shape of the patient's head. If it is desired, an assistant can direct the needle from the anterior view while the surgeon watches the needle from the lateral position. After the foramen is entered the needle is pushed 1.5 cm. further when, as a rule, paræsthesias along the other divisions of the nerve are observed. If blood or cerebrospinal fluid comes out of the cannula, the solution should not be injected. If this occurs the needle should be withdrawn slightly and the solution should be injected only if the operator is convinced that the point of the needle is outside of the subarachnoid space and not in a

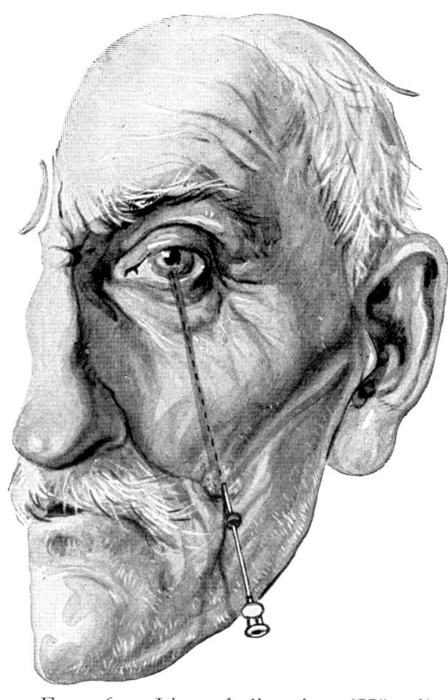

FIG. 162. Line of direction (Härtel), for injecting the Gasserian (semilunar) ganglion (anterior view). The anterior line of direction goes from the point of insertion through the pupil.

blood vessel. Before injecting alcohol for trigeminal neuralgia, 1.0 to 1.5 cc. of a 2 percent solution of novocain is injected, and after 5 minutes at most, the entire trigeminal area should be anæsthetized, if the needle is in its proper place. It is recommended by some to inject novocain also around the ganglion. After the injection the patients should be kept quiet and under no circumstances should they be permitted to lower their heads. The simultaneous injection of both Gasserian ganglia is permissible.

There are no serious complications connected with the injection of novocain solution into the ganglion if properly carried out. Only occasionally nausea, vomiting, rapidly disappearing abducent paralysis and pupillary dilation may occur. However, permanent changes may be produced by the injection of alcohol if this is not entirely confined to the ganglion. Blindness,

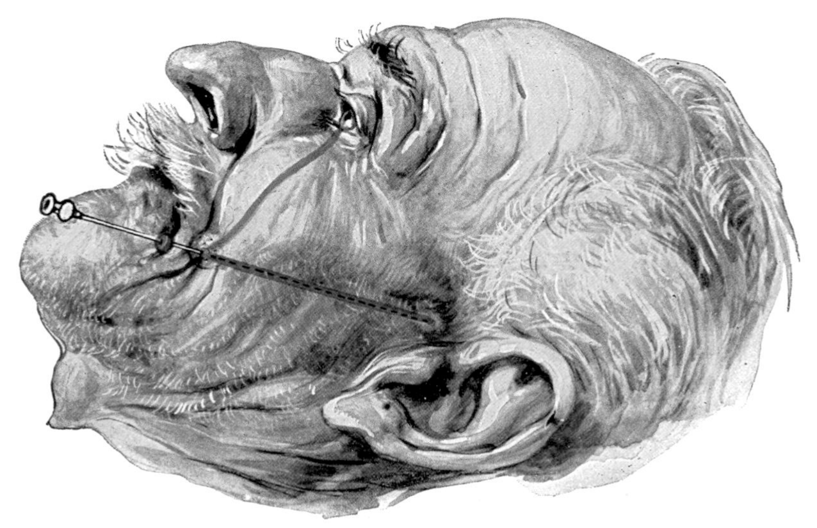

Fig. 163. Lines of direction (Härtel) for injecting the Gasserian (semilunar) ganglion, (lateral view). The lateral line of direction goes from the point of insertion through the articular tuberosity.

paralysis of the ocular muscles, of the facial and acoustico-vestibular nerves have been reported. Kulenkampff believes that he can avoid accidents of this character by very slow injection of the alcohol, which should take at least fifteen minutes, so that at the first appearance of disturbing signs the injection can be stopped. (Furthermore, alcoholic injection of the ganglion may lead to corneal ulceration just as avulsion of the ganglion or division of the sensory root may result in this very refractory lesion. Alcoholic injection of the ganglion makes later operative removal of the ganglion or division of its sensory root much more difficult. I. S. R.)

(2) Blocking of the First or Ophthalmic Division of the Trigeminal Nerve.

The injection of all branches of the first division of the trigeminal nerve is of importance where general anæsthesia is to be avoided in operations within the orbit. The branches (Fig. 159) which have already been given

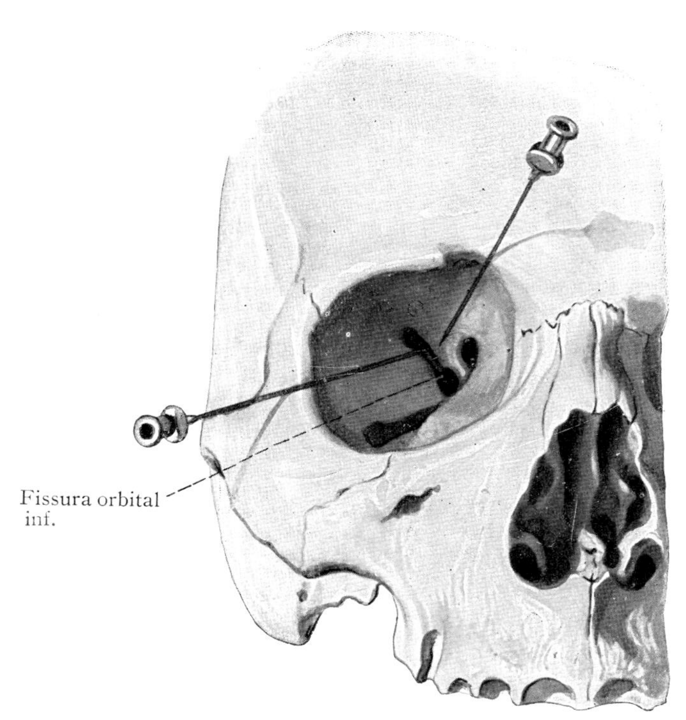

FIG. 164. Medial and lateral position of the needle for blocking the branches of the first division of the trigeminal nerve.

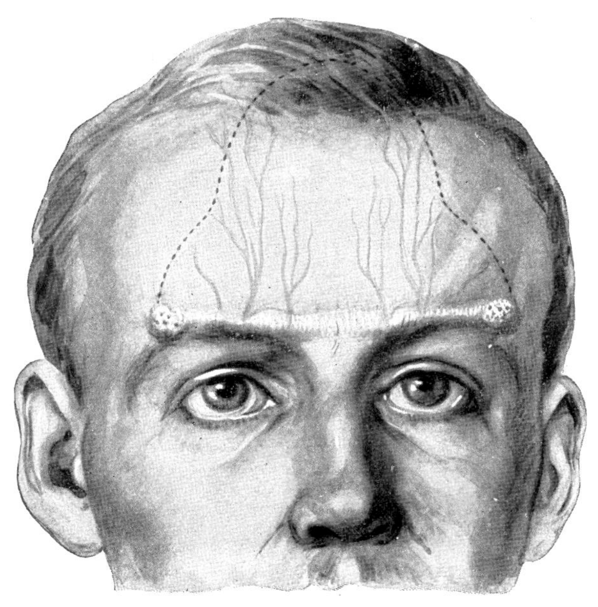

FIG. 165. Bilateral blocking of the frontal nerve by subcutaneous infiltration across the forehead at the height of the eyebrows. Boundary of the zone of anæsthesia.

off before the main nerve reaches the orbit, run on the outside of the ocular muscles. They consist of a medial pair, the anterior and posterior ethmoidal nerves, and a lateral pair, the frontal and lacrymal nerves, which supply also the mucous membrane of the ethmoid bone, the frontal sinus and part of the nose.

These four nerves can be reached through a medial and a lateral orbital injection.

For the **medial orbital injection** the needle is inserted a finger's breadth above the medial canthus of the eye, where the medial margin of the orbit meets the superior margin. It is kept in constant contact with the osseous wall of the orbit for about 5 cm. where 2.5 cc. of a 2 percent novocain solution are injected (Figs. 160, 161, 162).

For **lateral orbital injection** the needle is inserted just above the lateral canthus of the eye. It is kept in constant touch with the bone until it strikes the bony roof of the orbit at a depth of 4.5 to 5 cm. Here it is in the superior orbital fissure (Figs. 160, 161 and 164). Into this area are injected 3.5 cc. of a 2 percent novocain solution.

For the injection or **blocking of the terminations of the frontal nerve** (Fig. 165), a subcutaneous injection of 10 cc. of a 1 percent novocain-adrenalin solution is laid down at the height of the eyebrows. If the block is successful there will appear a triangular area of anæsthesia. The base of the triangle is the eyebrows and the apex in the midline reaches above the hair line. This method of injection has no considerable practical significance, since the block method gives better results in this area.

(3) Blocking of the Second or Maxillary Division of the Trigeminal Nerve.

Injection in the Pterygopalatine Fossa. The second division of the trigeminal passes through the foramen rotundum and divides into a number of branches, one going to the sphenopalatine ganglion (Fig. 159). The injection of the main division can be accomplished by infiltration of the fossa or, if the anatomy of the bony structure permits it, even in the foramen itself. The pterygopalatine fossa is reached with a needle either from the side of the face or through the orbit.

(a) Lateral approach. On the lower border of the zygoma where this meets the maxilla is found the zygomatic tubercle. It can also be found by dropping a perpendicular line from the external border of the orbit to the lower border of the zygomatic arch. With this tubercle as the landmark the needle is pushed upward and inward. After piercing the masseter muscle it comes in contact with the bone, just skirting the superior maxillary tubercle (Figs. 160, 161 and 166). At about 4 cm. the bony wall is no longer felt and the needle is then inserted about 1 cm. further, when it is in the pterygopalatine fossa. It is stopped by the bony wall of the fossa. If the needle is withdrawn slightly and the angulation changed, the foramen can often be entered, but a bony ridge may prevent this. The penetration of the nerve by the needle will be indicated by pain in the distribution of the second division in the upper jaw. Whether the needle can enter the foramen rotundum or not it should never be inserted more than 6 cm., and this length should have been previously marked on the needle. Five cubic centimeters of a 2 percent solution of novocain are distributed in and around the nerve, and an additional 2 cc. in the region of the maxillary tubercle as the needle is withdrawn.

If the nerve can not be reached due to the wing of the sphenoid, the needle should be inserted further laterally. If the needle is carried at too

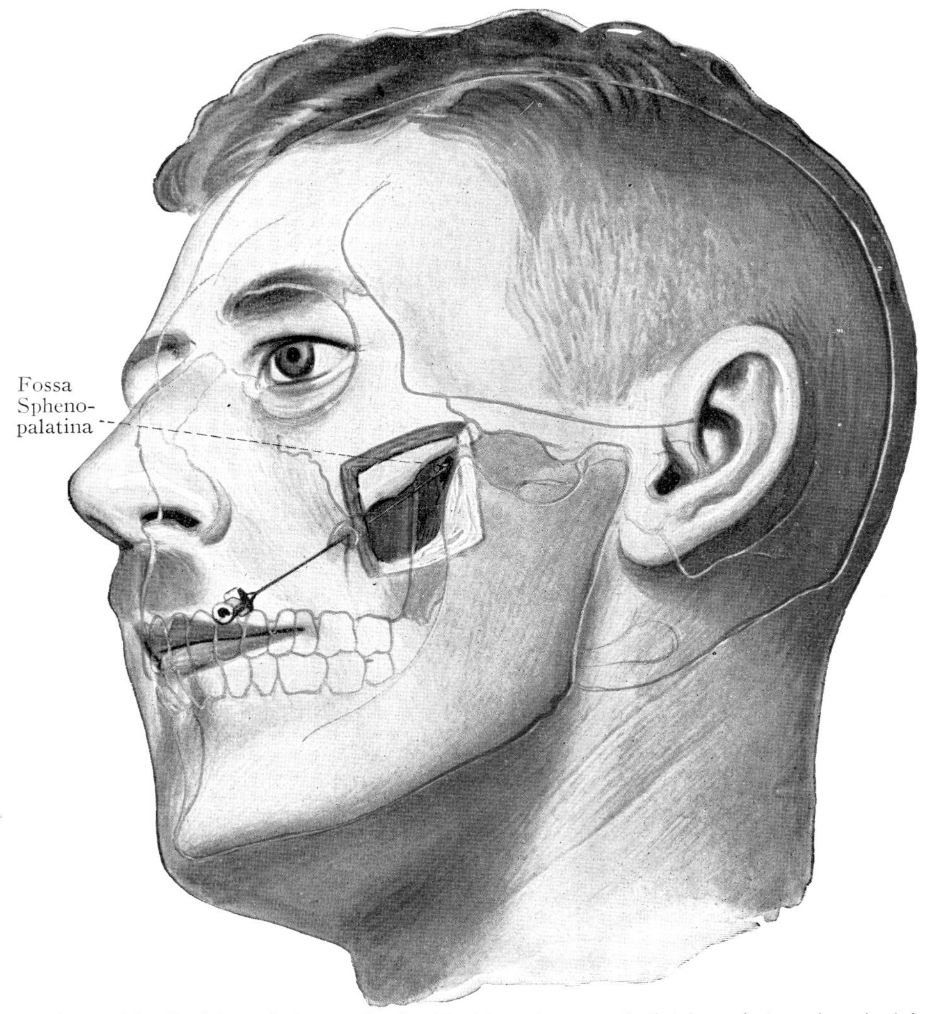

Fig. 166. Position of the needle for blocking the second division of the trigeminal in the pterygopalatine fossa from the side of face. The needle is inserted below the angle of the zygomatic arch and is carried medialward by keeping in touch with the maxillary tubercle.

great an angle or too far medially, it may find its way through the inferior orbital fissure or into the nose.

(b) Approach through the orbit. The inferior orbital fissure is used in approaching the nerve. The direction of the needle when properly inserted, is, when viewed anteriorly toward the medial-superior orbital angle. When viewed laterally it points toward the helix of the ear. The point for insertion of the needle, according to Braun, is at the point of intersection of the

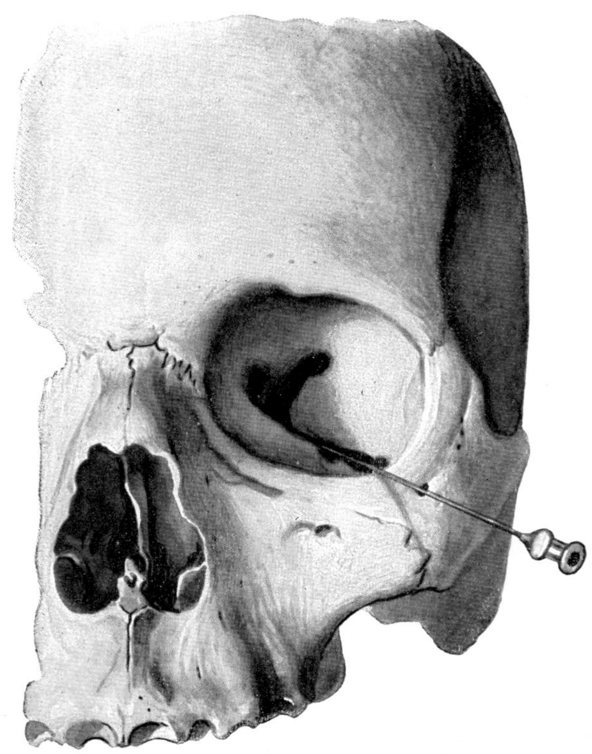

Fig. 167. Position of the needle for blocking the second division of the trigeminal in the pterygopalatine fossa through the orbit. The needle is inserted in the inferior orbital fissure.

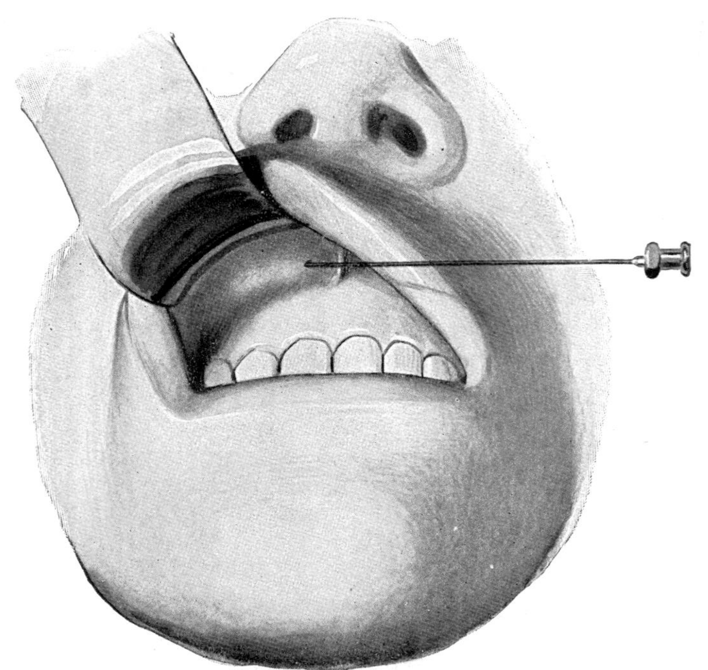

Fig. 168. Position of the needle for blocking the nerve of an upper tooth. It is inserted in the fold of the mucous membrane parallel to the masticatory surface.

prolongation of the upper margin of the zygomatic arch with the orbital margin. This corresponds to the point where the lateral orbital margin crosses the inferior orbital margin (Figs. 160, 161 and 167). The needle is inserted with its outer portion inclined slightly upwards so that the point is directed almost vertically upon the bony orbital floor. The outer portion of the needle is brought down to an almost horizontal position as its point is carried along the bone, until one feels the resistance of the fibrous tissue of the inferior orbital fissure. The needle should be directed through this area of resistance, pointing in a direction toward the center of the skull.

If properly directed paræsthesias appear just after the needle passes through the inferior orbital fissure. Two or three cubic centimeters of novocain should be injected at this point. At a depth of 5 cm. the needle should be in the foramen rotundum and there meet the bony resistance of the base of the skull. Five cubic centimeters of a 2 percent solution of novocain should be injected.

The lateral approach is more suitable for the injection of alcohol, but the orbital method is also used. Two cubic centimeters of absolute alcohol should be injected.

Blocking the Terminal Branch of the Infraorbital Nerve. This portion of the infraorbital nerve can be injected in the infraorbital canal. The injection is made after the needle is inserted into the canal at the center of the lower border of the orbit. By careful palpation with the point of the needle constantly against the bone the canal (Fig. 167) is found and 1 cc. of a 2 percent solution of novocain is injected into the nerve. The anæsthesia, if a bilateral injection is made, affects the anterior part of the nose, the upper lip and the cheek up to the lower eyelid.

Blocking of the Superior Alveolar Nerve. The branches of the infraorbital nerve which supply the upper teeth (Fig. 159) run posteriorly-anteriorly on the lateral side of the maxilla. They are partly just inside of the bone, partly on the bone, under the mucous membrane. The angle of the mouth should be retracted with Roux's hooks, and a needle is then inserted in the fold of the mucous membrane along the superior alveolar margin. This is kept parallel to the masticatory surface of the teeth, and the solution is injected as the needle is inserted further and further (Fig. 168). In order to eliminate pain from a tooth the anæsthetizing solution must extend between the teeth on either side of the tooth to be operated on. For anæsthesia of the last molars, the needle must be inserted in the fold in front of the epiphysis of the zygomatic arch and pushed inward and backward under the mucous membrane covering the maxillary tubercle. It should be mentioned that painless extraction of the upper teeth necessitates the simultaneous injection of the mucous membrane of the palate adjacent to these teeth.

(4) Blocking the Third Mandibular Division of the Trigeminal Nerve.

Injection at the Foramen Ovale. The third division of the trigeminal nerve can be injected at its exit from the foramen ovale. This is in the vicinity of the otic ganglion and successful injection results in anæsthesia of the mandible and tongue. (Fig. 159.) The needle is inserted vertically under the middle of the zygomatic arch (Figs. 160 and 161) in the direction

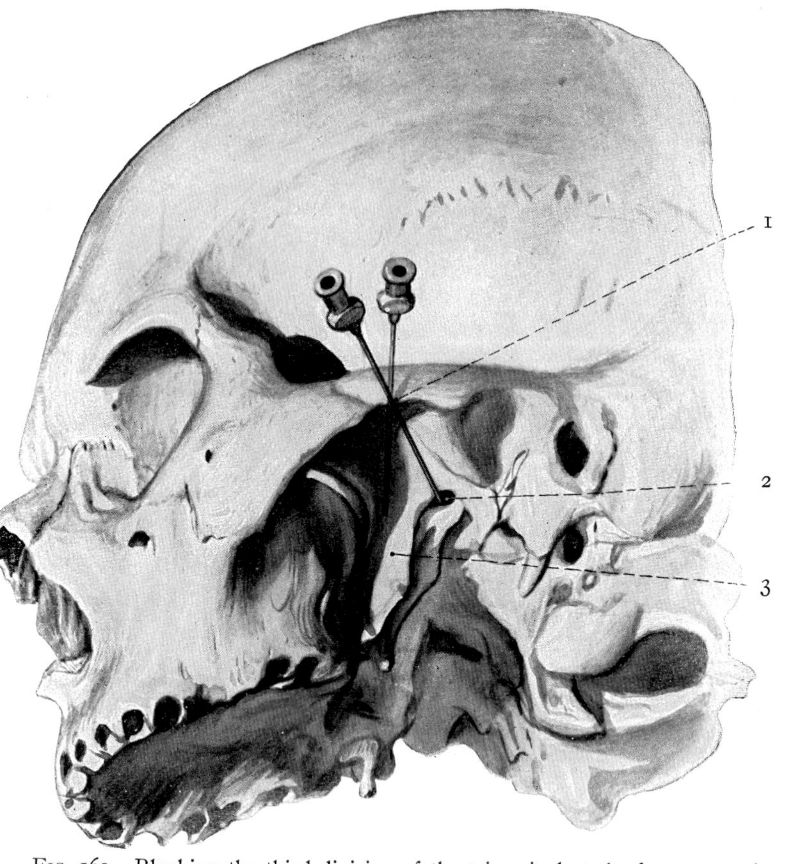

Fig. 169. Blocking the third division of the trigeminal at the foramen ovale. The needle, directed slightly forward, is inserted at the center of and under the zygomatic arch. It strikes at first the outer lamella of the pterygoid process, and is then slightly withdrawn and directed backward, where it enters the foramen ovale. (2) (The rubber marker which indicates the usual depth of insertion of the needle is not shown in the illustration.) 1. Insertion point at the middle of the lower border of the zygomatic process. 2. Foramen ovale. 3. Ext. lamina of the pterygoid process.

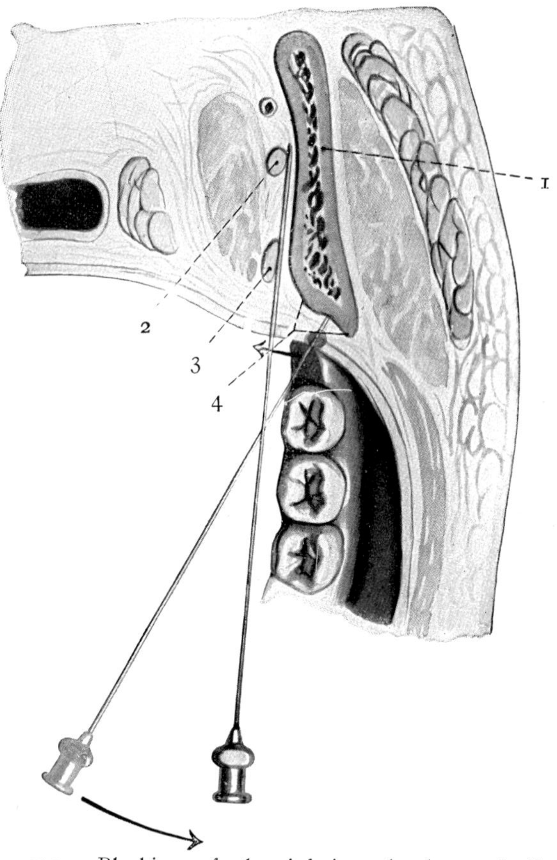

Fig. 170. Blocking of the inferior alveolar and lingual nerves. Horizontal section somewhat above and parallel to the masticatory surface of the lower teeth. The point of insertion of needle lies in the center of the retromolar trigon (Braun), which is bordered laterally by the margin of the coronoid process. The needle is directed from the opposite angle of the mouth and inserted into the trigon until it touches the mandible. It is slightly withdrawn, brought parallel to the teeth and then pushed backward along the bone until it comes in contact with the interior alveolar and lingual nerves. 1. Cross-section of the ascending ramus of the mandible. 2. Lingual nerve. 3. Inferior alveolar. 4. Retromolar trigon.

of the corresponding point of the opposite side. It is important to maintain the proper direction of the needle, and numerous devices have been employed to assist in this. At a depth of from 4 to 5 cm. the point of the needle strikes the outer lamella of the pterygoid process. At this point it is about 1 cm. from the foramen ovale (Fig. 169). The marker on the needle is placed 1 cm. from the skin. The needle is then withdrawn slightly and directed somewhat backwards. If the direction is correct the needle will miss the lamella of the pterygoid process and at the depth of the marker should enter the nerve. It may be necessary to insert it a few millimeters deeper, but no more. Five cubic centimeters of a 2 percent solution of novocain are then injected. For trigeminal neuralgia 2 cc. of absolute alcohol are injected.

The **Combined Injection of the Alveolar and Lingual Nerves on the Mandible.** The combined blocking of the inferior alveolar and lingual nerves which supply the mandible and tongue is carried out on the medial aspect of the ascending ramus of the mandible according to Braun's technic. A line of the anæsthetizing solution is placed just above the lingula and obliquely over the nerves (Fig. 172).

A long needle is used so that the syringe attached to it remains outside of the oral cavity. With the mouth open one palpates on the ascending ramus of the mandible, about 1 cm. lateral to and behind the last molar, a sharp bony ridge, the margin of the coronoid process. One half centimeter medial and posterior to this lies a second less prominent ridge (Figs. 170 and 171). These ridges enclose a small triangle of mucous membrane to which Braun has given the name of the retromolar trigon. One must observe continuously two things: first, the needle must remain parallel to a plane drawn through the crowns of the lower teeth, which plane in a sitting patient deviates more and more from the horizontal the wider the patient opens the mouth; secondly, the external extremity of the needle must always lie at the opposite angle of the mouth, so that the imaginary prolongation of the needle passes through the mastoid process of the side to be injected. In this way only can the needle point remain in constant bony contact with the slightly laterally directed mandible.

While the patient holds his mouth wide open (Fig. 171) the needle is inserted, keeping in mind the above directions, 1 cm. above the masticatory surface of the last molar in the center of the retromolar trigon. It should strike bone immediately under the mucous membrane, otherwise the point of insertion has not been correct. Frequently this is too far medially. The needle is carried further along the medial aspect of the mandible (Fig. 170), the bone being felt continually. As soon as the medial margin of the trigon is passed, the needle suddenly passes into the tissues. The external portion of the needle should then be carried to the opposite angle of the mouth so that the point again comes in contact with the bone. While the needle is being inserted and withdrawn (a distance of 2 to 3 cm.) 5 cc. of a 2 percent solution of novocain are injected.

(B) BLOCKING OF THE SUPERIOR LARYNGEAL NERVE

Injection of the superior laryngeal nerve causes anæsthesia of the larynx and the epiglottis. With the left index finger on the greater cornu of the

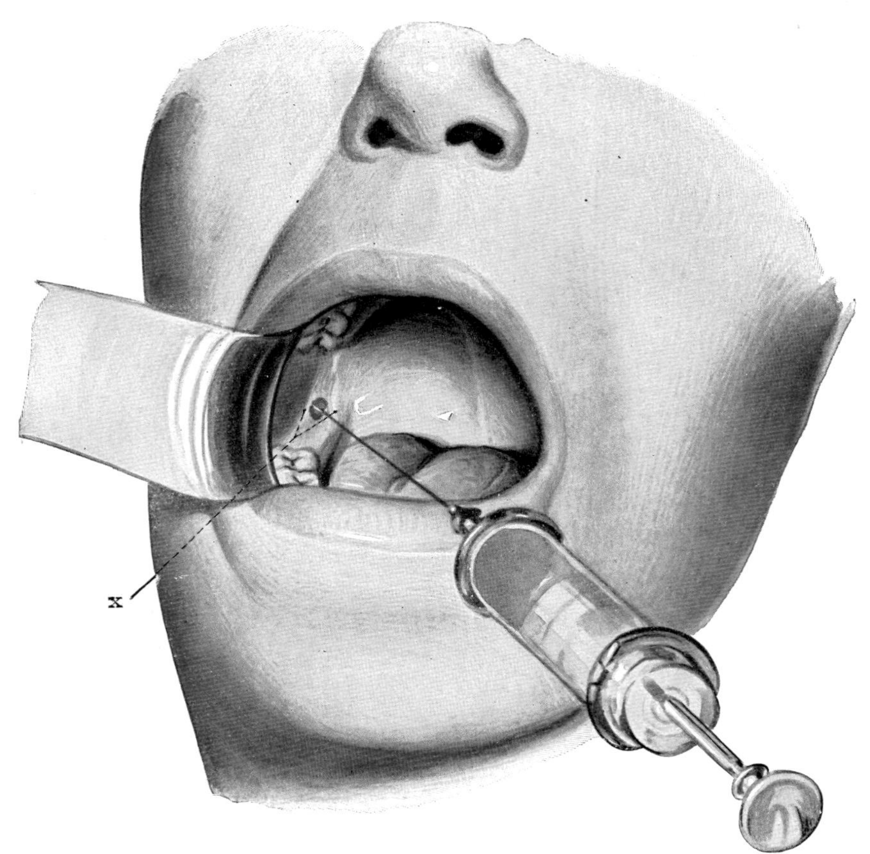

Fig. 171. Position of syringe in blocking the inferior alveolar and lingual nerves. The needle is inserted in the region of the retromolar trigon as illustrated in figure 170.

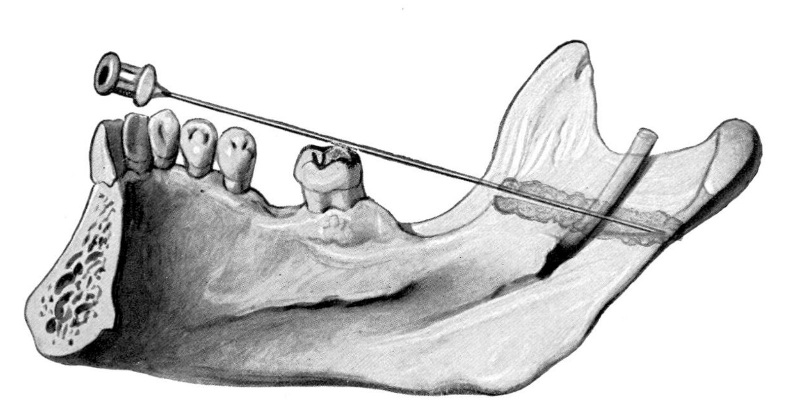

Fig. 172. Blocking the inferior alveolar nerve. The illustration shows the type of infiltration that results from injection of the solution while the needle is being carried backwards.

hyoid bone, a needle is inserted in the midline between the superior laryngeal margin and the hyoid bone and is carried laterally through the thyrohyoid ligament which offers considerable resistance, towards the cornu of the hyoid bone. While the area is being traversed 5 c.c. of a 1 percent solution of novocain is injected (Fig. 173). The procedure is repeated, on the opposite side, from the same point of insertion of the needle.

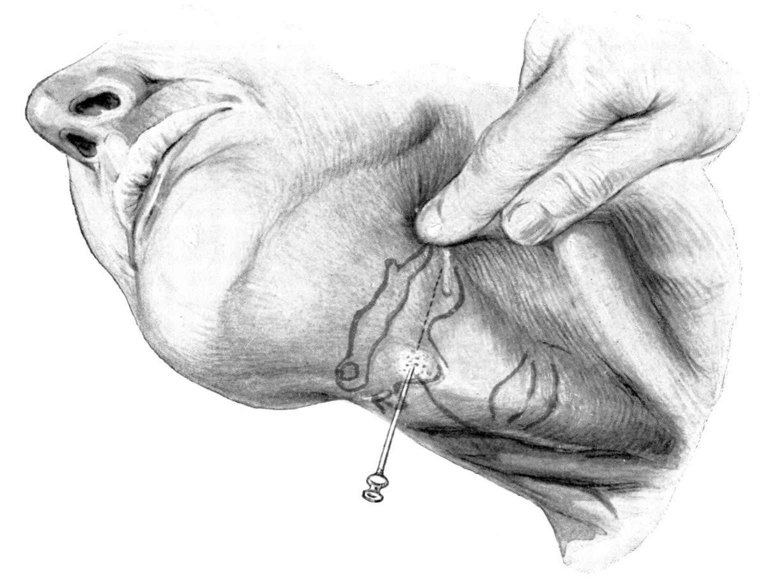

FIG. 173. Blocking the superior laryngeal nerve. The needle is inserted in the midline between the larynx and hyoid bone through the thyrohyoid ligament and is then pushed against the great cornu of the hyoid bone, which can be ascertained by palpation with the index finger.

(C) BLOCKING THE SPINAL NERVES AND THE SYMPATHETIC NERVES

After the posterior root of the spinal nerve has formed the spinal ganglion and has united with the anterior root in the intervertebral foramen, the combined trunk gives off anteriorly a branch running to a ganglion of the sympathetic chain, and then divides into a posterior and an anterior branch (Fig. 174). The posterior branch need not be considered in conduction anæsthesia, because the regions of the neck and back supplied by it can be anæsthetized much more easily by infiltration anæsthesia. Only in the interruption of the **greater occipital nerve,** which ascends back of the base of the mastoid process toward the vertex, may this method of anæsthetization be of any use for the posterior branches. This may be accomplished by placing an oblique line of 1 percent novocain-adrenalin solution cranially across its place of exit. However, it is advisable to add to this infiltration of the solution around the field of operation.

Sympathetic rami do not come off from the cervical spinal roots, but these nerves receive communications from the sympathetic trunk which ascends from the thorax. The anæsthetization of the sympathetic nerves in the neck is not necessary in operations in this area, but for the complete elimination of pain in cervical operations it is necessary to block the anterior branches of the spinal nerves which unite to form the cervical plexus. In the chest and abdomen sensory nerve block is not sufficient. In these areas the somatic sensory (spinal) nerves supply the parietes and the sympathetic nerves supply the viscera. In these areas, therefore, the sympathetic nerves carry the pain stimuli. Both nervous systems must be interrupted at the same time, if one desires to operate painlessly under local anæsthesia within the body.

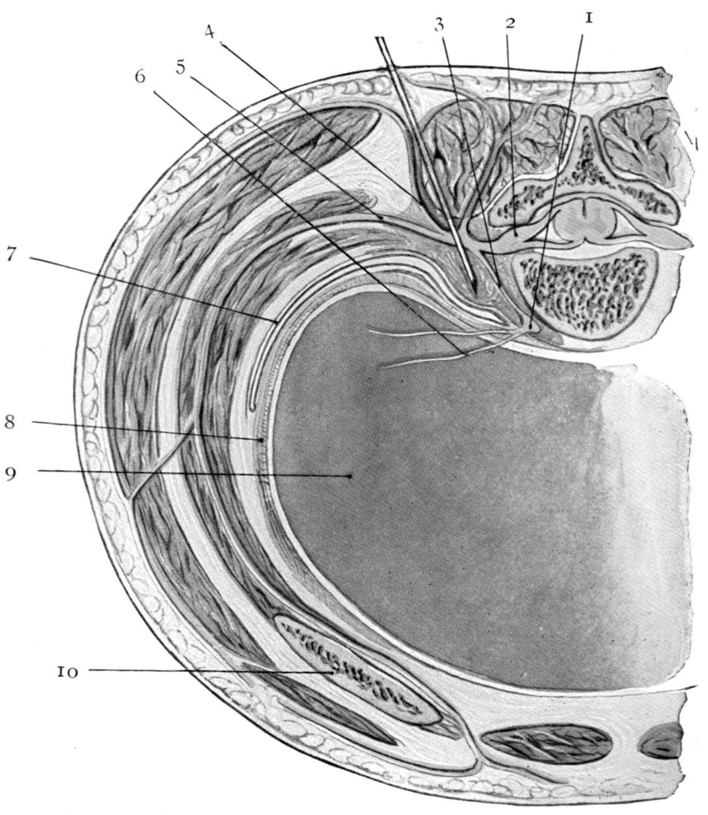

FIG. 174. Cross-section at the level of the eleventh dorsal vertebra (diagrammatic) showing the arrangement of the somatic nerves and the position of the needle and solution in paravertebral block. The needle is inserted through the back about 5 cm. from the midline at an angle of 60°. 1. Sympathetic ganglion. 2. Spinal ganglion. 3. Ramus communicans. 4. Posterior branch of a spinal nerve. 5. Anterior branch of a spinal nerve. 6. Sympathetic visceral branch. 7. Pleura. 8. Diaphragm. 9. Liver. 10. Rib.

In the thorax blocking of the nerves supplying the pleura and lung is without any great practical significance, since nearly all intrathoracic operations require general anæsthesia. Injury to the pleura, and pulling on the root of the lung or compression of it cause dyspnea and reflex inhibition of the heart's action and of respiration. Furthermore, opening of the free pleural cavity for other than the drainage of purulent or ascitic collections is fraught with danger unless positive pressure is used. Hence local anæsthesia is applicable only in operations on the chest wall, and conduction anæsthesia is used in this area for its effect on the spinal nerves. (White has recently described the method whereby paravertebral nerve block with alcohol in this area can be used for the relief of the pain of angina pectoris. I. S. R.)

The blocking of the sympathetic pathways is of importance chiefly in abdominal operations. If it is desired to carry out intra-abdominal operations painlessly under local anæsthesia, both the spinal nerves and the sympathetic nerves must be interrupted. The interruption of both systems can be accomplished in common at a site central to the nervus communicans, or separately in two places peripheral to the ramus communicans (Fig. 174). Since the anæsthetic which affects both systems simultaneously is injected just lateral to the vertebral column, it is designated as **paravertebral nerve block.**

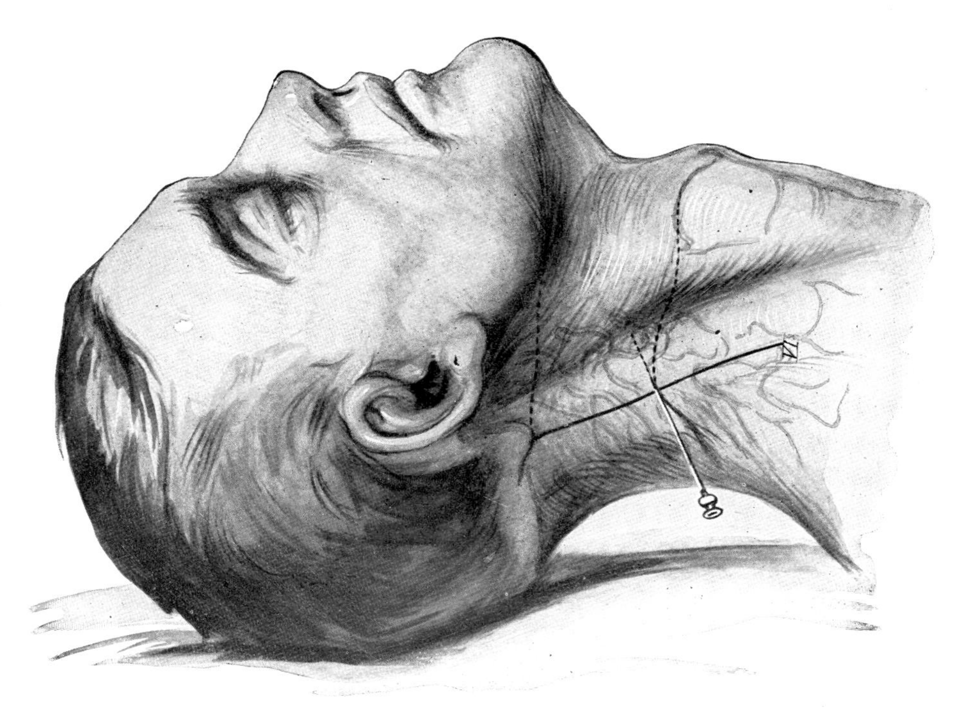

Fig. 175. Point of insertion of the needle for blocking the anterior branches of the third and fourth cervical nerves. The point lies in the middle of a line connecting the lower margin of the mastoid process with the carotid tubercle on the transverse process of the sixth cervical vertebra.

If the splanchnics alone are blocked, the abdominal wall must be injected with local anæsthesia at the site of the incision, or general anæsthesia can be used and paravertebral nerve block used merely to prevent visceral stimuli from reaching the cerebrum. The nerves of the anterior abdominal wall can be blocked and the intra-abdominal portion of the operation carried out under general anæsthesia or analgesia, since the visceral stimulus for pain is tension and mere handling or cutting of the viscera do not in themselves produce pain. The disadvantages of either method alone can be overcome by combining local and general anæsthesia in operative procedures.

(1) Anterior Spinal Nerve Block in the Neck

The nerves forming the cervical plexus, originate from the anterior divisions of the 2nd, 3rd, and 4th cervical nerves. These can be blocked on either side, with a single injection, by injecting an anæsthetic in front of the transverse processes of the 3rd and 4th cervical vertebræ. The point of insertion of the needle is determined according to the following scheme (Fig.

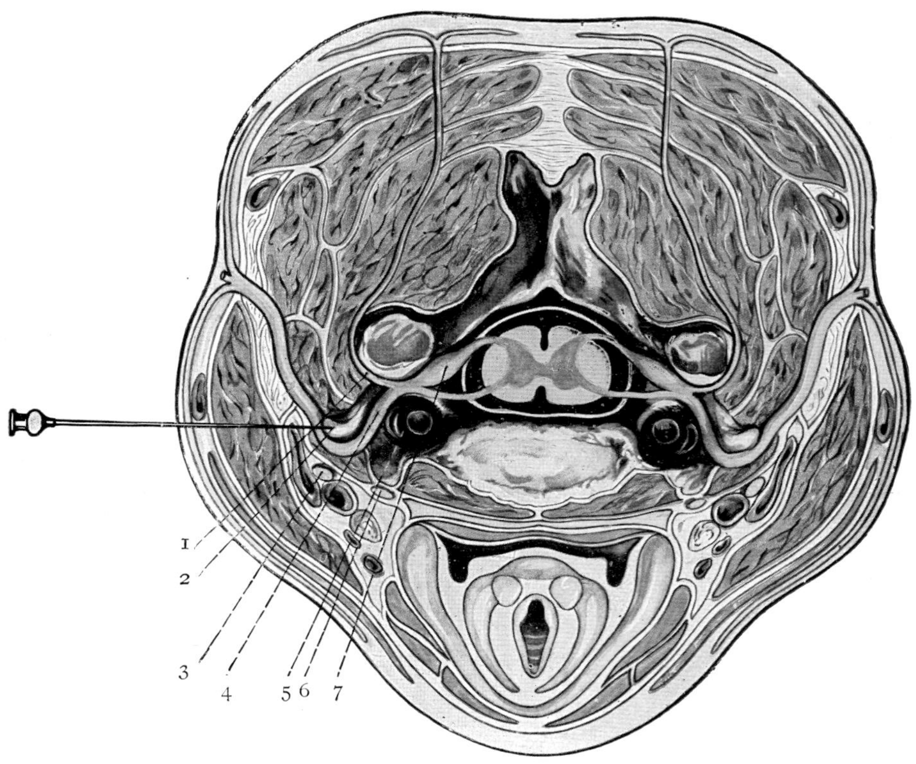

Fig. 176. Blocking the anterior branch of a cervical spinal nerve. Cross-section at the level of the third cervical vertebra (Härtel). The needle is carried through the sternocleido-mastoid muscle to the transverse process, where it meets the anterior branch of the spinal nerve. 1. Posterior branch of the spinal nerve. 2. Transverse process of the third cervical vertebra. 3. Vagus nerve. 4. Anterior branch of spinal nerve. 5. Vertebral artery. 6. Cervical sympathetic. 7. Spinal ganglion.

175). A line is drawn from the posterior margin of the mastoid process to the transverse process of the 6th cervical vertebra (carotid tubercle). This is approximately the line of the tips of the transverse processes. The point of insertion of the needle lies in the center of this line. If the head is extended the mid-point of a line joining the lower margin of the angle of the mandible and the upper margin of the thyroid cartilage may be taken as the point of insertion of the needle. If at this point the relaxed sternocleido-mastoid muscle is pushed forward, one can feel fairly close under the skin the transverse processes of the 3rd and 4th cervical vertebræ, if the patient's neck is not too thick. With the head slightly flexed and turned toward the opposite side, the needle is inserted through the sternocleidomastoid muscle, perpendicular to the adjacent transverse process, which should be reached at a slight depth (Fig. 176). The transverse process must be felt. The needle must not be carried in front of the transverse process, since in the latter area the vertebral artery, the great vessels of the neck, or the vagus nerve may be encountered. It is better to keep the point of the needle slightly behind the tip of the process. The dural sac of the cord may even be punctured with grave sequelæ. If after attempted aspiration no blood or cerebrospinal fluid is recovered the injection should be carefully begun. A 0.5 percent novocain-adrenalin solution is used.

After the injection of about 20 cc., the needle is withdrawn slightly and is then carried obliquely upward towards the head, but with no change in the direction. When the next transverse process is felt 20 cc. are again injected and the same procedure is repeated once more after carrying the needle obliquely downward towards the trunk. By this means one obtains anæsthesia in a few minutes of the antero-lateral soft parts of the neck. However I always inject subcutaneously some of the solution around the area of operation. In operations that extend beyond the midline the injection is done bilaterally.

Simple infiltration block anæsthesia permits one as a rule to carry out the majority of cervical operations painlessly. Since a number of catastrophies have followed the use of paravertebral cervical nerve block, I rarely use this method for cervical operations.

(2) Anterior Spinal Nerve Block (Intercostal Nerves)

Block Adjacent to the Vertebral Column. It must now be evident that blocking the anterior spinal nerves is sufficient to permit of painless operations on the thoracic or abdominal wall. Since every intercostal nerve supplies only a narrow area of the chest wall, or chest and abdominal walls, and in this area is not absolutely uniform in its course and extent, and since, furthermore, the individual nerves overlap in their distribution, it is necessary even for limited operations to interrupt more than one nerve. It may prove necessary in extensive operations to have as many as 20 injection points. Block anæsthesia in such an operation requires a great deal of time and attention, and causes the patient considerable discomfort. It requires the introduction of large quantities of an anæsthetic, and the failure to block properly a single nerve may mar the success of the entire procedure. Therefore, this form of anæsthesia is not ideal.

I use Braun's method for blocking the intercostal nerves without the rami communicantes (Fig. 177): The patient is placed in the sitting position with the body inclined forward and with the arms crossed and hanging down between the legs so as to separate the scapulæ as much as possible. A skin wheal is made 5 cm. distant from the spinous process of either the first or twelfth thoracic vertebra. With a long needle a narrow strip of skin parallel to the spinous processes at this distance is anæsthetized with 0.5 percent novocain-adrenalin solution. The lower border of a rib lies at a distance of 5 cm. from the midline, exactly at the level of the corresponding spinous process. If it is desired to interrupt the first intercostal nerve also, a 6 cm.

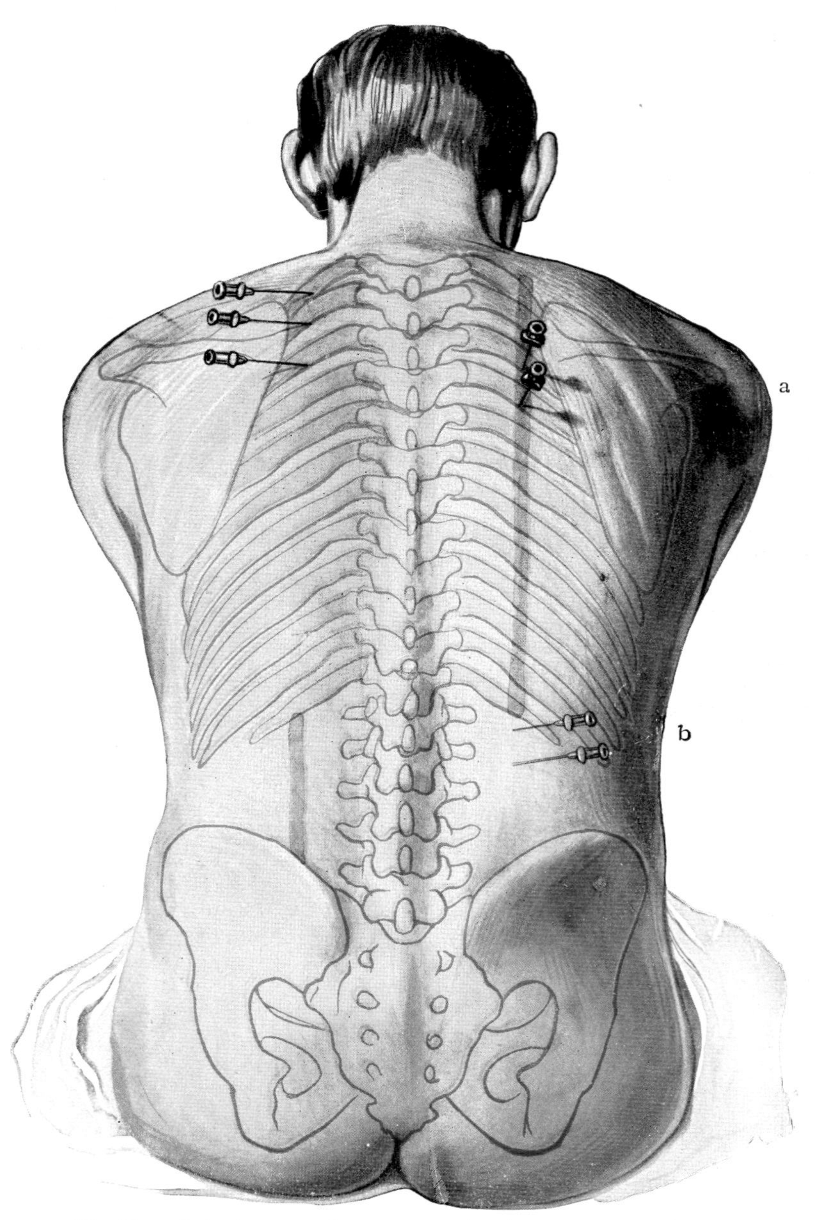

FIG. 177. Blocking of the intercostal nerves. a. A subcutaneous wheal, or series of wheals, is made five centimeters from the midline of the back. The needle is inserted vertically through this area at the desired height until it comes in contact with the lower border of the rib. It is slightly withdrawn, pointed caudally and then pushed one centimeter further. In this manner each intercostal space can be injected.

b. Paravertebral nerve block. The needle is inserted as above and then directed at an angle of 60° in the direction of the vertebral column.

needle is inserted vertically in the area of the infiltration-strip at the level of the 1st thoracic spinous process. The point of the needle should strike the first rib if the needle has been properly inserted. When the rib is felt the point is directed under the lower border of the rib, and a small amount of the anæsthetic solution is injected so as to push away the parietal pleura. The needle is then directed medially and caudally 0.5 to 1 cm. and the intercostal space is saturated with 15 cc. of a 0.5 percent novocain-adrenalin solution. While this needle remains inserted, a second needle is inserted about 3 cm. further caudally (the exact measure adjusts itself to the distance between the spinous processes), in the same manner, and 15 cc. of novocain-adrenalin solution are injected again. When this has been done the first needle is removed while the second remains in place, and the 3rd intercostal space is injected with the former. This procedure is repeated until the required number of intercostal spaces have been blocked.

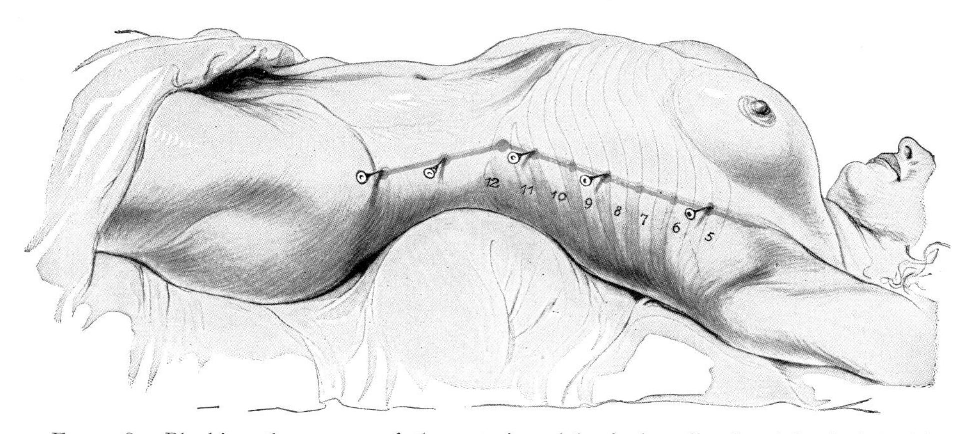

FIG. 178. Blocking the nerves of the anterior abdominal wall. In abdominal incisions above the umbilicus it is necessary to block the 5th to the 11th intercostal nerves; for abdominal incisions below the umbilicus it is necessary to block the nerves between the 11th rib and the crest of the ilium.

If one wishes to start with the 12th intercostal nerve, the 12th rib, which is always palpable laterally, is outlined. The point where this line crosses the area of skin infiltration is taken as the point for insertion of the needle. In a similar manner the injection can proceed upward. The sympathetic nerves are encountered in this type of injection (Fig. 174).

In operations on the upper part of the thorax, it is important to block the supraclavicular nerves in addition to the upper intercostal nerves. This can be done with a subcutaneous infiltration of a 0.5 percent solution of novocain-adrenalin. The nerves run from the back along the spine of the scapula over the shoulder and along the clavicle to the sternum.

For abdominal incisions above the umbilicus block of the 5th to the 12th intercostals is sufficient; for abdominal incisions below the umbilicus the 8th to the 12th intercostal nerves and the ilio-hypogastric and ilio-inguinal nerves should be blocked; while for abdominal incisions above and below the umbilicus it is necessary to interrupt all of these twenty nerves, so that twenty injections are necessary.

Block of the Spinal Nerves at a Distance from the Vertebral Column

Blocking the Nerves of the Abdominal Wall. If it is desired to anæsthetize the anterior abdominal wall only, which of course suffices for most abdominal wall incisions, the intercostal nerves can be more easily injected along the lateral chest wall. Here the ribs are more easily palpated and distinguished (Fig. 178).

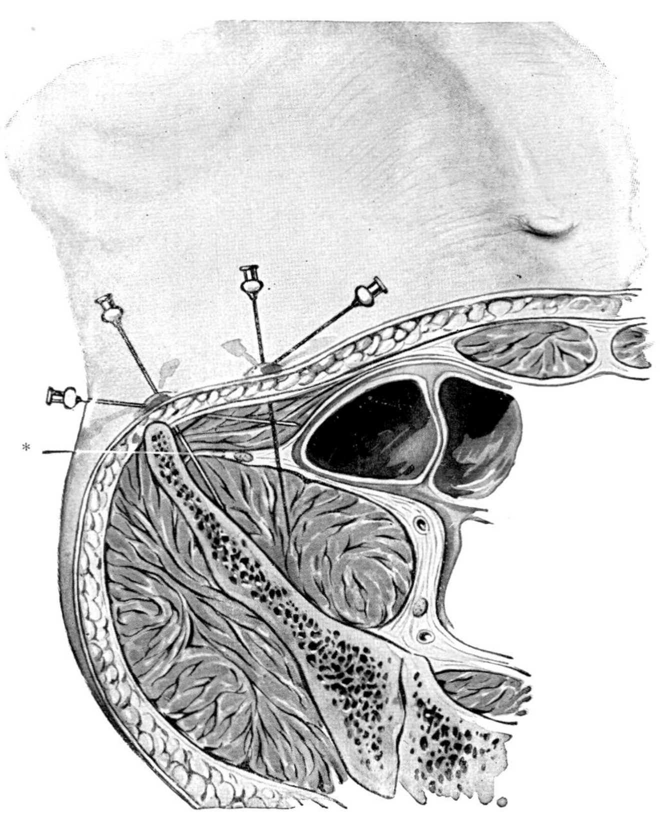

FIG. 179. Blocking of the ilio-hypogastric* and ilio-inguinal nerves The infiltration of the soft parts containing the nerves is done in a fan-like area through a puncture close to the anterior superior iliac spine (Härtel) or by a puncture 3 cm. medial to this (Braun).

The upper extremity of the patient, who lies on his back, is placed above his head. Just above the tip of the 12th rib and under the margin of the 11th rib lies the first point for insertion of the needle. The second point of insertion of the needle for blocking the nerves supplying the abdominal wall below the umbilicus lies on the highest part of the crest of the ilium. The fairly thick muscle-mass and the subcutaneous tissues between these two points, are infiltrated with at least 50 cc. of a 0.5 percent novocain-adrenalin solution. For abdominal incisions above the umbilicus, the intercostal nerves lying above the first point of injection are injected. The line of injection extends from the tip of the twelfth rib to the anterior axillary fold. Ten cubic centimeters of a 0.5 per cent novocain-adrenalin solution are injected under each rib margin. The injection continues upward and should include the 5th intercostal nerve. The blocking of all the intercostal nerves lying between the fifth rib and the ilium on both sides and the ilio-inguinal and ilio-hypogastric nerves will result in a loss of sensation on the entire anterior abdominal wall.

Block of the ilio-hypogastric and the ilio-inguinal nerves alone has a special significance because of the frequency of operations for inguinal herniæ under local anæsthesia. Since the upper end of the incision does not extend above the anterior superior iliac spine, the interruption of these two nerves suffices.

The nerves run, in the field of the operation, in the direction of the fibers of the external oblique muscle. They pass towards the external inguinal ring, piercing the transversalis, interior oblique and external oblique muscles diagonally, from within out. For blocking these nerves, the cross-section of the muscles at the level of the anterior superior spine is saturated thoroughly with the anæsthetizing solution (Fig. 179). The muscles are either saturated from an insertion point placed at the level of the anterior superior iliac spine in a fan shaped area toward the umbilicus (Härtel), or they are saturated through an insertion point placed three fingers breadth medial to and in a fan shaped area toward the spine (Braun). In both of these methods the needle is first inserted perpendicularly so as to infiltrate the muscles of the abdominal wall in this area. After this has been done the needle is withdrawn somewhat and pointed more superficially so as to infiltrate successive levels. Several shifts of the needle may be necessary, and in Braun's method the point of the needle should eventually touch the iliac bone. Finally the needle is directed toward the median line under the external oblique aponeurosis where in a fan shaped area the solution is deposited. During each shift in direction of the needle 10 cc. of a 0.5 percent novocain-adrenalin solution are injected. In Härtel's procedure, which I prefer, the needle is at first inserted adjacent to the spine, at which time the needle is carried deep. It is then inserted in subcutaneous tissue about 5 cm. medially and from both of the points of insertion the surrounding tissues are infiltrated.

In addition to the foregoing should local anæsthesia be chosen for the operation for inguinal hernia circuminjection is necessary. The injection is done in the following manner (Fig. 180). A point (point 1), somewhat above the upper end of the planned skin incision, and which is approximately the point of insertion for Braun's conduction anæsthesia, is marked. Then two points are made on either side of the site where the spermatic cord crosses the horizontal ramus of the pubis (points 2 and 3). After this the ilio-hypogastric and ilio-inguinal nerves are blocked as described by Härtel (Fig. 179). Then we join point 1 with point 2 and with point 3, by infiltrating the local anæsthetic subcutaneously in narrow strips. A 0.5 percent novocain-adrenalin solution is used. In the area of circuminjection a number of injections under the external oblique aponeurosis are made at suitable intervals after inserting the needle vertically through the subcutaneous tissues. In reducible herniæ we place from points 2 and 3, two more subcutaneous strips of anæsthesia toward the scrotum. In irreducible herniæ the entire scrotum is circuminjected at its base, from points 2 and 3, with a 0.5

percent novocain-adrenalin solution, as will be described under anæsthesia of the scrotum

Blocking the Nerves of the Spermatic Cord. After the method of Braun, a wheal is placed at the point where the spermatic cord leaves the horizontal ramus of the os pubis (Fig. 181). Through this wheal, the cord which is prevented from slipping away by grasping it between the thumb and index finger of the left hand, is injected. The needle is inserted at first

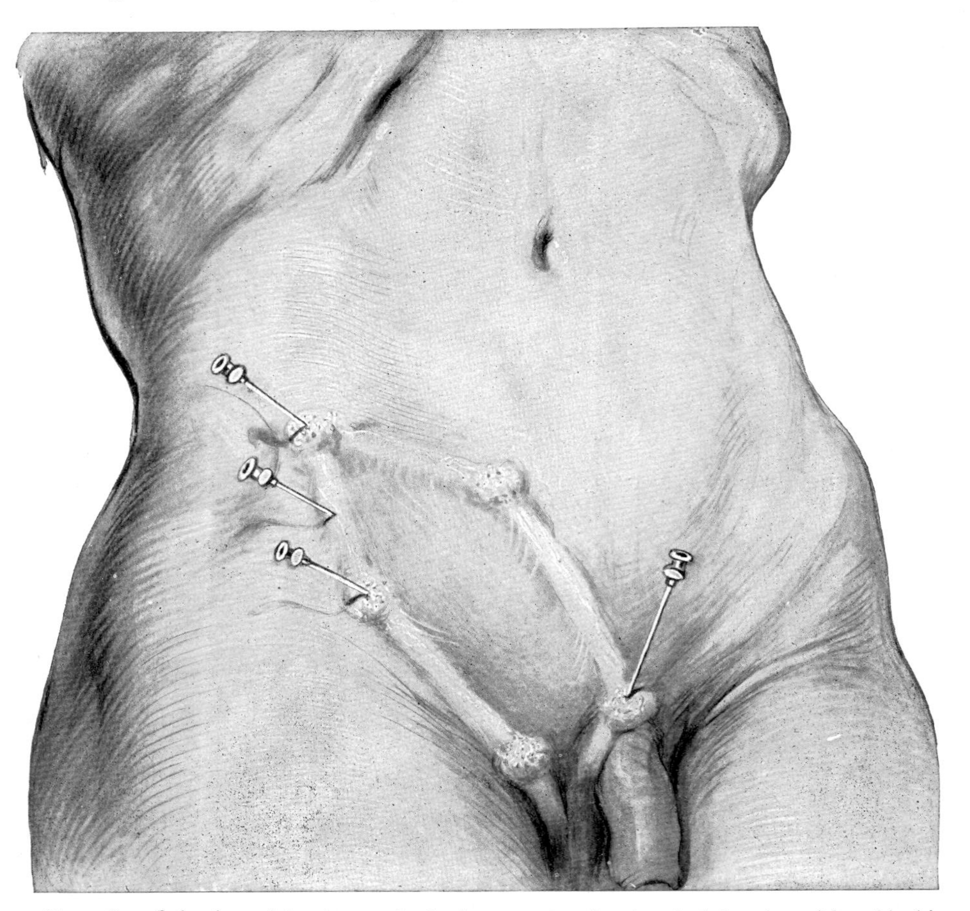

FIG. 180. Injection of local anæsthesia in operation for inguinal hernia. After blocking the ilio-hypogastric and ilio-inguinal nerves (figure 179) the field of operation is injected first subcutaneously and then under the aponeurosis of the external oblique.

perpendicular, and then to either side of the cord until the bone is felt. Each time 5 cc. of a 0.5 percent solution of novocain are injected. By this means the spermatic cord, the epididymis and the testis are rendered insensible to pain. Should the spermatic cord be followed further proximally, a little of the anæsthetizing solution is injected from the same place under the aponeurosis of the external abdominal oblique, in the inguinal canal.

Blocking the Nerves of the Scrotum. The line of attachment of the scrotum to the trunk is circuminjected with a 0.5 percent novocain-adrenalin solution. In fat individuals one must inject particularly thoroughly, infiltrating the fat as well as the several layers of the perineum (Fig. 182). It is not necessary to anæsthetize the penis if this is not desired. If it is desired to combine infiltration anæsthesia of the scrotum and penis with conduction

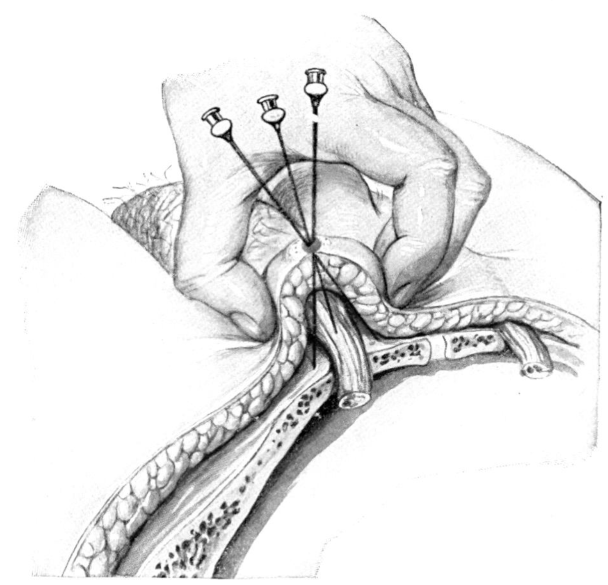

FIG. 181. Blocking the nerves of the spermatic cord. The point of insertion of the needle which is located where the spermatic cord crosses the horizontal ramus of pubis is grasped with the fingers and the anæsthetic is injected in several directions as illustrated.

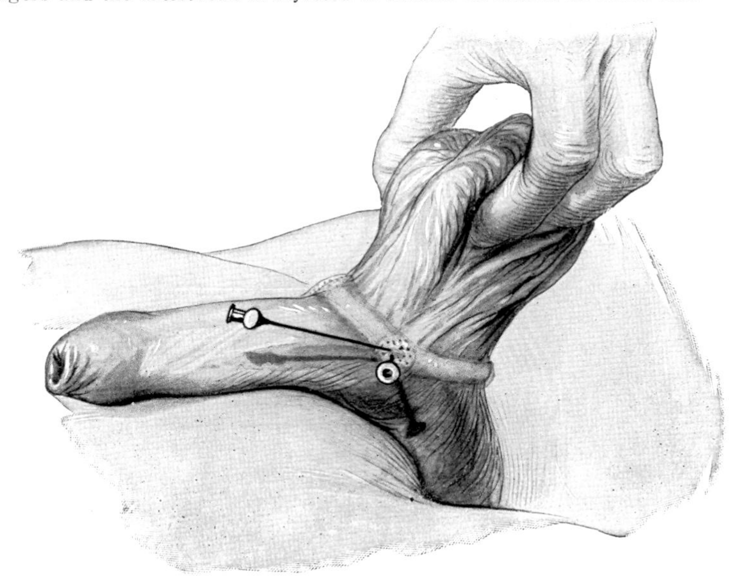

FIG. 182. Line of injection for scrotal anæsthesia.

anæsthesia of both spermatic cords, we insert the needle as shown previously for the injection of the nerves of the spermatic cord and use these entrance points for the block of the scrotum. The insertion points of both sides are then connected by an infiltration strip above the penis.

Blocking the Nerves of the Penis. Because of the occasionally observed disturbances which have occurred following circular infiltration of the shaft of the penis, Braun has advised that the anæsthetic solution be injected in the region of the base of the penis (Fig. 183). A point of insertion is marked on the side of the root of the penis, at the place where the spermatic cord crosses the os pubis.

While the penis is stretched vertically upward, the base of the penis is deeply infiltrated from the points where the corpora spongiosum of each side come out from under the symphysis and attach themselves to the shaft of the penis. The diagram for injection resembles a fan on each side beginning at the suspensory ligament of the penis and continuing to the insertion of the scrotum. Then a subcutaneous ring of anæsthetic solution is placed around the base of the penis from both points of insertion. In all some 100 cc. of a 0.5 percent novocain-adrenalin solution are needed.

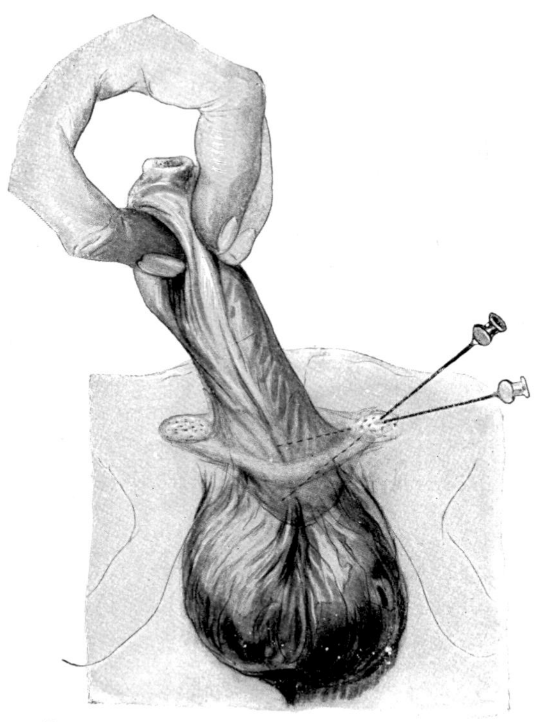

FIG. 183. Blocking the nerves at the base of the penis. The anæsthetizing solution is injected in a fan-shaped area on either side, from the point where the spermatic cord crosses the os pubis.

(3) Paravertebral Nerve Block. (Intercostal and Sympathetic Nerves.) (Sellheim, Läwen)

Paravertebral anæsthesia (Fig. 174) in which the anterior spinal nerves are interrupted central to the sympathetic ramus communicans, gives anæsthesia not only of the abdominal wall but also of the abdominal viscera. This type of anæsthesia has been widely used for abdominal operations. Each anterior spinal nerve lies ventral to the corresponding rib. For blocking the nerves a technic somewhat different from that described for intercostal injection is necessary. A narrow strip of skin about 5 cm. from the spinous processes, and for a distance necessary for the number of nerves to be blocked, is anæsthetized. This is similar to intercostal nerve block. The needle is inserted through this area on to the corresponding rib. However, instead of carrying the needle parallel to the median plane but slightly caudally around the rib, as in intercostal nerve block, it is withdrawn slightly and directed toward the vertebral column at an angle of 60° with the tissues of the back (Fig. 174). In this direction it is directed about 2 cm. along the lower rib margin. The point of the needle comes to rest on the lower border of the ventral aspect of the rib, just beyond the angle and between this and the pleura. The needle may come in contact with the transverse process. If this occurs its angle is to be increased so that it may pass anterior to it. During the insertion of the needle, after the rib is reached, 0.5 percent novocain-adrenalin solution should be injected continuously, in order to separate the pleura from the inner surface of the rib so as to prevent piercing it. In all, 20 cc. of the solution are injected for each nerve. While the first needle remains in position, the procedure is repeated in the next intercostal space (Fig. 174), so that gradually the injections are completed. With proper technic, the injected solution finally results in a continuous subpleural pool ventral to the ribs, so that the space lying between the pleura and ribs, through which the intercostal nerves pass, is completely saturated.

(4) Simple Block of the Sympathetic Nerves in the Abdomen

The sensory pain perceiving paths running in the sympathetic trunk for the viscera of the upper abdomen, the liver, the gallbladder, the stomach, the duodenum, the pancreas, the spleen, the upper part of the small intestine and the transverse colon, unite at the level of the origin of the celiac artery to form the celiac plexus and the paired celiac ganglia. The centripetal fibers of these ganglia run for the most part in the major and minor splanchnic nerves, which enter the abdomen through the diaphragm in the immediate vicinity of the aorta. If one can successfully introduce a sufficient quantity of an anæsthetic solution in the region of these nerves, the structures which they supply become insensible. The injection can be made through a needle inserted through the soft parts of the back (dorsal or Kappis' route), or, in the manner which I always use, from the front after opening the abdominal cavity (ventral or Braun's route) (Fig. 184).

Splanchnic Anæsthesia by the Dorsal Route (Kappis). The patient lies on his side. The point of insertion of the needle is located on each side, 7 cm. distant from the midline, and under the margin of the twelfth rib. A 12 cm. long needle is inserted diagonally forward and medially in the direction of the body of the 1st lumbar vertebra (Fig. 184). After the vertebral body has been reached, one feels along its lateral wall, until the needle slides past it. After the last bony resistance has been felt the needle is carried another centimeter deeper. Its point lies now just above and in front of the 1st lumbar vertebra adjacent to the insertion of the diaphragm on the vertebral column and in the immediate proximity of the splanchnic nerves. Kappis injects about 30 cc of a 1 percent novocain-adrenalin solution at this level and then carries the needle a little more caudally along the lateral surface of the vertebra and injects 20 cc. more. The procedure is repeated on the opposite side. One can distribute the solution solely on the sides of the first lumbar vertebra, inject there 70 to 80 cc. of a 0.5 percent solution of novocain-adrenalin.

Following this method of inducing splanchnic anæsthesia, collapse and isolated deaths have occurred. I prefer the ventral route.

Splanchnic Anæsthesia by the Ventral Route (Braun). After the abdominal cavity has been opened through a midline incision above the umbilicus under local or preferably general anæsthesia (infiltrating the sides of the incision with 0.5 percent novocain), the left lobe of the liver is lifted very gently with a retractor, and the stomach retracted downwards by making tension on the lesser omentum. The operator palpates with the left index finger the pulsating aorta on the first lumbar vertebra which lies at the level of the ensiform process (Figs. 184 and 185). The index finger is placed firmly in the center of the 1st lumbar vertebra, which pushes the aorta to the left. With the right hand, a 12 cm. long needle is introduced along the left index finger to its point of contact with the vertebral body. It should strike bone directly after penetrating the thin posterior peritoneum, otherwise the path of insertion of the needle is incorrect.

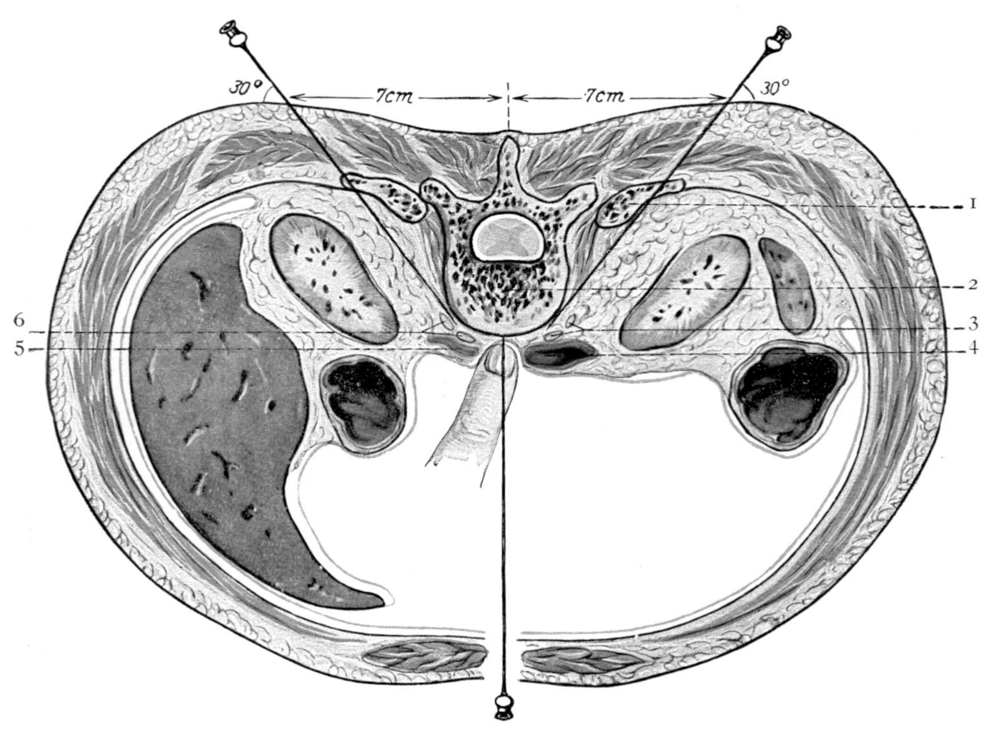

Fig. 184. Splanchnic nerve block. Cross-section at the level of the first lumbar vertebra. (a) Method of Kappis. The needle is inserted 7 cm. from the midline and carried forward into the retroperitoneal space in touch with the body of the vertebra. (b) Braun's method. After the completion of the medial abdominal incision the point of the left index finger is placed on the center of the first lumbar vertebra by holding apart the viscera and along it the cannula is inserted to the bone between aorta and inferior vena cava. 1. Cross-section of rib. 2. Cross-section of lumbar vertebra. 3. Left splanchnic nerves. 4. Aorta. 5. Vena cava. 6. Right splanchnic nerves.

After one has convinced himself that a vessel has not been punctured, the syringe is attached and the tissues saturated with 100 cc. of a 0.5 percent novocain-adrenalin solution. The anæsthesia occurs within a few minutes. Although failures occur also with this method, Braun has had no catastrophes nor have I.

(5) Parasacral Conduction Anæsthesia (Braun)

Parasacral conduction anæsthesia is merely paravertebral nerve block of the nerves emerging through the sacral foramina. By this block it is possible to eliminate pain from the perineum, rectum, urethra, bladder, pelvic floor, scrotum (except its contents), the penis, prostate, and to an extent from the vagina, uterus and parametrium. The anæsthesia is free from danger, but is detailed, and in my experience somewhat uncertain. We use the method of Braun, which is as follows: With the patient in the lithotomy posi-

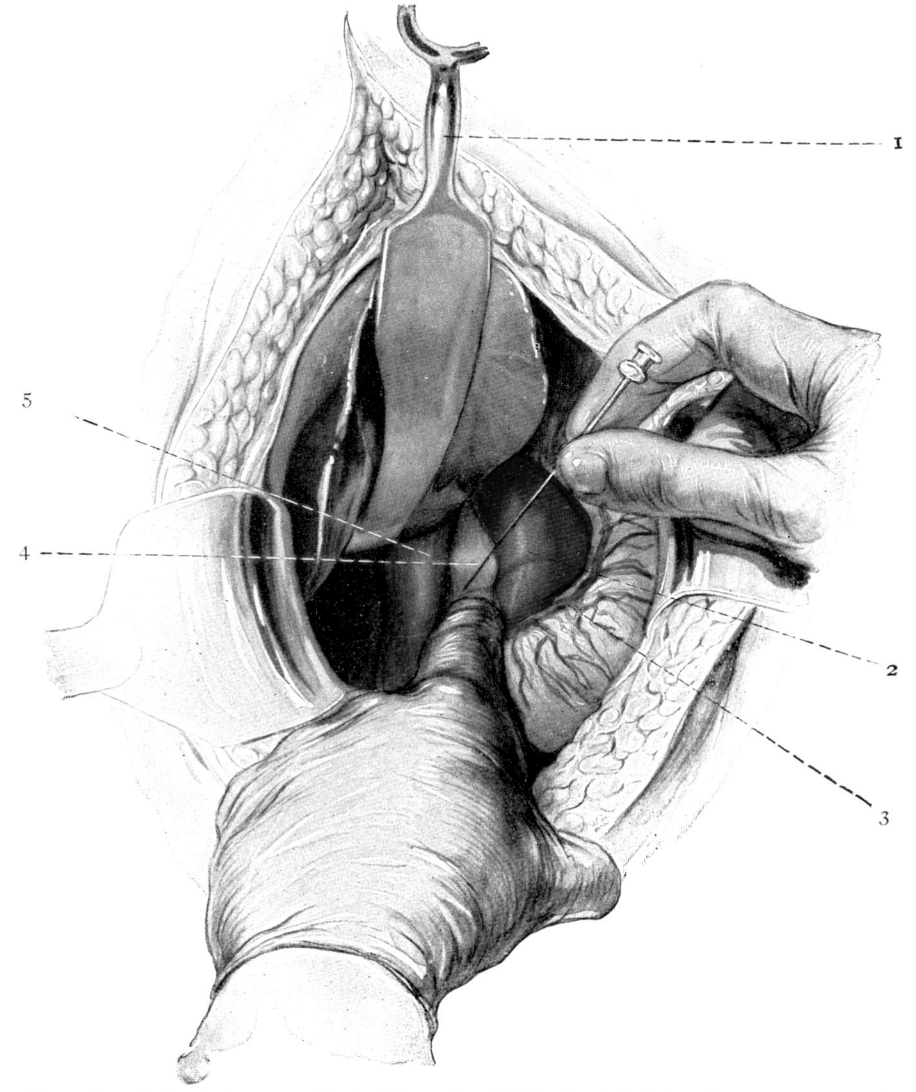

FIG. 185. Splanchnic nerve block (Braun). While the left index finger separates the inferior vena cava and the abdominal aorta at the level of the first lumbar vertebra the needle is pushed against the vertebra. 1. Retractor for retraction of the liver. 2. Aorta. 3. Stomach. 4. First lumbar vertebra. 5. Inferior vena cava.

tion, points are marked 1.5 to 2 cm. to the right and left of the tip of the coccyx. With a 12.5 cm. long needle inserted parallel to the sagittal plane, the point is carried to the lower border of the sacral bone (Fig. 186). The needle is pushed anterior to this border parallel to the sagittal plane along the arched anterior surface of the bone, for a distance of 6 or 7 cm. where in the region of the 2nd sacral foramen the needle again strikes bone. As the needle is slowly withdrawn, about 50 cc. of a 0.5 percent novocain-adrenalin solution are injected along the inner surface of the sacrum. The needle is then withdrawn until the point is in the subcutaneous tissue, it is then reinserted parallel to the sagittal plane, but the point is slightly more ventral, which directs it more toward the linea innominate, and the external portion of the

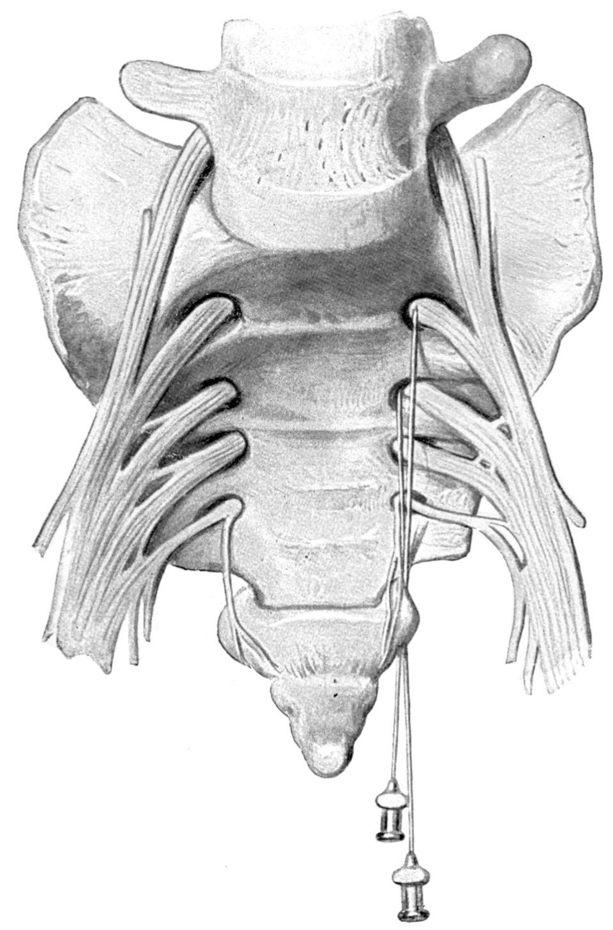

FIG. 186. Parasacral nerve block. The needle is inserted about 1.5 cm. from the tip of the coccyx. It is then slipped anterior to the lower border of the sacrum, parallel to the sagittal plane to the second sacral foramen. It is then slightly withdrawn and carried up to the first sacral foramen by changing the direction of the tip of the needle.

needle is slightly more dorsal. At a depth of from 9 to 10 cm. the needle strikes bone in the vicinity of the 1st sacral foramen. At this level about 30 cc. of a 0.5 percent novocain-adrenalin solution are injected. The same procedure is repeated on the other side. To block the superficial nerves of the coccygeal plexus, which supply the skin around the anus and perineum, a layer of the solution is laid down for a distance of about 5 cm. between the tip of the coccyx and anus, and a subcutaneous strip is infiltrated ventrally, parallel to the midline from the point of insertion of the needle to the top of the proposed skin incision.

(D) BLOCKING THE NERVES OF THE UPPER EXTREMITY

(1) Blocking the Brachial Plexus

In the upper extremity we have the happy situation of being able to deposit the anæsthetic in one place and thereby block the entire brachial plexus so that anæsthesia of the entire extremity is obtained. I find Kulenkampf's method satisfactory for this. The anæsthetizing solution is injected into the brachial plexus, just above the middle of the clavicle. At this point the plexus is close under the skin, and just lateral to the subclavian artery. The first rib at this point lies in approximately a sagittal direction, posteriorly it is above this plane, while anteriorly it is below it. Its wide surface just above the middle of the clavicle forms the floor of the region of operation. I adhere closely to Kulenkampf's technic as far as the injection is concerned, but I believe that it is better to have the patient in the recumbent position instead of having him sit erect. The head is turned to the opposite side and extended, a roll being placed under the shoulders.

In this position one sees, in very thin individuals, the plexus in the form of a series of cords in the supraclavicular fossa, so that one may inject directly into it. As a rule the plexus is not visible and must be sought with the point of the needle. The patient is instructed to say "Now," as soon as he notices tingling in the hand or forearm. The anæsthetizing solution should never be injected unless paresthesias are definitely perceived. The point of insertion of the needle is determined as follows. The pulsation of the subclavian artery is palpated above the clavicle. This point usually corresponds to the prolongation of the line of the external jugular vein, and it is marked with colored solution. As a rule it will correspond to the middle of the clavicle. About 0.5 cm. lateral to this a skin wheal is made and a small gauge needle 6 cm. long is slowly directed toward the spinous process of the 3rd thoracic vertebra (Figs. 187 and 188). The mistake is easily made, from fear of striking the artery, of inserting the needle too far laterally. The needle should be kept close to the artery, for the plexus lies directly against it, and puncture of the artery is not followed by any serious consequences, if a fine enough needle is used. The needle is carried further in the same direction, until tingling in the hand or forearm is observed or until the needle meets the first rib. If the latter occurs, the needle must be withdrawn and reinserted in another direction, usually closer to the artery. If distinct paresthesias set in and no blood runs out the needle, 15 cc. of a 4 percent novocain-adrenalin solution are injected without changing the position of the needle. The pulsation of the subclavian artery is much more noticeable after this injection. A few cubic centimeters of the solution are distributed slightly deeper and a few somewhat more superficially. After 30 minutes at the latest, a more or less impressing motor paralysis and a complete sensory paralysis of the upper extremity is observed, with the exception of the skin around the shoulder and the outer proximal third of the upper arm. If the operation extends to this area also, it is blocked by subcutaneous cir-

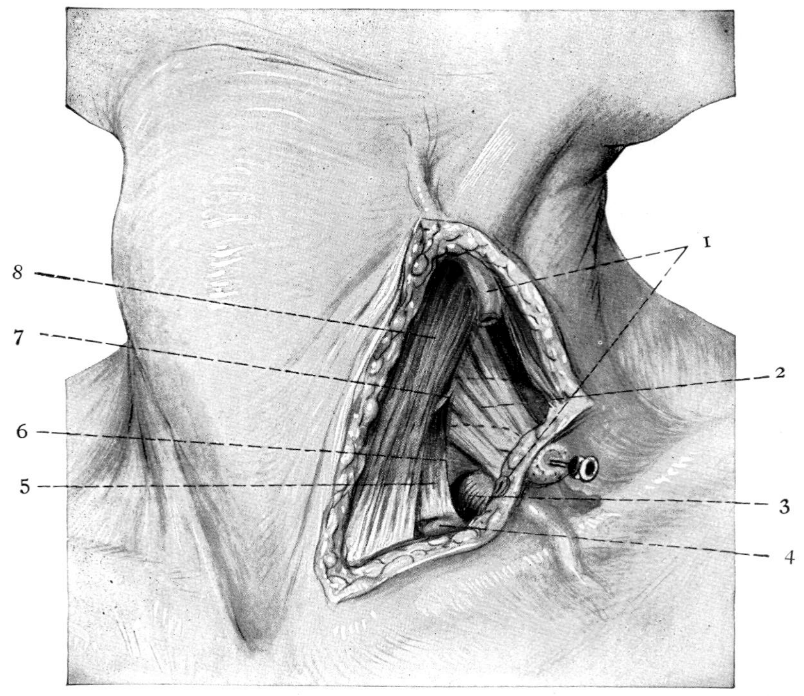

FIG. 187. Blocking the brachial plexus above the clavicle. The needle is inserted into the plexus just above the clavicle, lateral to the pulsation of the subclavian artery in the direction of the spinous process of the third thoracic vertebra. It is important to keep in mind the close relation of the subclavian artery, the pleura and the phrenic nerve. 1. Ext. jugular vein (severed). 2. Brachial plexus. 3. Subclavian artery. 4. Subclavian vein. 5. Anterior scalene muscle. 6. Pleura. 7. Phrenic nerve. 8. Sternocleidomastoid muscle.

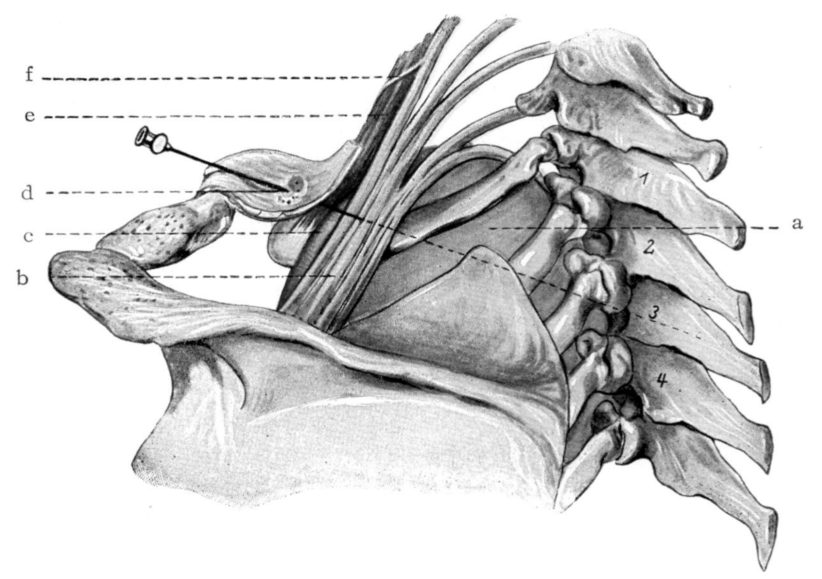

FIG. 188. Blocking the brachial plexus above the clavicle. The needle is introduced in the direction of the spinous process of the third thoracic vertebra. The relation of the pleura is important. a. Pleura. b. Brachial plexus. c. Subclavian artery. d. Point of insertion above the clavicle lateral to the pulsation of the subclavian artery. e. Anterior scalene muscle. f. Phrenic nerve.

cuminjection proximal and at right angles to the axis of the extremity. Although I do not, as a rule, use an Esmarch bandage for brachial plexus anæsthesia, I see no objection to the use of hyperemia, which many surgeons use for this anæsthesia.

In brachial plexus anæsthesia by this method there occurs regularly a transitory block of the phrenic nerve and with it paralysis of that half of the diaphragm, which is unnoticed and of no significance to the patient. The same applies to the frequently encountered sympathetic paralysis (Horner's symptom-complex). On the other hand, puncture of the pleura may give rise to very disagreeable symptoms, even to the state of collapse. The patient complains of severe pains in that side of the chest. In some cases an extensive pneumo-thorax may result, which may be fatal; in others the pain may be the result of a hemothorax. I am of the opinion that these unfortunate accidents are avoidable if the technic of the injection is good, and that they should not prevent one from using this method of anæsthesia which is so simple, and should be safe.

(2) Blocking the Ulnar Nerves at the Elbow

The little finger and the hypothenar eminence is made anæsthetic by blocking the ulnar nerve at the elbow. With the elbow-joint in extension, the nerve can be rolled in back of the median condyle with the palpating index-finger. It is held firmly with the thumb and index-finger of the left hand and a fine needle is inserted in it (Fig. 189). As soon as the characteristic tingling pain is experienced, 5 cc. of a 2 percent solution of novocain-adrenalin are injected.

(3) Blocking the Nerves of the Hand

For anæsthesia of the entire hand the following nerves must be blocked; (1) the trunk of the ulnar nerve, (2) the median nerve, and (3) the end-branches of the radial (musculo-spiral) nerve. The injections are preferably done at the level of the wrist (Fig. 190). The ulnar nerve is blocked by injecting 5 cc. of a 2 percent novocain-adrenalin solution on the radial and the under surface of the tendon of the flexor carpi ulnaris muscle a few centimeters proximal to its insertion in the pisiform bone. The needle is inserted on the radial side of the distinctly palpable tendon and the solution distributed on the radial side and under the tendon. The median nerve is sought just above the wrist, as the needle is inserted obliquely radially into the tissues on the ulnar side of the palmaris longus muscle, until paresthesias occur in the hand. Here also 5 cc. of a 2 percent novocain-adrenalin solution are injected. At the same level a subcutaneous ring of 0.5 percent novocain-adrenalin is placed around the forearm, to which is added a sub-fascial half-ring on the extensor side of the wrist. By this means, the cutaneous nerves, as well as the terminal branches of the radial (musculo-spiral) nerve are interrupted.

(4) Blocking Separate Portions of the Hand and of the Individual Fingers

The elimination of pain in parts of the hand together with the adjacent fingers is not true conduction anæsthesia inasmuch as the nerve block depends more on general circumjection than on systematic block of certain nerves. The block is obtained by infiltrating the anæsthetic solution in a very definite manner (Figs. 191, 192 and 193). If these patterns are followed the many nerves in the interosseous spaces can be blocked by infiltration. This may be done by using a needle of suitable length, inserting it through the webs of the fingers, and carrying it proximally through the interosseous space (Figs. 192 and 193), or by inserting the needle through the dorsum of the hand in the proximal portion of the interosseous space and then volarward

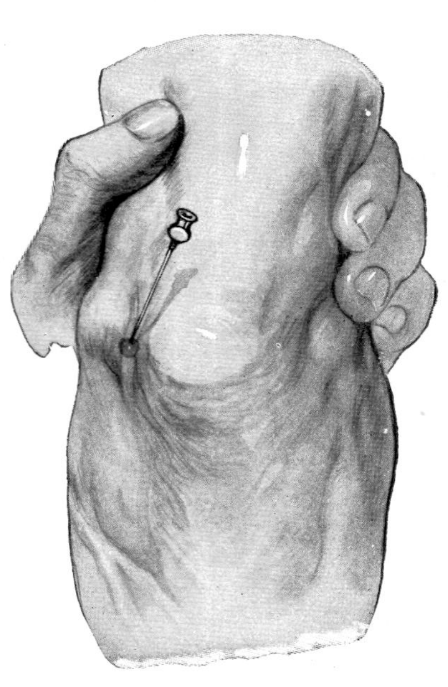

FIG. 189. Blocking the ulnar nerve at the elbow. The elbow is held in nearly full extension. The needle is inserted in the ulnar nerve at the point where it can be palpated between the medial condyle and the olecranon.

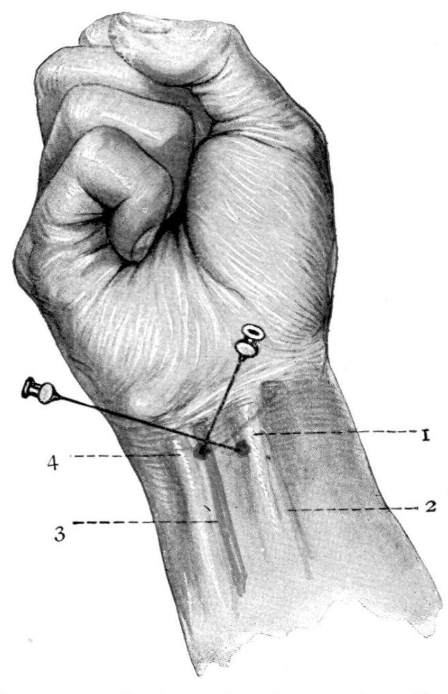

FIG. 190. Blocking the ulnar and median nerves at the wrist. To inject the ulnar nerve the needle is directed toward the ulnar side from its point of insertion at the radial side of the tendon of the flexor carpi ulnaris. To inject the median nerve the needle is directed toward the radial side from its point of insertion at the ulnar side of the tendon of the flexor palmaris longus. 1. Tendon of the palmaris longus. 2. Median nerve. 3. Ulnar nerve. 4. Tendon of the flexor carpi ulnaris.

into the palmar space, where the palpating finger should feel the tenseness caused by the injected fluid (Fig. 192). The points of insertion for subcutaneous injection of the dorsum of the hand may be chosen as desired. For subcutaneous injection of the palmar surface of the hand one uses, because the tension of skin and fascia makes needle puncture more difficult, the webfolds, making exception for the outer side of the skin of the thumb and of the 5th finger. A 0.5 percent novocain-adrenalin solution is used for injection. Anæsthesia of the entire finger should be obtained if the injection has been successful.

The anæsthetization of the individual fingers alone is obtained by plac-

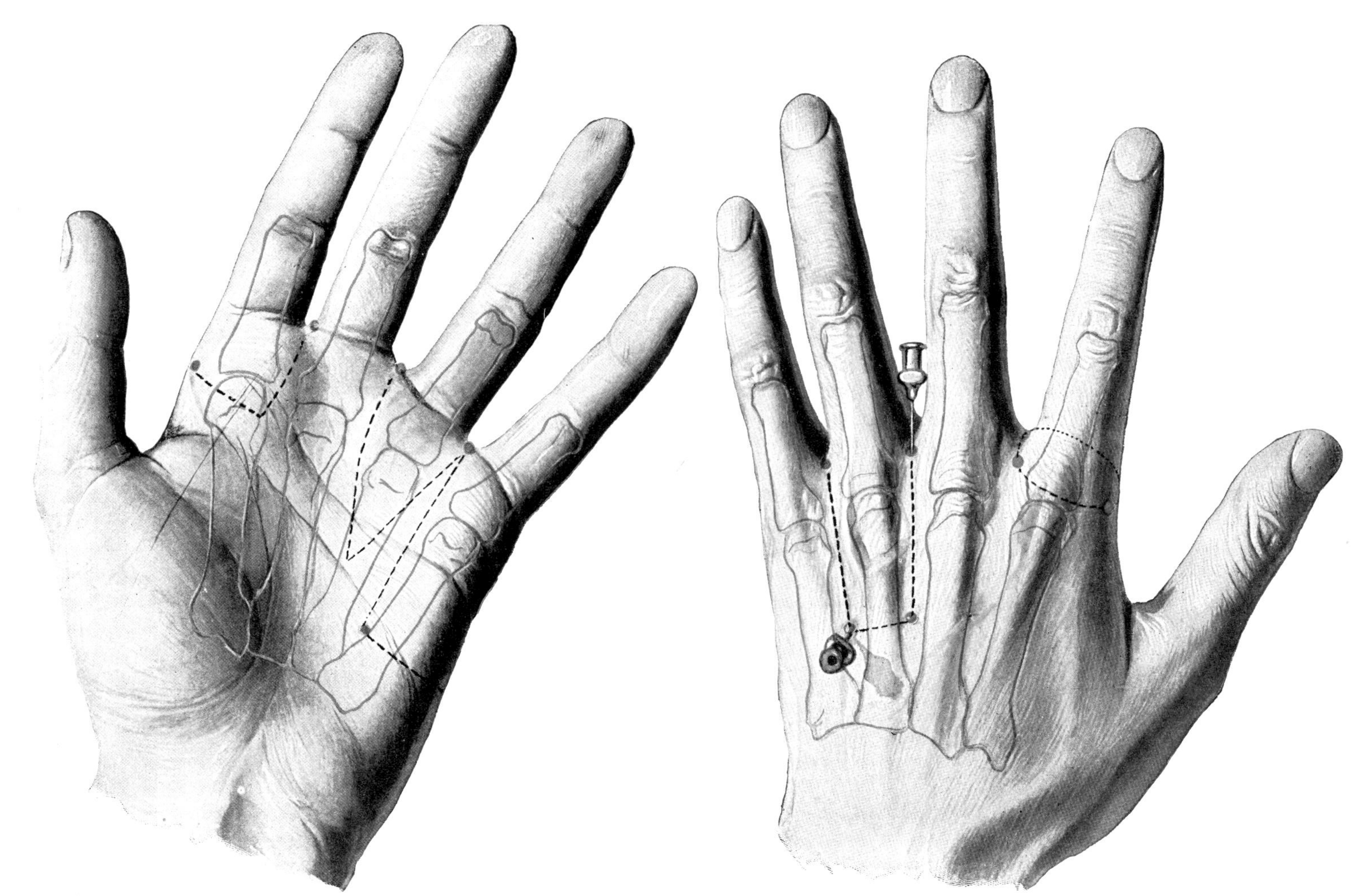

Fig. 191. Points of insertion of needle and lines of direction for anæsthetization of the index finger, ring finger and little finger, including the adjacent parts of the hand.

Fig. 192. Points of insertion of needle and lines of direction for anæsthetization of the index finger and ring finger, including the adjacent parts of the hand.

ing a subcutaneous ring of the anæsthetizing solution around the base of the finger, wherein we differ from Oberst who injected merely along the lateral sides of the fingers. (Fig. 192.) I do not use a ligature around the finger as suggested by Oberst, but use adrenalin in the anæsthetizing solution. To prevent the frequently experienced post anæsthetic pains I have adopted Braun's suggestion of using small quantities of a stronger solution, 3 to 4 cc. of a 2 percent novocain-adrenalin solution, and of placing the injection ring proximal to the web-folds rather than distal to them. As a rule two points of insertion on the dorsum of the hand are sufficient for the injection. The gradually advancing insensibility reaches the finger tips in from 5 to 10 minutes.

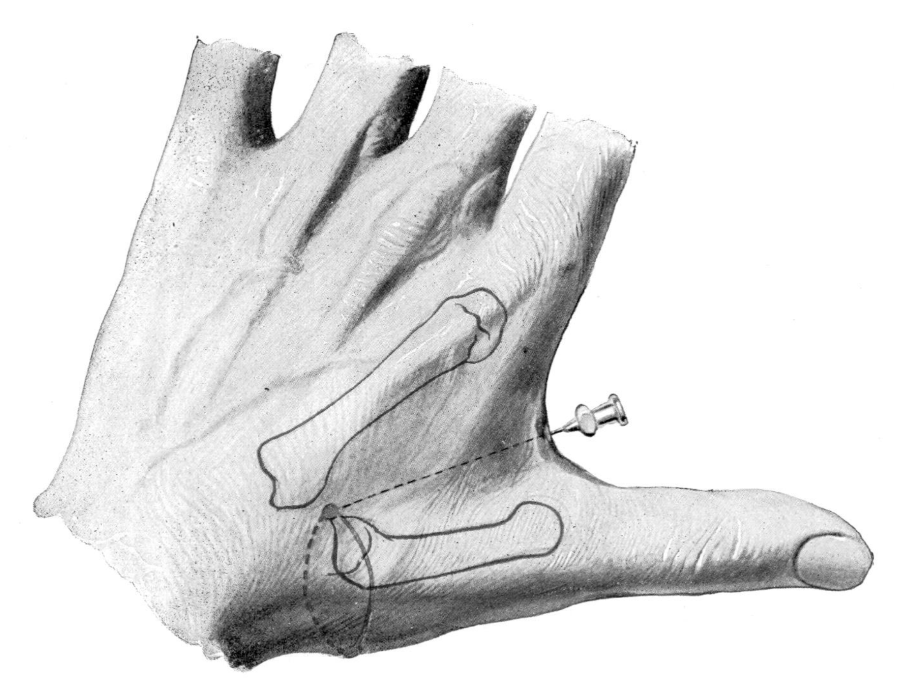

FIG. 193. Points of insertion of needle and lines of direction for anæsthetization of the thumb, including the adjacent metacarpal bone.

(E) BLOCKING THE NERVES OF THE LOWER EXTREMITY

In the lower extremity it is not possible to obtain complete anæsthesia of the entire member from one point of injection, because the leg is supplied by a number of sensory nerves which do not enter the thigh at one site. The following nerves must be considered: (1) sciatic, (2) femoral (anterior crural), (3) lateral femoral cutaneous, and (4) obturator. Blocking of these nerves is tedious, time consuming and uncertain. Furthermore it is only possible with large quantities of the anæsthetizing solution. Obviously, therefore, conduction anæsthesia of the lower extremity has found no enthusiastic supporters. Nevertheless, block of the individual nerves possesses some practical significance.

(1) Blocking the Sciatic Nerve at its Exit from the Pelvis (Keppler) (Fig. 194)

The nerve fibers which make up the sciatic nerve are spread out like a fan in the small pelvis. After emerging from the sciatic notch, they join above and lateral to the ischial spine above the lower bony margin of the

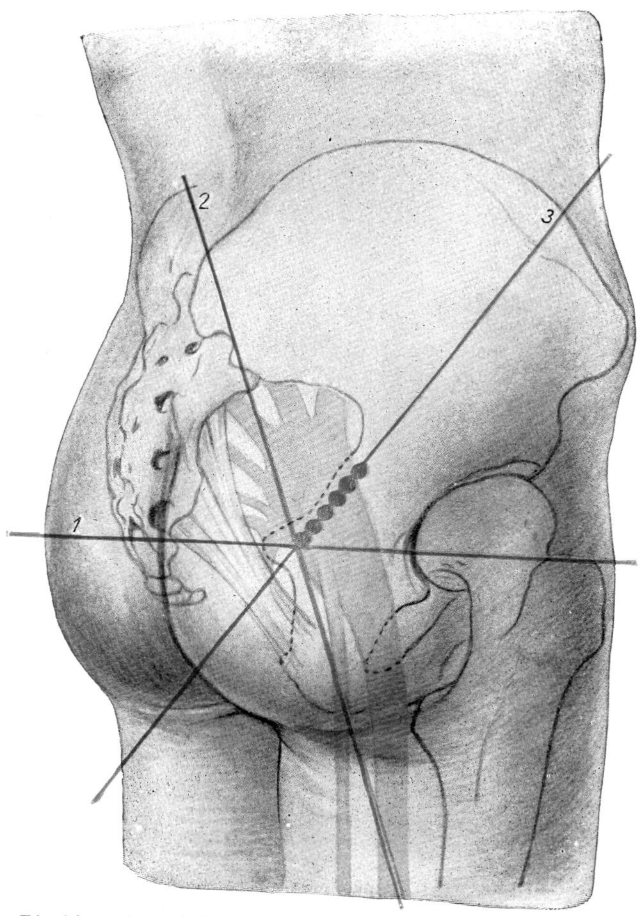

FIG. 194. Blocking the sciatic nerve. Line 1 runs transverse to the axis of the body through the proximal point of the greater trochanter. Line 2 runs from the posterior superior iliac spine to the outer margin of the tuberosity of the ischium. Line 3 runs from the intersection of Lines 1 and 2 to the gluteal tubercle on the crest of the ilium. The injection is made in the area indicated by the blue dots.

notch. The nerve then passes in a latero-distal direction along the posterior aspect of the thigh. The nerve is preferably blocked as it lies on the bony margin of the notch. This point is preferable to a more distal point. In order to ascertain the medio-distal terminal point of this several centimeter long line, the following lines are drawn as suggested by Keppler. The patient lies on his abdomen or on the unaffected side with the hip-joint flexed. A line is drawn transversely (line 1) (Fig. 194) from the proximal point of the greater trochanter to the proximal end of the anal groove. A second line which runs approximately in the long axis of the body (line 2) is drawn from the posterior-superior iliac spine to the lateral margin of the tuberosity of the ischium. At the crossing point of these two lines lies the medio-distal point of the line of injection. In order to find the direction of this line, the crossing point of lines 1 and 2 is united with the anterior gluteal tubercle of the crest of the ilium, which is perceptible along the anterior segment of the crest of the ilium (line 3). A needle at least 12 cm. long is inserted vertically into the tissues at the point of junction of these lines. The needle is inserted until the bony margin is felt and paresthesias occur in the testicle, penis or perineum. The bone is then palpated a few centimeters further along latero-proximal direction of line 3, when paresthesias are observed in the thigh and

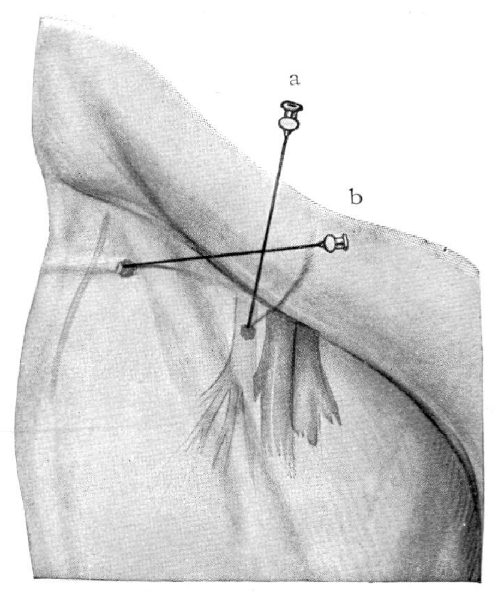

FIG. 195. a. Blocking the femoral (anterior cural) nerve under inguinal (Poupart's) ligament, lateral to the point of pulsation of the femoral artery. b. Blocking the lateral femoral cutaneous nerve by a subcutaneous and sub-fascial line of infiltration, distal to the anterior superior iliac spine and transversely across the thigh.

leg. After the first onset of paresthesias, the area along line 3, extending 4 cm. from the point of junction of lines 1 and 2, is saturated with 30 cc. of a 2 percent novocain-adrenalin solution. The posterior side of the thigh, the leg, with the exception of the inner side and the foot, become insensible in a short time.

(2) Blocking the Femoral (Anterior Crural) Nerve (Läwen) (Fig. 195)

Immediately under the inguinal (Poupart's) ligament the left index finger is placed over the point where the pulsation of the femoral artery is palpable. A fine needle is inserted vertically 1 to 1.5 cm. lateral to this until the fascia lata, which is easily felt, is penetrated. Gentle exploration with the needle should be continued until paresthesias are produced and then 5 to 10 cc. of a 2 percent novocain-adrenalin solution are injected as the needle is pushed another centimeter deeper during the injection. The midportion of the anterior surface of the thigh and the inner side of the leg, become insensible, the exact extent and degree being variable.

(3) Blocking the Lateral Femoral Cutaneous Nerve (Nystrom) (Fig. 195)

This nerve enters the thigh by passing the inguinal (Pourpart's) ligament medial to the anterior superior iliac spine, and penetrates the fascia lata from inside out at a variable distance below the ligament. It innervates the skin of the lateral side of the thigh for a varying extent. Its interruption alone frequently suffices for the removal of Thiersch grafts from the lateral surface of the thigh. The needle is inserted two finger breadths distal and medial to the anterior superior iliac spine. From this point the subcutaneous, as well as the subfascial tissues are injected transversely outward and below the spine, with 30 cc. of a 0.5 percent novocain-adrenalin solution.

(4) Blocking the Obturator Nerve.

The nerve, as suggested by Läwen, is blocked by injecting subcutaneously and subfascially 30 cc. of a 0.5 percent novocain-adrenalin solution across the medial aspect of the thigh at the junction of its middle and upper thirds. Insensibility to pain is obtained for a variable distance along the medial aspect of the thigh below the point of injection.

(5) Blocking the Nerves of the Foot

For the elimination of pain in the foot the following nerves must be blocked: (1) tibial, (2) deep peroneal, (3) the cutaneous branches of the superficial peroneal nerve, and (4) the termination of the saphenous nerve.

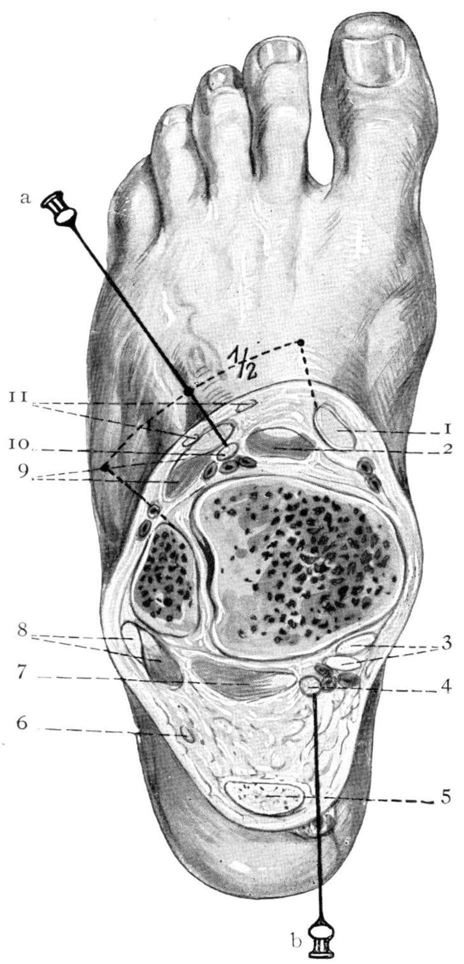

Fig. 196. Blocking all the nerves of the foot just about the ankle joint. a. The deep peroneal nerve is reached by inserting a needle midway between the tendon of the tibialis anticus muscle and the anterior margin of the lateral malleolus. b. The tibial nerve is reached by inserting a needle in a sagittal direction from a point 1 cm. medial to the tendon of Achillis. 1. Tendon of the anterior tibial muscle. 2. Extensor hallucis longus muscle. 3. Tendons of the posterior tibial muscle and the flexor digit. longus muscle. 4. Tibial nerve. 5. Tendon of Achillis. 6. Suralis nerve. 7. Flexor hallucis longus muscle. 8. Peroneal muscles. 9. Extensor digit. longus muscle. 10. Deep peroneal nerve. 11. Superficial peroneal nerves.

The Tibial Nerve is found behind the medial malleolus with the posterior tibial artery. It lies directly on the bone and between the flexor hallucis longus tendon on the one side, and the tendon the flexor digitorum longus and the posterior tibial artery on the other side. As suggested by Braun a needle is inserted at the level of the thickest portion of the medial malleolus, 1 cm. medialward from the medial margin of the tendon Achillis. It is inserted forward until the posterior surface of the tibia is felt (Fig. 196). If blood appears the needle should be withdrawn slightly and pointed more laterally. The search should continue until paresthesias appear in the toes and then 5 cc. of a 2 percent novocain-adrenalin solution are injected.

The Deep Peroneal Nerve lies at the level of malleoli, on the anterior lateral aspect of the ankle, diagonally opposite the tibial nerve, and between the extensor digitorum, and extensor hallucis longus tendons. It is directly over the lower end of the tibia. The point of insertion of the needle is at

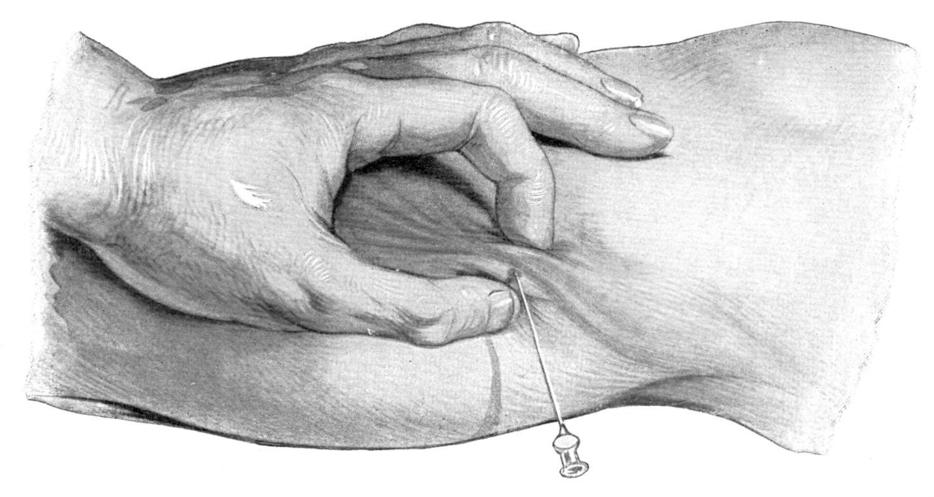

Fig. 197. Blocking the trunk of the common peroneal nerve. The injection is made below the head of the fibula, where the nerve can be felt as it crosses the bone.

the level where the fibula begins to flare into the lateral malleolus, in the center of the line of union between the lateral margin of the tendon of the anterior tibial muscle and the anterior border of the fibula. The needle is inserted vertically down to the bone and this region is infiltrated with 10 cc. of a 0.5 percent novocain-adrenalin solution (Fig. 196).

The Saphenous Nerve and the **Superficial Peroneal Nerve** run in subcutaneous cellular tissues, the first on the medial, and the second on the lateral aspect of the ankle. They can be blocked by a ring of anæsthetic solution placed around the lower leg just above the malleoli. About 75 cc. of a 0.5 novocain-adrenalin solution are required.

Instead of blocking the deep and superficial peroneal nerves in the manner indicated, the **common nerve trunk** can be blocked just below the head of the fibula (Fig. 197). At this site the nerve can be rolled under the finger, when it is sought with a fine needle, until paresthesias set in. Five cubic centimeters of a 2 percent novocain-adrenalin solution are injected.

(6) Blocking Individual Sections of the Foot Together with the Individual Toes

Conduction anæsthesia of individual sections of the foot is done in the manner already given for the hand. Since the foot is considerably thicker than the hand, it is necessary to use more fluid for the injections.

(F) VENOUS ANÆSTHESIA (BIER)

Instead of carrying the anæsthetizing solution to the nerves by injecting it into the interstitial tissues, it may also be conveyed to the nerves through the veins, presuming, of course, that it is possible to shut off by an Esmarch band the veins of the region of operation.

There are two forms of venous anæsthesia. They can be classified as direct, or immediate venous anæsthesia, or venous infiltration anæsthesia; and as indirect, or collateral venous anæsthesia, or venous induction anæsthesia.

In direct venous anæsthesia as much blood as possible is expelled from a section of a limb, the limits of which are fixed by two sterile Esmarch bandages (Fig. 200). The area between these tourniquets is disinfected. In anæsthetizing the distal portion of a limb, as the hand or foot, the distal bandage is omitted, and the proximal one should not be placed further proximally than the middle of the forearm or the calf of the leg (Figs. 198 and 199). In the bloodless area bounded by the tourniquets, a previously marked superficial vein, such as the cephalic, basilic or saphenous is exposed under local anæsthesia. Its proximal end is ligated and a cannula is inserted in the lumen of the distal portion where it is securely tied. The cannula is connected with a Bier venous anæsthesia syringe.

It is possible to use any 100 or even 50 cc. syringe in the event that a Bier syringe is not available. A section of rubber fitted with adapters may be used to connect the syringe and the cannula. Under powerful pressure, 40 to 50 cc. of a 0.5 percent novocain solution, without adrenalin, are injected if anæsthesia of the forearm is desired, while 70 to 100 cc. of the solution are injected in the saphenous if anæsthesia of the lower leg and foot is desired. If the injected fluid is seen to run out of the wound, either one or more small veins may have been opened, or the cannula is not securely fixed in the vein. In either event these defects should be corrected. At the conclusion of the injection the cannula is removed, and the distal end of the vein is ligated. The skin wound is then sutured.

Within a few minutes the portion of the extremity between the tourniquets is anæsthetic. The anæsthesia lasts until the proximal tourniquet is removed. The distal bandage may be removed as soon as anæsthesia sets in If the proximal tourniquet causes pain, another may be placed just distal to it within the area of anæsthesia, and the one causing pain can then be removed.

Within about 15 minutes, that portion of the extremity distal to the lower tourniquet becomes insensible as the result of anæsthetization of the nerves passing through the zone of injection. This is known as indirect venous anæsthesia (Fig. 200). Its systematic carrying out will give results.

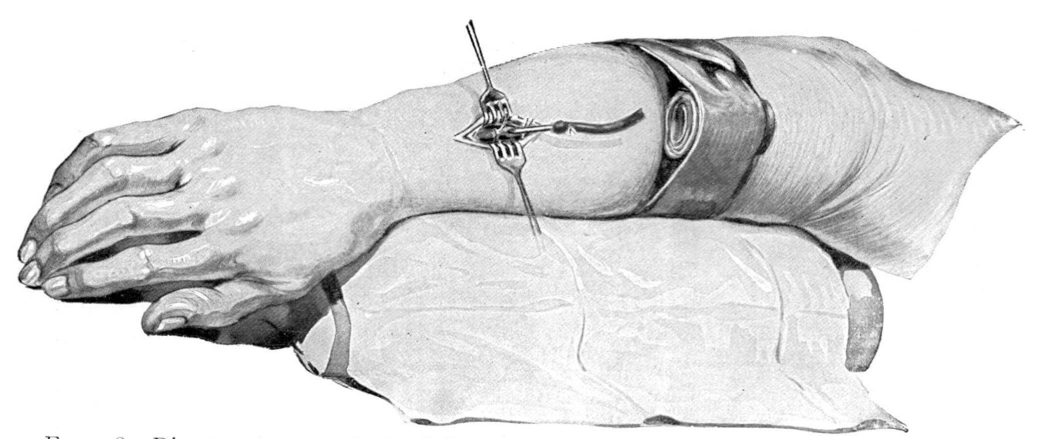

Fig. 198. Direct venous anæsthesia of forearm and hand. After constricting the forearm, the anæsthetizing solution is injected into a superficial vein in the region of operation.

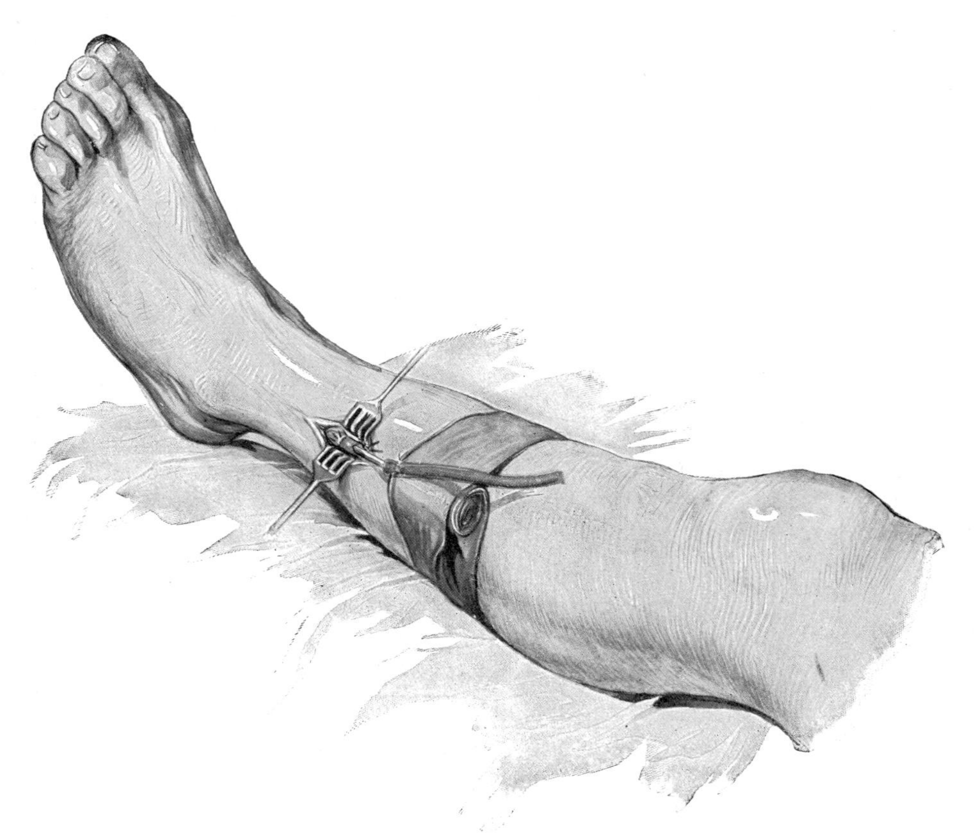

Fig. 199. Direct venous anæsthesia of leg and foot. After constricting the leg, the anæsthetizing solution is injected into a superficial vein in the region of operation.

Apart from the consideration of technical formalities and the fact that the prolonged use of an Esmarch tourniquet on the upper extremity may cause pressure palsy, venous anæsthesia is reliable and safe. If one considers the danger of injury to the vessels which may occur during forcible dilatation, venous anæsthesia is contraindicated in arteriosclerosis, diabetes and other nutritional disturbances.

One should also be warned against its use around inflammatory lesions. Since pain returns almost instantaneously after removing the proximal tourniquet, and since in extensive operations, especially major amputations, one can hardly find and control all bleeding points before the tourniquet is re-

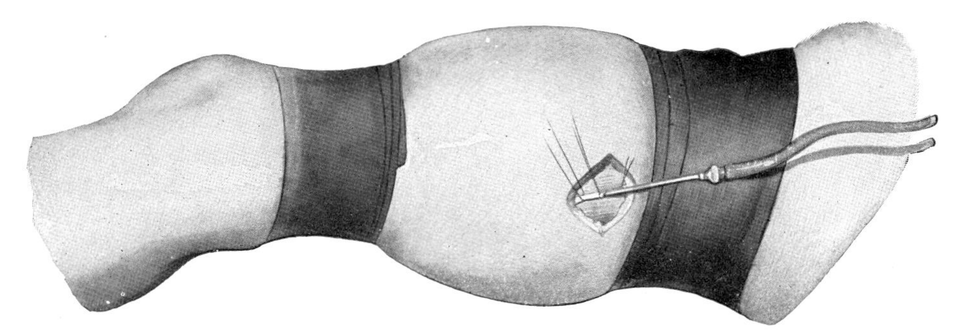

FIG. 200. Direct venous anæsthesia of the thigh, and, at the same time, indirect venous anæsthesia of the leg and foot. The anæsthetizing solution is injected into a superficial vein between two bands constricting the limb. If the field of operation is located between the two bands, the venous anæsthesia is direct. If it lies distal to the distal band, the venous anæsthesia is indirect, for the conduction of the nerves supplying the area of operation is interrupted at a distance from the field of operation.

moved, this method is open to certain serious limitations. The method has, therefore, up to the present time not found many enthusiastic supporters.

(G) SPINAL ANÆSTHESIA (BIER)

In spinal anæsthesia the anæsthetic is placed in the spinal subarachnoid space so that the nerve roots are bathed in the anæsthetic solution (Fig. 201). A variety of substances have been used for injection, but my experience with this method of anæsthesia has been, more or less, limited to two substances. I have found Tropacocain 0.06 to 0.07 gm. very satisfactory. This is put up in ampoules, each ampoule containing 1 cc. of a 10 percent sterile solution. Novocain solutions have been very widely used in recent years. Some preparations are already in solution, and others must be dissolved in cerebrospinal fluid. The amount to be injected varies with the size of the patient and the height of the anæsthesia desired. Although much larger doses of this drug are used apparently safely, I use 0.001 gm. (1 mgm.) of novocain for each kilogram of body weight. This is always injected as a 1 percent solution. This dilution factor is very important in the use of such small amounts of the drug. Adhering strictly to this technic I have had no untoward accidents. For operations in the upper abdomen or thorax twice or even three times this amount has been used.

For the spinal anæsthesia one should have two lumbar puncture needles made of platinum-iridium. The gauge should be from 0.7 to 1.2 mm. and the needles should be fitted with a stylet. The bevel should be short. A 10 cc. record syringe should be filled with the required quantity of anæsthetic solution, and a 5 cc. record syringe fitted with a fine needle which should be used to inject a 1 percent novocain solution subcutaneously. As a rule I insert the needle between the 3rd and 4th lumbar spinous processes. If difficulty is encountered in its introduction, or if the anæsthesia is to extend above the umbilicus, I insert the needle between the 2nd and 3rd lumbar spines and at times even between the 12th thoracic and the 1st lumbar spinous processes. I do not believe it is safe to inject the solution between higher segments because of the danger of medullary center paralysis, although I am aware that higher injections are often recommended. The height of the anæsthesia can be controlled by the pressure of the injection, the amount of the solution and the position of the patient.

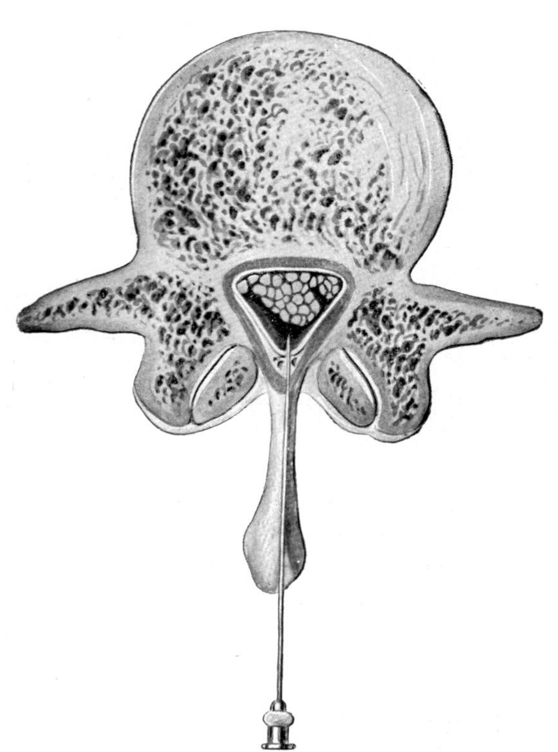

FIG. 201. Position of the needle in puncture of the dural sac for spinal anæsthesia.

The spinous process of the 4th lumbar vertebra lies on a line joining the highest points of the two iliac crests (Fig. 202). It is best to mark the spinous processes before preparing the skin, but after placing the patient in the desired position. The 3rd lumbar vertebra should be marked with a larger dash to distinguish it. I prefer the sitting position for the insertion of the needle and the injection of the solution. The patient sits across the operating table. The legs hang down on one side of the table, and the arms hang freely between the legs flexing the spine. One should be careful in regard to the exact horizontal position of the pelvis and accordingly of the table as well (Fig. 203). Shifts from the desired position may readily occur, since the position is not comfortable for the patient, and with the light thrown on the back this shift may not be recognized. Should the patient not be able to sit, he should be laid on his side on a flat support, and the spine flexed so that the knee and chin approximate each other (Fig. 204). The operator sits facing the back of the patient. The skin over the area is prepared with ether and alcohol. I do not use iodine or other disinfectants for fear of carrying some in on the needle. After rubbing the skin with these solutions the individual spinous processes stand out more distinctly. The point of insertion lies exactly in the mid-line, and I prefer to insert the needle along the upper margin of a spinous process. Here, with a 5 cc. syringe an intracutaneous skinwheal is made, after which the needle is inserted vertically for a distance of 2 or 3 cm. during which time novocain is injected. After a few moments the lumbar puncture needle is inserted in the same place and directed perpendicular to the surface of the back. Employing both hands one should be careful that the needle during its insertion through the easily moved skin is being inserted at the level of an interspinous ligament. Since the interspinous ligament offers a very definite

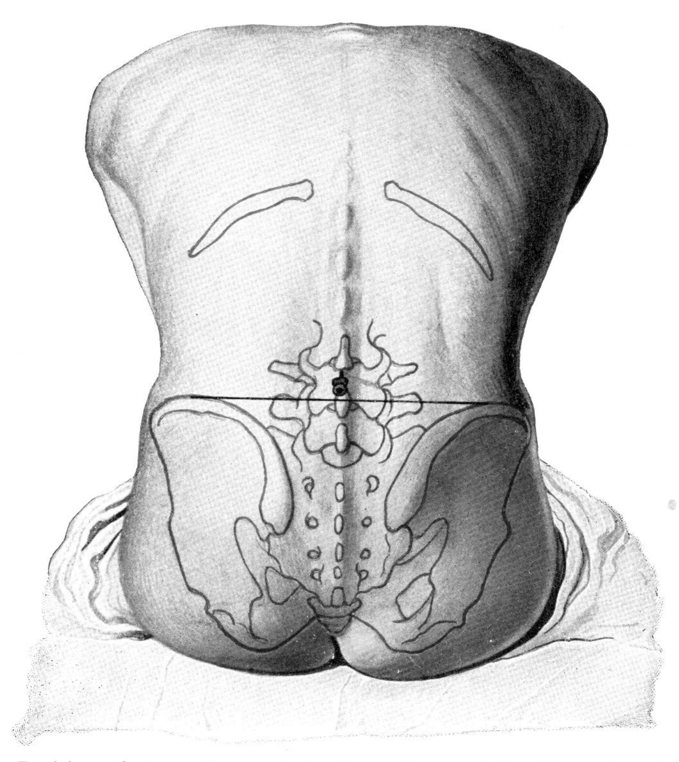

FIG. 202. Position of the patient and location of the point of insertion of the needle for lumbar anæsthesia, in the sitting posture. The line connecting the iliac crests passes through the spinous process of the fourth lumbar vertebra, above which the needle is inserted.

resistance against the progress of the needle it is best to support the needle as it is forced through this layer with an anatomical forceps (Fig. 203). The needle is pushed further, millimeter by millimeter, always perpendicular to the surface of the back, at that level. The hands of the operator are firmly supported against the back, so that in spite of the resistance offered by the ligamentous structures the needle can be safely forced home. If the needle strikes bone it should be withdrawn for a short distance and its direction altered in the sagittal plane. As the needle passes through the spinal theca the resistance disappears and a slight click off is felt in the hand guiding the needle. Withdrawal of the stylet will be followed by the appearance of a water clear fluid, if the point of the needle has reached the subdural space

The needle must not be carried further. If the patient experiences pains in a leg, the point of the needle is in too deep and has probably deviated to one side. It should be withdrawn somewhat, and reinserted in a better direction. If in spite of a supposedly proper insertion of the needle no fluid flows from it, the needle should be rotated, gentle suction should be made or the needle should be very slightly withdrawn. It may be necessary to withdraw it entirely and re-insert it. It is fairly easy, even though the needle is inserted in the mid-line, to glide off to the right or left of the dural sac as it pierces the intraspinous ligament. A "dry tap" is practically always due to an error in technic. If the fluid drops very slowly, one should attempt to increase

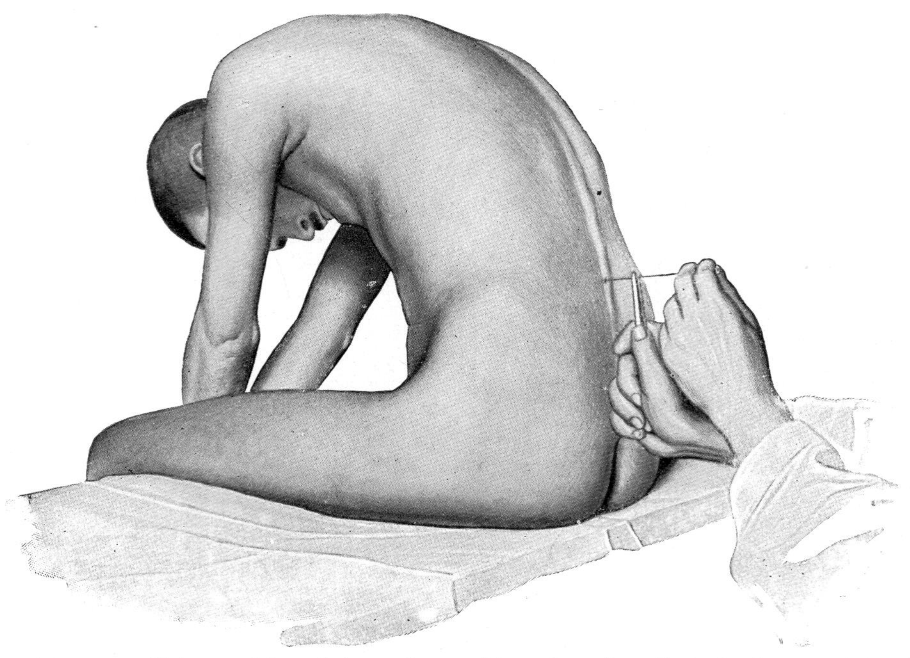

FIG. 203. Sitting position of the patient and insertion of needle in lumbar puncture. The patient sits relaxed with his back flexed, allowing his hands to hang down between his legs. The fine needle is supported by forceps during insertion.

the rapidity of the flow by very slightly shifting the position of the needle. As long as the cerebrospinal fluid macroscopically contains blood, the anæsthetic should not be introduced. If bloody fluid continues to flow, or even after shifting the position of the needle a free flow of fluid does not result, or if a "dry tap" seems inevitable, the needle should be withdrawn and reinserted at a higher level, or this type of anæsthesia should not be used.

I always remove more fluid than the amount I wish to inject. It is better accurately to measure the fluid removed in a calibrated test tube. When the amount desired has been removed, I attach the syringe containing the anæsthetic solution and aspirate slowly 5 to 10 cc. of cerebrospinal fluid into it. The total contents of the syringe are then slowly injected without undue pressure. When the syringe is empty, the needle and syringe as one are withdrawn with a jerk, and the patient is straightened out from his flexed position. This serves, as a rule, to close the puncture hole by shifting the tissue layers. The puncture point in the skin is covered with a sterile dressing. The patient is then placed horizontally on the operating table, and prepared for the contemplated operation. Within about five minutes there occurs sensory and motor paralysis up to the umbilicus, which persists for from ½ to 1½ hours. I do not believe it is possible to attain higher anæsthesia by placing the patient in the Trendelenburg position. The assumption that this can be attained can be seen to be unwarranted when it is known that even a Stovaine solution for example has the same, or even a lower specific gravity than the cerebrospinal fluid. Therefore, in Trendelenburg's position it should flow not towards the head, but towards the pelvis, if the

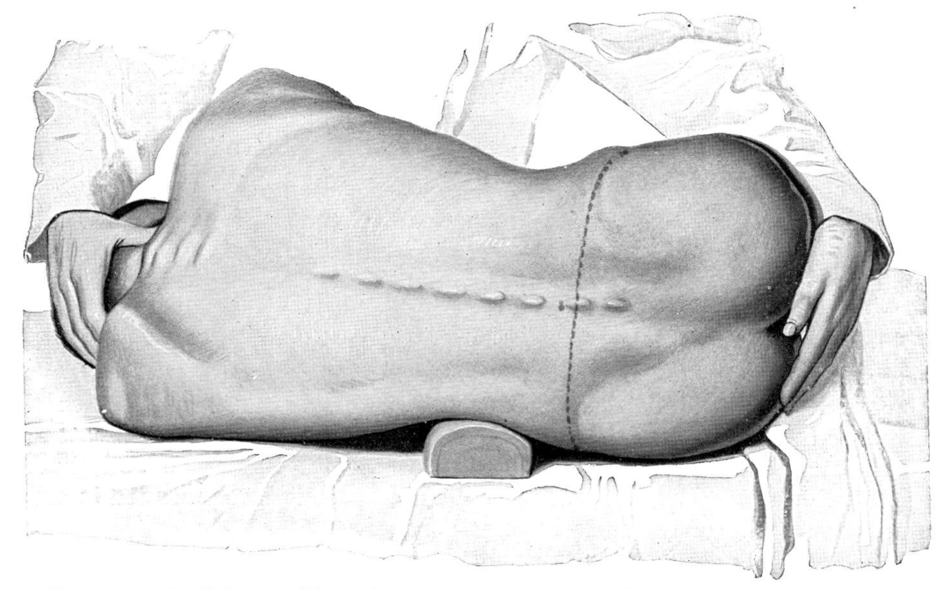

FIG. 204. Reclining position of patient and location of the point for insertion of the needle in lumbar puncture. The patient lies with a pillow under his side in order to have the bodies of the vertebrae in a straight line. The line between the iliac crests passes through the fourth lumbar vertebra and the needle is inserted just above this point.

distribution of these solutions in the subdural space would follow merely the laws of gravitation. The height of the anæsthesia, as I have said previously, will depend on the dosage, the amount of solution, and the pressure with which it is injected. The solution will diffuse in the cerebrospinal fluid and the Trendelenburg position will tend to prevent too high a level of anæsthesia rather than favoring it. Because of this I have no scruples in employing a steep Trendelenburg position, if this is desirable, in fact this position is being used more frequently than ever in conjunction with spinal anæsthesia.

Spinal anæsthesia in itself is a simple, ideal method of eliminating pain for all operations below the umbilicus. (Increasing experience, especially in the United States, has broadened its indications so that it is now used in many clinics for upper abdominal operations. I. S. R.) Unfortunately, the frequency with which accidents occur following its use, even though the method has been carefully controlled, makes it the most uncertain and dangerous method of anæsthetization which we know of. That it is most satisfactory for the surgeon can not be questioned, but that it is far from safest for the patient is also beyond question. Its use in our clinic is therefore limited to a few cases where the often insignificant disadvantages of another method of anæsthesia appear greater in a given disease than the rarer but greater dangers of spinal anæsthesia (See 1, B: "The General Examination and Preparation of the Patient"). It is particularly useful in the aged, and in patients suffering from cardiac, pulmonary or metabolic diseases in association with a surgical lesion. It should not be used in diseases of the central nervous system. Occasionally anæsthesia may not be attained, or collapse associated with marked vasomotor depression may occur, or even paralysis of the respiratory mechanism. These conditions are as a rule not associated with errors in technic. In my experience it makes little difference which substance is used for the anæsthesia nor whether or not adrenalin is used with them; whether much or little cerebrospinal fluid is permitted to escape; whether or not after the injection the patient is rapidly placed in the horizontal position; or whether or not and to what a degree the Trendelenburg position is assumed. It is the very occasional catastrophe, which comes without previous warning, in an otherwise series of perfect anæsthetizations that makes me wary of its use. In some instances the anæsthesia is not of sufficient degree or not to a sufficient height to permit operative interference. If the degree of anæsthesia is not sufficient within 10 minutes after the injection, it should be reinforced with some other type of anæsthesia, preferably of the inhalation type. Generally only a small amount of ether is necessary.

Vasomotor and respiratory collapse are supposedly associated with the contact of the anæsthetic with the medulla. If the collapse is threatening and persistent, immediate measures for resuscitation should be undertaken. Lumbar puncture and drainage of the subdural space is recommended in order to remove as much of the anæsthetic as possible.

Spinal anæsthesia is practically always associated with a fall in the blood pressure, in which, according to investigations conducted in our clinic, it differs very markedly from other forms of local anæsthesia. (König, German Surgical Congress, 1922.) This drop in pressure is frequently associated with nausea, vomiting, and profuse perspiration. Cardiac failure may occur. Spinal anæsthesia should not be attempted unless provision is made for the repeated estimation of the blood pressure. (The vasomotor depression may be to a degree prevented by the simultaneous administration of adrenalin or by the previous administration of 50 mgm. of ephedrine. These may be repeated after injection of the anæsthetic if the fall in blood pressure is alarming. I. S. R.) The inhalation of carbon dioxide for short intervals tends to elevate the pressure, to stimulate respiration, and to overcome the tendency to nausea and vomiting. In cardiac collapse I have found the intravenous injection of 1 cc. of adrenalin (1:1000) almost a specific, although there is no contraindication to any cardiac stimulant. I have often used cardiazol.

In some cases paralysis of respiration overshadows everything else. The patients complain, even though the pulse is still good, of a sensation of pressure in the chest; and of inability to breathe. They become cyanotic, call for air, and finally are unable to carry on respiratory movements. With failing respiration comes a failing blood pressure. When respiratory distress is marked artificial respiration should be begun and should be continued until the patient can again breathe easily. For the relief of respiratory disturbances I have found that the intravenous injection of lobelin (0.01 gm.) is often efficacious.

A frequent extremely unpleasant after effect of spinal anæsthesia is headache. This may be very severe, and may last for weeks, or even for months. These may be associated with symptoms of meningismus. I have been unable to confirm the usefulness of large quantities of fluid given by mouth, by vein, or by rectum in combating this complication. Antipyretics, hypnotics, or even narcotics may be necessary for relief. Likewise we do not possess a prophylactic remedy for the fortunately exceptionally rare and obstinate paralyses, amongst which abducent paralysis predominates.

If a needle is broken during the injection of the anæsthetic and a piece remains in the tissues, the intervertebral space should be marked at once, and the fragment should be removed, as a rule, immediately after the primary operation has been completed. A small incision rarely suffices, unless the needle breaks just under the skin. If the needle breaks deep in the tissues it is better to make a long medial longitudinal incision and to remove both spinous processes limiting the intervertebral space. It may even be necessary to remove the posterior vertebral arch. However it is better to remove the fragment at some time before the patient is discharged from the hospital in order to avoid a malpractice suit.

SUPPLEMENT

Puncture of the Subarachnoid Space for Other Purposes

Spinal puncture is done not only for anæsthetization, but also to obtain spinal fluid for examination for blood, pus, globulin content, cytologic examination, or for the various tests for cerebrospinal syphilis. It is also done for injecting sera and antitoxins; for estimating the pressure of the cerebrospinal fluid; for injecting air for encephalography; and for injecting radio opaque substances for roentgenographic exploration. The technic of the puncture itself is the same as that described for spinal anæsthesia. The same careful asepsis must be maintained. Fluid for examination should be collected in sterile tubes.

If the pressure of the fluid is to be measured, a glass manometer should be attached to the needle before any fluid, or at most a few drops, escape. These tubes are calibrated and the readings can be made direct. If a non-calibrated tube is used the distance between the needle and the height of the fluid is measured with a sterile millimeter rule (Fig. 205). The resultant figure indicates the fluid pressure in millimeters of cerebrospinal fluid. The manometer should be of small bore, 1 mm., so that too much fluid does not escape. Cardiac pulsations and respiratory waves should be transmitted to it. Pressure on either jugular vein will cause a rise in the pressure if there is no obstruction in the spinal sac and the jugulars are patent (Queckenstedt).

For encephalography an exacting technic is necessary. The air may be injected after ventricular, cisternal or lumbar puncture. Several technics are used, but I will describe that which I use and have found very satisfactory. Ten cubic centimeters of fluid are first aspirated with the patient in the sitting position. The syringe which is used should have the piston and barrel greased with sterile vaseline, and the needle should be fitted with a stop-cock. After removing 10 cc. of fluid 10 cc. of air are injected, and this procedure is repeated until fluid is no longer obtained. If this method is followed the

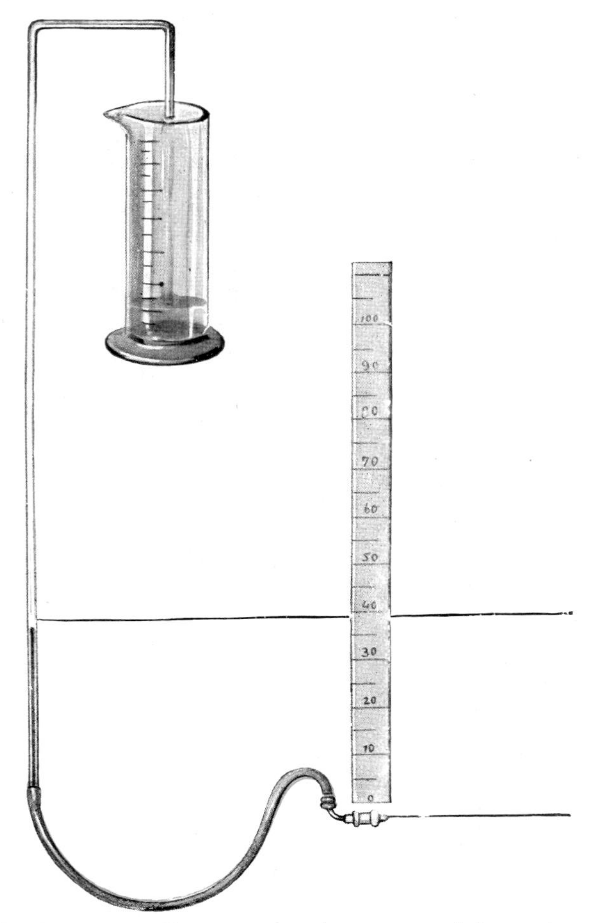

FIG. 205. Simple apparatus for measuring the pressure of the cerebrospinal fluid.

quantity of air introduced can never exceed the quantity of fluid removed and a rise in pressure will not ensue. In all from 40 to 80 cc. of air are gradually introduced. As a rule I prefer ventricular puncture to encephalography.

Puncture of the Cisterna Magna (Cisterna Cerebello-medullaris)

While an x-ray contrast medium, air, is used in encephalography, this being lighter than the cerebrospinal fluid rises in the subarachnoid space with the patient in the sitting position. It also enters the ventricular system. In the iodized oils we possess roentgen opaque substances which generally are heavier than the cerebrospinal fluid. Iodipin is an iodized oil which when injected into the spinal subdural sac gravitates toward the most dependent part of the sac. Under normal conditions with the patient in the upright position the most dependent portion of the sac is the lumbar extremity. If, however, a lesion of the cord exists which obstructs the free flow of fluid the iodized oil remains at the level of the obstruction, entirely or in part, temporarily or permanently, depending on the degree of occlusion. By this means

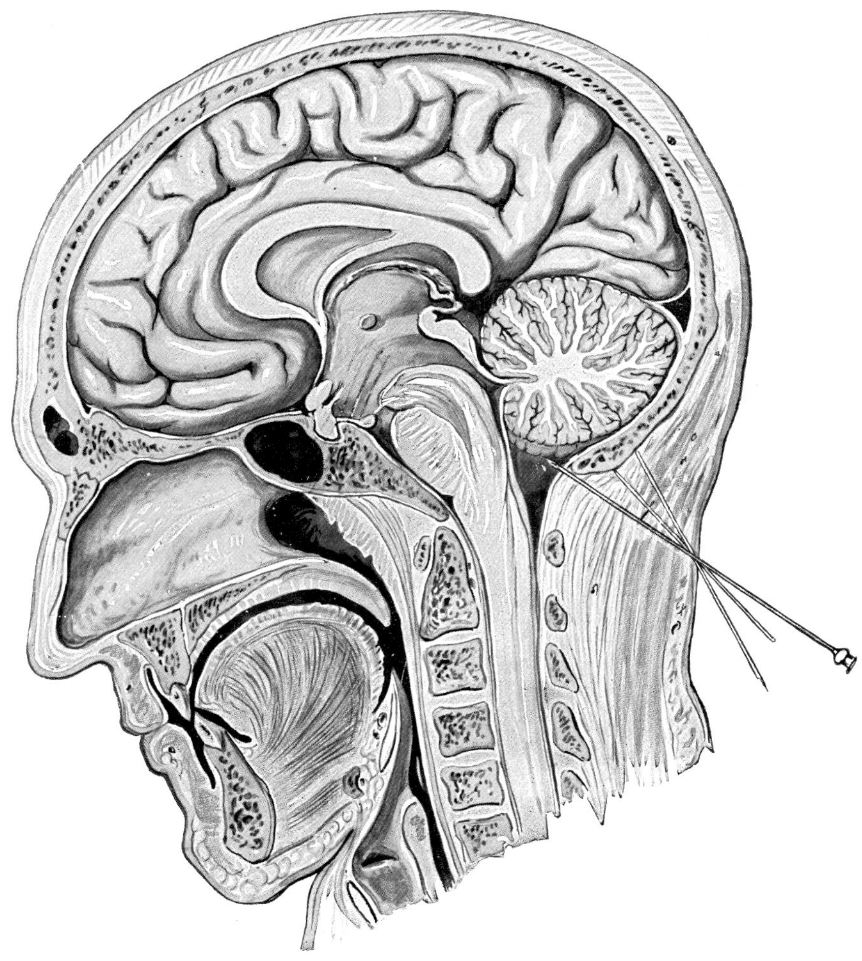

FIG. 206. Puncture of the cisterna magna. The head is acutely flexed, the needle is then inserted in the midline in the groove under the inferior occipital protuberance. It at first touches the occipital bone when its point is withdrawn and carefully depressed until the margin of the foramen magnum is felt. It is then slipped into the cistern.

important data may be obtained in cases where the neurological findings are not sufficient to enable accurate localization of a lesion. As a rule, Iodipin (Merck), which is a 40 percent solution of iodine in oil, is introduced after cisternal puncture with the patient in the sitting position. One or two cubic centimeters are injected and the flow of the oil is watched under the fluoroscope with shifts in the patient's position. X-ray pictures should also be made for a permanent record. Iodipin is quite viscid so that it can not be injected unless it is warmed. Iodipin is also made in a form which is lighter than the cerebrospinal fluid. This form of Iodipin is usually injected by lumbar puncture, the same amount, 1 or 2 cc., being used. If both forms are used, the heavy by cisternal puncture and the light by lumbar puncture, one can obtain information not only of the location, but of the extent of a lesion.

Puncture of the cisterna magna is performed between the tabular portion of the occipital bone and atlas. The head is flexed and a lumbar puncture needle is introduced in the midline in the groove between the skull and the first cervical vertebra. The needle is directed obliquely upwards until the tabular portion of the occipital bone is felt; when it is slightly withdrawn and

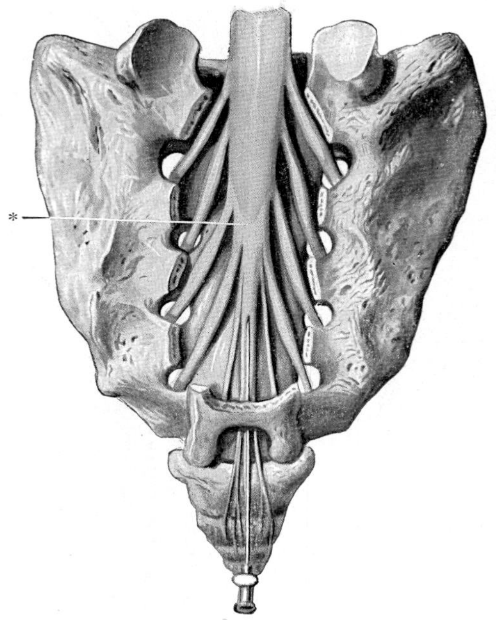

FIG 207. Position of the needle in sacral anæsthesia. The needle is carried through the hiatus in the sacral canal, where its point lies extradural. *Caudal end of the dural sac.

reinserted in a more nearly horizontal direction. This is repeated until the point slips past the rim of the foramen magnum and pierces the atlanto-occipital membrane, if the puncture has been successful, when cerebrospinal fluid will escape after the stylet is withdrawn (Fig. 206). The cerebrospinal fluid pressure can be estimated, fluid removed for examination, or medicaments introduced.

(H) SACRAL ANÆSTHESIA AND EPIDURAL INJECTION (CATHELIN, LÄWEN)

The nerve trunks of the sacral plexus, after they leave the subdural space, can be interrupted in the sacral canal which is extradural by injecting an anæsthetic solution into the canal (Fig 207). If successful anæsthesia of the parts surrounding the anus is produced, the perineum, gluteal region, scrotum, penis, the lower portion of the rectum, vagina, urethra, prostate, and anus become insensible. The technical difficulty of the method lies in reaching the sacral canal, which may be nearly impossible in very stout indi-

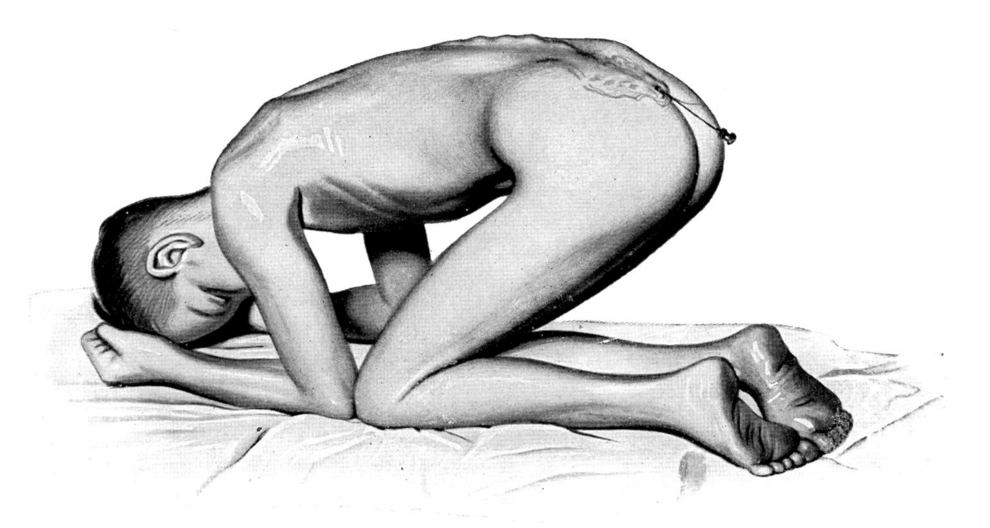

FIG. 208. Knee-elbow position for insertion of the needle in sacral anæsthesia.

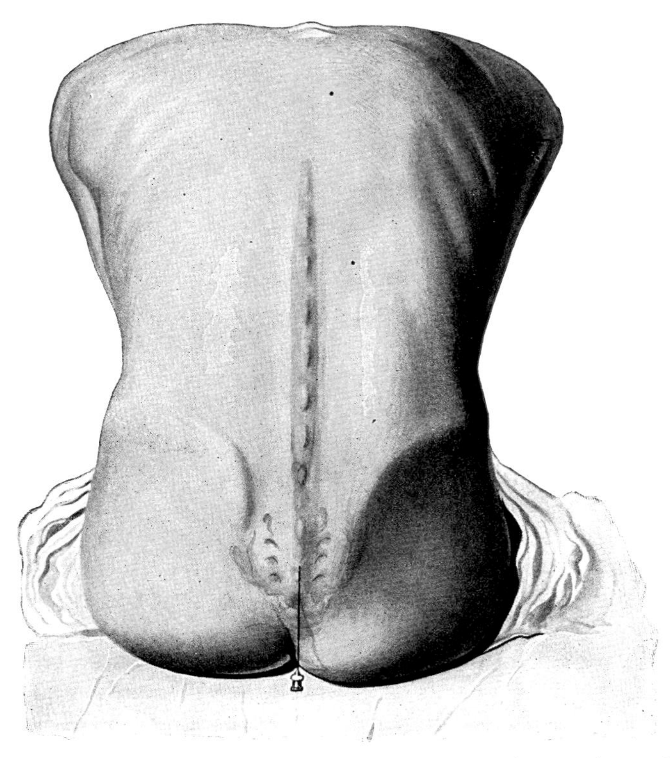

FIG. 209. Sitting position for insertion of the needle in sacral anæsthesia.

viduals. In performing sacral puncture, the patient is placed either in the knee-elbow position (Fig. 208), or he is placed on a high operating table, so that his buttocks extend beyond the table margin (Fig. 209). Only when necessity demands it is the lateral position used. In finding the hiatus of the sacral canal, the operator palpates the last projection of the medial sacral crest, and below and lateral to this, the two sacral cornua. Between the two bony prominences stretches the membrane covering the opening (Fig. 207). The site is marked with a colored solution, and the area is prepared with alcohol and ether. A wheal is made with novocain and a lumbar puncture needle provided with a stylet is inserted exactly in the midline over the fontanelle. It is directed perpendicularly to the bone (first position of the needle). The needle is withdrawn slightly and the external portion of the needle is carried anteriorly (second position of the needle), so that when it is again introduced it will be carried into the sacral canal. It should be inserted 5 to 6 cm. (Fig. 210). If blood appears after the stylet has been removed, the method should be given up. If cerebrospinal fluid appears the needle should be withdrawn a little. I use for this injection 20 cc. of a 2 percent novocain-adrenalin solution. The injection must be done slowly. Twenty minutes at least elapses before complete anæsthesia results, during which time the patient is laid down with the upper part of the trunk elevated. Good anæsthesia is not always obtained, and failure to obtain it has been ascribed to errors during the injection of the solution, and to anatomical variations. Because of its uncertainty and because of the limited extent of the anæsthetic field the procedure is not widely used.

Epidural Injection. It is possible to reach the lower spinal nerves by a second route, by injecting between the spinal membranes and the wall of the vertebral canal, after introducing a needle through the intervertebral foramina of the lumbar region.

Patients so injected have paræsthesias and sensory disturbances, but complete anæsthesia such as is necessary for major operations does not occur even if novocain is used. This procedure is therefore not applicable for the elimination of pain during operations, but it is excellent for controlling pain in severe sciatica. In the latter it may be repeated as often as ten times, the injections being given at weekly intervals.

The following describes the technic of the epidural injection. The patient should receive a hypodermic of 0.01 to 0.02 gm. of morphine one-half hour before the injection. For the injection the patient is laid on the well side, a pillow supporting the lumbar region. As in lumbar puncture one ascertains the spinous process of the 4th lumbar vertebra by drawing a line joining the highest points of both iliac crests. After anæsthetizing the place of puncture a lumbar puncture needle is inserted a good hand's breadth lateral to the spinous process of the fourth lumbar vertebra. The needle is introduced vertically at an angle of 160° to the surface of the back in the direction of the body of the fourth lumbar vertebra (Fig. 211).

If the needle point strikes the body of the vertebra, a slight change in its direction is sufficient to permit it to penetrate the epidural space through the 4th lumbar intervertebral foramen. This foramen is easily recognized, since as soon as it is entered the needle can suddenly slide several centi-

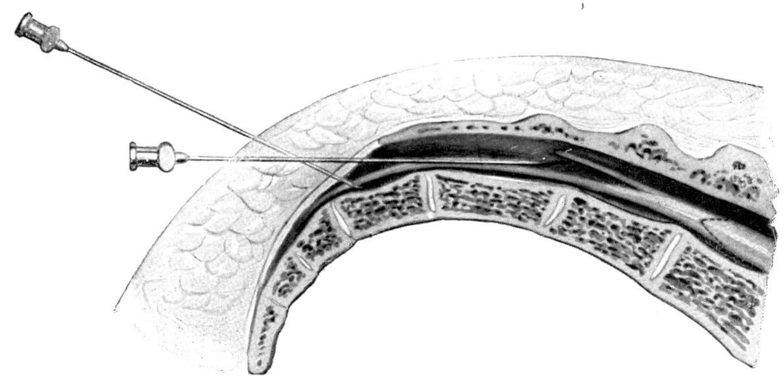

Fig. 210. Introduction of needle into sacral canal. The needle is inserted through the hiatus in the fifth sacral vertebra, the outer end being then depressed until the needle can be pushed upward several centimeters in the canal.

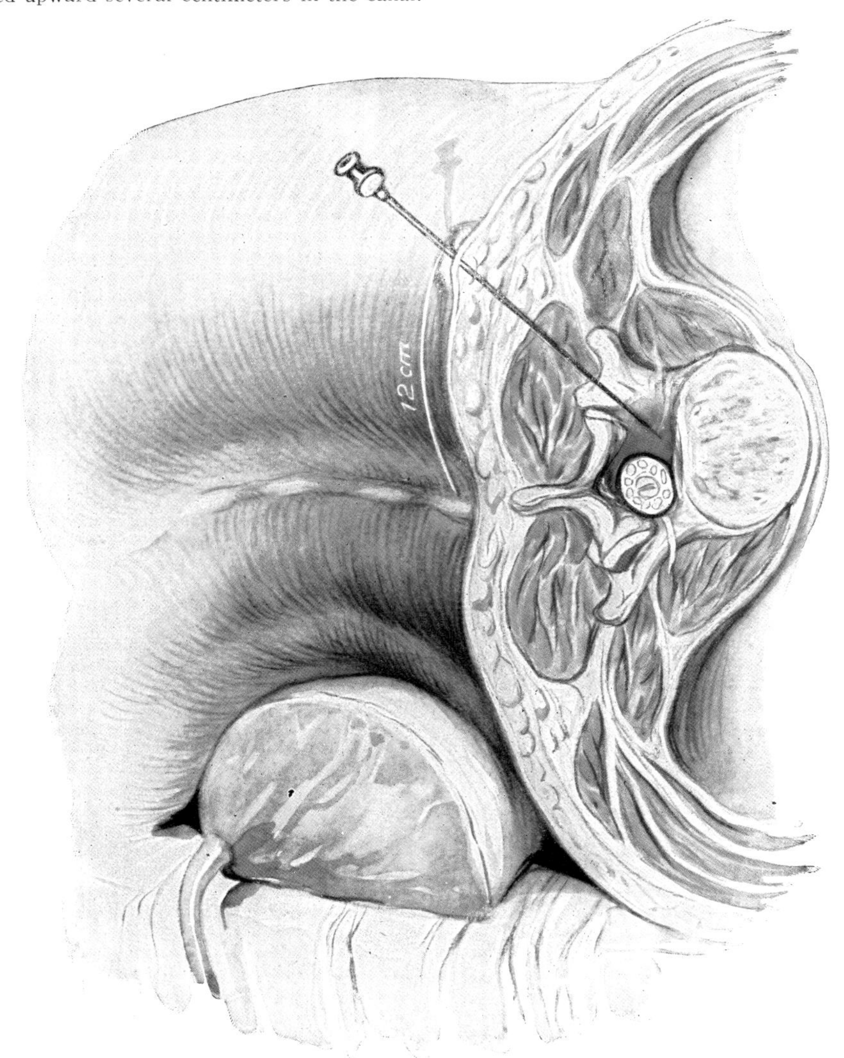

Fig. 211. Epidural injection in the lumbar region. The needle, inserted about twelve cm. from the midline, slips through the intervertebral foramen into the vertebral canal, so that its point lies between bone and dura mater.

meters deeper. If spinal fluid escapes from the needle, it has been introduced too far and it should be withdrawn slightly before the solution is injected. If during the introduction of the needle the patient complains of pain, a little 0.5 percent novocain-adrenalin solution is injected.

When the needle is in position 10 cc. of a 0.5 percent novocain-adrenalin solution is injected in the epidural space. After a few minutes have elapsed physiologic salt solution is gradually injected. If the patient experiences pain on the healthy side during the injection, the needle must be slightly withdrawn. If severe pains occur in the back or in the region of the sciatic nerve on the diseased side during the injection, the injection is delayed or it is continued while ethyl chloride is sprayed over the painful area. Some patients during the injection show sudden signs of increased intracranial pressure: headache, unconsciousness, cramps, cyanosis, slowing of the pulse, dilated and fixed pupils. In such cases the injection should immediately be discontinued. Under ordinary circumstances 100 to 200 cc. of saline solution can be injected. If it is impossible to pass the needle through the 4th lumbar intervertebral foramen, or there is cause to favor another site, the injection can be performed through a higher intervertebral foramen of the lumbar spine. It is possible to use several intervertebral foramina at the same sitting, but this seems unnecessary since the injected fluid spreads over a wide area between the spinal membranes and the bone.

CHAPTER III

THE CONTROL OF INFECTION

Until well in the second half of the last century infection of operative wounds was the rule rather than the exception. In fact the absence of a severe infection after operation was considered an anomaly. As a result of these infections the postoperative mortality was appalling. In the years 1868-1869, at the Berlin Bethany Deaconess Hospital, Küster reported that of 26 amputations 20, or 77 percent, died from pyemia. In a report covering 5 years during the first half of the 19th century, in the Paris hospitals Malgaigne found 300 deaths out of 560 operations, a mortality of 54 percent. The mortality after child birth was equally as high. Indeed, the observation was general that the mortality from purulent infections subsequent to operation, especially the much dreaded "hospital sepsis," was low if the patients were kept in private houses or in newly built hospitals, while with the accumulation of patients, particularly in the army hospitals, and in the hospitals which had been used for many years, it mounted gruesomely. We know today, that this difference in morbidity and mortality depended upon carrying of infection from patient to patient, the virulence of the infecting organism increasing through transmission. We still observe infections of a similar type in the extensive phlegmons. In those days, however, the etiology remained unknown and for several hundred years it destroyed, to a great degree, the surgeon's opportunity for success. Pirogoff, from the facts at hand, concluded very ingeniously that it was better to lodge his operative cases in peasants' huts. It is not surprising that under such circumstances so many young physicians broke down. They were unable to continue this branch of medicine with its incalculable results and therefore abandoned surgery, towards which they had turned in happy ignorance. The depletion of the ranks can surprise no one (Küster). While we wonder today that one had the courage to undertake an operation, the surgeons of that time seemed satisfied with their failures. Nevertheless few had the ego of Boyer, who in 1820 wrote these amazing words: "The surgery of our day has made the greatest advances, so that it appears to have reached the highest or almost the highest degree of perfection, of which it is capable" (from Küster).

Today the infection of an operative wound, after an aseptic operation, is the exception rather than the rule. The occurrence of an infection in a previously clean case demands an investigation for the "break in the asepsis." This remarkable change in such a short period of time, without interfering with the simplest safeguards in our operative management, is connected with the names of Semmelweiss and Lister, Pasteur and Koch. During the year 1922, when I was director of the Surgical Clinic at Königsberg we had 3.13

percent of wound infections in the aseptic operations, while in the year 1923, we had 1.34 percent, an average therefore of 2.23 percent (Teichert, Zentralbl. f. Chirurgie, 1924, 39, 2121).

A. THE ASEPTIC OPERATION

By far the most important and decisive measure for controlling post-operative infection is prophylaxis. It is much more important to prevent infection than to combat it successfully, and every modernly conducted surgical clinic has as its corner stone the impress of prophylaxis.

The surface of the earth, all living creatures and objects, are covered with countless germs, whose penetration into wounds may bring about wound infection; without the presence of such germs, which may also occasionally be carried to the wound by the blood, wound infection can not occur.

The art of asepsis consists in carrying out an operation so that no, or at most very few, pathogenic or virulent organisms come in contact with the operative wound. It would be ingenious if in this germ containing world it would be possible to reserve a germ free area for the operative wound and the structures which surround it.

This is to a degree possible, for the bacteria adhere to objects and they do not possess the power of motility in space. Furthermore, air is of subordinate importance as a conveyor.

Only when the air becomes polluted with an abundance of germ-laden dust particles or droplets, as may occur after coughing and sneezing, can it be considered practically as a means of infection. Hence, when previous to operation, the materials which are to come in contact with the wound are sterile, they may remain so during the operation.

Unfortunately it is not possible to have complete sterility. Only that which can be boiled or that which can be heated by steam to 120° C. can be rendered sterile (physical sterilization). For the skin of the hands and the skin around the field of operation, we must be content with a reduction in the number and virulence of the organisms by chemical disinfection. It is easy to see therefore, that in spite of so-called asepsis we can never fully guarantee the complete aseptic course of an operation. This is even more true when one considers that a wound infection may result from bacteria which have come through the blood stream from the tonsils, intestinal canal, or distant furuncles. Since physical sterilization, when properly carried out, surpasses by far chemical disinfection in safety, we prefer physical sterilization whenever this is possible, and consider chemical disinfection merely a makeshift. The experimental measures for the efficiency of bacterial sterilization must take into account the power of resistance of the anthrax spore.

Instruments made of metal, glass, porcelain, hard and soft rubber become sterile after five minutes of boiling. Soda in the proportion of about 1 to 100 is added to the water, so that the boiling point is raised. Furthermore this prevents the rusting of metal instruments. Because of the repeated boiling to which instruments must be subjected I have mine made of metal whenever possible. So that they may be more easily cleansed, they have flat surfaces, and in most instances they can be taken apart. Rustless and stainless steel is excellent, except for knives. Instruments made of ordinary steel should be either nickel-plated, or better, chromium-plated, in order to prevent rusting.

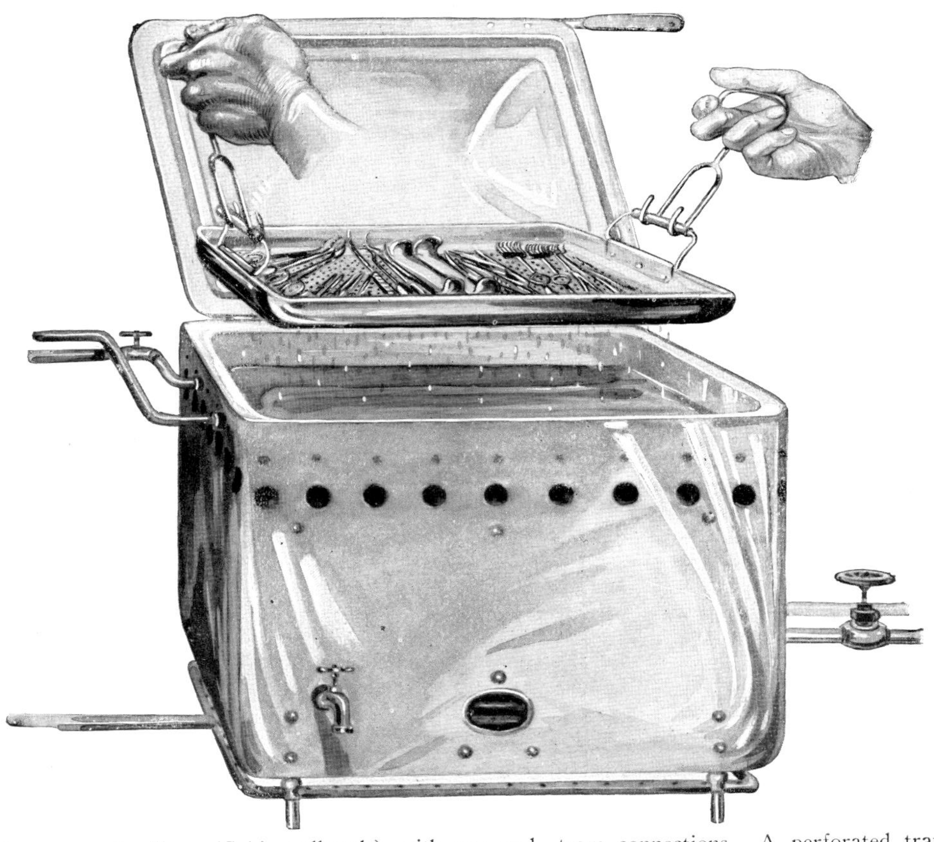

FIG. 212. Sterilizer (Schimmelbusch) with gas and steam connections. A perforated tray holding the boiled instruments is being lifted from the boiler by two handles.

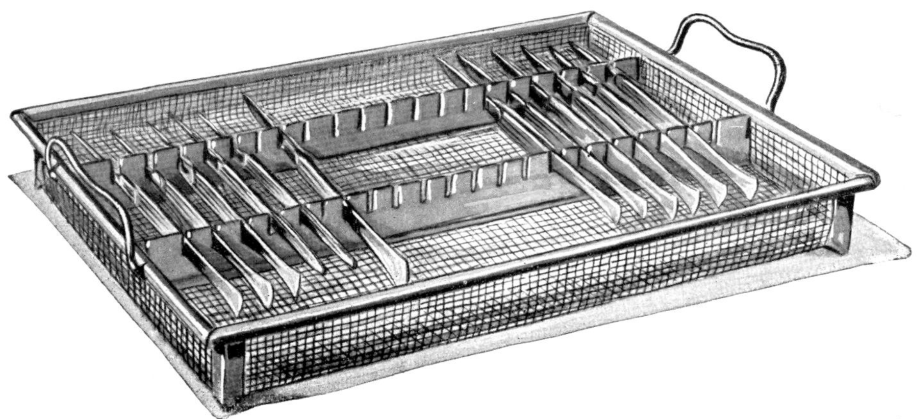

FIG. 213. Knife tray, in which the knives may be sterilized without damaging their edges.

The few instruments in which it is difficult to replace wood, such as the mallet, can readily be boiled.

Likewise all articles made of glass and porcelain are boiled. Some substances may preferably be sterilized by dry heat. If this is done they should

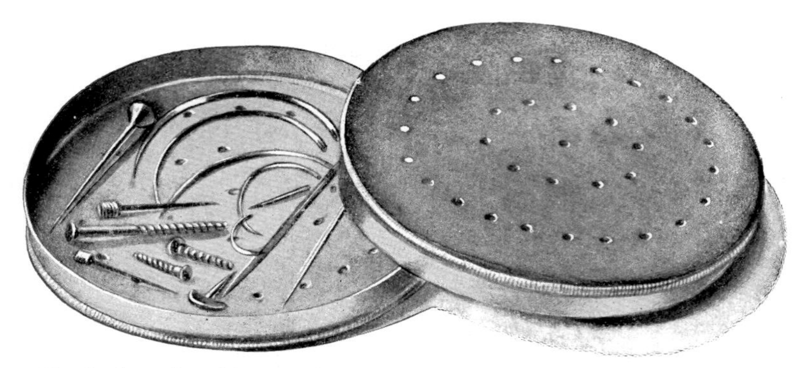

Fig. 214. Needle box, in which needles and other small articles are placed for sterilization so they will not be lost.

be subjected to a heat of 200° C. for one hour. After use every instrument is boiled and then mechanically cleaned by washing and polishing. For this washing running water should be at one's disposal. The instruments are then resterilized.

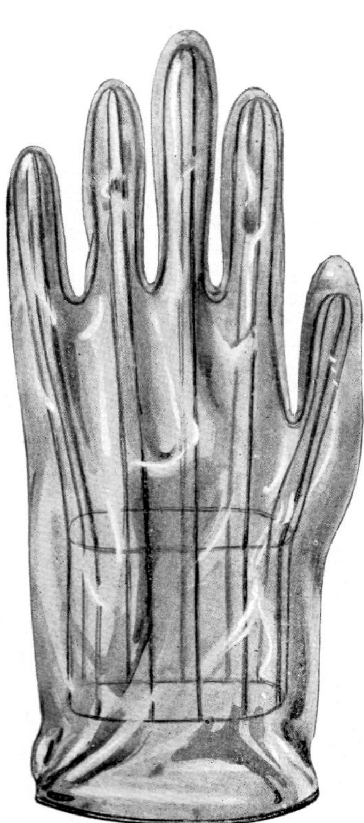

Fig. 215. Wire frame placed in rubber glove during sterilization.

For boiling instruments I have found the Schimmelbusch sterilizing apparatus (Fig. 212) quite efficient. The steam developed in this apparatus is partly condensed by a cooling coil which surrounds the brim, and the remainder escapes through a vent leading to the exterior. With the aid of a tray, which can be grasped with two handles, the instruments are lifted from the sterilizer after boiling, and are placed on a sterile frame to drain and cool. They are removed from this by the instrument nurse in a manner which will be described later.

Especially good care must be taken during the sterilization of knives because of their sensitive edges. So that the cutting edge may not be damaged by knocking against the other instruments, they are placed in a special tray for boiling. In this the cutting edge is free (Fig. 213). The frequently observed custom of protecting the edge of the knife with a cotton wrapper is bad, since the wet cotton offers a very definite resistance during its removal and thus dulls the knife. It is preferable to boil the knives in distilled water for 5 minutes, since water containing

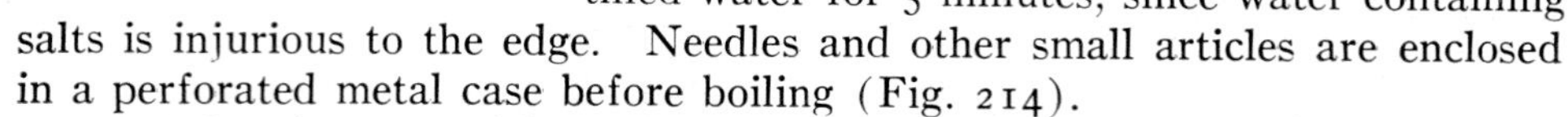

salts is injurious to the edge. Needles and other small articles are enclosed in a perforated metal case before boiling (Fig. 214).

All dressing materials, such as cellulose, cotton, tampons, compresses, sponges, bandages, the linens, such as gowns, towels, mouth masks, cotton gloves, rubber gloves, and brushes are sterilized in an autoclave at a temperature of 110 to 138° C. and a pressure of 10 to 35 pounds for a period of from 15 to 60 minutes depending upon the temperature and pressure.

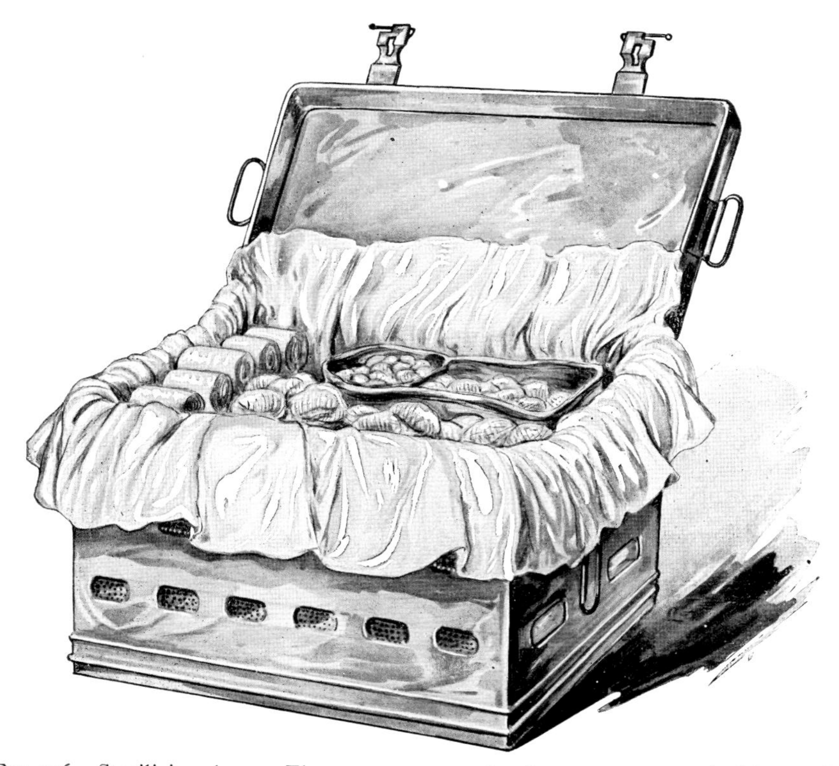

Fig. 216. Sterilizing drum. The gauze sponges, bandages, etc., are packed in muslin bags. This drum is more convenient than the round one previously used. It has adjustable openings which permit of ready access of the steam during sterilization.

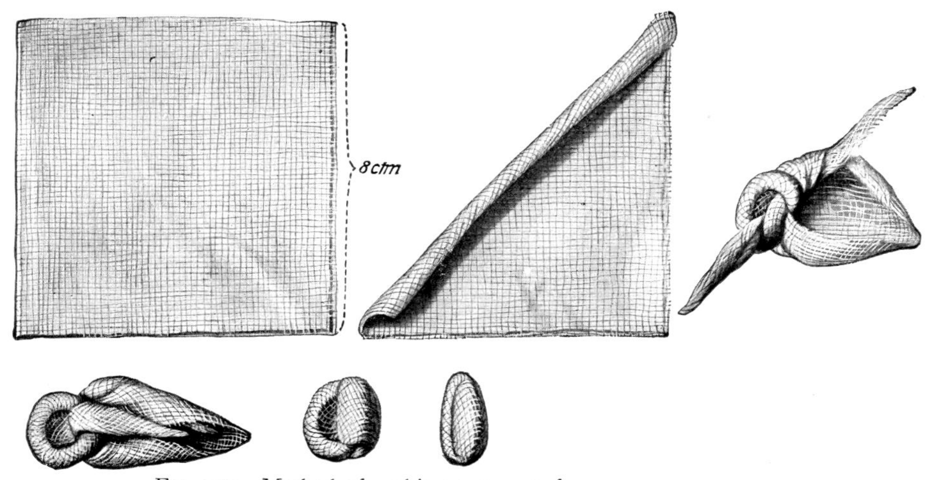

Fig. 217. Method of making a sponge from a gauze square.

One must be especially careful in the sterilization of rubber gloves. In my clinic these are placed on a wire frame (Fig. 215) which is protected with a linen glove and sterilized in the autoclave for one-half hour at a temperature of 110° C.

The dressings and the linens are packed in special cases and placed in a Schimmelbusch drum, so that the steam has ready access to them (Fig.

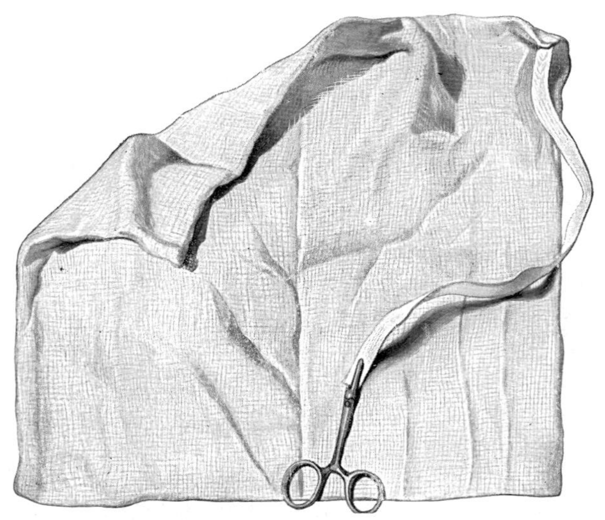

FIG. 218. Laparotomy pad with tape and clamp attached.

216). The drums are exposed to the steam of the autoclave with the slits open. After the sterilization is terminated hot dry sterile air is turned on so that the materials in the drums may be dried. When the autoclave is opened the slits in the drums are closed. The drums are opened just before they are to be used. The sacks are then carefully opened with sterile instruments, and the contents taken out with sterile instruments by a nurse who has previously

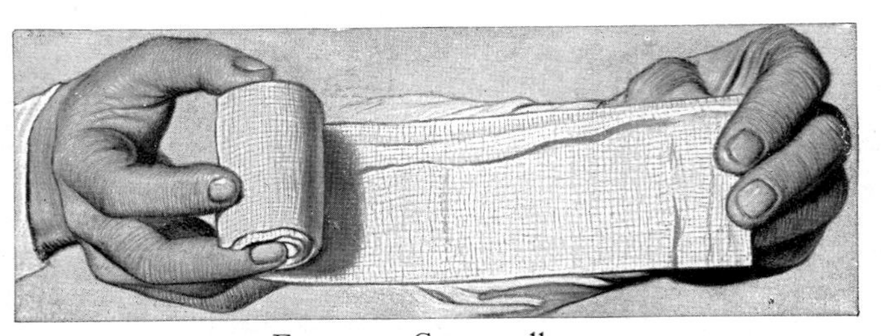

FIG. 219. Gauze roll.

scrubbed up. Once a drum is opened it should be used and any materials left in it should be resterilized. From time to time, to convince myself of the safety of my sterilization, I employ v. Mikulicz's controls. These consist of a strip of blotter which is placed at the bottom of the material to be sterilized. The blotter is thickly covered with a 3 percent starch paste, which is partly dried and then immersed in a solution of potassium iodide, after which it is dried. The bluish black colored blotter becomes discolored if sufficient heat is present. One may also use commercial paper strips, on which as the result of a similar chemical reaction the word "sterilized" appears when they are exposed to sufficient heat. It is well to have the autoclave checked from time to time to assure oneself of its efficacy. The autoclave may also be tested by placing cultures of anthrax spores in it, but a better method is the use of a thermometer which will accurately register the maximum degree of heat attained.

In case of necessity the operative linens and the dressings can be sterilized by boiling. If this is done they should be used while still wet. If it is impossible to autoclave these materials I prefer the ironing of the freshly washed materials.

For tampons I use folded gauze 12, 30 or 50 cm. square. As tampons for the dissecting forceps I use doubled gauze, 8 cm. square, which is folded together as shown in illustration 217.

For sponges I use a sewed 45 cm. square of gauze of four thicknesses (Fig. 218). In order not to overlook their position, an occurrence which is very serious in abdominal operations, I place a hemostat on the tape which extends out of the wound. Or these may come with a large glass bead already attached to the tape.

By roller-gauze we mean a rolled piece of gauze folded six-fold, 1 m. long and 5 cm. wide (Fig. 219).

We prefer to use cellucotton as a material for absorption and for padding since it is both excellent and cheap.

Our iodoform gauze is prepared as follows: rolls of gauze are saturated with a solution consisting of iodoform 200 parts, ether 1600, alcohol (96%) 1600, glycerin 200. The wet gauze is placed in a sterile bucket, and covered with a sterile cloth, wherein it soon drys. Before it is used, it is packed in a Schimmelbusch drum and separated from its walls with a layer of cotton 2 cm. thick. It is then sterilized for a half hour, at 100° C. Because of its offensive odor I have for some time given up the use of iodoform in my clinic, and have replaced it with the equally efficient vioform. The vioform packs are made by saturating the gauze rolls in the following solution: vioform 10 parts, absolute alcohol 50, glycerin 25, refined sugar 10, distilled water 500.

The dressing materials made of gauze, and the bandages, may be used over again several times, providing they are not too soiled. For this purpose, after being used, they are boiled for a half hour in soapsuds and then washed in a washing machine, after which they are dried and worked over as new material. Dressing material that is not to be used again should be burned in an incinerator.

Silk and linen sutures are wound around porcelain bobbins (Fig. 220) and boiled for 5 minutes in distilled water. In doing this care is taken to cover the reel with a piece of rubber tubing or to place on it a removable wire rod, so that the sutures are not unduly stretched when wet, which would make them fragile. The water is removed and the silk or linen is then boiled again for 2 minutes in 0.5 percent corrosive sublimate solution. It is left in this last solution until it is used. Silk rolls which have been used can be reboiled in the sublimate solution. Of course the sutures must be tested for their strength.

Suture material made of metal and silkworm gut are boiled with the instruments in the usual manner. Horsehair is boiled for 3 minutes in distilled water and then placed in sterile oil.

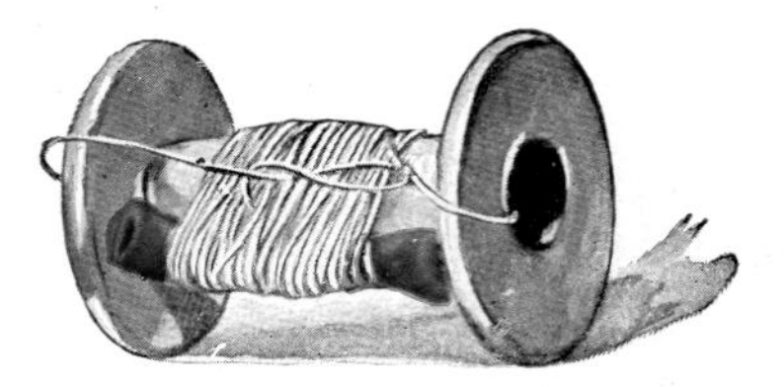

Fig. 220. Silk and linen sutures are wrapped on a porcelain spool over a piece of small rubber tubing to prevent weakening from tension.

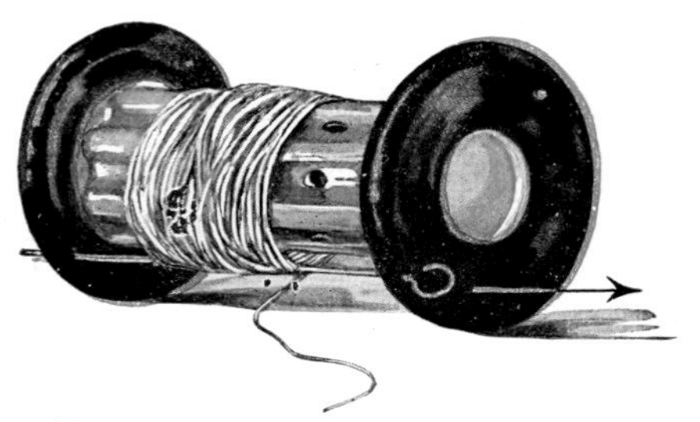

Fig. 221. Porcelain spool for silk with a removable wire rod which prevents overstretching of the moist silk.

In Germany catgut is obtained in sterilized dry balls which are kept in receptacles filled with 96 percent alcohol. The catgut balls must remain in the receptables for at least two days to become pliable. It is regrettable that most of the catgut manufactured in balls lacks tensile strength. (In the United States the majority of clinics use catgut put up in glass tubes. These may nor may not be boilable. The manufacturers use various processes for sterilization and various solutions for surrounding the gut in the tubes. The most frequently used catguts are the plain, the iodine and the chromic gut. These resist absorption for variable periods when buried in the tissues. The tubes are kept in sterile containers surrounded by one of the antiseptic solutions (Fig. 222). The tubes containing the same size of gut are surrounded with rubber bands. I.S.R.)

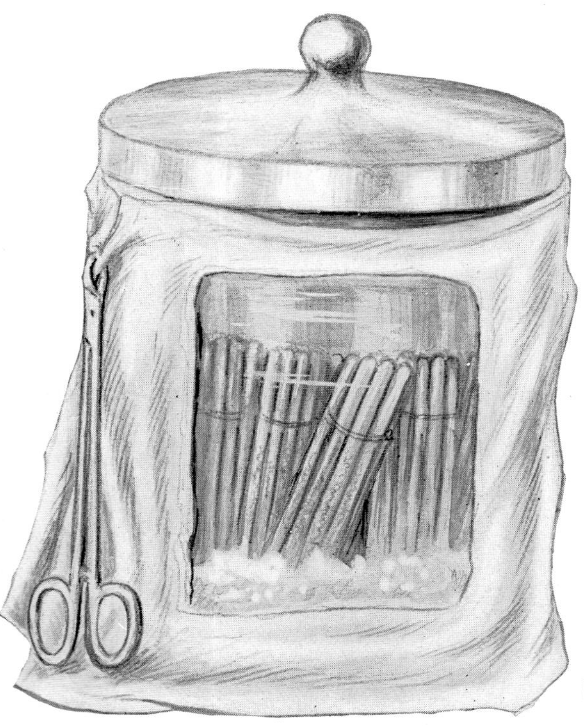

Fig. 222. Container for storing sterile catgut in an antiseptic solution.

Operating gowns should fasten in the back. They should have long sleeves which fit tightly around the wrists, over which the gloves are drawn (Figs. 223 and 224). If the sleeves are too short, or tend to slip from beneath the glove, the space between the sleeve and the glove should be covered by a special rubber or knitted cuff (Fig. 225). The operating gown should reach to about the middle of the leg.

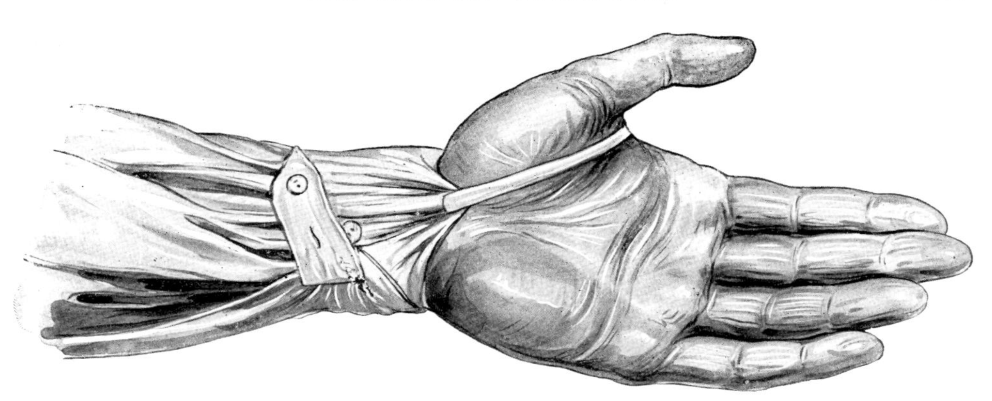

FIG. 223. The loop on the sleeve of the operating gown prevents the sleeve from slipping back from the glove.

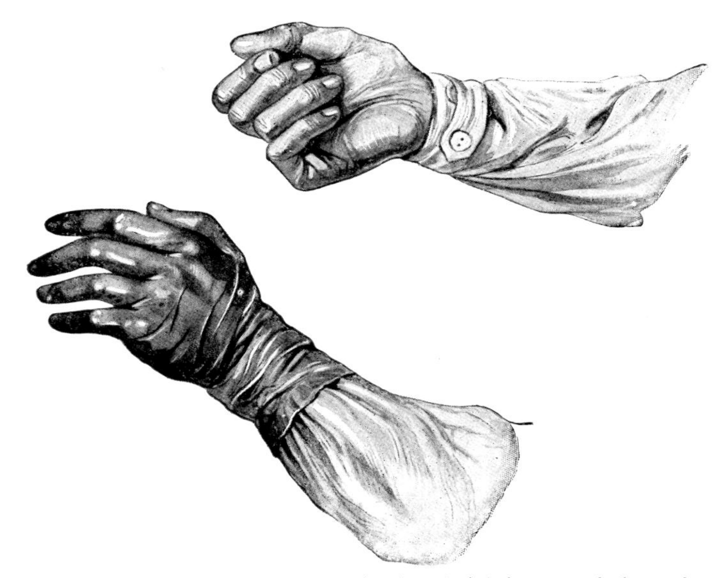

FIG. 224. The sleeve of the operating gown is closed tightly around the wrist (right arm). The rubber glove is drawn over the cuff for greater protection (left arm).

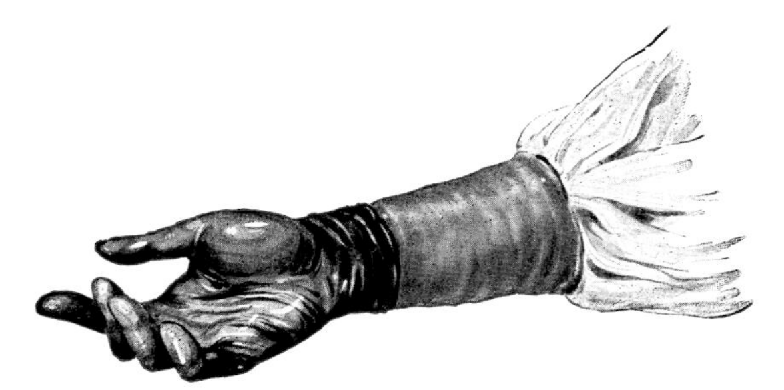

FIG. 225. A rubber cuff covers the space between the sleeve of the gown and the glove, when the sleeve is too short.

Although speaking should be limited during the operation, it can not be entirely avoided. Mouth-masks are therefore used for protection against droplet infection. These are made out of four thicknesses of gauze in a rectangular shape, the sides being provided with tapes (Fig. 226).

I believe that a full beard is hazardous. I permit my staff to have a short-trimmed moustache. As a rule we use a head band around our closely cut hair, or a cap made of a loosely woven material such as gauze (Figs. 226 and 227), and I am of the opinion the operator and his assistants are in need of a clear and cool head, which can not be the case when the entire head is covered with a tight cap in an exceedingly warm operating room, as is customary in many clinics. The nurses' hair should be covered by complete masks (Fig. 228). I believe that the large hoods worn by some orders of nuns are handicaps during the operation both as regards asepsis and illumination.

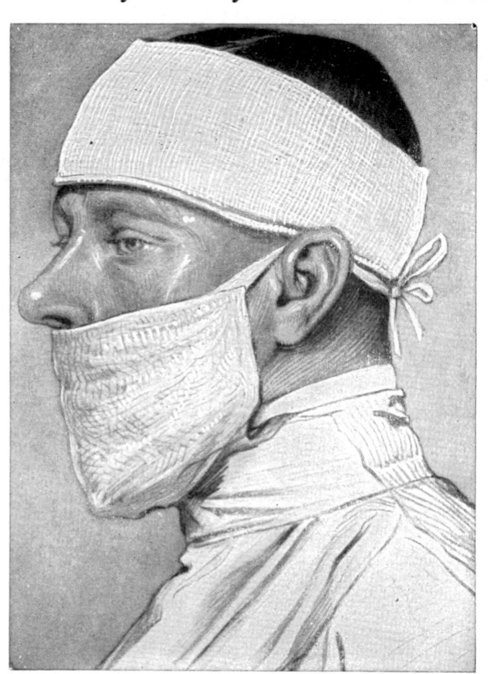

Fig. 226. Face mask and forehead band (Kirschner).

Our cotton gloves are marked on their backs with stars, the left with a red one and the right with a green one. In this way the proper glove can be easily placed on the correct hand.

Rubber gloves are washed in running water immediately after they are used. They are hung up and turned inside out and dried on both sides, after which they are sprinkled on both sides with talcum powder. After they are packed or drawn over cotton gloves on a wire frame, they are sterilized by steam. If need be, the rubber gloves may be sterilized by boiling. If this is done they must be used wet. Before slipping on dry gloves, the hands should be powdered with sterile talcum. The right glove is put on first.

Hand brushes should be sterilized by steam and should then be kept in an antiseptic solution. I use a 2 percent Sagrotan solution. One should beware of brushes with stiff bristles. We use brushes only in scrubbing the fingernails. The rubber sponges which we use routinely for scrubbing the hands, are boiled in a solution of soda.

Silk catheters are sterilized much the same as the dressing materials in the autoclave. Every catheter should be wrapped in a special cloth or in a special paper case, otherwise the catheters will stick together. They may also be boiled for several minutes in glycerine.

The cystoscope, with the exception of the lens, is boiled. The lens is disinfected by immersion for an hour in a 2 percent Sagrotan solution, or any other suitable solution.

I use only two sizes of "drapes"; a small one 1 m. square; and a large one, 1.40 m. x 1.80 m., the shorter side being marked with a red edge I do not use fenestrated linen or angular sheets.

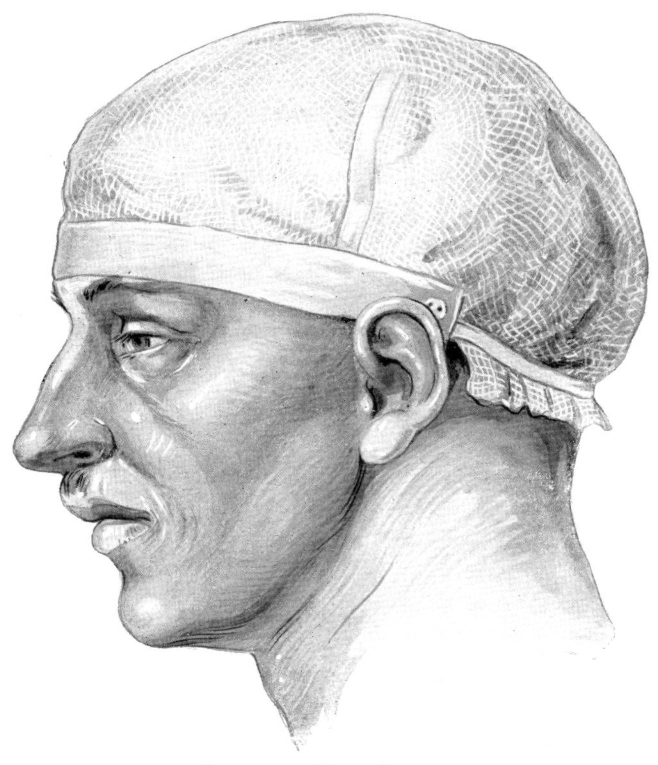

FIG. 227. Operating cap.

The skin of the human body can not be rendered germ free. Our methods of chemical disinfection effect only a reduction in the number of germs and an attenuation of those which remain.

THE DISINFECTION OF THE FIELD OF OPERATION

Every detailed preparation of the field of operation which subjects the patient to undue exposure, or injures the skin, should be condemned. The site of the field of operation should be shaved the day before operation after the skin has been thoroughly cleansed. A cleansing bath is given if the patient's strength permits it and if this is not contraindicated by the lesion. In other cases a sponge bath is given. In emergency operations, the patients are shaved and cleansed immediately before the operation. My method of skin disinfection consists in one thorough painting of the skin at the site of operation with tannin-alcohol (denaturated alcohol 1000, tannic acid powder 75, fuchsin, a few granules). (See Reports, German Surgical Congress, 1922, Kirschner, Noetzel.) The addition of fuchsin is merely to show how much of the skin has been prepared. In those operations in which it is not desirable to discolor the skin, as well as in infectious processes, the fuchsin is omitted. The painting should be done with sponges well saturated with the solution and sufficient solution should be used to paint the area thoroughly. In many clinics, 5 percent tincture of iodine is used. The area of operation is painted twice. This procedure is more expensive; it is more apt to irritate the patient's skin and mucous membranes; it obliterates the color of the skin and affects the texture, which is of importance in infectious processes. It may give rise to adhesions from contact of the intestines with the painted skin (Propping). These disadvantages are not met with in the tannin-alcohol method of disinfection.

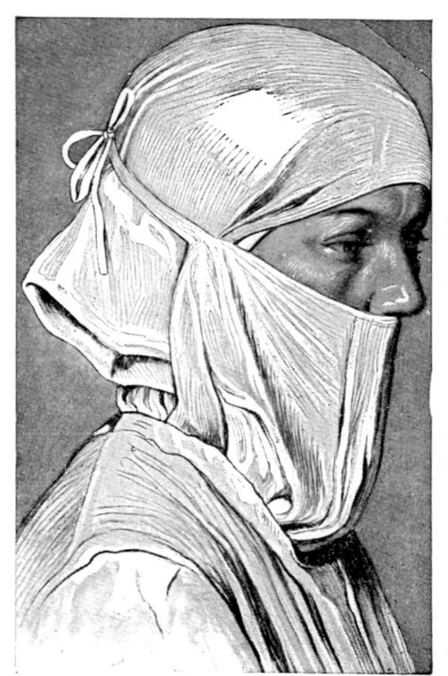

Fig. 228. Complete head and face mask.

To protect ourselves we use a rubber apron while scrubbing and during the operation. I also use white rubber shoes. These are easier to clean than are those made of leather. The surgeons' and assistants' suits are made of white cotton material. The sleeves of the shirts should be short.

The Disinfection of the Hands. Even in the disinfection of the hands the simplest methods are often the most efficient. The hands and forearms, up to the elbows, are washed for from 3 to 5 minutes in warm running water with soap, using a soft brush. In about the middle of the scrubbing the fingernails should be cleaned with a boiled orange wood stick, or one made of celluloid. The use of metal nail cleaners should be condemned, since any material harder than the nail itself will scratch the nail, leaving grooves in which dirt can later accumulate. After the soap and water, the hands and forearms are washed for five minutes with 60 percent denatured alcohol. This solution is placed in basins and the washing is done with sterile rubber sponges. Figure 229 shows the type of basin in ordinary use, while figure 230 illustrates the one I have found most satisfactory.[1] After the alcohol wash, the hands should be held up above the level of

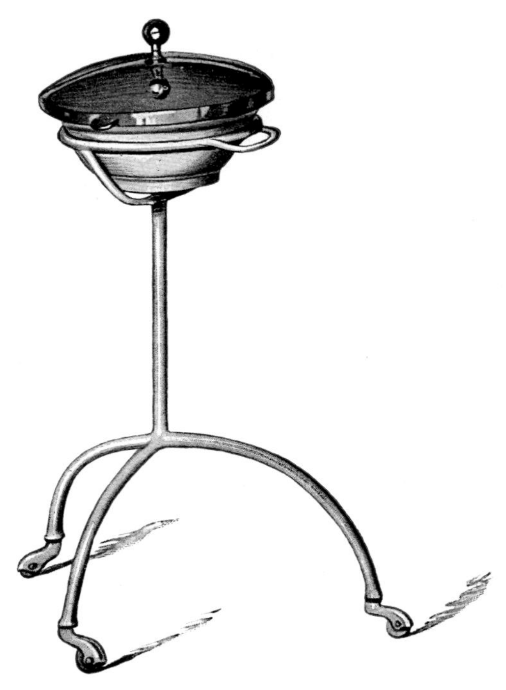

Fig. 229. Bowl for solutions with stand and cover, for disinfection of the hands.

[1] The alcohol which has been used for disinfection of the hands can be used over again after it is filtered and sufficient fresh denatured alcohol is added to make this a 60 percent solution. We have used since 1916 commercial denatured alcohol and never have noticed the slightest damage to our hands.

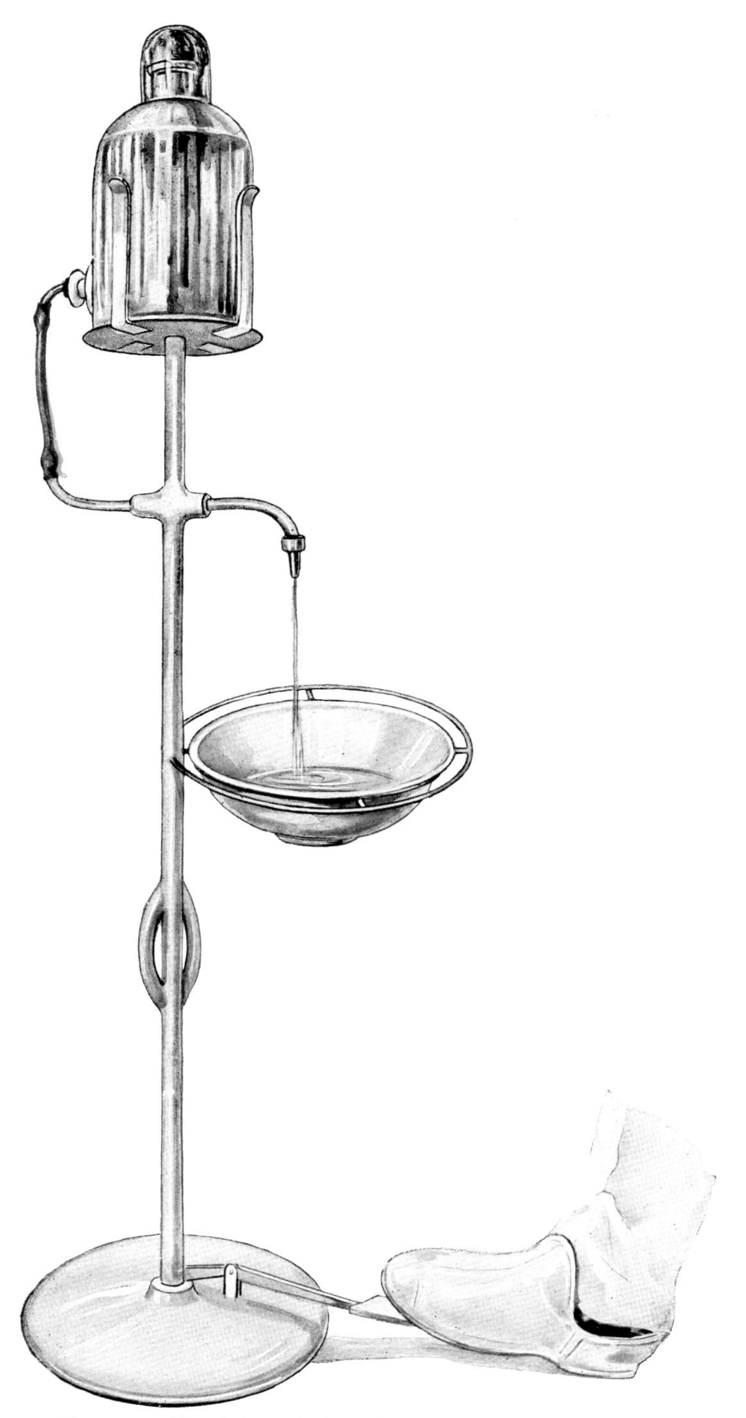

FIG. 230. Stand for solutions for disinfection of the hands.

the elbows, so that bacteria-laden droplets may not drip on them from above the elbow toward the prepared forearm and hand (Figs. 231 and 232). The hands are dried with a small sterile towel, which is either handed to the surgeon or assistant with a sterile forceps, or is picked up from a sterile towel pile in such a way as not to touch or moisten the others in the pile. The hands are dried first and then the distal portion of the forearms. The proximal half of the forearm is not dried. With this, the hand disinfection is completed. The gloves are put on after the gown has been put on and after the field of operation has been prepared.

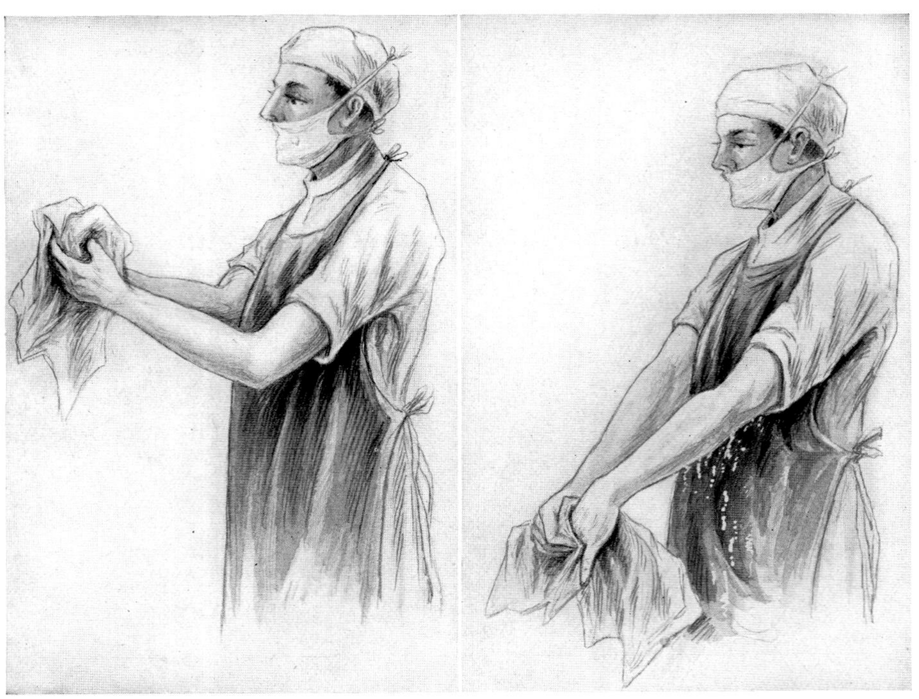

Fig. 231. Drying the hands, after rinsing in alcohol. The sterile towel is held away from the unsterile apron and the hands are held above the level of the elbows to prevent drops of alcohol from the arms running over the hands.

Fig. 232. Two errors frequently made: The sterile towel that is used for drying the hands brushes against the contaminated apron. The hands are held lower than the elbows, so that drops run to the hands from the arms.

This simple method of alcohol disinfection suffices, according to our experience. Under certain conditions the easily evaporating alcohol can not be kept in readiness for a long period, nor can it be carried in large quantities. This makes its use unsatisfactory in military work. It is of great practical importance to find a substance which is not easily altered and which can be carried in a small volume. I believe I have found such a substance in Sagrotan. (Rauch, German Surgical Congress, 1925.) A 2 percent solution of Sagrotan can take the place of 60 percent alcohol for hand disinfection. I have used it successfully for one year at the Königsberg Clinic instead of alcohol.

The surgeon must take constant care of his hands, in order to prevent contamination and infection. His whole life is an uninterrupted, conscious, effort at prophylaxis. He must not let his hands, while practicing surgery or in private life, touch unclean or purulent material; and he must protect them against injuries and chapping. In changing dressings two forceps, "the long, easily boiled fingers," should take the place of the hands. This is an evidence of care, training, and dexterity. In septic operations, in the examination or dressing of purulent wounds, in examinations of the rectum or oral cavity, the surgeon should protect his hands with good rubber gloves. "I wear rubber gloves all day, and I take them off when I operate" (Kocher). One may operate more safely without washing the hands which have been kept clean and have not been contaminated with virulent organisms, than with an infected hand after a careful disinfection! Semmelweiss has said: "It is safer not to dirty the finger, than to do so and clean it again." As we enter a ward, the nurse in charge hands us a pair of rubber gloves.

When it was ascertained that it was impossible to render the hands germ-free, Friedrich in Germany and Halstead in America introduced the use of rubber gloves in surgery. This provided a valuable means for enhancing aseptic surgery, but even then it did not always provide a bacteria-free hand. The numerous minute perforations which are often present in the very thin rubber gloves often prevent a completely aseptic operation. Later development has given the rubber glove an entirely new and perhaps even a higher importance; namely, to protect the hands against soiling during septic operations and other unclean work. Today, rubber gloves are indispensable in surgery. In a septic operation they protect the clean hand from the infected wound, in aseptic operations they protect the clean wound from the contaminated hand! I insist on the use of rubber gloves in every operation. The assistants in abdominal operations frequently use cotton gloves over rubber gloves, in order to hold firmly slippery viscera.

For particularly delicate work, as for example in the suture of blood vessels, I remove the rubber gloves, without fear of endangering the asepsis. The hands must be washed in alcohol, after the rubber gloves have been taken off. When cotton gloves are saturated with blood and tissue fluid, when one shifts from an infected area to a relatively sterile one, or when a rubber glove is torn, the hands should be rapidly disinfected and the gloves replaced by sterile ones.

The modern surgeon, who is conscious of the fact that the best disinfection of the hands, with the addition of gloves, is not the ideal, avoids as much as possible getting his hands in contact with the wound and attempts to work in the wound only with instruments. The hands do not belong in the wound. It must be understood, however, that these efforts are successful only to a degree, since in the placing of ligatures, for instance, it is impossible to keep the hands out of the wound.

The Operating Room. Since bacteria are deposited on objects, and can not really be conveyed except by contact, any room may be made suitable for operation after the most careful preparation, providing it is thoroughly cleaned, flies eliminated, and it is rain proof. This is often necessary during military action. Under normal conditions major operations are naturally undertaken in specially equipped rooms, in which not only the most minute asepsis is guaranteed, but the illumination, temperature, ventilation, and equipment have been considered.

To provide a greater aseptic security it is advantageous to divide the operating clinic into an aseptic and a septic section, each section having its own instruments, linens, tampons, dressings, etc. This separation, however,

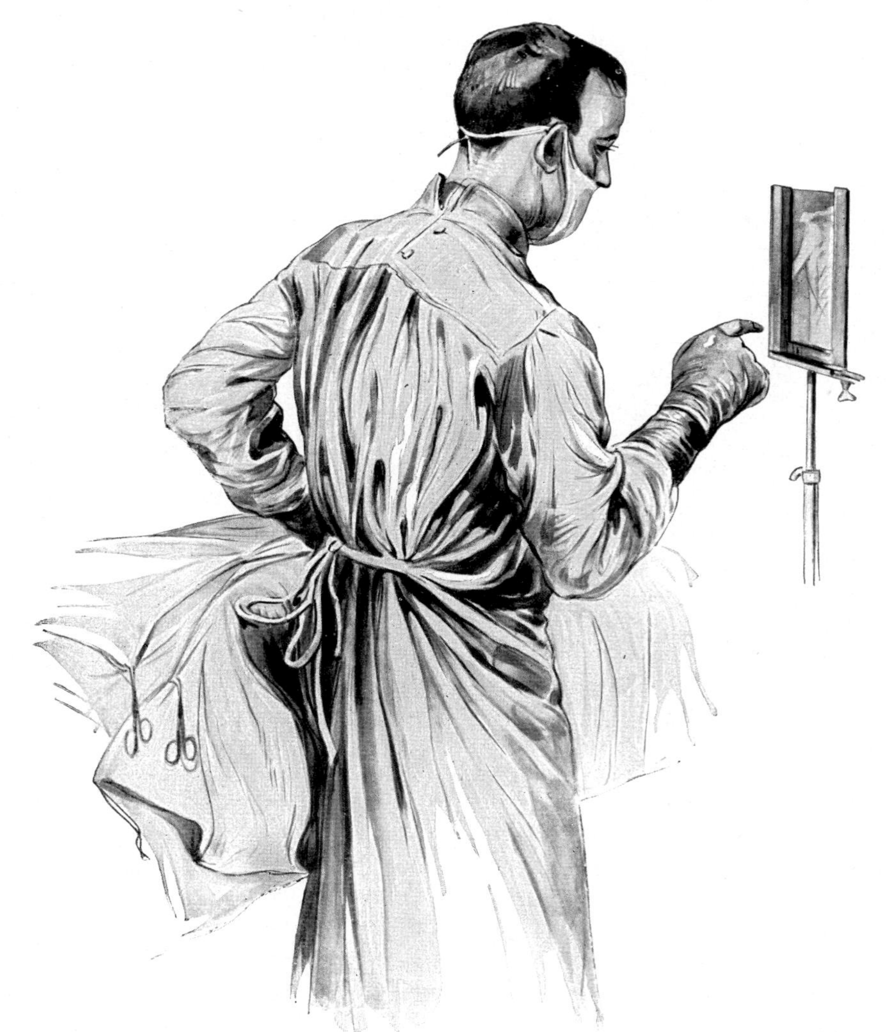

FIG. 233. A mistake often made: The operator touches the sterile linens with the non-sterile back of his gown.

is not complete and is not entirely effective unless the operators, assistants and personnel are divided at the same time. Theoretically this is ideal; practically it is impossible. It is impossible always to draw a sharp line between aseptic and septic cases, since every operation for intestinal resection must be considered septic. In reality, the separation of the operating rooms and their divisions is a suggestion only, since the practise of operating on severe purulent, phlegmonous cases in an operating room directly connected with the septic wards amounts to approximately the same thing. At the Königsberg Clinic for some years, as a result of building alterations I operated on all patients in one room, and did not have separate wards for septic and non-septic cases, without noticing any deleterious results as far as the operative asepsis was concerned. I have never seen the transmission of an infection, as for example erysipelas. For this, direct contact is necessary.

As a model for a modern Surgical Clinic I will describe and sketch the plan which is at present being carried out at the Tübingen Clinic under my direction.

I have provided for four operating rooms. It can no longer be doubted that several small operating rooms are preferable to one large operating room in which several operations can be done simultaneously. Only in this way can one separate patients, odors and operative materials. In this way, too, it is possible to operate upon each case in a freshly prepared room without the loss of time.

Between each two operating rooms is a sterilization room. The three rooms constitute an operating suite. The two suites are connected by a scrub-up room, which provides room for the surgeons and nurses to scrub and disinfect their hands, and to put on their sterile gowns. They can then enter the operating room ready to operate. Each operating room has a push door, near the windows, which opens into the sterilizing room from which the operating room is constantly supplied with its sterile necessities. This door is away from the operating table so that entrance and exit from the operating room does not affect the operating room team.

The plan of the sterilizing rooms is similar on each side. It is so arranged that the sterilization of instruments, their transportation to the operating room, their use, their return to the sterilizing room, and their cleansing and resterilization can be done with a minimum of work. The used instruments are passed through a window from the operating room into the sterilizing room, where they are placed in a sterilizer and boiled. From this they are lifted and cleansed under running water, and then placed in a second instrument sterilizer. When sterilized they are removed and taken through the push door to the general instrument table. From this they are passed on to the operating table, and when used they are again passed out through the window, and the process is repeated.

In the sterilizing room is also found an electric sterilizer with distilled water for sterilizing syringes, an autoclave, an electrical basin sterilizer, and a warming cabinet for storing intravenous solutions. It also has a spigot from which flows distilled water. The physiological salt solution is kept in small individual flasks. The use of solutions from a general supply tank, even though originally sterile, is open to many disadvantages in that it can rarely be kept sterile and the danger from reactions following its use intravenously is greater.

Each operating room has its own operating table, instrument tables, and a rack for the sterile drums. At the entrance of each operating room is a table which contains the necessities for anæsthetization. All other apparatus which may be necessary during the operation are kept in four specially provided rooms which open off the main hall and are directly adjacent to the operating rooms. These can be seen in the plan (Fig. 234).

For illumination each operating room is covered with a glass skylight. The glass is frosted, so that the direct rays of the sun are not admitted. Light is also admitted from the windows in the north wall. The use of arti-

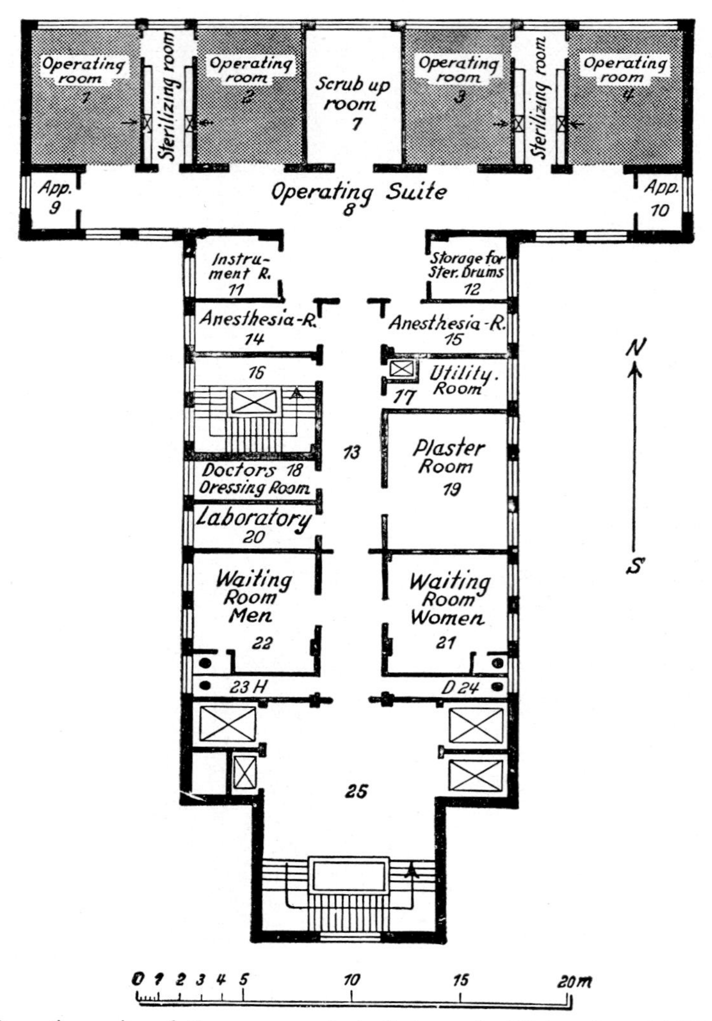

FIG. 234. Operating suite of the new surgical clinic at the University of Tübingen. The cross shading indicates the overhead lighting of the operating rooms by a skylight.

ficial light in the day is not interfered with by the natural light which comes through the glass.

For artificial illumination we use a fixed ceiling light and a standing lamp which can be moved and is adjustable. The illumination in both types may be transmitted directly from individual points, or indirectly through reflectors. In both types of lighting shadows are apt to be present. In some of the newer lights the reflection is obtained from a series of mirrors which are inserted in the crown of the lamp and the light can be adjusted so as to minimize the shadow. The Pantophos-Zeiss lamp (Fig. 235) is an excellent example of these. The Asciatique and Scialytique lamps are based on very similar principles. The light may be thrown a greater distance by a single mirror (Zeiss-Siedentopf).

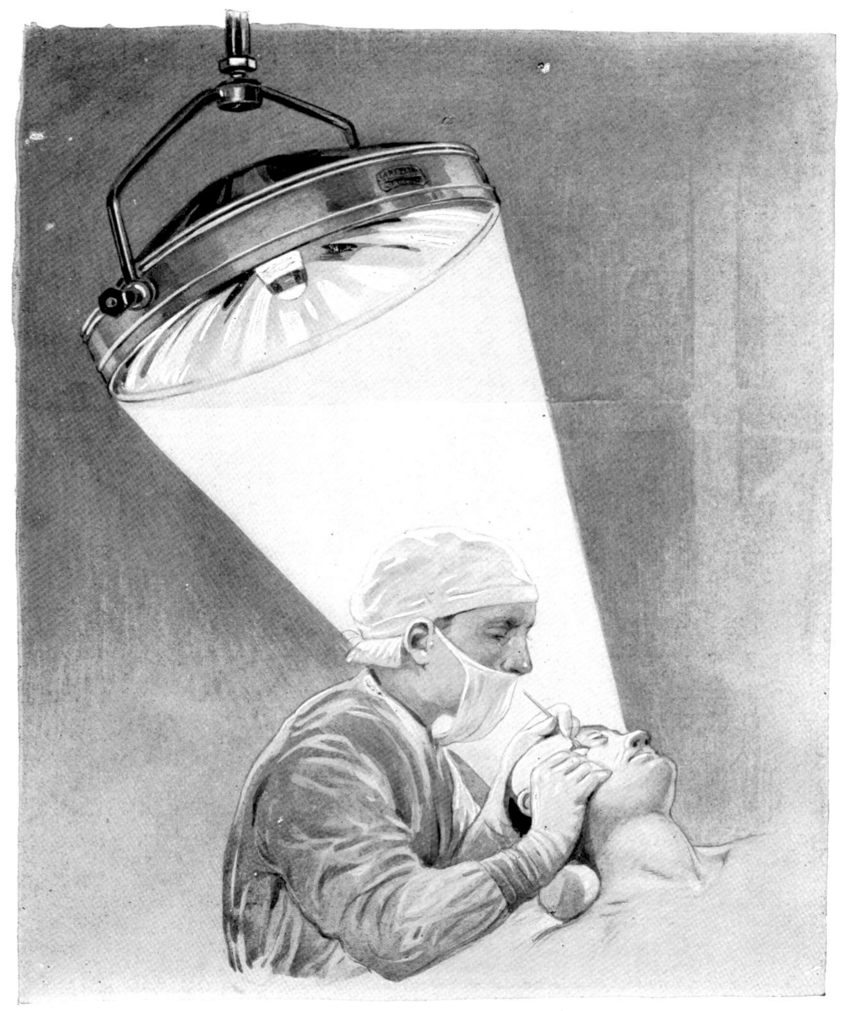

FIG. 235. Pantophos light (Zeiss).

In lighting the field of operation by rays of light falling from different directions, the putting out of one or of a few bundles of rays causes but an imperceptible obscuring of the field of operation—shadowless light. If the rays of light touch the head of the operator, it develops considerable heat, so that it is quite desirable to interpose heat-filters.

A fixed lamp or mirror, whether standing or suspended, sends its best light principally along a narrow circumscribed shaft, so that in order to obtain good illumination of the operative field, the operating table must often be moved. Objections can be raised against the horizontal displacement of lamps or mirrors serving for ceiling illumination, as in Schubert's lamp, where the sliding is done on iron rails, because of the possibility of falling dust. It is not possible in these lights to change to any considerable extent, the direction of the rays, so that they can not be made to come from the side to illuminate properly the perineum. The only type of lamp which permits one to obtain the light from any direction is the standing lamp (Fig. 236).

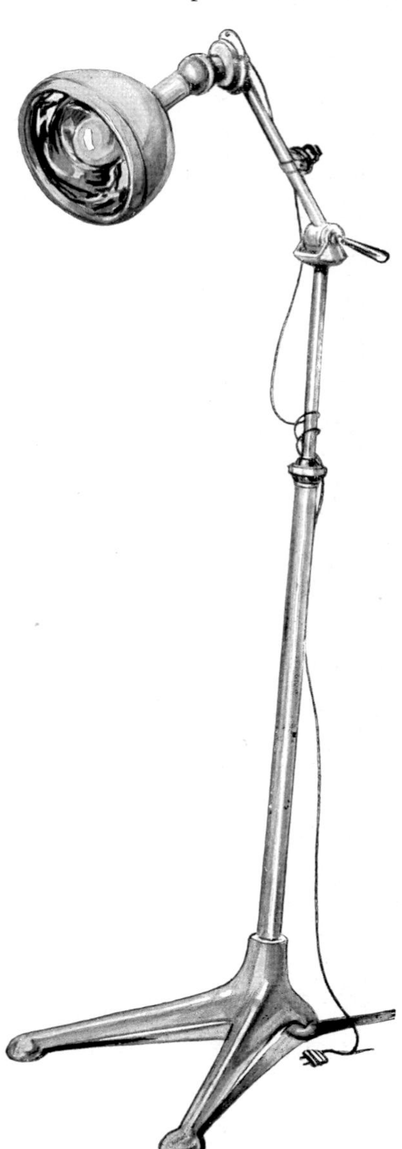

Fig. 236. Portable lamp (Zeiss).

It is practical to have the electrical illumination supplied by two separate sources, so as not to encounter difficulties in case one source of electrical current should become temporarily impaired.

In spite of this it is not always possible, with any of these devices adequately to illuminate the depths of a wound, as for example the depths of the opened urinary bladder. Adequate illumination is however often necessary for proper orientation. In such instances it is preferable to use a light which can be introduced into the wound. For this surgeons are now using small electric lights which are similar to those used in cystoscopy and bronchoscopy. These are made in various shapes and are indeed very useful. They are sterilizable (Fig. 237). The lights which are attached to various instruments such as knives, scissors, and forceps I have not found practical.

Although I believe that the displacement of white by color in the operating room has been overdone, still I believe it advisable to use gray for the floors and the walls up to an angle of 45° above the direct line of vision. Above that the walls may be white.

The removal of air by suction at the point of origin of the anæsthetic vapors and of unpleasant odors has not proved successful. In order to make these fumes harmless it is only necessary to provide for their rapid dissemination throughout the operating room. I accomplish this by suitably placed electric fans (Fig. 238). It is necessary to provide a method for replacing the air of the operating room. The source should not be close to the operating table. The ventilating methods which utilize long conduits or air shafts are not dependable, nor are they clean. I believe that the best system for ventilating the operating room consists of inlets directly through the outer wall and of similar outlets which are regulated by efficient fans. If fresh air is available it is not always necessary to suck out the air in the room, since the incoming fresh air will force out the contaminated air.

For heating, only steam or hot-water should be considered, the radiators being placed beneath the windows. The radiators must be accessible from all sides so they may be cleansed daily. Large operating rooms can be heated rapidly in case of an emergency by open-flame alcohol burners. The procedure may have to be repeated since the air cools rapidly. Extreme caution must be exercised in any operating room where an open flame exists. The temperature of the operating room, considering that the patient is only

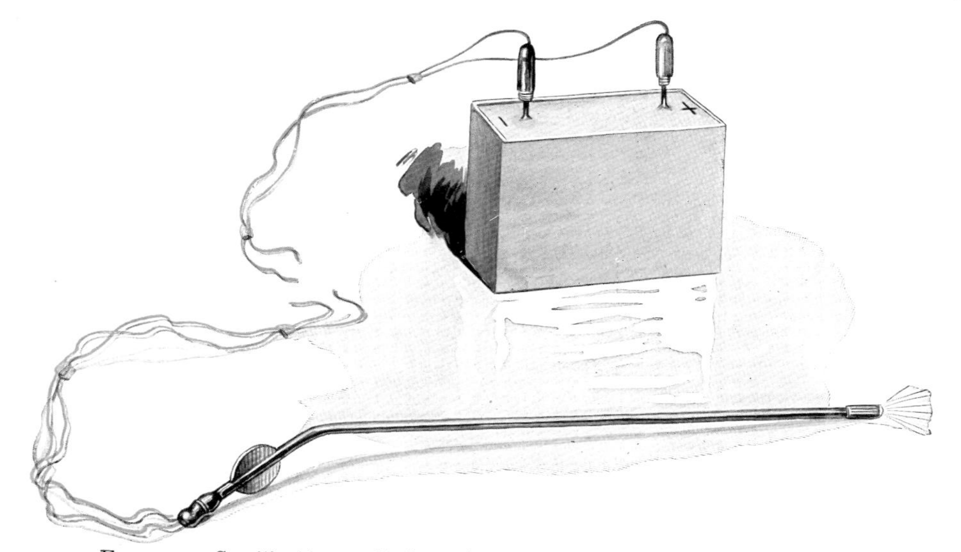

FIG. 237. Sterilizable small light for illuminating the depths of wounds.

partly covered and that the general anæsthetic lowers the body temperature, should be 25°C. By means of electrically controlled thermometers the temperature in the operating room is indicated in and controlled from the power plant. A moist temperature of 25°C. is tolerated with difficulty by the surgeon, his assistants, and the nurses within the operating room. Small electric fans placed at strategic points help to cool off the individual persons and provide for them a cool area in an otherwise over-heated room. Care must be exercised so that the draught does not strike the field of operation or the patient. Bacteriological researches have shown us that by using such ventilators there is no greater precipitation of bacteria.

The soiled linens are dropped through a trap which is placed just above the floor in the wall adjacent to the sterilizing room. The chute takes the soiled laundry to a collecting room on the floor beneath. The linens drop into boilers which soak and boil them so that they are not touched until they are sterilized. After being boiled they are dried in a built-in turbine. They are removed from the apparatus through a door and are received in the laundry room sterilized and nearly dry. In this way other materials in the laundry never come in contact with the soiled linens of the operating room until these are sterilized.

Along the passageway leading to the operating rooms are found a plaster room; a surgeons' dressing room; a laboratory where smears and frozen sections may be prepared; four rooms for apparatus and storage; a splint room; large waiting rooms, and special rooms for the staff and its personnel.

The instruments are kept in built in cabinets which are in the rooms just outside of the operating rooms. The volatile anæsthetics are kept in an electric refrigerator.

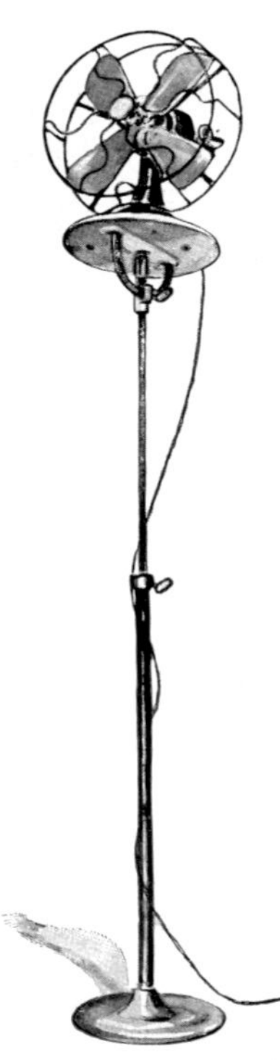

FIG. 238. Electric fan with stand for use in the operating room.

The operating suite is situated at the top of the nine story building so that it is above the street dirt and noises. I believe this is the proper location for the operating room. Furthermore, any noise which may originate on the operating room floor is not apt to get to the wards, private rooms, or into the gardens surrounding the hospital.

In the operating room we attempt to get along with as few persons as possible, not only for economy's sake, but also because the fewer workers the more quiet it is and the less danger there is of a slip in technic. It is necessary to have present for every operation, the surgeon, his assistants, the anæsthetist, and one or two sterile nurses. Besides these there should be at least one or preferably two non-sterile aids, who place the patient on the table, tie the gowns on those wearing them, bring and take away instruments, apparatus, dressings, solutions, medicaments, service the electrical apparatus, lamps, ventilators, etc. When more than one operation is performed in the same room, two or three helpers suffice for both operations, and a further helper for every additional operating table. Our appliances are so arranged that many of them can be used by individuals prepared to operate. The faucets in the sinks can be operated with the head or with the foot. All the operating room doors and those of the adjoining rooms can be opened with the foot from either side. For this purpose, they are provided on both sides, about 20 cm. from the floor, with iron brackets (Fig. 239). The doors close automatically, noiselessly, and without catching. To lessen the noise in the operating room as much as possible, all objects which stand have rubber caps on their legs and rubber wheels are provided on all tables. The buckets are made noiseless by using rubber covers over their bottoms. The handles are covered with rubber. Noises in the operating room are not only disagreeable, but they are also injurious. They annoy the unanæsthetized patient, and they disturb the operator. They cause orders to be given in a louder tone of voice, and they distract the operating personnel from the patient.

It is of advantage to have provision for fluoroscopy in the immediate vicinity of the operating room. We have in our x-ray department a special operating room with an under-table tube, where bone operations and the removal of foreign bodies, etc., can be undertaken. There should also be a small laboratory near by, but this should not be connected with the operating room. In this tissues and fluids can be examined while the operation is in progress. This is frequently of great help. This laboratory should be equipped to prepare histological frozen sections, so as to determine within a very short time whether the surgeon is dealing with a benign or malignant tumor. In this laboratory, specimens may also be kept under glass until the completion of the operation. Such a laboratory is a source of considerable aid and comfort to the surgeon, especially if it is in charge of a competent pathologist.

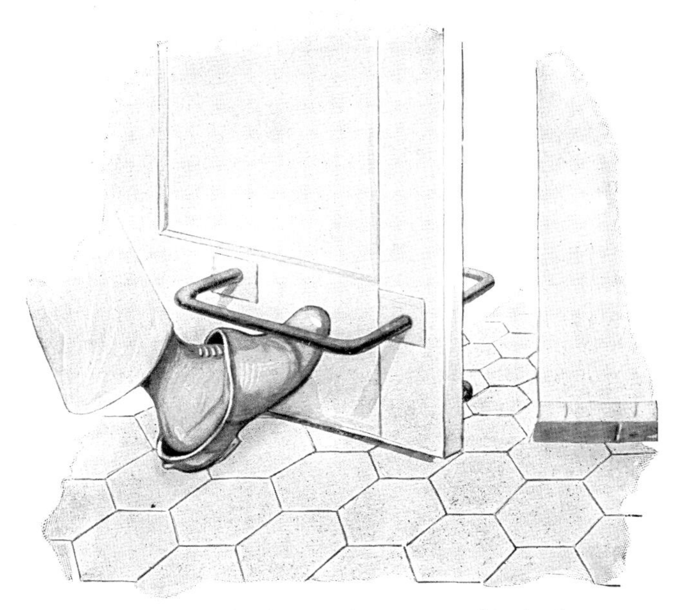

FIG. 239. Device for opening a door with the foot.

Apparatus for Aspiration of Fluids. The need for aspiration of fluid frequently arises in the operating room and in the sick room. In the operating room it is often necessary for the removal of ascites or collections of pus; for the aspiration of blood during operations; for clearing the field of operation as in suprapubic cystotomy, or cholecystotomy; for evacuation of the contents of portions of the intestine or stomach; during esophagoscopy or bronchoscopy. At the bedside we need continuous aspiration mainly for drainage of the bladder and the stomach, and for the drainage of empyema cavities. In the latter cases it can be used to maintain a subatmospheric pressure.

For suction the following materials are used: 1. A common syringe. 2. Syphonage. 3. The drop-aspirator. 4. The bottle-aspirator. 5. Potain's apparatus. 6. The water pump. 7. The electric suction pump. These apparatus are interchangeable in their use, but for certain uses one of them may be superior to the others.

1. The employment of the syringe for aspiration has its chief field of usefulness in exploration for collections of fluid or pus. The syringe is attached to a hollow needle. The barrel of the syringe should never be pulled out further than three-quarters the length of the cylinder. When syringes are used for emptying cavities, as for instance the pleural cavity, care must be taken to provide a method which will prevent air from entering the cavity while the syringe is connected and disconnected. This can be accomplished by means of a compressible short rubber tube inserted between the syringe and the cannula, or by means of a stop-cock.

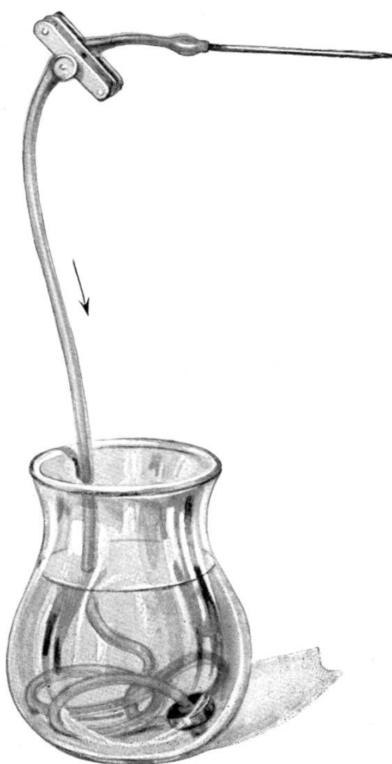

Fig. 240. Continuous syphon drainage (Bülau). The needle is connected with a tube on which is a screw clamp and which is weighted at its end with a metal weight. The end of the tube is placed in a vessel partially filled with an antiseptic solution. The needle is inserted with the tube filled with solution and the cock closed. This prevents air from entering and tends to maintain the normal pressure of the space into which it is inserted.

2. Syphonage is easily obtained by attaching a hollow needle to one end of a rubber tube and a weight with a hole in it at the other end. The tube is filled with a sterile or antiseptic solution and a clamp is placed on the tube close to the needle. The weighted end is placed in a glass vessel partly filled with sterile water or an antiseptic solution (Fig. 240). When the tube is raised it remains filled with fluid. After the cannula is inserted by puncture into the fluid collection which is to be aspirated, the clamp is opened and syphonage begins. The collecting receptacle should be at a lower level than the position of the needle. The suction pressure developed is proportional to the perpendicular distance between the two fluid levels and can thus be graduated at will by raising or by lowering the stand which holds the collecting receptacle.

3. The drop-aspirator (Hartert) (Fig. 241) employs the suction created by the dropping of water through a specially made glass bulb. A Martin drop-bulb (Fig. 242) is connected above with a bottle filled with water. The tube carrying the water into the bulb is adjusted for a slow drop of the water into the bulb. The outlet tube is 1.3 mm. in diameter so that the drops fill the entire cross section of the tube as they flow out. The tube varies in length from 1 to 2 meters, depending on the suction desired. It ends in a collecting vessel. Coming from the side of the drop-bulb is a glass tube for attaching the suction tube which is connected to an aspirating bottle. The water is regulated so that a drop falls about every second. Since the dropping of the water is not dependent upon the quantity of the aspirated fluid, and since it is not dependent on atmospheric pressure, the apparatus may be used to advantage for aspirating fluid from an enclosed cavity which is not air-tight.

4. The Bunsen bottle-aspirator creates suction by the flow of water

from an elevated container to a lower one. As the fluid flows from the upper bottle a subatmospheric pressure is created in the upper container

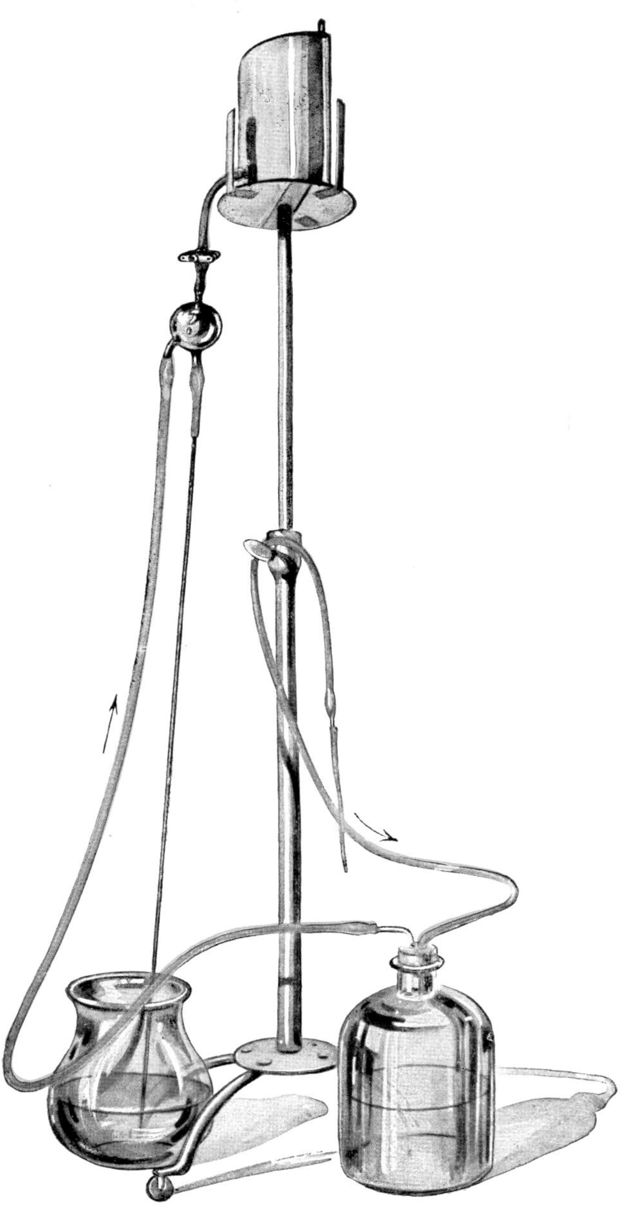

FIG. 241. Drop-aspirator (Hartert). When the drops fall from the irrigator through the thin glass tube, air is sucked from the large tube, so that a subatmospheric pressure is established in the collecting receptacle.

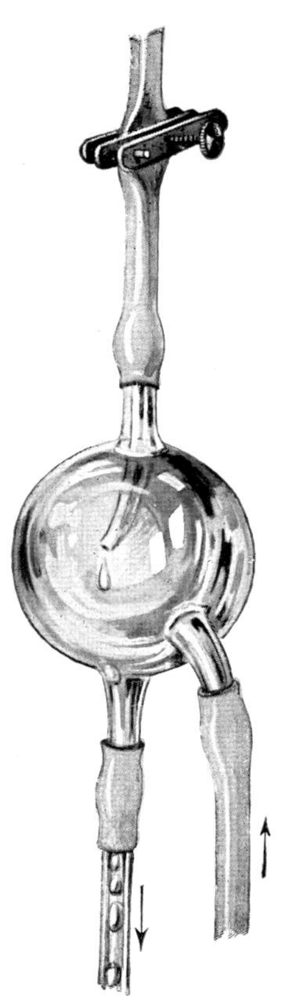

FIG. 242. The glass bulb of the drop-aspirator, with outlet at side, and screw clamp on tubing.

which is transmitted to the collecting receptacle (Fig. 243). The disadvantage of this method is that after the upper receptacle is emptied the bottles must be transposed in order to maintain suction. For this reason the containers should be large. Since only that much water can flow from the upper bottle into the lower one as there is fluid aspirated by the suction tube, and since the negative pressure in the suction tube depends upon the distance

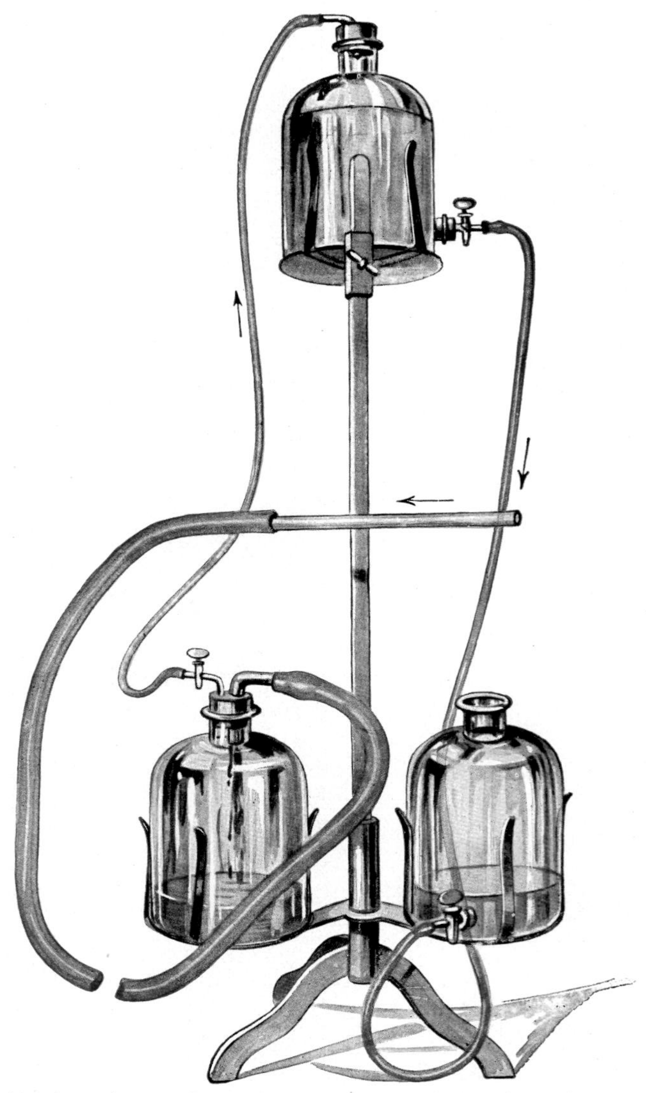

FIG. 243. Bottle-aspirator (Bunsen). The water flowing from the upper bottle into the lower bottle, creates a subatmospheric pressure in the upper bottle, that is conveyed by another tube to the collecting vessel and thence to the heavy suction tubing. This tubing is connected to a 2 cm. glass tube which serves to empty the intestine.

between the fluid surface of the bottles, the apparatus has its greatest field of usefulness in those cases in which a subatmospheric pressure of varying degree is required, as for example in the management of empyema. (The Deryl Hart apparatus used in the United States makes use of this principle. I.S.R.)

5. The Potain aspirator (Fig. 244) consists of a bottle with a two-hole

cork, through one opening of which passes the suction tube and through the other a tube connected to an aspirating pump. Each tube is provided with a stop-cock. By keeping the stop-cock on the suction tube closed, while the one leading to the pump is open, the air in the bottle can be exhausted by the pump. The stop-cock on the tube connected to the pump is closed after creating a subatmospheric pressure in the bottle and the cannula is inserted in the cavity to be aspirated, as for instance, in the pleural cavity. When the stop-cock of the suction tube is opened, the fluid flows into the bottle. When the suction is exhausted, the stop-cocks are again set so that the air in the bottle may again be removed to a point where suction is reestablished. The apparatus is adaptable for only short periods of aspiration.

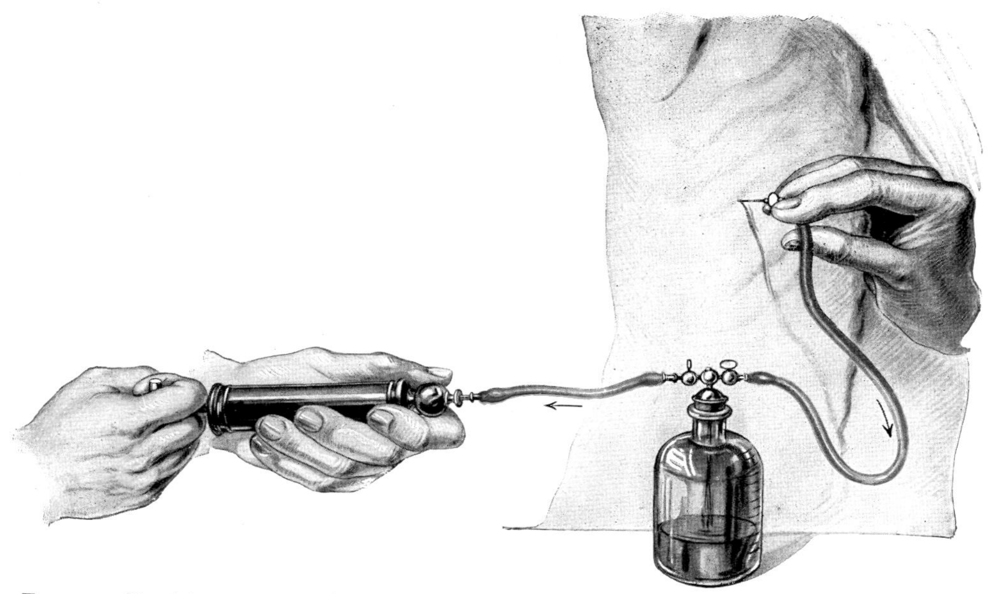

FIG. 244. Potain's apparatus. By pumping out the air, a subatmospheric pressure is created in the collecting bottle. This is maintained by adjusting the stop-cocks.

6. With the water pump (Fig. 245) a stream of water flows with great rapidity through a glass tube, which is provided with a side arm. As the water flows rapidly through the tube it carries air with it thus creating suction in the side arm connection. This apparatus must be connected with a water faucet, so that frequently long tubes are necessary to bring the suction tube to the place where it is desired. The force of aspiration can not be well controlled unless it is possible to regulate the water pressure. Considerable variations in this pressure will affect the suction. This method is applicable to the aspiration of open cavities.

7. The most efficient apparatus for creating suction is undoubtedly a well made electric pump. There are numerous varieties of these. If the pump is to be used for long periods the motor should be of a type which does not heat easily. It should also be easily regulated so that varying degrees of suction can be obtained. A variety of suction tips can be used with this apparatus (Fig. 246).

In all these aspirating apparatus the fluid aspirated is collected in a collecting receptacle.

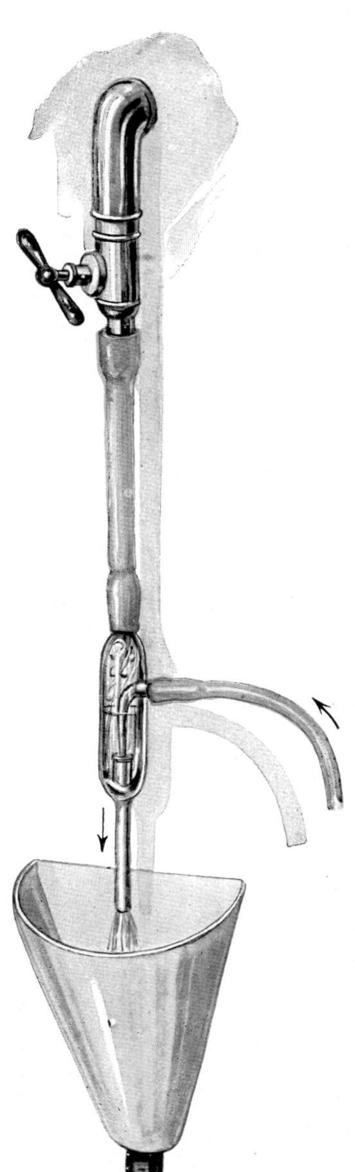

FIG. 245. Suction pump connected to a water tap. The water running through the glass cylinder draws air from the side arm, so that suction is created in the rubber tube attached on the side.

It is important that all tubing, connections, and stoppers be air tight if proper suction is to be obtained. The apparatus should always be tested before using it. Rubber stoppers are more satisfactory than are those made of cork. The stoppers should be placed in hot water just before their use.

Cannulæ, glass and rubber tubes, should be of a size suitable to the type of fluid to be aspirated. The tubing should be thick enough to withstand suction, otherwise it will collapse. For removing the contents of the intestine, a tube of a minimum diameter of 2 cm. is best.

Of considerable importance in the outcome of any operative procedure is the **transport of the patient** to and from the operating room. This fact should be given careful consideration in planning the construction of a surgical clinic. The patient should be transported from the ward or room in his bed and the distance to be traversed should be as short and as direct as possible. The corridors through which the patient is taken should be warm and the elevators should be provided with electric heaters. The patient should not be jarred and there should be no delay in transport. In order to obtain these conditions the relatively narrow, but high buildings which are provided with sufficient elevator service are far superior to the buildings which spread out over a large area.

These provisions were taken care of in building the new surgical clinic at the University of Tübingen. The plan of this clinic is illustrated in figures 247a and 247b.

B. ASEPTIC TECHNIC OF THE OPERATIVE SET-UP AND OF THE WOUND DRESSING

On the day before, the time for the operation should be scheduled and if several operations are contemplated the time for the first one should be scheduled. The list of operations and the time should be placed on a bulletin board, so that every one connected with the operating room knows what is to be done and may prepare for it. A clock should be found in every operating room.

In arranging the operative schedule, one should bear in mind the assignment and rotation of the assistants as regards infected and non-infected cases, and the advisability of starting with the non-infected and extensive opera-

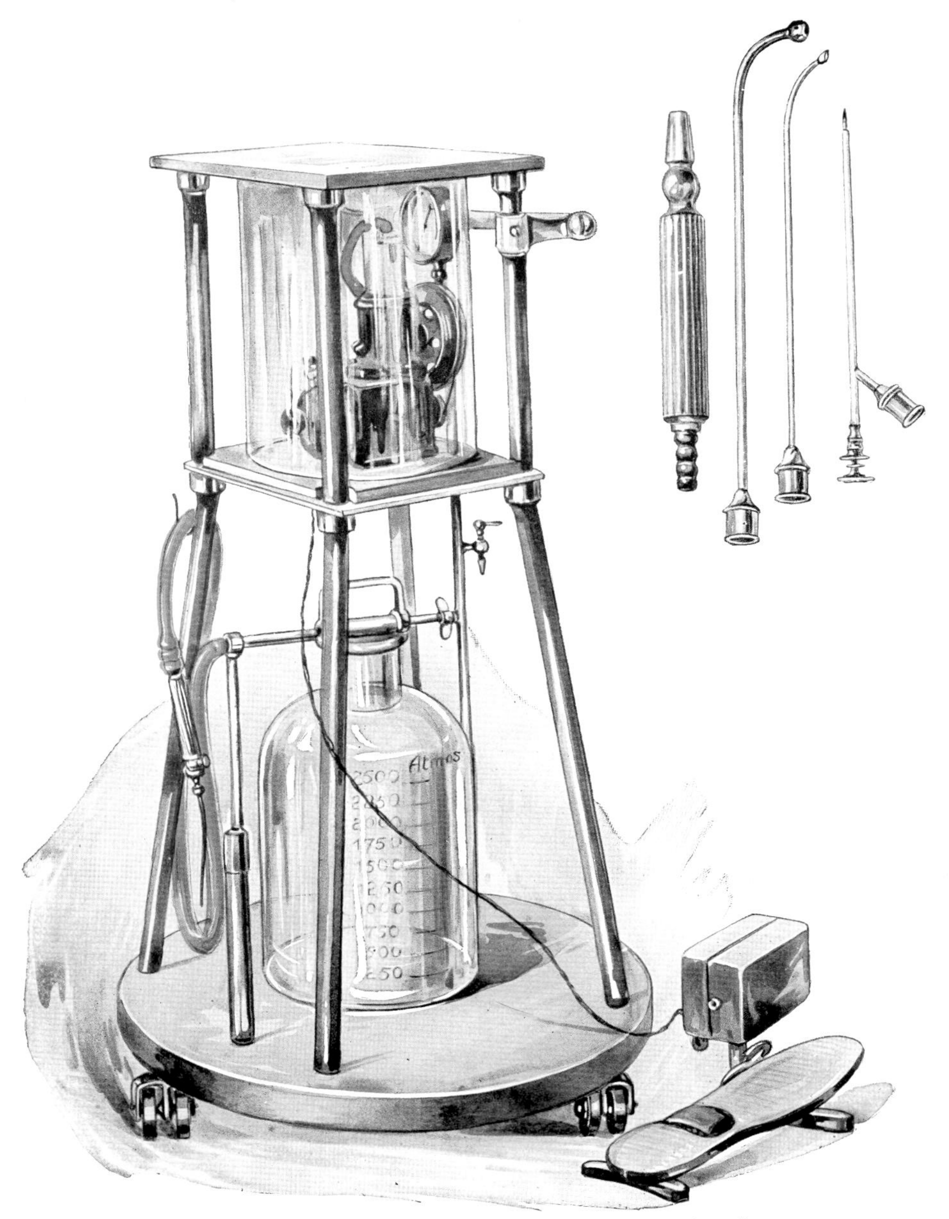

FIG. 246. Electric suction pump with various suction tips.

tions, while the obviously infected cases are left to the end. Below is the type of schedule which I use.

The operating room nurses must first prepare the operating room. They place all necessary instruments in the sterilizer, and put the sterile sponges.

dressings and linen-drums in their proper places without opening them until the contents are to be removed by a sterile nurse. A trained instrument nurse begins scrubbing up with soap and water about 30 minutes before the time set for the skin incision. She first puts on the cap and mask, then after

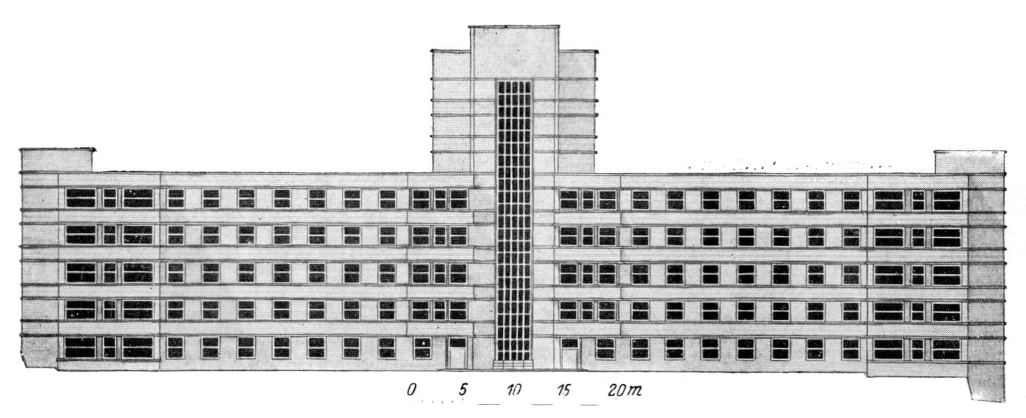

Fig. 247a. View of the new Surgical Building at the University of Tübingen, from the south. In the center is the administration unit with the main stairs and elevators. In back of this are the laboratories and the clinics. On the top floor of this wing are the operating rooms. On both sides facing the south are the wards.

scrubbing and disinfecting her hands, a sterile gown and gloves. With sterile forceps she unfolds the drum covers and takes out of them whatever is necessary.

No.	Station	Name	Operation	Operator	Assistants	Anæsthetist	Instrument Nurse	Operating Room No.
1	Female	Meyer	Removal of a loose body in a joint	A.	B.C.	D.	E.	1
2	Child	Ernest	Radical operation inguinal hernia	G.	H.J.	K.	L.	2
3	Female	Miller	Thyroidectomy	B.	A.E.	C. (Local)	C.	1
4	Male (1)	Kraus	Removal of lipoma	G.	L.J.	K. (Local)	Etc.	3
5	Male (2)	Smith	Opening of a closed tuberculous abscess	G.	K.	R.		3
6	Etc.	Etc.	Appendectomy	Etc.	Etc.	Etc.		2
7			Gastro-enterostomy					1
8			Resection carcinoma of the sigmoid fixture					2
9			Tracheotomy					3
10			Resection of tuberculous knee fistula			D. (Narcylen)		4
11			Sequestrectomy for chronic osteomyelitis			E. (Lumbar)		5
12			Drainage of pleural empyema →	→	→	C. (Positive pressure)		5
13			Incision of suppurative infection of the hand					5
14			Incision of superficial abscess					5
15			Amputation for gas gangrene					5

If the operation is to be performed under local anæsthesia, my instrument nurse prepares the solutions for the anæsthesia, and places them on a special sterile table, together with the necessary syringes, needles and sponges. The instrument table is then arranged. The nurse in charge of the instruments covers a large glass-top table with a double layer of sterile towels, or

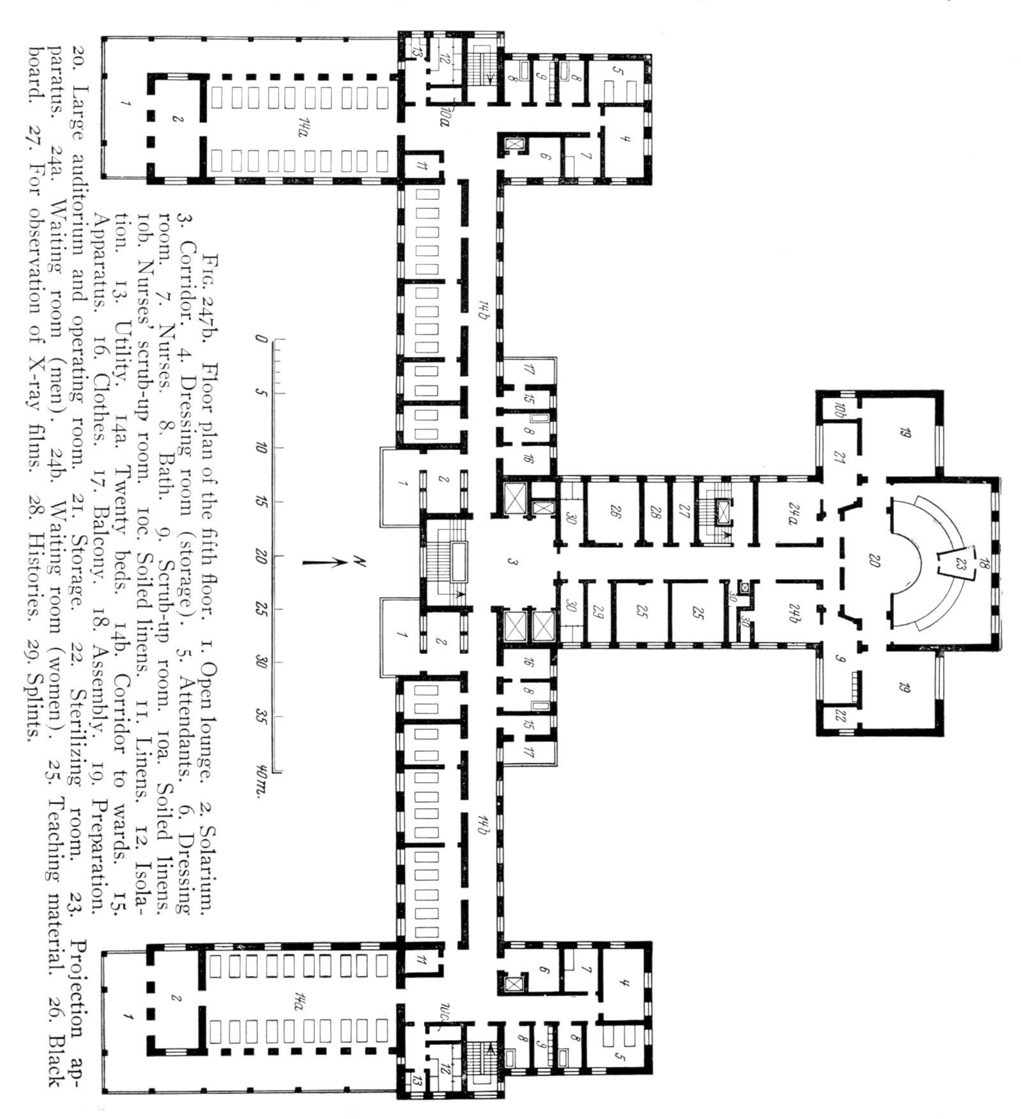

Fig. 247b. Floor plan of the fifth floor. 1. Open lounge. 2. Solarium. 3. Corridor. 4. Dressing room (storage). 5. Attendants. 6. Dressing room. 7. Nurses. 8. Bath. 9. Scrub-up room. 10a. Soiled linens. 10b. Nurses' scrub-up room. 10c. Soiled linens. 11. Linens. 12. Isolation. 13. Utility. 14a. Twenty beds. 14b. Corridor to wards. 15. Apparatus. 16. Clothes. 17. Balcony. 18. Assembly. 19. Preparation. 20. Large auditorium and operating room. 21. Storage. 22. Sterilizing room. 23. Projection apparatus. 24a. Waiting room (men). 24b. Waiting room (women). 25. Teaching material. 26. Blackboard. 27. For observation of X-ray films. 28. Histories. 29. Splints.

a sterile rubber sheet over which sterile towels are placed. She then covers the Mayo stand with a rubber cover over which she draws a sterile linen slip (Fig. 248a and b). On the large table are arranged the boiled and cooled instruments, the suture material and the ligatures, while on the stand are placed the instruments immediately necessary. Every surgeon has his own method of placing these but the arrangement should be such as to minimize time in searching for them. The sponges and the dressing drums are opened, small quantities are taken out with a sterile forceps and are placed on a small sterile covered table in a sterile wire basket. Only a sterile nurse not directly connected with the operation should remove sponges, dressings or linens from the drums once the operation has begun.

When a number of major operations are to be done they are conducted in a large operating room where two or even more operations may be performed at the same time or in individual operating rooms. There can be no doubt but that the latter arrangement is preferable. If several operations are to be done simultaneously in one room the necessary instruments are placed by the head instrument nurse on a large supply table. It is the duty of this

a

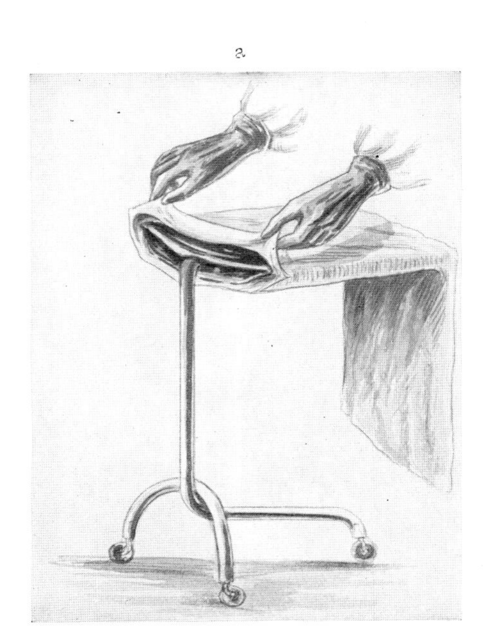

b

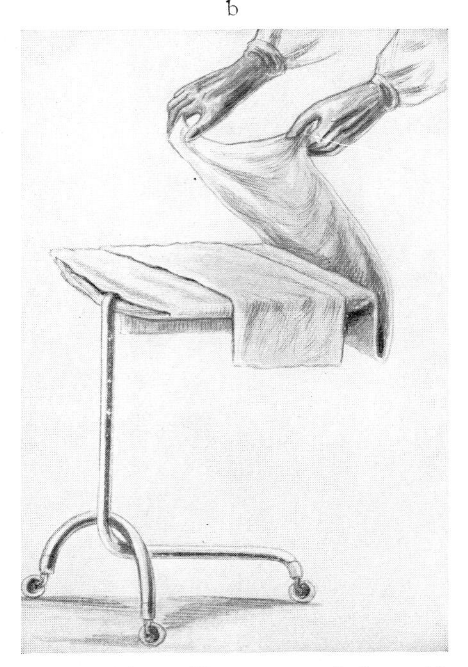

Fig. 248 a and b. The instrument table is first covered with a rubber cover and then with a sterile slip, both of which cover the under surface of the table as well.

head nurse to supply the individual small instrument tables with the required instruments, sponges, suture material and ligatures. She must keep them constantly supplied, but at no time come in contact with the individual spheres of operation (Fig. 249). She remains continuously sterile, even when septic operations are performed, for she has nothing to do with the individual operation. The assistant instrument nurses do not come in direct contact with her; they ask her for what they need, and they in turn furnish the operator with the instruments, ligatures, sutures, etc. When the instruments have been used they are placed on basins which are passed into the sterilizing room by an attendant. In this way the supply table is constantly replenished. When only one operation is conducted in the room at a time the problem is simpler, but a major and minor instrument table should still be used (Fig. 250).

The Arrangement of Instruments on the Mayo Stand. The instruments are always placed on the small table in the same order, and this arrangement is maintained throughout the operation (Fig. 251). If a constant arrangement is maintained the operator and assistants can reach for instruments with the same certainty that a piano-player or typist touches his keys. The general plan of arrangement is such that the instruments used with the right hand are placed on the right side of the table, and those used by the left hand on the left. The more frequently used instruments are placed to the front, and those used less frequently to the back.

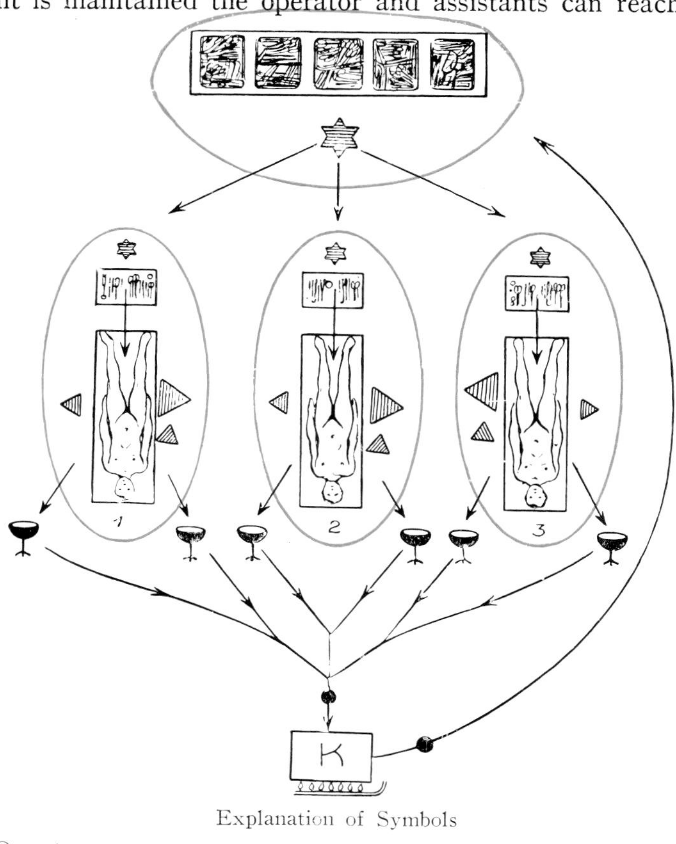

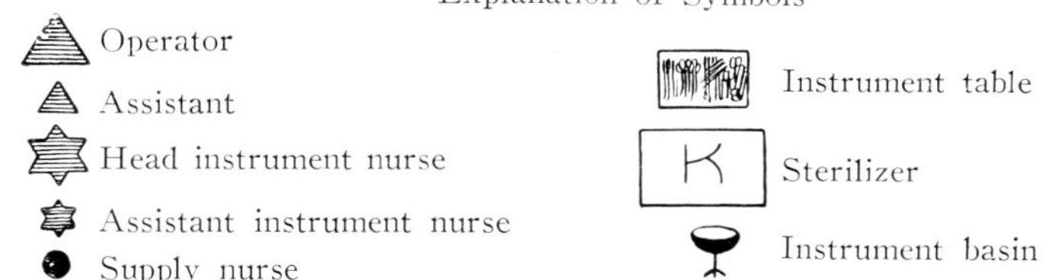

Fig. 249. Provision for the conduction of three operations at the same time, to maintain asepsis.

The head instrument nurse arranges the large glass table so that it forms an independent unit, and from it the individual instrument tables are supplied. The assistant instrument nurses take care of their individual spheres of activity in connection with their operating tables and instruments, without coming in contact with the head instrument nurse or the other assistant instrument nurses. All instruments used in the individual operations are discarded into the instrument basins, from which they are removed by a non-sterile attendant and placed in the sterilizer. After sterilization they are brought back and placed on the large sterile glass-top table.

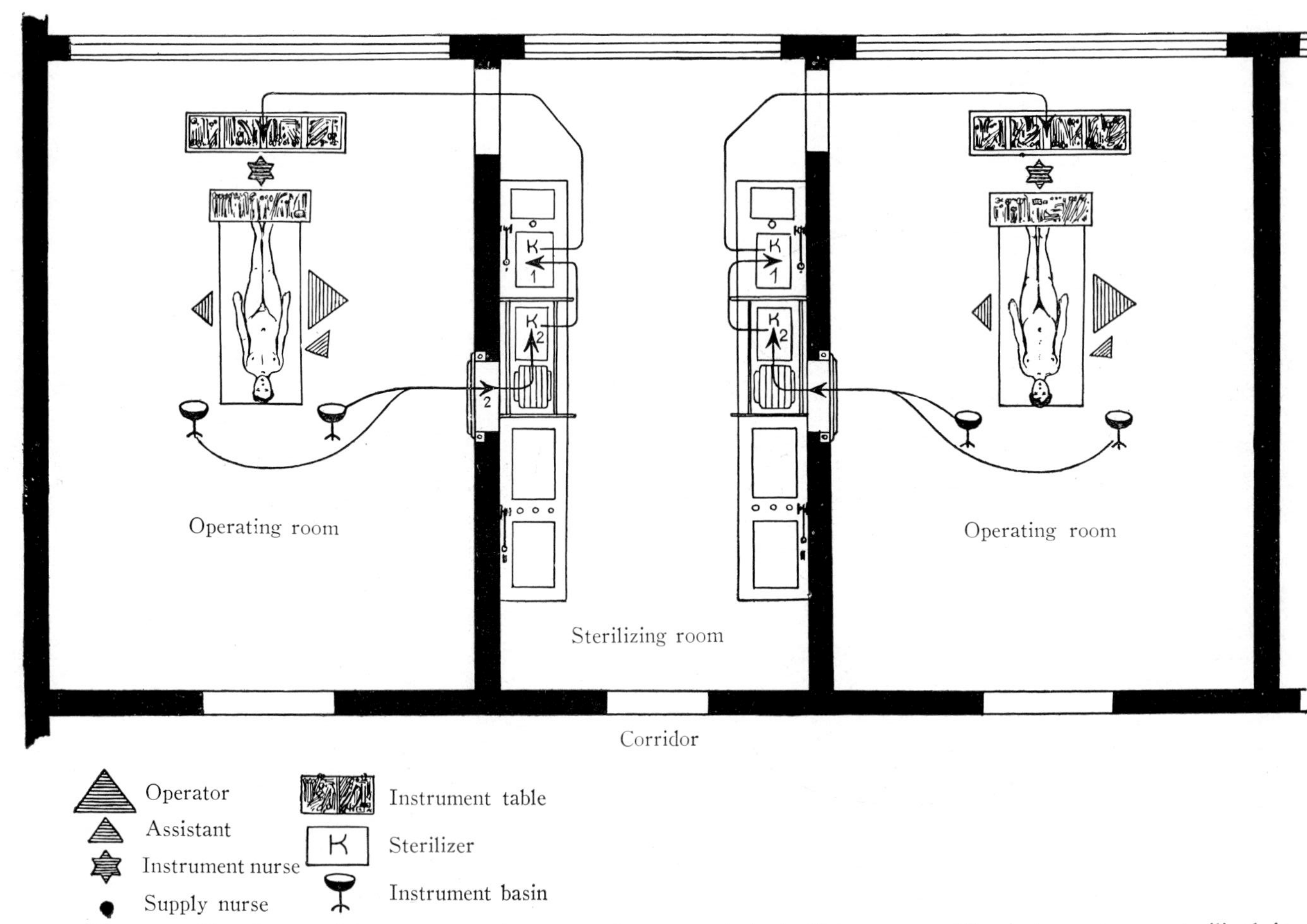

FIG. 250. Plan for supplying two operating rooms from a central sterilizing room. The instruments are sterilized in sterilizer No. 1 and are then taken to the supply table in either operating room. After being used in the operation they are passed through a connecting window into sterilizer No. 2, washed and cleaned and then resterilized in sterilizer No. 1.

In my set-up I have a rubber mat in the center front, on which the instruments used are put back, if they are not thrown into the instrument basin to be resterilized. On the edge of the mat lies the scalpel, to the right of it, a curved and a straight scissors, a little further to the right are the hemostats, further back, long Billroth clamps, and in the back right corner

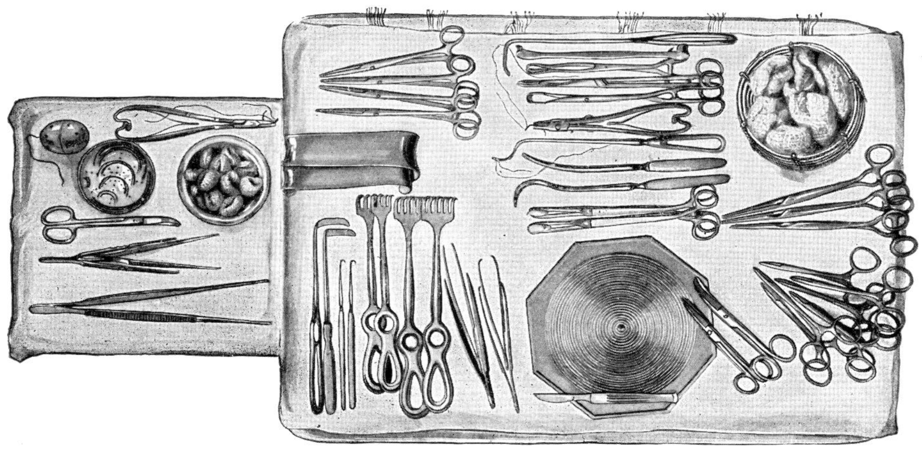

FIG. 251. Arrangement of instruments on the small instrument tables (Kirschner).

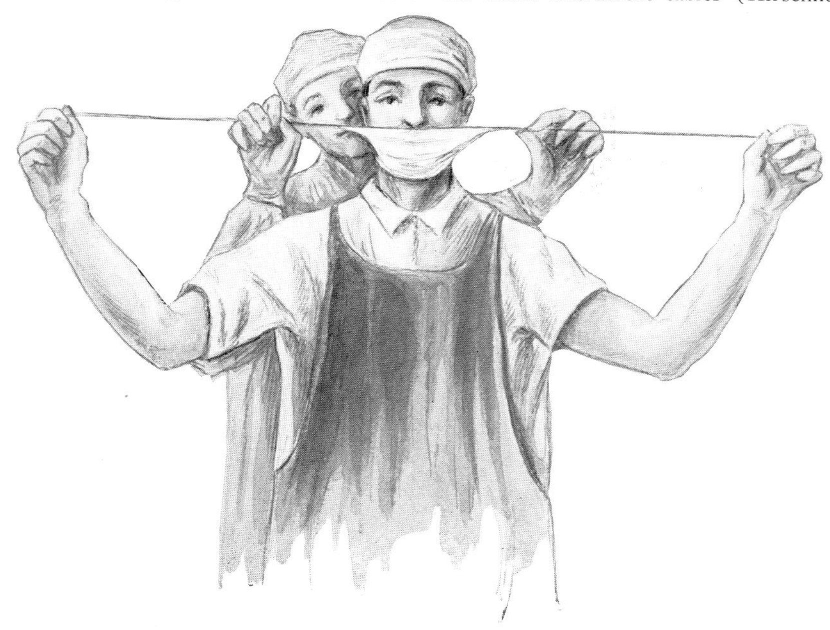

FIG. 252. Putting on the mouth mask.

there is a wire basket with small sponges. To the left of the mat are placed first the surgical, then the anatomic forceps, next the hook retractors, behind these are two Roux, or abdominal wall retractors. In the back left corner are placed the Kocher clamps. Back of the rubber mat, in the space between the sponge-basket and the Kocher clamps, we place two tissue forceps, the aneurism needles, the needle holders, and other special instruments, such as dressing forceps, bone instruments, etc.

Ordinarily I have the instrument table placed to the right of the operator. The handles of all instruments are directed to the right. If the table should occasionally have to be placed to the left of the operator, the handles are turned to the left, without changing the place or order of the instruments.

A small tray is attached to this table, on which the instrument nurse places her needles, suture material, and anything else she may need during the operation.

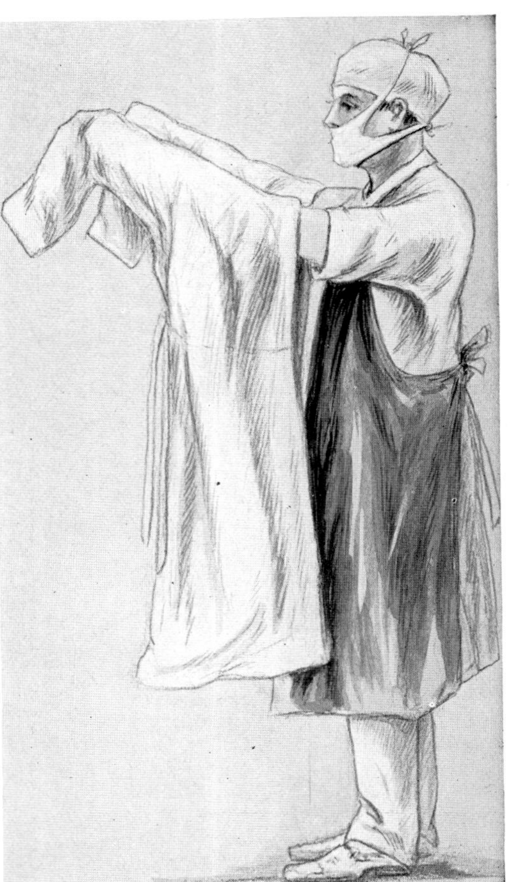

Fig. 253. The proper way to put on an operating gown.

The operator and assistants have been provided with caps before scrubbing up. After they have finished scrubbing with soap, water, and alcohol, they dry their hands and lower forearms. The rubber apron is carefully dried with a towel by an attendant, or it is removed. A nurse assists the surgeon in putting on the mouth mask and gown. If the mask is sterile the surgeon grasps the two upper tapes by their extreme ends in such manner that the upper border of the mask lies directly under the nose, while the nurse grasps the tapes as shown in figure 252, carries them over his ears and ties them over the vertex. She then ties the lower tapes. In putting on the gown one must be careful to place both arms in the sleeves at the same time and the nurse then ties it in the back (Fig. 253). The mistake is frequently made of inserting first one arm, which allows the inner side of the gown to come in contact with non-sterile clothing. When the second arm is inserted it must touch the contaminated sleeve inlet and thus the hand is no longer sterile (Fig. 254). Every surgeon and assistant prepared to operate, should so train himself that there is no necessity of consciously maintaining this asepsis. It should be a reflex mechanism. Due to the imperfection of our methods and because of our unintentional mistakes, the "aseptic" surfaces of men and objects can not be called germ-free but "germ-poor." The border-line area of asepsis, as for example, the area where the prepared skin meets the non-aseptic skin, or the outer margin of the sterile covers, should be given a wide berth. It is understood that a person dressed to operate should not come in contact with non-sterile objects. It is our rule to keep at a distance of one meter from them.

Aseptic objects, such as the patient's skin, the covers, the instruments and the wound, should not be touched more than is absolutely necessary.

Certain areas which may appear to be sterile are in reality contaminated. Thus the back of a sterile gown is no longer sterile when it has been tied by unsterile hands. It is unfortunately not uncommon to see an individual in a sterile gown lean his back against a sterile table (Fig. 233), which must later be touched by the operator, his assistants, or a nurse. Thus the instruments become contaminated and the aseptic technic has been sacrificed.

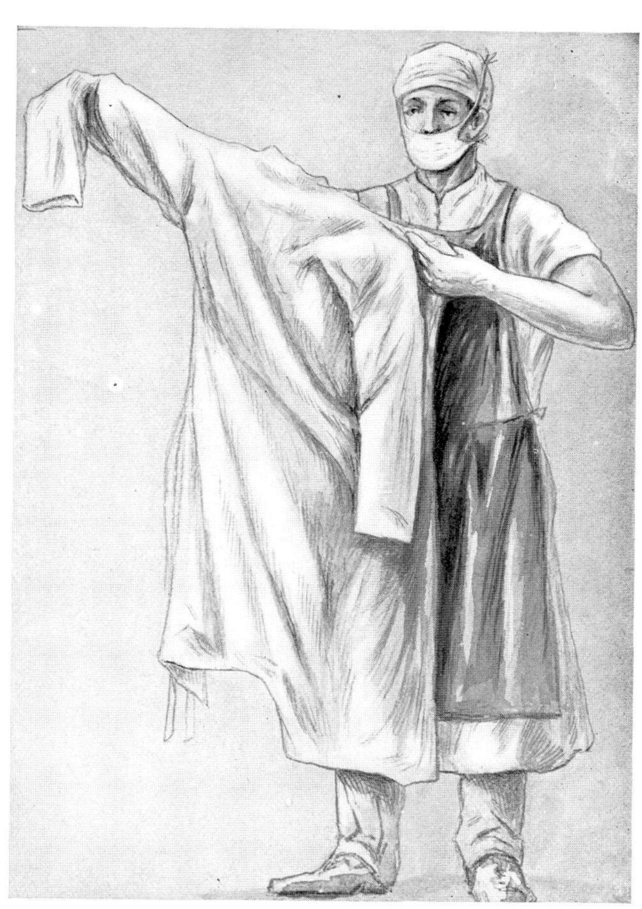

FIG. 254. The wrong way to put on an operating gown.

The following rule should therefore be observed by every aseptically dressed person: avoid contact with anything but the aseptic sphere, which you must touch only when absolutely necessary!

Should a patient's legs have to be moved during an operation, they should be carefully covered with sterile covers fastened on with towel clamps, or safety pins, and then wrapped with gauze bandages. When the area of operation is limited to the amputation of a limb, the limb is to be protected above and below with sterile towels, leaving exposed only the field of operation.

If the operation involves individual fingers or toes or is just proximal to them, that portion of the extremity below the site of the incision should be covered with a sterile rubber finger-cot.

In regard to asepsis, we believe it is important that after the operator has disinfected his hands and put on his gown and gloves, and the field of operation is fully prepared, he should not palpate the region to determine the line of the skin incision. Whenever it is necessary to determine by palpation the line of incision or other topographical points, the operator should do this before preparing for the operation. At that time the skin may be marked with an indelible coloring solution[1] (Fig. 255). This skin marking may also be done after the sterilization of the operator's hands. The pre-operative marking is important also in that it limits the area which need be exposed. The marking is also of great aid in difficult plastic operations, indicating exact locations and measurements of areas involved in the plan of operation. (E. König, Zentralbl. f. Chirurg., 1920).

After the patient is placed on the operating table and the straps are fastened, the area of operation is thoroughly painted with an alcoholic solution of tannic acid. A layer of mastisol is put on the skin with a sterile

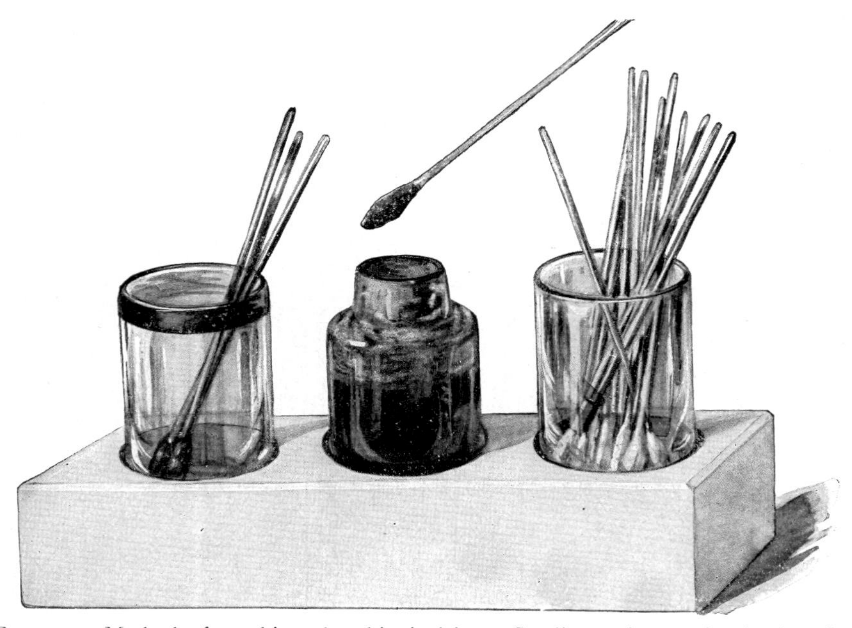

Fig. 255. Method of marking the skin incision. Sterile swabs are in the last jar, the second jar contains the colored solution for marking the skin, and the first jar, with a black band around the top, is for the used swabs.

sponge forceps about 2 cm. from the intended line of incision. With the aid of an assistant, folded sterile covers are placed over the mastisol and close to either side of the line of incision. They are further fastened to each other and to the skin with towel clamps (Fig. 257). When local anæsthesia is being used care must be taken that the towel clamps are not attached to a non-anæsthetized portion of the skin. The towels can also be fastened together and to the skin by sutures, or by safety pins. Besides the commercial mastisol, I have found the following mastic preparation very serviceable: mastic 20 gms., rosin 10, dissolved in benzol 50 cc., Venetian turpentine 5 cc., linseed oil 20 drops.

If the field of operation reaches up to the chest or neck, a wire semicircle is fastened across the operating table, so as to separate the anæsthetist

[1] The composition of our coloring solution: violet (ether-soluble) 2.0, benzol 100.0, benzoin-resin 10.0.

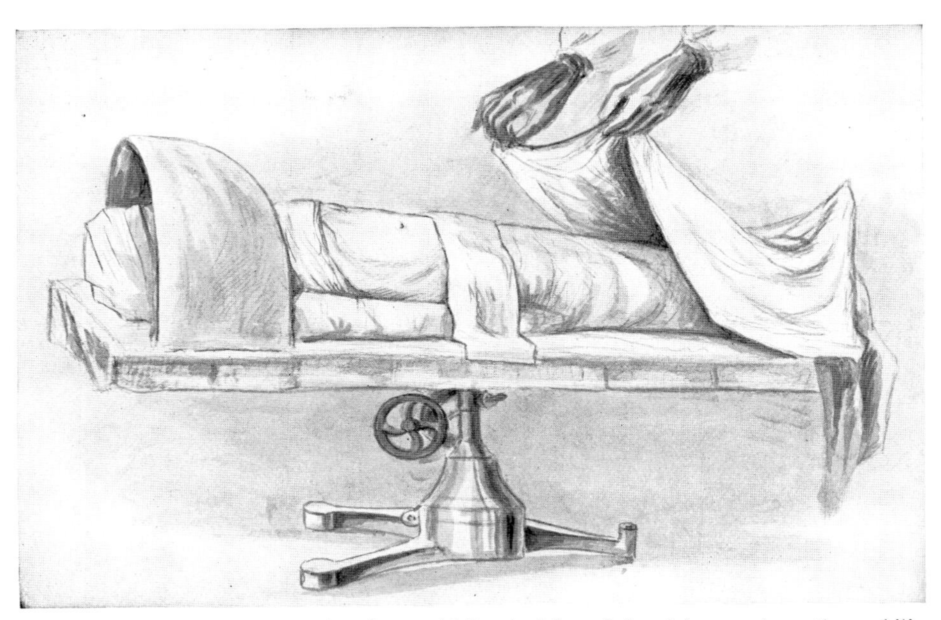

FIG. 256(a). Complete covering for a mid-line incision of the abdomen above the umbilicus. The upper part of the covers are fastened over a frame so that the anæsthesia can be carried on without danger of interfering with the asepsis.

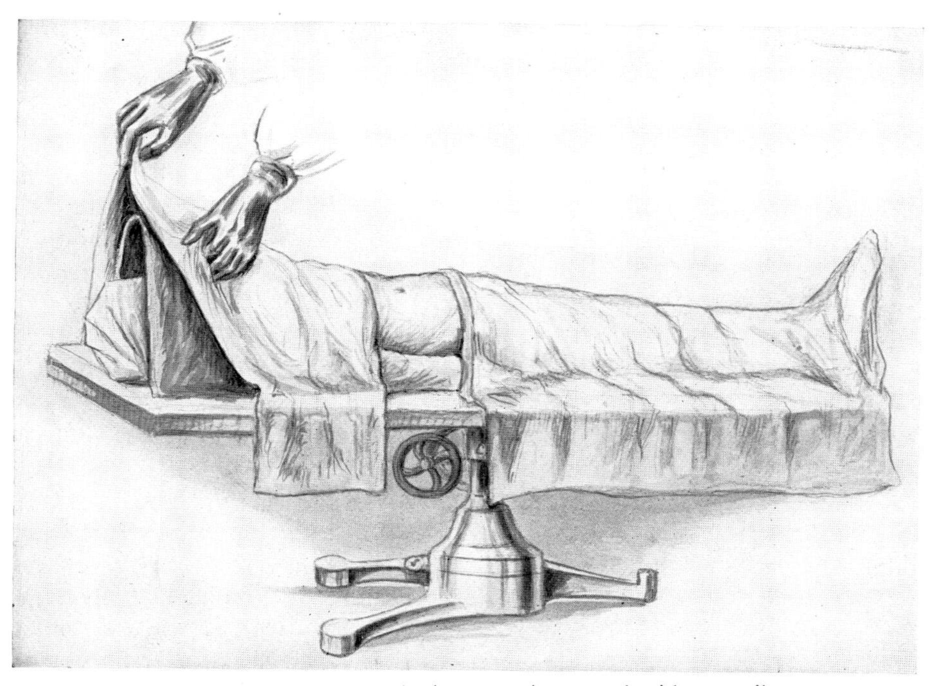

FIG. 256(b). The anæsthesia screen is covered with a sterile cover.

from the field of operation (Figs. 256 a and b). The head of the patient lies under a sterile tent, opened towards the anæsthetist, so that the asepsis is not endangered by the patient's respiration and at the same time the anæsthetist has ready access to his mouth (Fig. 258).

When the patient's sterile drapes have been applied the small instrument table is pushed to its proper place. In some clinics the operator and assistants put on their gloves after placing the sterile covers, while in others the gloves are put on before this is done. The rubber gloves are grasped by the instrument nurse from the outside, with the cuff turned back (Fig. 259). The right glove is always put on first. The surgeon slips his hand

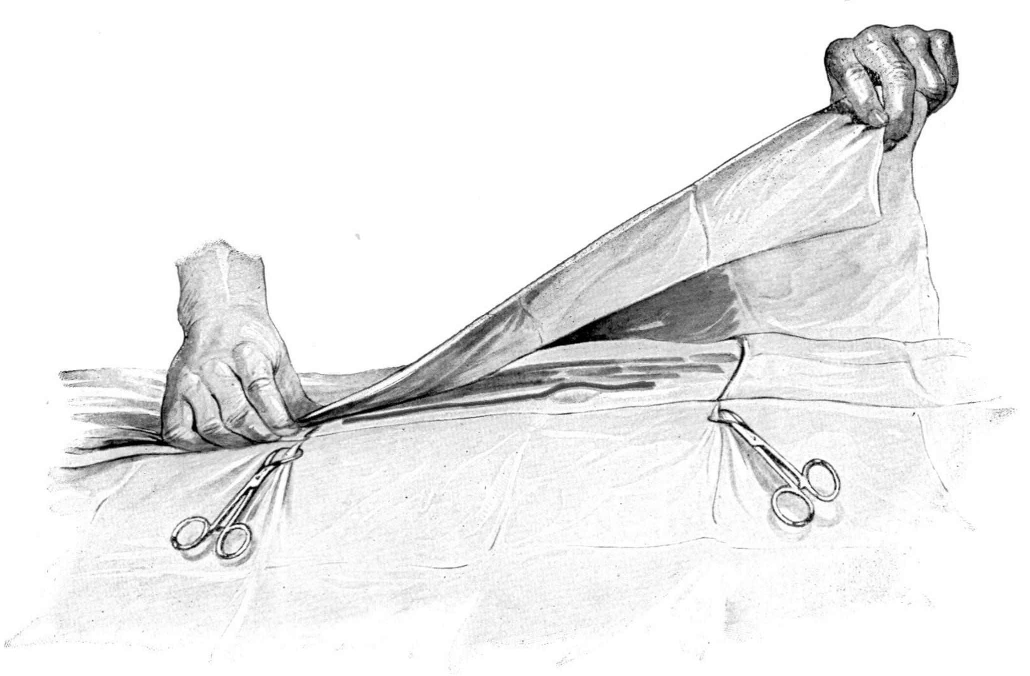

Fig. 257. Covering the field of operation. After the skin is painted with disinfecting solution, and the area covered with mastisol, the sterile covers are put on and fastened with towel clamps.

into it without touching the outside or coming in contact with the nurse. The glove is drawn over the cuff of the sleeve so that no space is left uncovered. (Figs. 224 and 225). An instrument basin (Fig. 260) and a bucket are placed on either side of the operating table. If additional illumination is necessary this is provided before the operation is begun.

When the operation is to be performed under local anæsthesia, the surgeon should first scrub up with soap and water, and rinse his hands with alcohol. He then paints the area of operation with the alcoholic tannin solution, covers one side of the area with a towel, and proceeds to inject the local anæsthetic. When he has finished the injection he should then go through the formal preparation of his hands and forearms. Spinal anæsthesia is performed by us immediately after disinfecting the hands, but before putting on the sterile gown. The advantage of this procedure is that it permits

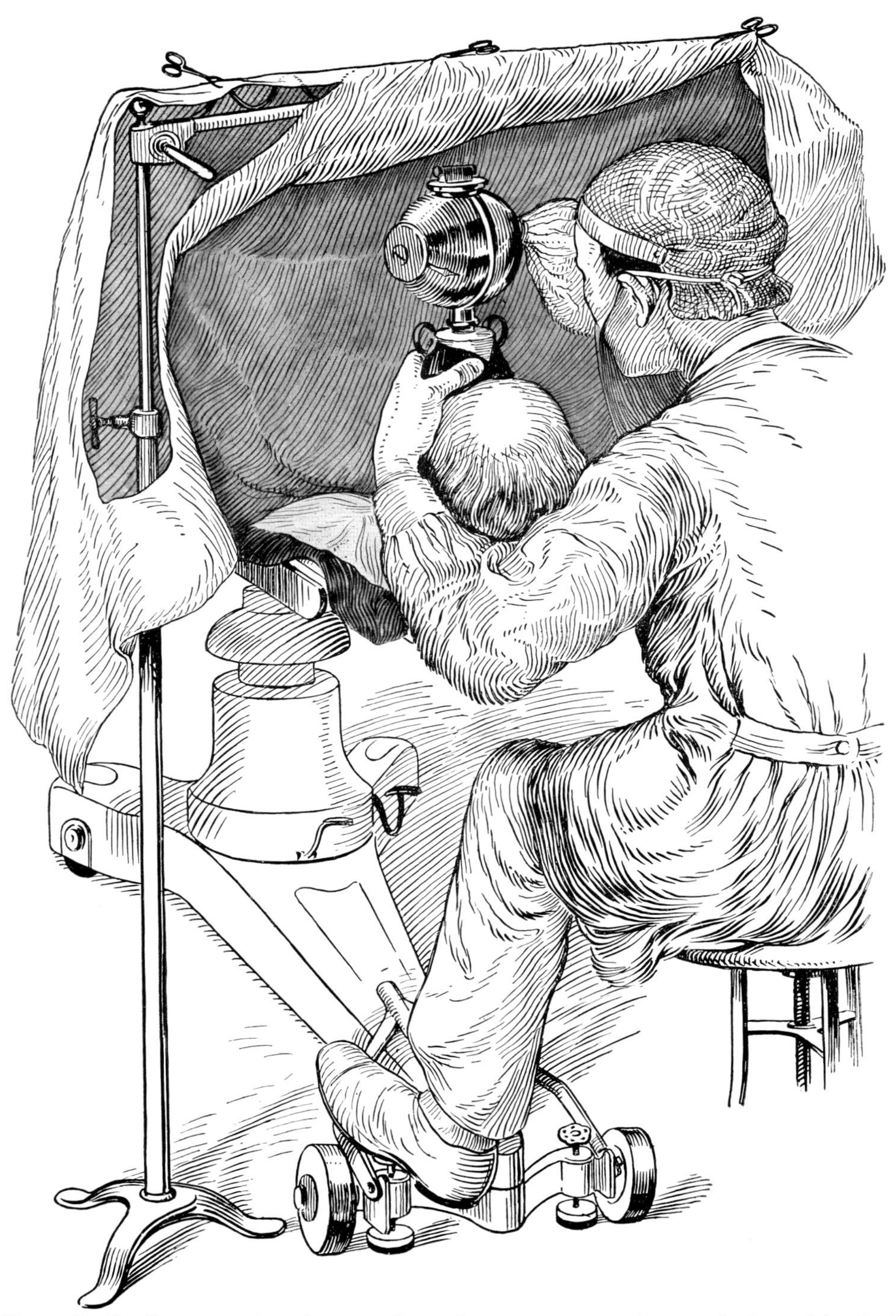

FIG. 258. Sterile covers draped over a frame form a tent over the anæsthetist and head of the patient.

sufficient time to elapse, while the surgeon is finally preparing himself, for the anæsthetic to take effect.

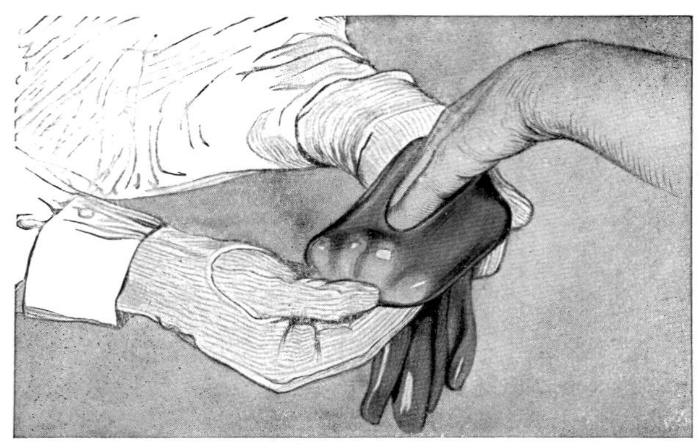

Fig. 259. Putting on a sterile rubber glove. A sterile assistant holds the glove by the cuff in such a way that the hand may be inserted without touching the outside of the glove.

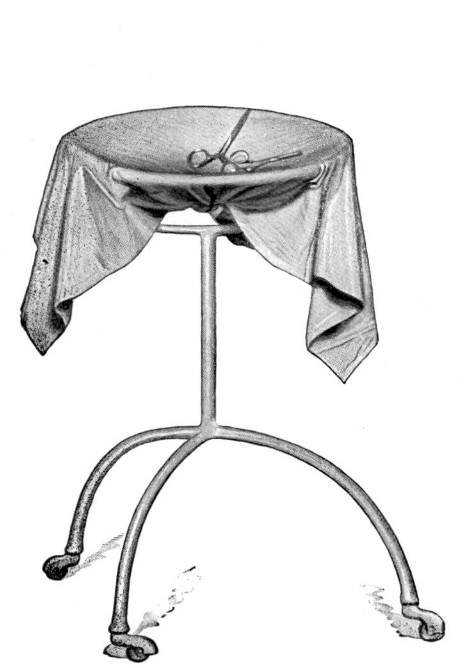

Fig. 260. Frame covered with a towel which is used as a receptacle for instruments that are no longer needed or are to be resterilized.

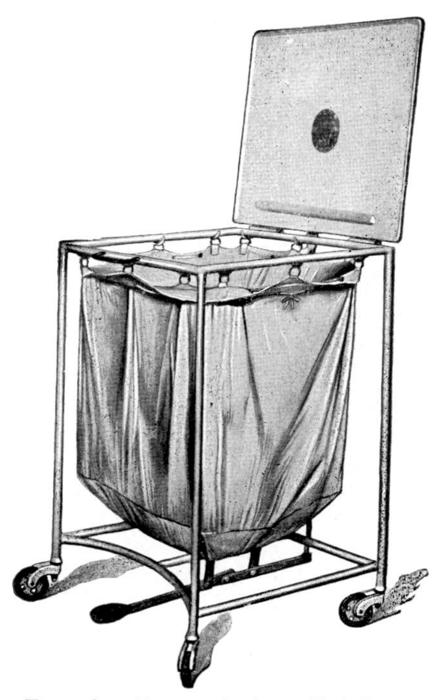

Fig. 261. Receptacle for soiled linens.

All instruments which are not to be used again in the operation, or which must be resterilized before use, should be immediately thrown into the instrument basin. This basin consists of a towel, thrown over a frame (Fig. 260).

I consider it best to replace all used instruments by freshly boiled ones, as long as this does not interfere with the course of the operation. For instance, I use hemostats but once, after which they are discarded and the instrument nurse replaces them with others. It is absolutely necessary to change all instruments, disinfect the hands, change gloves, and put on fresh covers to obtain an aseptic field following an infectious part of an operation, as for instance, in abdominal operations after having finished an intestinal resection and anastomosis.

The soiled linens should be placed in large, open, suspended bags which can be kept in a room adjoining the operating room (Fig. 261), unless a shaft for soiled linens is provided in the plan of the clinic. In my new

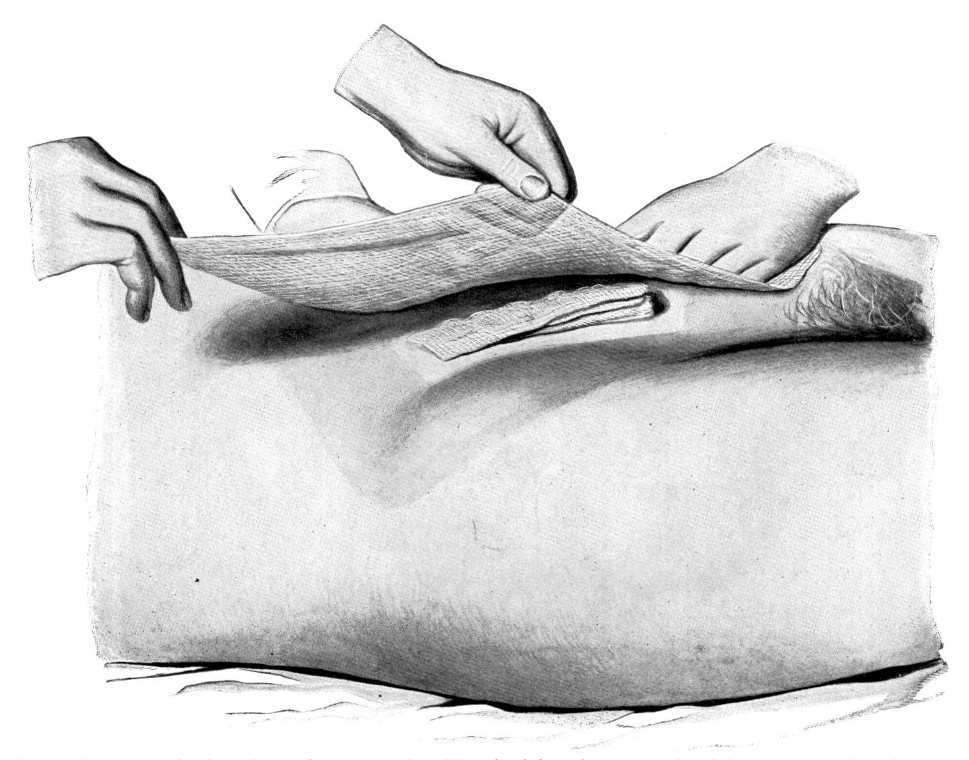

FIG. 262. Mastic-dressing of a wound. The incision is covered with a gauze dressing, the area around it is then painted with mastic and a single layer of gauze pasted on.

clinic in Tübingen I have provided a chute for linens. This chute leads to a boiler which washes, sterilizes and then dries by centrifugalization.

The Sterile Wound Dressing. After the operation is finished I cover the incision with sterile gauze, and place a coating of mastic around this. A large piece of gauze is then put on, which is held by the mastic (Fig. 262). The mastic may tend to come through the gauze and cause the patient's gown to stick to the dressings. This can be prevented by rubbing some cotton over the gauze. Adhesive plaster is widely used in America instead of mastic (Fig. 263). In the case of a draining wound, we put on a larger amount of gauze, and cover this with several layers of cellucotton, the entire dressing being held on with adhesive plaster and bandages. A circular bandage on an anæsthetized patient, unless carefully applied, may cause

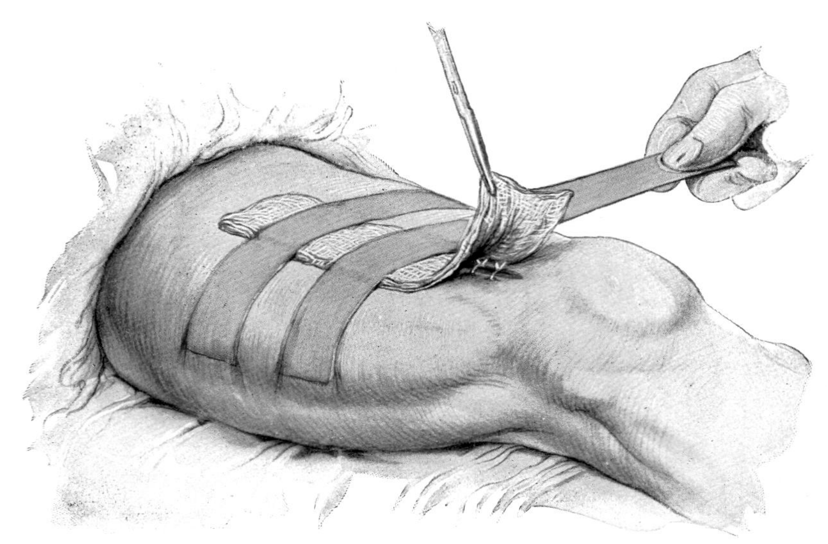

Fig. 263. Dressing a wound with adhesive plaster.

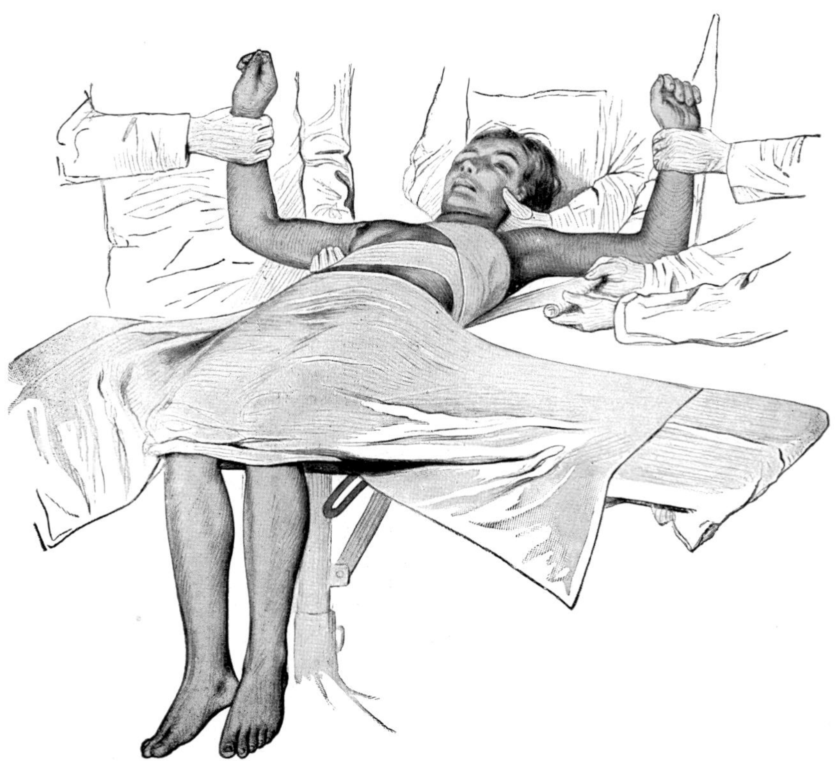

Fig. 264. Bandaging the chest of an anæsthetized patient. The patient is laid across the operating table so that the upper part of the body projects beyond the table and the legs hang down. The body is supported under the head and arms.

considerable discomfort. In bandaging the chest (Fig. 264) the patient is placed across the operating table with his legs hanging down, while the upper part of the body is freely movable, three helpers holding the head

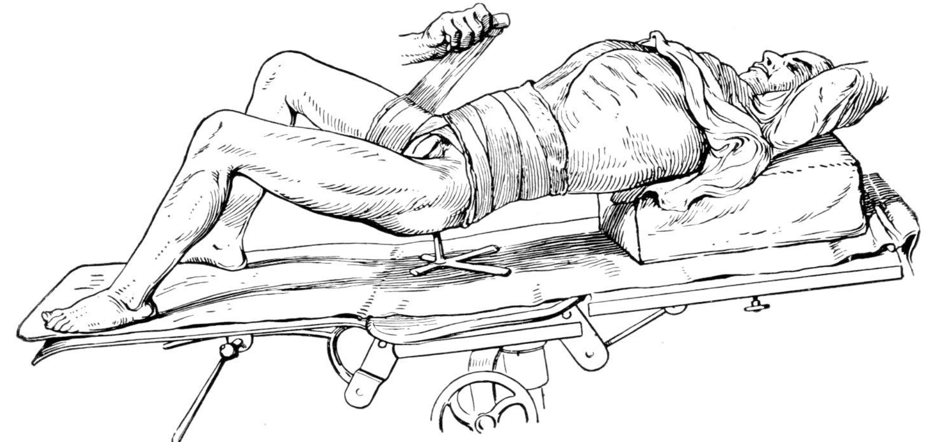

FIG. 265. The patient is supported on pelvic rest during application of bandage to the abdomen, pelvis, groin, or thigh.

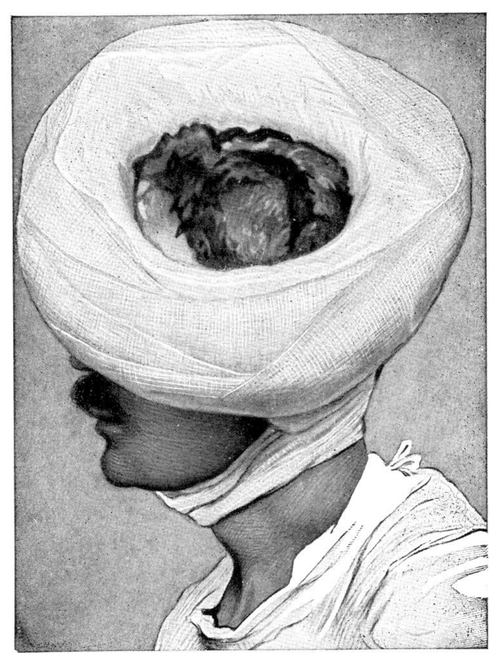

FIG. 266. Cellucotton ring for protection of wound from pressure.

and the arms while the bandage is applied. When a circular abdominal bandage is to be applied (Fig. 265) the patient is placed on a pelvic rest which is withdrawn after the bandage is finished.

Wounds closed without drainage, in which there is danger of contact with infectious fluids, such as feces, sputum, or even urine, can be protected by a coating of flexible collodion, zinc paste, or rubber dam which is fastened around the wound dressing. The part operated on should if possible be kept at rest and elevated. Special regions which have been operated on and which are subjected to pressure should be protected by a cellucotton ring (Fig. 266) or by a wire mesh such as is used for cutaneous plastic operations (Fig. 385). The cellucotton ring is fastened around the wound with mastic or adhesive plaster and reinforced with bandages.

It is necessary, in certain instances where the patient is uncoöperative, delirious, or exceedingly nervous, to restrain him so that he can not touch his

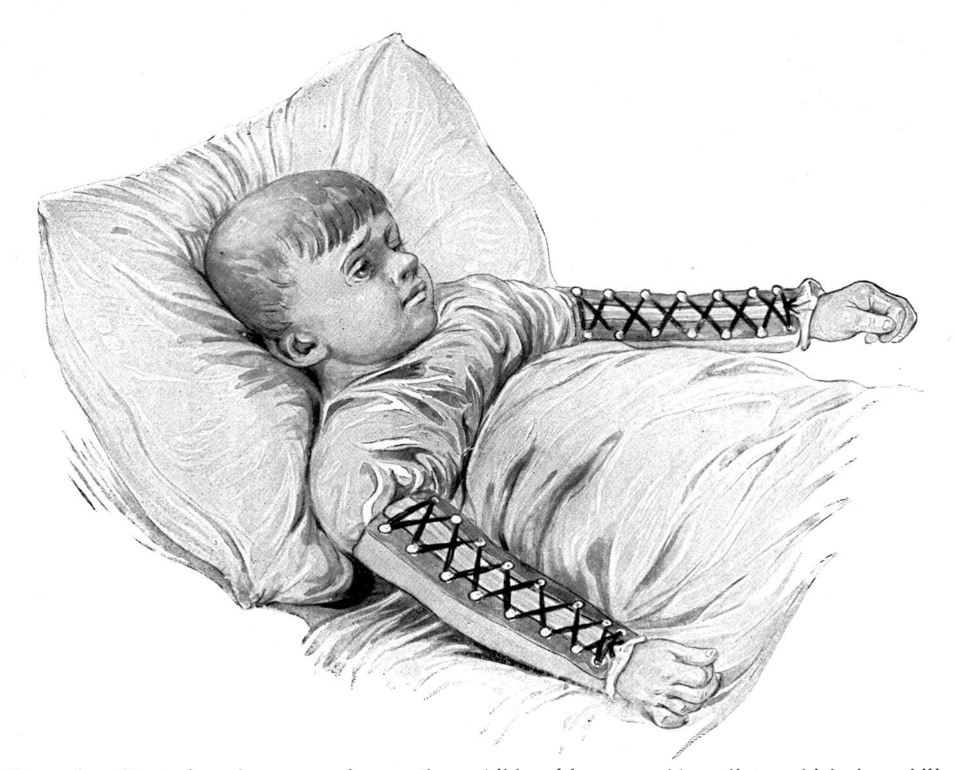

Fig. 267. Fastening the arms of a restless child, with removable splints which immobilize the elbow-joints.

dressings or wound. This is especially true in children. It is often impossible to control a patient, in spite of careful watching. This forced restriction of movements must be instituted with care so that the patient is permitted a certain amount of freedom. Laced splints are effective for the arms (Fig. 267). With these, the patient can not reach the head, neck, or body with his hands. Suitable splints applied to the knee joints in extension, prevent the patient from standing up. Such splints are taken off every two hours, the limbs are moved and massaged, and the splints are then replaced. For this reason removable splints are preferable to the plaster cast bandages recommended by many surgeons.

I do not dress a clean wound for eight days, if there are no indications of infection. The stitches or the clamps should be removed on the eighth day, although some surgeons prefer to remove the skin sutures on the fifth or sixth day and the tension sutures on the tenth day. If the wound has healed by primary intention, a small protective gauze dressing should be put on after removal of the sutures.

It is a valuable rule, never to drain a wound which is not infected or contaminated. Errors in asepsis, excessive duration of an operation, a wound which can not be closed without leaving pockets, or the presence of excessive fat may make drainage advisable. No special rules can be given for this, since the conditions are so variable. The surgeon must use his judgment, and if there is any doubt it is safer to drain. When in an aseptic operation a drain is inserted for safety, it should be removed in one or two days without disturbing the rest of the dressing. If no evidence of infection occurs the dressing is not removed until the sutures are to be taken out on the eighth day.

It is customary in some clinics to place the patients freshly operated upon in a special section for a few days, removing them to their original ward later. This arrangement has the great advantage that these patients can be given the very best attention by the nurses and the surgeon and his assistants can visit them much more frequently than if they were scattered all over the hospital. Furthermore, patients to be operated on are spared the sight of the distress of the fresh-operatives.

C. CONDUCT OF THE OPERATION IN AN INFECTED FIELD AND THE PRIMARY CARE OF TRAUMATIC WOUNDS (FRIEDRICH)

When the surgeon is compelled to operate in an infected area the same aseptic measures in preparation should be followed as for an aseptic operation. Even though the operative site may be primarily infected it is the surgeon's duty to prevent, if possible, the secondary invasion of other bacteria or the spread of the primary organisms to non-infected areas. If the asepsis is complicated by an open wound, sinus or intestinal fistula in the area of operation, precautions to prevent gross contamination must be taken before the operation is begun. The focus should be sterilized, if possible, by cauterization and the leaking of infectious material should be prevented by packing the sinus or fistula with iodoform gauze, by securing a sponge over the opening, or by suturing it securely with silk or linen (Fig. 268). It is difficult, in spite of thorough mechanical cleansing and disinfection, to completely remove the bacteria of the skin adjacent to the fistula.

Sometimes a focus of infection is opened during the course of an otherwise aseptic operation, as for example the opening of the intestine during an intestinal resection. If the time at which the otherwise aseptic operation becomes contaminated can be accurately determined, all instruments used during this stage of the operation should be kept separate and should be discarded when asepsis is reestablished. In this way infection in an otherwise clean area may be prevented. The procedure may be carried out in one of two ways. The instruments to be used during the non-contaminated portion of the operation can be covered with towels, or, what is better, an entirely new instrument table can be used at this time. At the same time, the operator, assistants, and nurse, after a brief hand disinfection, change their rubber gloves, and when necessary, also their gowns. While this is being done an assistant should be delegated to watch the wound.

The Primary Treatment of Traumatic Wounds (Friedrich). Every traumatic wound may be regarded as primarily infected, since contamination always occurs. In the fresh wound the bacteria are merely on the surface and several hours must elapse before they invade the adjacent tissues (Friedrich). Theoretically, therefore, it is possible to remove entirely all infectious bacteria within the first few hours, if the wound, like a foreign body, can be excised. The earlier the excision of the wound is done, the better are the prospects for preventing subsequent infection. This method of wound re-

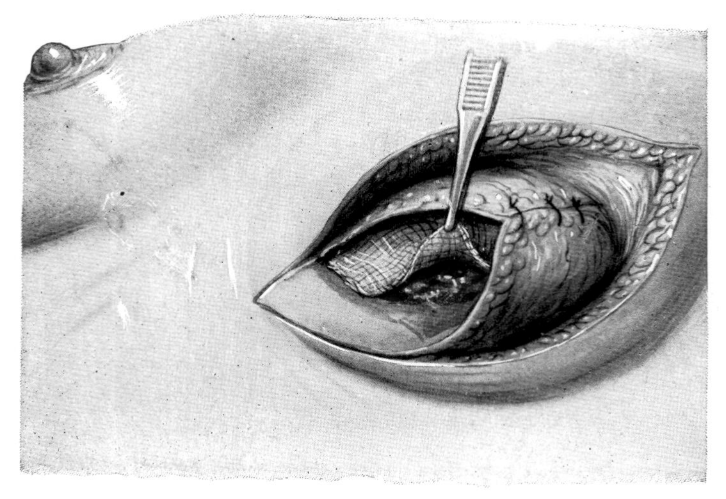

Fig. 268. Removal of an infected ulcer from the area of operation. The ulcer is cauterized and the skin incisions are made well away from the ulcer margins. The ulcer is then covered with iodoform gauze and the dissected skin margins are sutured over it so that the freshly exposed tissues are not contaminated.

vision is carried out in my clinic whenever a wound is seen within the first 24 hours, although we do not limit ourselves absolutely to this time. The advantage of excision is not only the elimination of bacteria, but also the removal of devitalized tissue which is a very favorable medium for bacterial growth.

The wound revision is begun by incising the skin margins at a distance of about 1 cm. around the wound, and the dissection is carried downward through all the tissue layers to the depth of the wound, so that the excised tissues, under the most favorable circumstances, are funnel or cylindrical shaped. In extensive, deep wounds with numerous sinuses this complete revision is impossible, just as complete excision of the margins of certain deep wounds cannot be carried out where important structures, such as nerves, vessels, and tendons, course through them. This is likewise true when the wound approaches one of the body cavities (joints, chest cavity, abdominal cavity, etc.), the opening of which would be an error in technic. The revision of certain wounds must therefore remain incomplete. In the badly contaminated wound, and in those wounds in which complete revision is impossible, drainage must be established and where multiple pockets exist the wound should be widely opened, counter drainage established, and loose gauze packing inserted. In my experience, the infiltration of the area surrounding

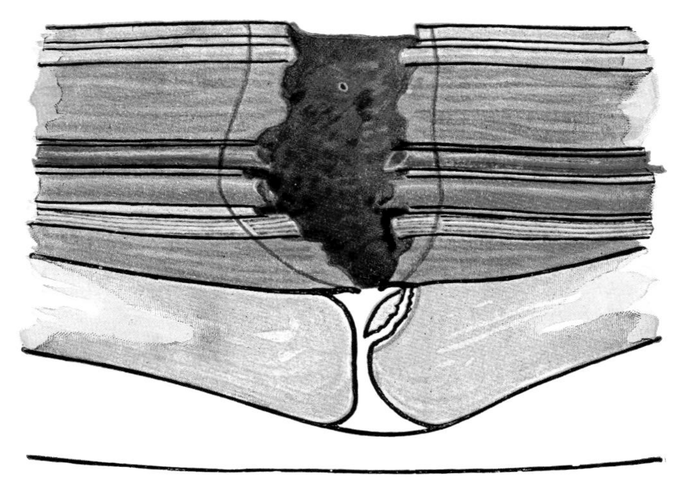

FIG. 269. Preparing a wound for primary repair (diagrammatic). The wound is excised by removing from one-half to two cm. of tissue from the edges, and at the same time, a bone chip is removed from the opened joint.

the wound with an antiseptic solution contributes nothing after a thorough wound revision. Tetanus antitoxin should always be administered in traumatic wounds. The prophylactic dose is 1500 units.

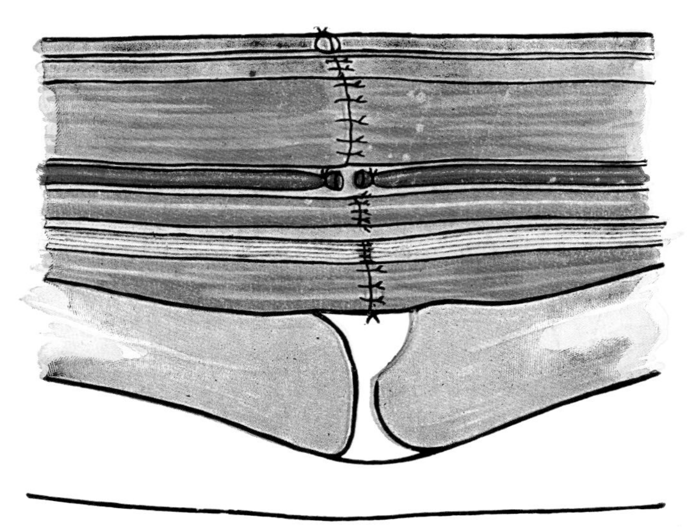

FIG. 270. Primary repair of a wound. The freshened wound is closed by suturing each layer, as in the original structure, after the joint capsule is closed.

An important aspect of wound revision is the control of hemorrhage. The smaller vessels are ligated, while the larger vessels may have to be sutured. Anatomical structures should be reunited in their proper planes and the larger nerves, as well as tendons, muscles, and bones should be restored in continuity. Any body cavity which has been partly opened, such as the peritoneal, pleural, pericardial, or the cranial cavity, as well as the joint cavities, should be closed so that infection in them is prevented.

D. THE OPERATIVE MANAGEMENT OF LOCAL INFECTION

In the operative management of local suppurative lesions I follow, as do most surgeons, the old dictum: *Ubi Pus, Ibi Evacua!* Only the technic varies, the principle remains the same. The measures for evacuation should not be limited to the simple removal of the pus, but they should be extensive enough to provide adequate drainage for the inflamed and edematous tissues surrounding the suppurative area. Unless adequate drainage is established the tissues become devitalized and necrotic, and further suppuration occurs. When tissues are under considerable tension from infection early incision will prevent tissue destruction, forestall abscess formation, and limit the progress of inflammation. The incision will relieve tension and permit the flow of lymph and tissue fluids to the exterior, thereby lessening the danger of bacterial extension and the absorption of bacterial toxins. This affords favorable conditions for limiting the inflammatory process to its original focus.

In contrast to physical measures for the control of infection, the use of chemical measures is not nearly so effective. After a few hours bacteria do not lie only on the surface of a wound, but also in the depths of the tissues. Thus it is frequently not possible to reach them with disinfectants introduced into the wound. When a disinfectant is put into a wound or injected into the tissues around a wound (deep antisepsis), the disinfectant is reduced in its bactericidal properties by the tissue fluids and the tissues are devitalized, thus lowering their power of resistance. The slight degree of hyperemia which results from their use does not seem to counterbalance these disadvantages. Similarly, in my experience, the injection of albumin, especially the use of blood (Läwen) in infections, is of little value although it is used by many surgeons.

The answer to the question whether it is possible to disinfect living tissue without injury, is a moot point among surgeons throughout the world. To many the affirmative answer is a part of their creed. I belong to the unbelievers.

Exploratory Puncture. It is possible, and at times highly desirable, to make an exploratory puncture before or during an operation, in order to determine whether there is an accumulation of fluid in a certain portion of the body; or whether the contents of a collection are pus, blood, serum, or some other type of fluid. It is immaterial whether the fluid is in a natural cleavage space, such as a joint, or the pleural cavity; or in the tissues, as an abscess, or a subcutaneous cyst. At the same time aspiration through a needle is the simplest therapeutic method for the removal of pathologic accumulations of fluid. It can be used either as a therapeutic procedure, when if necessary repeated punctures may be done, or it can be used as a preliminary stage of a complete operation. An example of the latter is the relief of tension in an empyema of the thorax before attempting rib resection. For aspirating large quantities of fluid, one of the methods of aspiration previously described should be used.

If the operator possesses sufficient skill, he may perform such a simple thing as a puncture without preparatory disinfection of the hands. In any event it is better to do a puncture without touching the place of insertion or the needle. It too frequently occurs in clinical practice that both are touched by imperfectly prepared hands. Therefore I wash my hands only superficially for the ordinary puncture, dry them carefully, and put on sterile rubber gloves. After the place for puncture is marked with a colored solution, the site of operation painted with alcoholic tannin solution, and the sterile covers are arranged, an anæsthetic wheal is raised at the point of puncture. When the puncture is deep I infiltrate the entire puncture tract with a 1 to 2 percent solution of novocain. I use a 5 to 10 cc. record syringe for exploratory puncture. The needle should not be too short, nor should it be unnecessarily long. The longer the needle the more difficult it is for the fluid to pass through it. The gauge of the needle must be suited to the anticipated thickness of the fluid to be removed. The mistake is frequently made of choosing so fine a needle that thick fluid such as pus can not be aspirated through it. My puncture needles have an outside diameter of from 1.8 to 3 mm. They are kept in all lengths. It may be necessary to have certain cannulæ made to order. If the syringe and needle are not united by a sterile instrument nurse before handing them to the surgeon, he can make this connection with a sterile forceps. Care should be taken to see that this union is tight. Before attempting the puncture, the syringe and needle should be tested by aspirating and expelling sterile salt solution. The syringe may be made more efficient by placing a small amount of vaseline on the plunger. The plunger must be completely inserted in the barrel before the puncture is made. Otherwise air will have to be injected before aspiration can be attempted.

After the anæsthetizing solution has had time to take effect, the operator pushes the needle, without touching it, through the tissues in a straight direction. If there is any doubt as to the depth of the fluid accumulation, he constantly makes suction by pulling on the piston of the syringe as it is slowly pushed through the tissues. If the syringe fails to work easily, especially when thick pus or blood has been aspirated, the needle is left in place, and the syringe is removed and cleansed with sterile saline solution, or it is replaced with another. In closed cavities, such as the pleural cavity, when the needle and syringe are separated an obturator is placed in the lumen of the cannula. In aspirating, as soon as fluid enters the syringe, the needle should remain stationary. If only exploratory puncture is desired, the cannula and syringe are removed at the same time. The punctured fluid is examined immediately after its removal from the syringe (cytologically, by culture, chemically, or by animal innoculation, as desired). When the puncture is done for evacuation of a collection, the syringe is removed from the cannula when it is filled, the contents expelled, and the syringe replaced. This is repeated until the desired result is obtained. Often after evacuation of an abscess the cavity is washed out thoroughly with physiologic salt solution which is introduced through the cannula that has been kept in place. The salt solution is allowed to flow in and then is aspirated.

In an attempt to sterilize the abscess wall, one may use for irrigation, instead of saline solution, certain of the antiseptic solutions: 3 percent phenol, 3 percent boric acid, or one of the newer organic mercurial preparations. Recently certain quinine derivatives have enjoyed particular favor in Germany; among them Vuzin, Eukupin and Rivanol (1 to 500 to 1 to 5000). We have not been able to detect any specific action in any one of them. Small quantities of these solutions may be left in the abscess cavity in the hope of prolonged action. A similar effect is anticipated from the introduction of 2 to 10 cc. of Chlumsky's solution (pure carbolic acid crystals 30, trit. camphor 60, absolute alcohol 10). The proprietary name of this solution is Erysol. Likewise 5 to 20 cc. of a 10 percent iodoform-glycerine mixture, which must be shaken well before using, or 2 percent tincture of iodine, have been used. None of these preparations can accomplish disinfection of tissues invaded by bacteria. At most they prevent bacterial

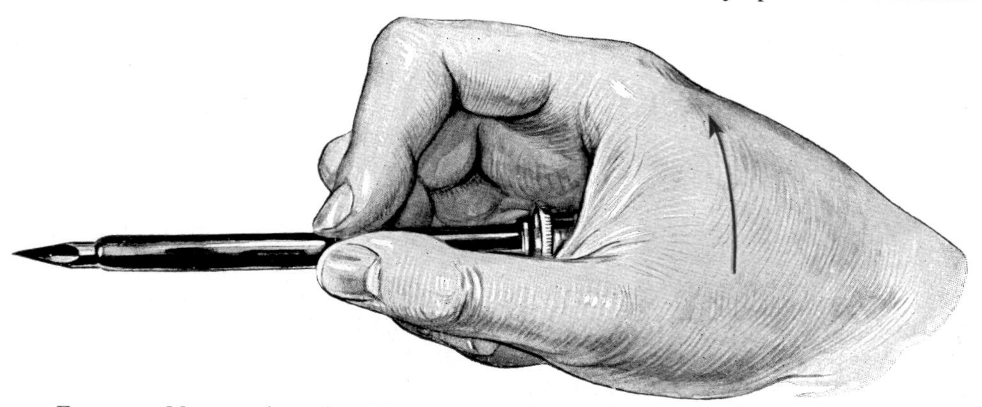

Fig. 271. Manner of holding a trocar while inserting it. The head of the trocar rests firmly in the palm, the depth of insertion is controlled by the index finger, and the trocar is rotated to the right as it is plunged in.

growth in the contents of the abscess cavity and in the dressings. Their bactericidal properties are negligible. They act on the tissue mainly as an irritant, causing hyperemia and stimulating the formation of granulation tissue.

For the therapeutic removal of pus from a thick-walled cavity or a cavity whose walls are friable, a trocar and cannula should be used. After anæsthetizing the line of puncture, the skin is incised, as is also any firm fascia underneath it, so that the trocar may be inserted without undue pressure. The trocar and cannula are grasped in the hollow of the hand so that the trocar is prevented from slipping back, and the index finger is used to limit the depth of insertion (Fig. 271). With a twisting movement it is inserted to the desired depth. If the cannula has entered the collection, the fluid escapes as soon as the trocar is withdrawn. Irrigation and the introduction of antiseptic solutions may be carried out in the same manner as described above. A tube may be inserted through the cannula for subsequent drainage, or, as is often done in tuberculous cavities, the skin opening is closed with a suture. If a suction apparatus is attached to the cannula, the pus can be removed without contamination of the surrounding field.

Evacuation of Tuberculous Abscesses. Aspiration is frequently used in cold or tuberculous abscesses. The needle should not be inserted directly through thin tissue layers covering the abscess or at a dependent point, but from above, diagonally through thick tissue layers, so that a fistula will not develop (Fig. 272).

I personally prefer, as a rule, incision for the emptying of tuberculous abscesses with immediate closure by suture. This requires the most rigid asepsis to prevent mixed infection. If it is desired to study the contents of an abscess bacteriologically or by animal innoculation, a small amount of pus may be obtained by aspiration with a syringe and needle. The line of incision should be similar to the line of puncture. After anæsthetizing the line of incision, the soft parts covering the abscess are incised until the abscess is reached, and the contents evacuated. By retracting the wound margins, the abscess wall can be carefully removed, if it can be loosened

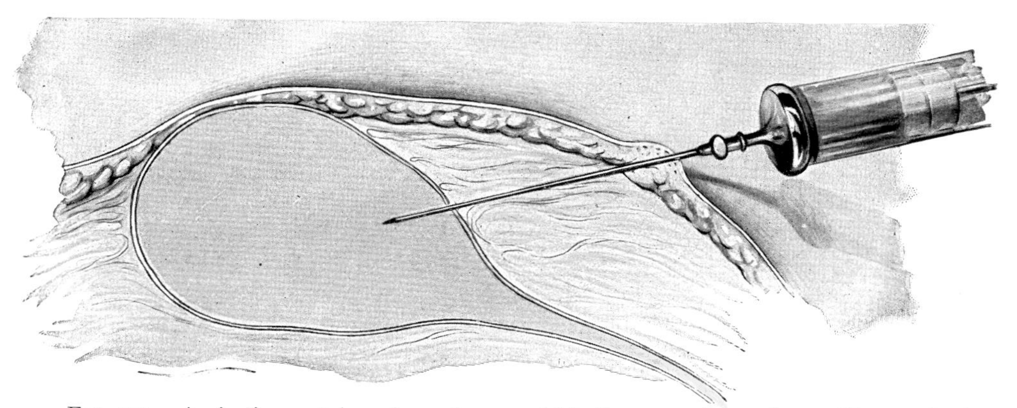

FIG. 272. Aspirating a tuberculous abscess which lies near the surface. The needle is introduced distal to the point where the abscess is pointing through a thick layer of tissue, after anæsthetizing the point of insertion.

without undue trauma, with a gall-stone curette or with a tampon. If the membrane can not be removed easily, force should not be used, nor should the curettement be too vigorous. Care should also be exercised in dealing with strands of tissue coursing through the abscess cavity. They may contain blood vessels, injury of which may result in severe hemorrhage. The abscess should be irrigated with a 3 percent phenol solution or some other suitable antiseptic. The line of incision should be carefully sutured in layers. Should one desire to leave an antiseptic in the cavity, such as iodoform-glycerine or Chlumsky's solution, as is often recommended, 10 to 20 cc. of either should be introduced before inserting the last suture in the tissues surrounding the abscess.

The Management of Phlegmons and Acute Abscesses. Wide incision of every suppurative area, to permit of unobstructed evacuation and the release of tension in the tissues, is the most effective means for controlling suppuration and its sequelæ. The ancient axiom, *Ubi Pus, Ibi Evacua,* is as true today as it was a century ago. The maintenance or restoration of function should be borne in mind during every operation, and those therapeutic measures should be chosen which will be adequate, but cause the least interference with later function.

The simple aspiration of an acute abscess should rarely be done, and then only in exceptionally mild infections where it is possible to repeat the procedure frequently. In all severe infections wide incision is to be preferred. This uncovers all the inflamed layers, be they suppurative or merely inflammatory, overlying a suppurative lesion. In these cases it is advisable to use general, in preference to local, anæsthesia. Even though general anæsthesia is preferable in extensive infections whose confines are not clearly demarcated, I prefer local anæsthesia in the limited infections where I can determine in advance the extent of the incision necessary. I have never observed any disadvantage from its use in properly selected cases. It is also possible to use conduction anæsthesia, but spinal anæsthesia should not be used since metastatic infections have been observed following spinal puncture. Hemorrhage should be avoided as much as possible.

The focus of infection should be incised at its most dependent portion, so that drainage by gravity will be favored when the patient is in the position which he will maintain for the greater part of the time. The overlying tissues should be sharply incised with a knife. Blunt dissection and tearing is not good surgery and is injurious. Such injury to tissues interferes with healing after the usual aseptic operation. How much more damaging must this be when it is inflicted on inflamed tissue. Rough procedures may force infectious material into previously unopened tissue spaces. Only when the abscess has a very thin overlying wall is it permissible to insert a blunt hemostat or dressing forceps and to enlarge the opening by withdrawing the instrument with the blades opened. If in making the incision, the surgeon is not sure of avoiding important structures, such as tendons, nerves, or blood vessels, these should be exposed and carefully protected by an incision which runs parallel to them. Should the infection be close to serous spaces or cavities which are themselves not infected, tendon sheaths, joints, pleura, peritoneum, pericardium, tunica vaginalis propria, these must be carefully protected from injury and subsequent infection. If doubt exists as to their inclusion in the inflammatory process, aspiration may be attempted through a non-infected area under the most rigid asepsis previous to making the incision. Overlying muscles should be retracted. They should only be nicked or divided when it is otherwise impossible to gain access to, or drainage from the infected area. Actively bleeding vessels should be ligated; oozing from inflamed tissues stops spontaneously or can be checked by loose packing.

If the area of infection is so extensive that it can not be adequately drained through a single incision or, if a large single incision may lead to mutilation or the division of important structures, multiple incisions should be made. The additional incisions may at times be made more easily by raising the subcutaneous tissues with a dressing forceps or hemostat inserted through the original incision. The second incision is made over the tip of the instrument and the new wound can then be enlarged either with a scalpel or by opening the blades of the instrument (Fig. 273). This procedure may also be used for inserting a through and through drain. The counter-opening must be large enough not only to permit the drain to pass through it, but also to allow the escape of pus around the drain.

It is frequently difficult to establish the exact extent of the purulent process and to expose each pocket. The difficulty can be largely overcome by careful sponging or aspiration of the purulent material so that one can observe small openings from which pus may exude when gentle pressure is made on the surrounding tissues. On the contrary, probing the wound with sounds or dressing forceps for tracts of infection (Payr's duct abscesses) should only be attempted with the greatest hesitancy. These instruments

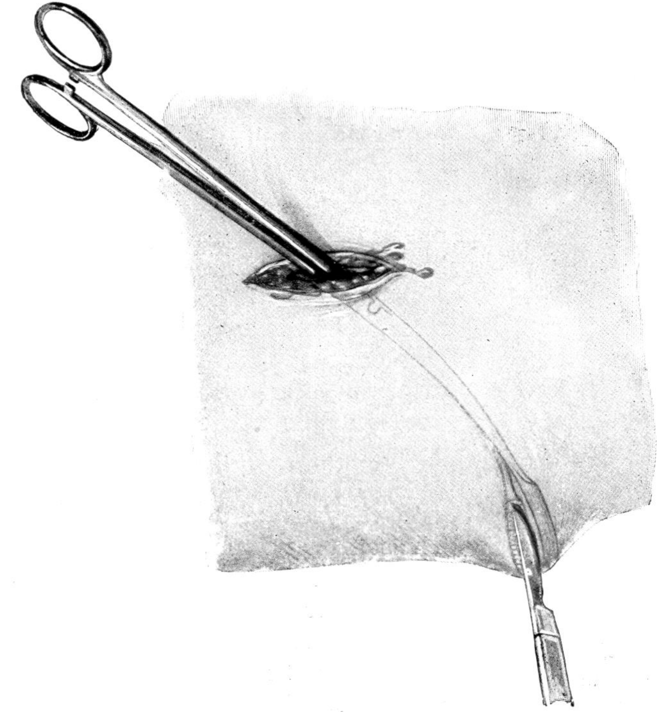

FIG. 273. A counter-incision may be made by inserting a dressings forceps into the abscess through the original incision, pushing it against the skin and then cutting down on the slightly opened points.

may very easily penetrate loose healthy muscle spaces, as in the forearm, where they can be advanced without resistance, leading one to believe that he is in a sinus when that is not really the case. When in doubt, it is much better gently to insert the gloved hand into the wound.

After finishing the operation the area is washed with sterile normal saline solution or with a mild antiseptic solution (2 percent Sagrotan, hydrogen peroxide, boric acid, potassium permanganate, 3 percent phenol) until all pus and blood are removed.

The management of the furuncle and carbuncle is described in Chapter V. B. 5, under: Operations on the Skin and Subcutaneous Tissue.

Drainage. With adequate incision of the foci of infection the operative task is not completed. One should make certain that any new collections can drain freely and continuously so that pus does not reaccumulate and form pockets which increase tissue tension. Simple incision is, as a rule, not sufficient since the majority of wound margins are inclined to fold up and close. We have found in our clinic that a very excellent means of maintaining drainage is the use of the "hole-incision" (Fig. 274). (Schubert: Zentralbl. f. Chirurg. 1923, p. 83.) It consists in excising a tissue cylinder which includes all the layers involved in the infection. The diameter of this cylinder depends on the severity and extent of the infection and on the length of time the drainage is intended to last. Zur Verth has suggested the excision of an elliptical piece of tissue. The use of stretching clamps to keep the incision open has not become popular. These must be kept in various sizes, which is in itself a nuisance, and furthermore they are apt to produce pressure necrosis. They are also easily dislodged. The suturing apart of the skin and deeper tissues is also ineffectual, since the tension sutures cut through after a very short time and the suture holes provide a means for carrying the infection. Erysipelas has been known to start in this way.

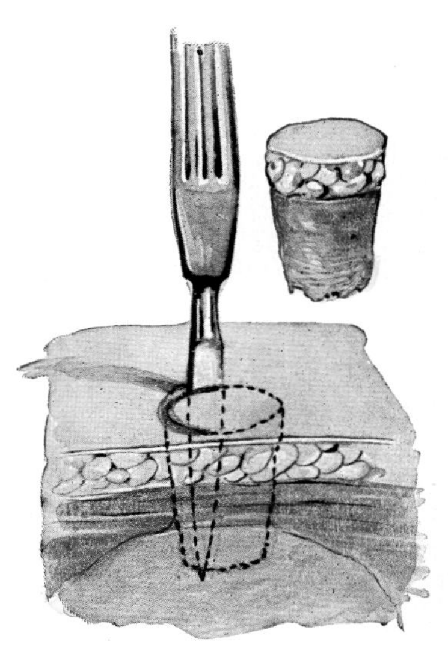

FIG. 274. Circular excision of tissue for drainage. A cylindrical plug of tissue over the abscess is removed, providing a gaping opening for drainage of the pus.

The most effective and most widely used measures for keeping a wound open are drainage and packing. Drains are made of rubber or of glass. Glass drains are changed more easily, but should be used only when pressure upon important structures, such as large vessels or nerves, can be avoided. Rubber drains have the great advantage of adaptation to the wound. The soft ones can hardly exert an injurious pressure on the tissues. They can be cut to suitable lengths and be provided with lateral openings where desired. Rubber drains may be shortened when the dressing is being changed without completely removing the drain, and they can be quickly sterilized in boiling water. Drains of elaborate shapes, which are frequently seen, are superfluous. The drains which are chosen should be wide enough for the pus to flow through unobstructed (Fig. 275).

Lateral openings in a rubber tube should be cut lengthwise with the scissors, since cutting the openings transversely causes a much weaker place in the rubber (Fig. 276). Drainage tubes should be inserted from the surface of the wound down to the deepest part of the wound in such a manner that if possible the pus will flow out by gravity (Fig. 277). If it is desired to maintain the drain at a definite place in an otherwise large wound the method illustrated in figure 278 may be used. The method is simple and permits one to change the tube with the assurance that the second tube will go to the desired spot. Drains should be prevented from coming out of or slipping into the wound by fastening them to the skin or to the dressings. Sutures may be used, but safety pins are suitable when rubber drains are used.

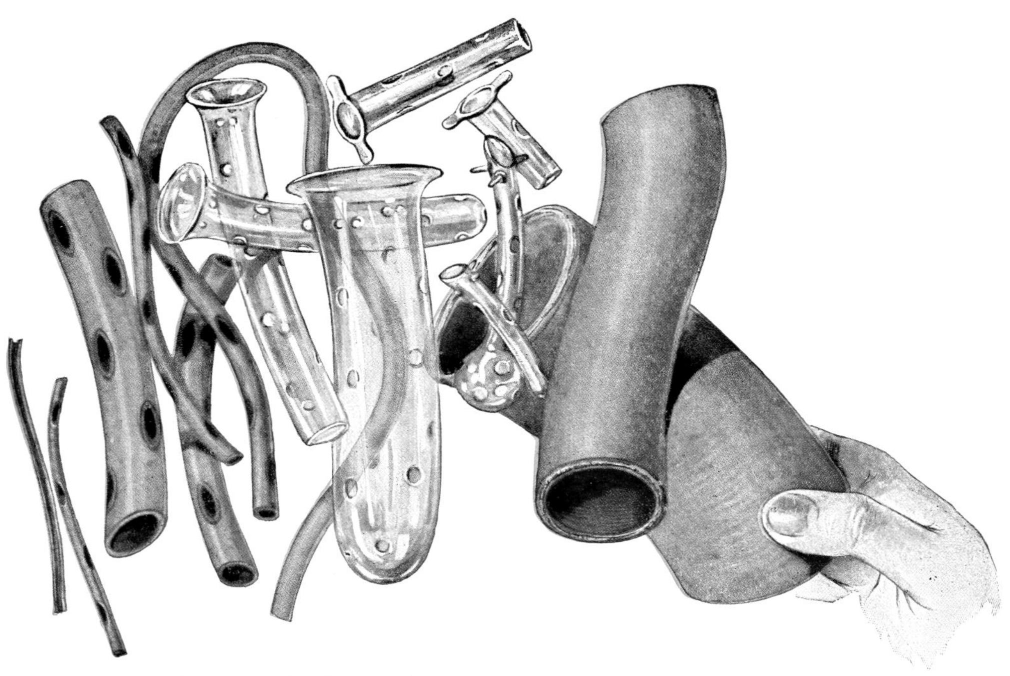

Fig. 275. Various kinds and sizes of rubber and glass drains.

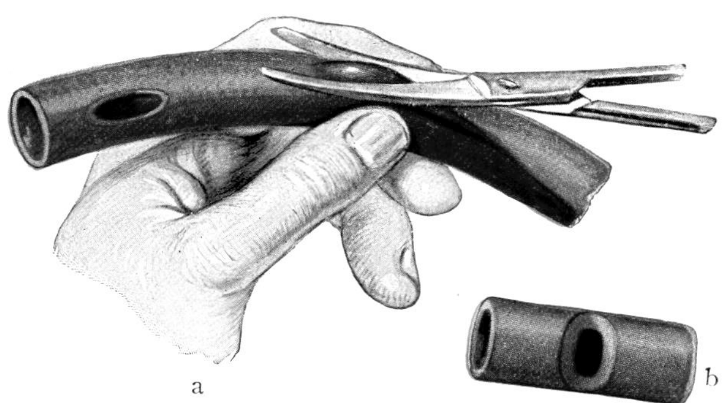

Fig. 276. a. Cutting a longitudinal opening in the side of a rubber drain. b. Incorrect transverse opening.

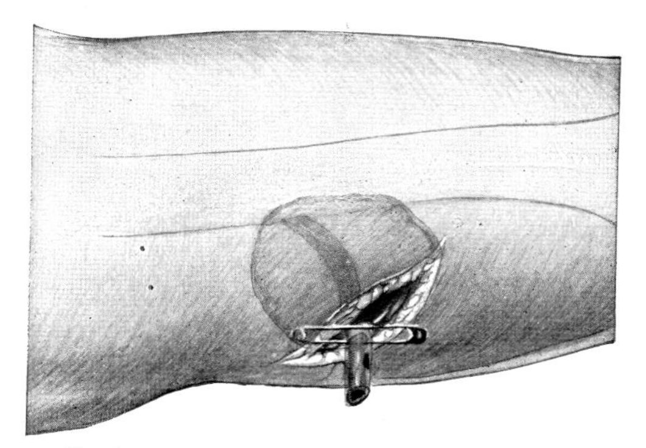

Fig. 277. Drainage at the most dependent part of an abscess.

To prevent pressure on the tissue by a safety pin, a piece of gauze is inserted under the pin (Fig. 279).

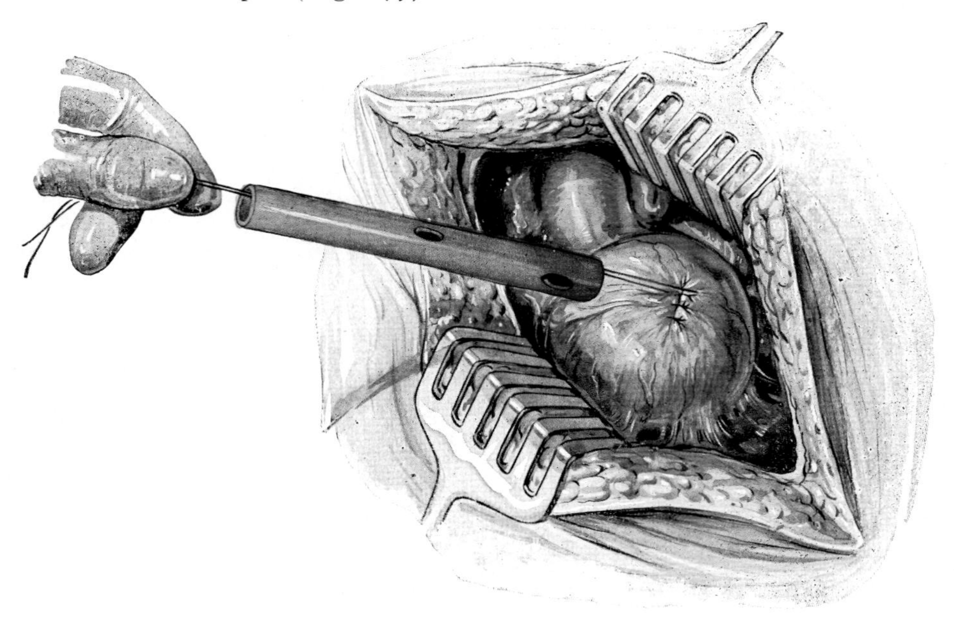

FIG. 278. The drain is directed to the desired point by being slipped over the long ends of the last suture.

In order to prevent a drain from slipping into a large cavity, such as the pleural cavity, a long silk thread is tied to the drain, and its ends are

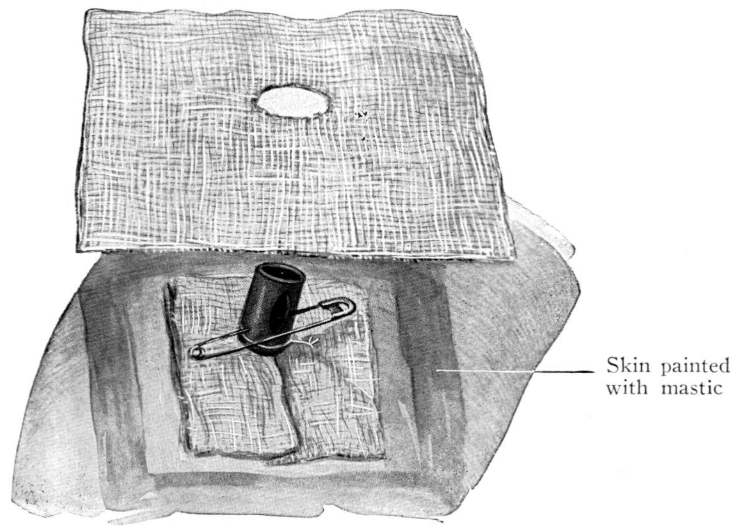

FIG. 279. Fastening a drain. A safety pin through the drain is held firmly in place by a piece of gauze over it which is fastened to the skin with mastic.

fastened some distance from the wound with adhesive plaster. If a drain should be lost it can be located by the x-ray.

It is necessary in certain cases, such as empyemata or enterostomies, to fasten the drainage tubes especially securely, so that the tubes will remain indefinitely in the cavity in which they are placed. The drains must be kept intact and protected against damage, so that they can be used over a long period. For this purpose a piece of rubber tubing 1 to 2 cm. in length and just wide enough to fit firmly around the drain is placed at the point where the longer tube will meet the skin. This rubber cuff may be changed when desired and therefore can be used for any method of retention. The cuff is put on as follows (Fig. 280): after the drainage tube is placed in its correct position, it is grasped securely with a hemostat where it meets the skin. A second hemostat, on whose tip is the rubber cuff, grasps the end of the exposed tube. The tube is stretched between the two hemostats and the cuff slips easily down the narrowed drainage tube which has been moistened with water. As soon as the tension is released, the cuff fits snugly against the drain, which has resumed its normal thickness. To fasten it, two large safety pins are put through the rubber cuff. A gauze pad is placed beneath the pins, and a perforated piece of adhesive plaster is used to fasten these to the skin (Fig. 281).

Long silk threads may be attached to the safety pins and fastened to a different place on the body. If the drainage tube, as in gastrostomy or cholecystostomy, is carried through the dressings the rubber cuff is fastened to the outside of these.

Packing. The term packing, or tamponing, when applied to a dressing which is used to keep a wound open, is a misnomer, since one does not wish to tampon the wound with the strips of gauze and thus dam back fluids. The actual purpose is to secure an open wound and to secure capillary fluid drainage from within outward. For this purpose the wound should be packed loosely and without pressure with the gauze strips.

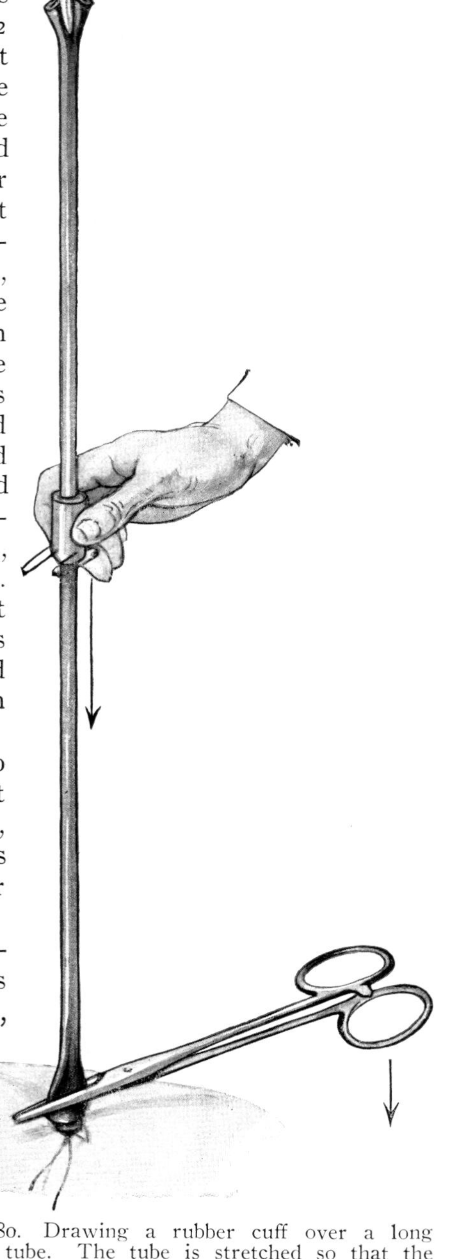

FIG. 280. Drawing a rubber cuff over a long drainage tube. The tube is stretched so that the cuff slips on easily, but fits firmly when the tube is relaxed. The cuff is used to fasten the tube after it has been inserted.

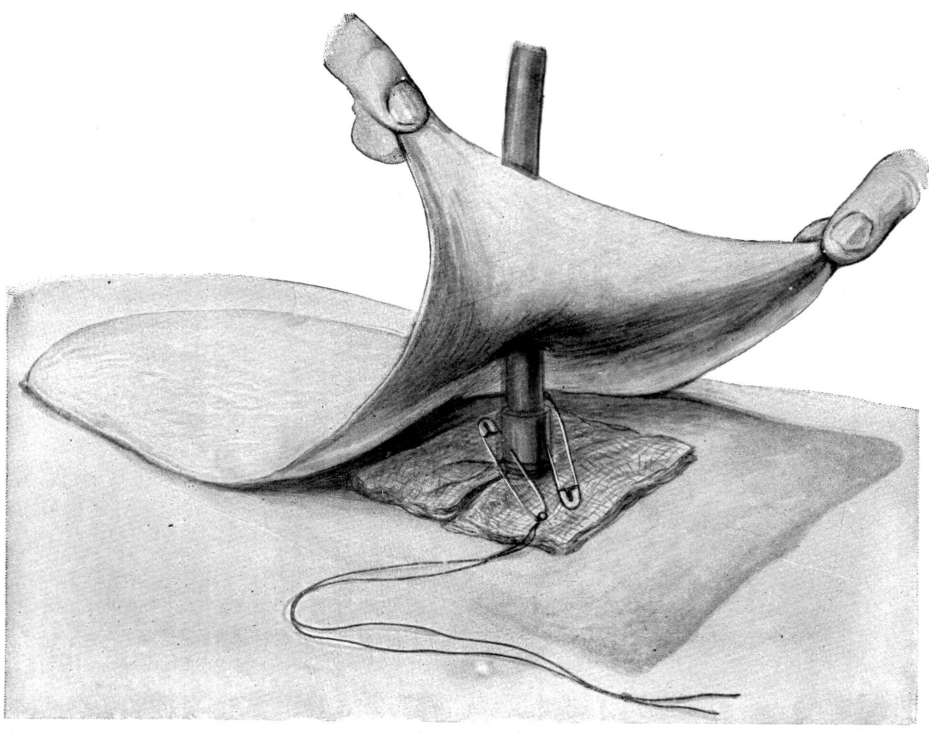

FIG. 281. Fastening the rubber tube by means of the cuff. A large piece of adhesive plaster is being applied.

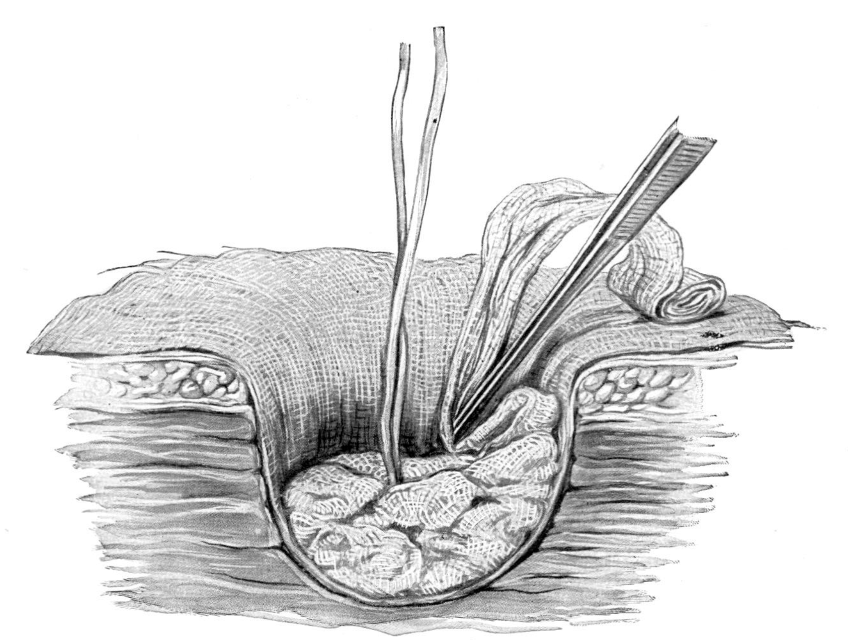

FIG. 282. v. Mikulicz' Tampon. The wound is covered with a large gauze pad to the center of which is attached a double tape. The inside of the pad is packed with gauze which can be changed as frequently as is desired. The gauze pad is removed by pulling on the tapes.

The pain and tissue damage which often results from changing packing which is adherent to the wound can be diminished by using v. Mikulicz' method. A large piece of gauze, to the center of which is attached a long tape, is placed in the wound so that it fills all the recesses (Fig. 282). The

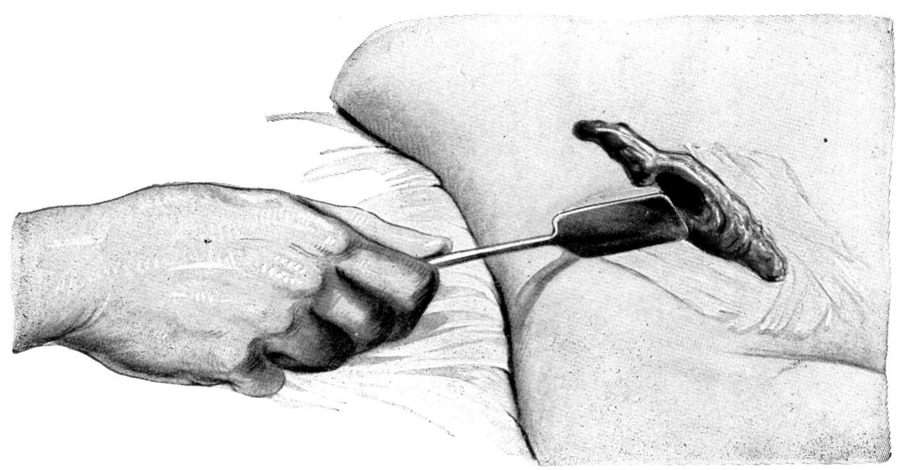

FIG. 283. Protection of the skin and young epithelium surrounding a drainage wound by a thick layer of zinc oxide ointment.

inside of this gauze layer is filled loosely with packing or cellucotton. When the dressing is to be changed it is only necessary to remove the packing. The large piece of gauze is left in and is gradually removed by pulling on the tapes as the wound diminishes in size.

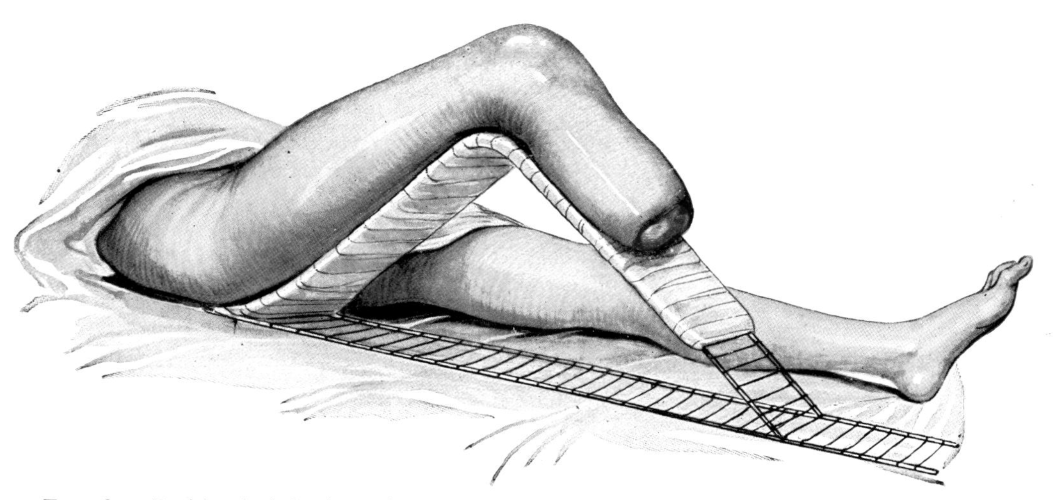

FIG 284. Position in infections of the foot and leg, here an infected amputation stump. The site of infection is elevated but without the danger of the pus burrowing upward.

Since the wound secretion in the gauze offers additional nutriment for bacteria growth, it is of advantage to impregnate the gauze with an antiseptic. I use vioform gauze exclusively. Other antiseptic gauzes may also be used. Pyoktanin gauze, which has been suggested by my former assistant Baumann, has the advantage of not adhering to the wound.

The value of packing as drainage is slight. As soon as the gauze strips become saturated with wound secretion, they tend to dam back the pus in the wound, therefore this method is being used less frequently for the drainage of suppurative wounds. The chief use of tamponage is to check parenchymatous hemorrhage, and to keep open the superficial layers of deep wounds so that they may granulate from the bottom. The technic for tamponage for the control of more serious hemorrhage is described in Chapter IV, A: "The Control of Hemorrhage."

To protect the skin surrounding a purulent wound from the irritating effects of pus, I cover the skin with Lassar's zinc paste (Fig. 283). Fluffed gauze is placed over the wound, the edges of which may be protected as has been previously described (Figs. 262 and 263). Over this wound dressing we place several layers of sterile cellucotton, which can be removed when they are saturated with wound secretion without changing the primary gauze dressings.

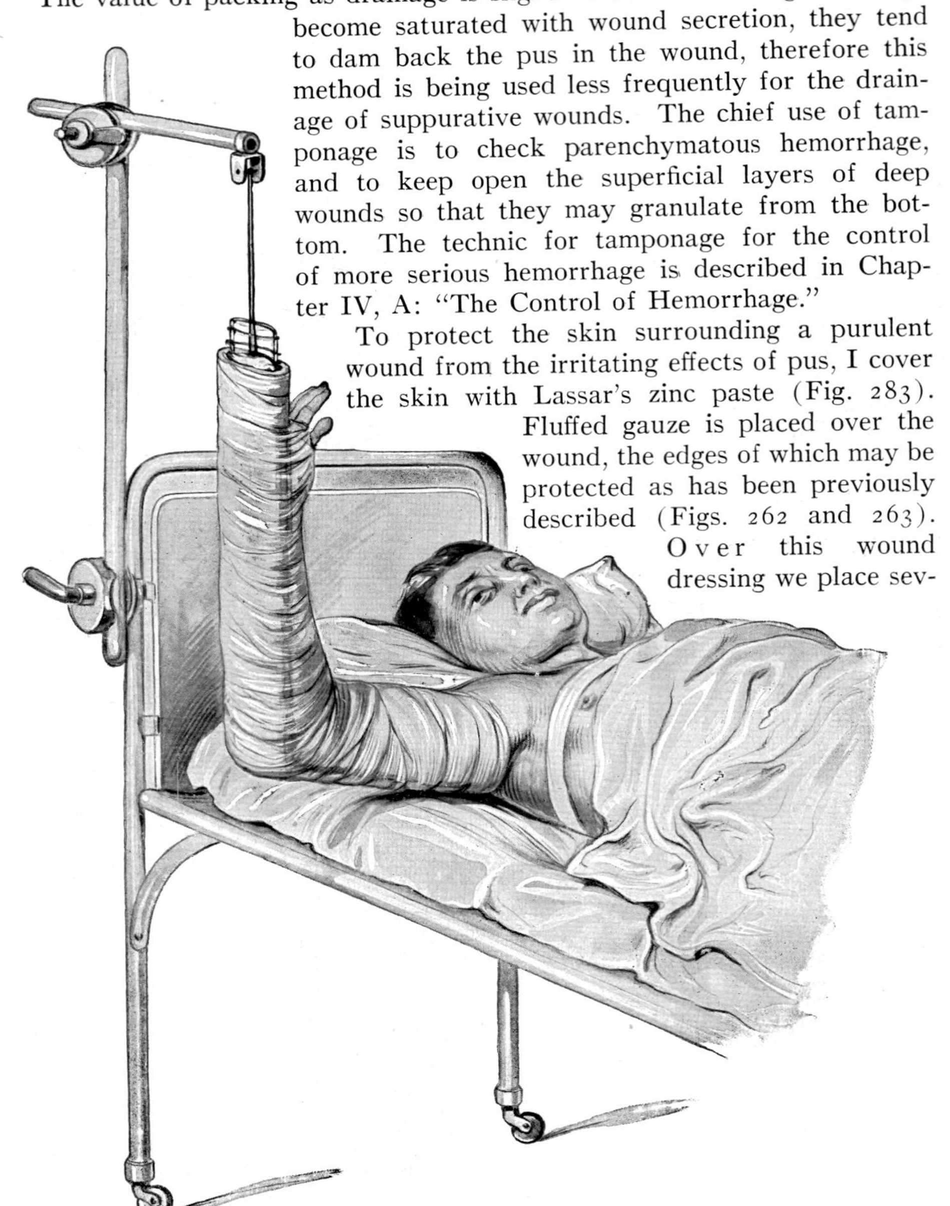

Fig. 285. Vertical elevation of the forearm, to promote healing in the absence of severe symptoms of infection.

Complete rest of the infected area is essential. This can be accomplished by various types of splints or bandages.

The question as to whether the infected area should be elevated or dependent should be considered from two points of view. The elevation of the distal portion of an extremity promotes the resistance of the tissues by favoring the flow of blood and lymph, thus overcoming stasis and reducing the swelling associated with inflammatory processes so that suppuration is less likely to occur. On the other hand, elevation favors the proximal extension of abscesses and infiltration, and may possibly aid in the spread of thrombi. The dependent position of the extremity produces an opposite effect (Fig. 284).

With these conflicting considerations, I use the following procedures in practice. The limb is placed in the dependent position in the stage of acute inflammation, when the virulence of the infection has not yet been controlled; in phlegmons; in infections where there is abundant wound secre-

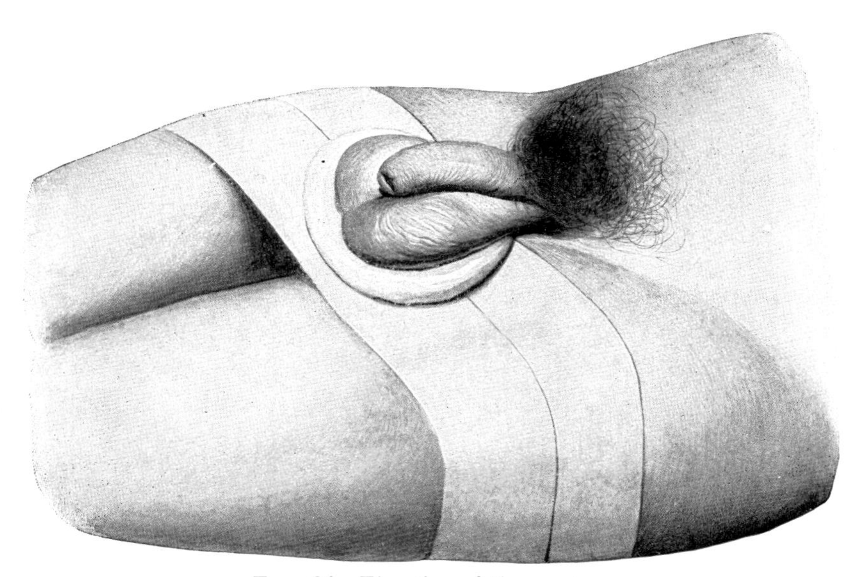

FIG. 286. Elevation of the scrotum.

tion; in multiple abscess formation; in lymphangitis; glandular swellings, and high fever. Later, when the virulence of the infection has subsided, when the suppuration has become circumscribed, and after the inflammatory symptoms and the fever have decreased, the limb is elevated.

The arm is elevated as follows: It is fastened to a splint with the elbow-joint bent at a right angle. When the forearm only is affected, the upper extremity is abducted and the forearm is held vertically (Fig. 285). When the arm also is affected it is placed in an oblique position resting on a large pillow.

To elevate the scrotum (Fig. 286), a pillow, a cup-shaped splint resting on both thighs, or strips of adhesive plaster fastened to both thighs may be used.

Figure 287 shows the splint used for the elevation of the entire lower extremity. The thigh is perpendicular and the leg is at an angle of 45° to the horizontal plane of the body.

The Braun splints which are excellent, simple and inexpensive are very useful for maintaining elevation of a part. I have modified the one for the lower extremity so that it can be adjusted for any position (Figs. 288, 289, and 290).

The special operative measures used in infection of certain highly developed tissues, are described with the surgery of these tissues. The principles

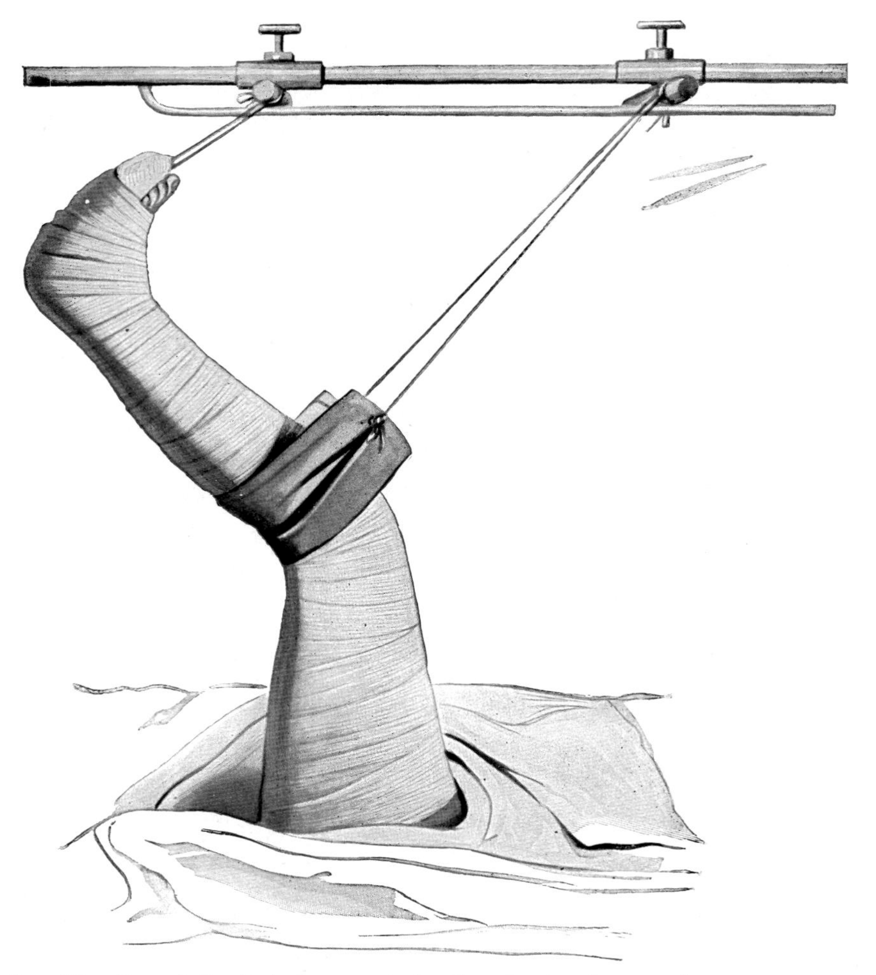

FIG. 287. Elevation of the limb to promote healing, in the absence of severe symptoms of infection.

for the amputation of limbs are discussed in Chapter XI. Amputation is a last resort in progressive, virulent infections that can not be otherwise controlled.

No attempt is made here to describe the general management of a local infection. It is worth while to remember that tetanus antitoxin should be used in all traumatic wounds, and in the revision of old wounds, whose freedom from a latent infection can not be guaranteed.

E. CHANGING OF DRESSINGS AND THE FURTHER CARE OF THE WOUND

Every change of dressing should be regarded as an operation and must be performed with the same painstaking aseptic precautions. Since it is,

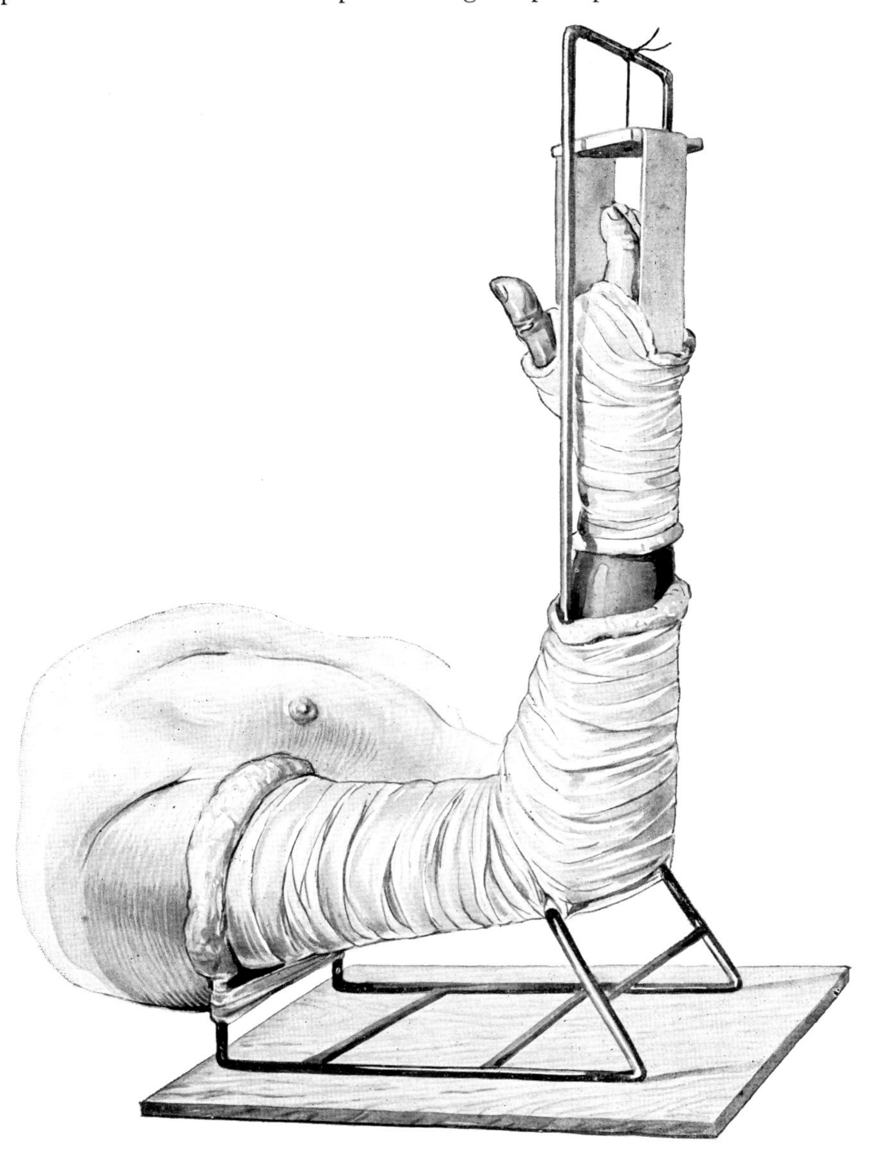

FIG. 288. Apparatus for elevation of the forearm.

as a rule, possible to change a dressing without touching the skin or dressings with the hands, it is not essential that the hands be thoroughly disinfected for every change of dressing. The surgeon may simply wash his hands and put on sterile gloves, but because of the contamination of his hands he should touch the dressings with sterile instruments only.

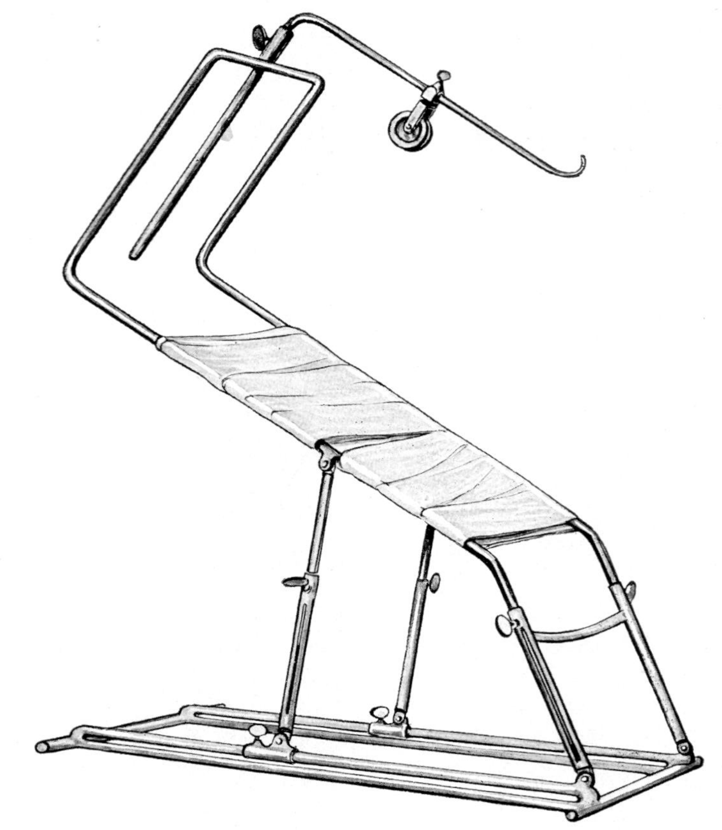

Fig. 289. Apparatus for elevation of the leg.

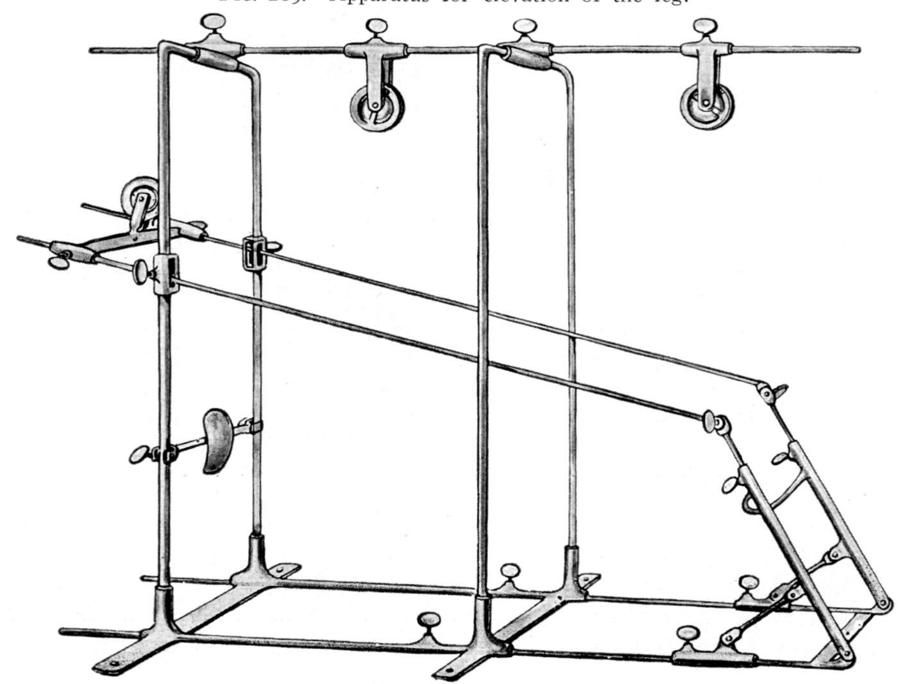

Fig. 290. Adjustable apparatus for elevation of the leg.

For the comfort of the patient, to save time, and to maintain the quiet of a hospital, it is best to leave the patient in his own bed in the ward and change the dressing there, instead of taking him in his bed or on a litter to a dressing room. Exceptions to this are difficult or painful dressings, those

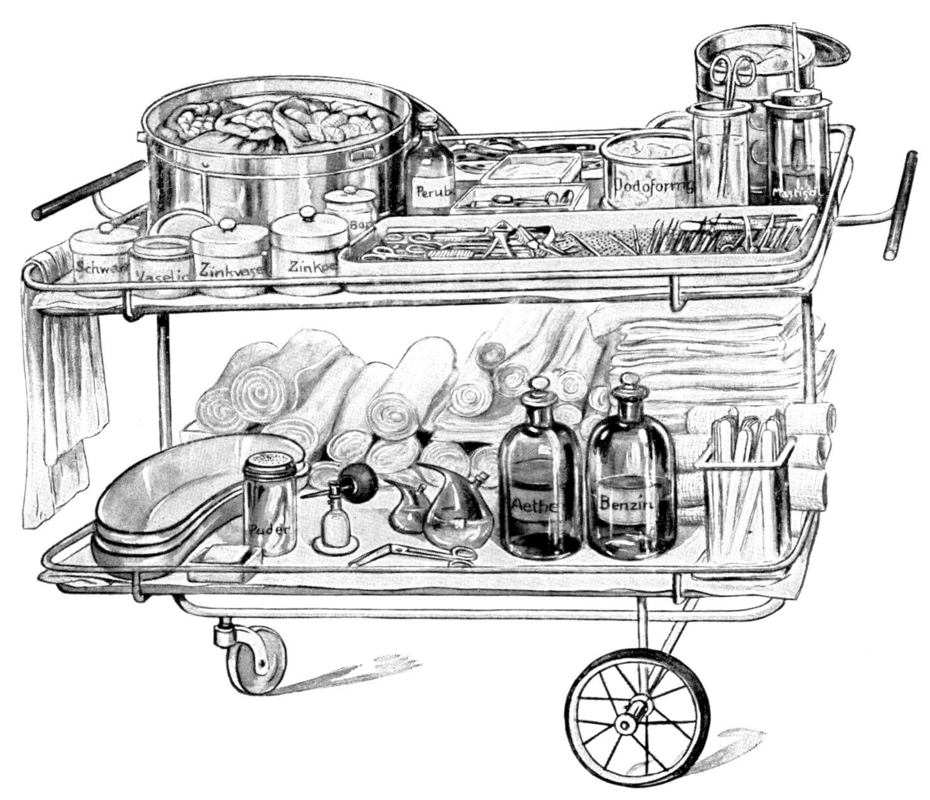

FIG. 291. Dressing-cart with the usual instruments, dressings and drugs.

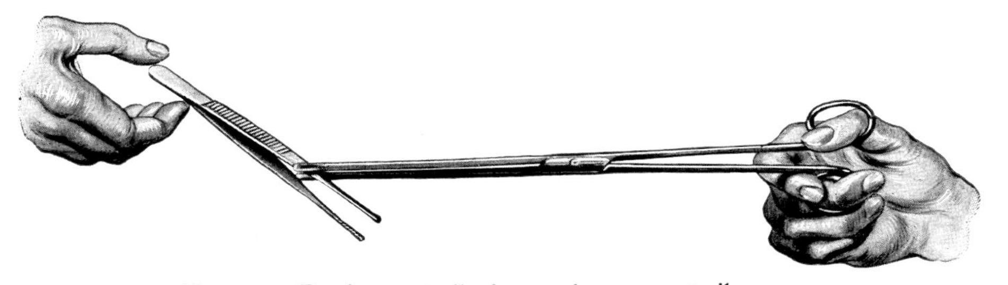

FIG. 292. Passing a sterile forceps by a non-sterile person.

which are repulsive, or those in which the patient may be unduly exposed. A dressing-cart with rubber wheels carrying all the necessary instruments, solutions, dressings, etc., should be used for the bedside dressing (Fig. 291). A patient should never be dressed sitting or standing. His eyes should always be covered with a cloth to prevent his seeing the wound.

When changing dressings, a non-sterile assistant should hand the surgeon the needed instruments from the sterile instrument tray with a sterile forceps (Fig. 292). The instrument forceps should be kept in a sterile dry glass cylinder or in a 2 percent solution of Lysol (Fig. 291). The surgeon uses tissue forceps, or at times a special dressing forceps. Naturally, one should always be careful that the instrument forceps does not become contaminated in passing materials from the tray to the dresser. The wound can be cleansed with a sponge held by a dressing forceps without danger to the surgeon's hands. To economize in trays and to save time, especially in large wards, the necessary sterile instruments, forceps, scissors, etc., for dressings may be hung on a sterile rack and taken off separately by the

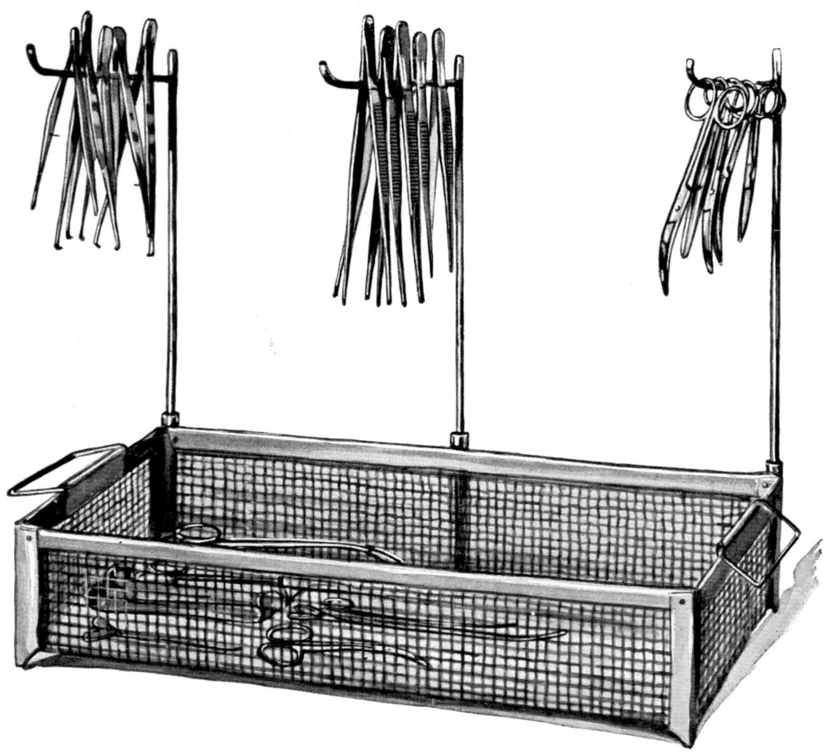

Fig. 293. Wire basket with racks for suspending sterile instruments so that they can be readily taken off by a non-sterile person with a sterile instrument forceps without contaminating other instruments. Particularly suitable for the outpatient department.

attendant (Fig. 293). Attention and discipline compensate for such assistance without endangering the asepsis.

Each change of dressing is an insult to the wound cells, and when painfully done, taxes the strength of the patient. This is evident from the rise in temperature and exhausted condition of the patient seen so frequently following extensive wound dressings. One should therefore be careful not to change dressings more frequently than is necessary. In the absence of any signs of infection, the dressings covering a supposedly clean wound should not be removed before the first sutures are to be taken out. In our clinic this is done on the eighth day. The stitches or clips should then be removed, and the wound which is clean should be protected with a small dressing for a few more days. Drains inserted as a precaution should be removed the 1st, 2nd or 3rd day after operation. In case of active local infection, or where it is deemed that a secondary operation may be necessary, the dressing should be changed daily and the wound revised as indicated. In the presence of gas gangrene the dressing should be done at least twice daily. With the abatement of the acute manifestations, the dressings need not be changed so often. When infection has subsided and the discharge has ceased, the dressings may be left on for two, three, four or more days. When there is a copious discharge which rapidly saturates the dressings it is only necessary to change the outer dressings at frequent intervals, while the entire dressing may be changed daily.

The greatest possible care should be exercised in changing the dressings. In fractures and diseases of the joints the removal or change of dressings should in no way interfere with the immobilization of the extremity. It is never permissible to use force in removing dressings, to separate roughly the edges of the wound, to rub the wound surface with sponges, or to do anything which may produce pain unnecessarily. When the dressings are adherent they should be softened with a 3 percent hydrogen peroxide solution, with luke-warm oil, or sterile saline solution. These measures should be instituted several hours before the dressings are to be removed. Packing in the wound should be removed cautiously, while the wound margins are gently retracted. Drains should not be changed unless it is desired to insert smaller ones or unless they are to be completely removed. They may be shortened daily and may be used to irrigate the depths of the wound. After the accumulated pus in the wound has been removed by irrigation with hydrogen peroxide or sterile saline solution, or by gentle sponging, the wound is examined for secondary abscesses, fistulæ, foreign bodies, etc. The greatest care should be exercised in this examination since the patient is not under the influence of an anæsthetic. In the majority of instances it is unnecessary to palpate the wound. The skillful can see at one glance what the unskillful can not find after a thorough examination. Only in the presence of distinct indications, such as poor general condition, rising temperature, etc., which can not otherwise be accounted for, is one permitted to act drastically and to make a detailed examination of the wound with the patient under the influence of an anæsthetic. In this way the necessity of a subsequent operation can be determined.

In the course of wound repair the skin surrounding the wound should be kept free of pus. The skin should be cleansed with dry sponges. If covered with scabs, these should be removed with benzine sponges. The area around the draining wound should be covered with a thick layer of Lassar's zinc paste. After thorough wound toilet any drains or packing which were removed should be reinserted if necessary, but as the infection subsides the drains should be shortened or completely removed. If a collection reaccumulates the drains should be reinserted. Deep wounds should be filled loosely with sterile gauze to facilitate healing from below upward. The packing and dressing gauze may be covered with a sterile ointment so that they will not adhere to the fresh granulations and injure them when the dressings are removed. When granulation tissue fills the wound packing should be discontinued and the wound covered with an ointment-covered gauze until healing is complete.

Among the numerous remedies, Lassar's paste (ac. salicylic 2, zinc oxide, starch aa 24.0, vaseline ad 100.0) has stood the test of time. Exuberant granulations should be cauterized with silver nitrate and covered with silver nitrate ointment (Billroth's black ointment: silver nitrate 1.0, balsum peru. 10.0, petrolat. ad 100.0).

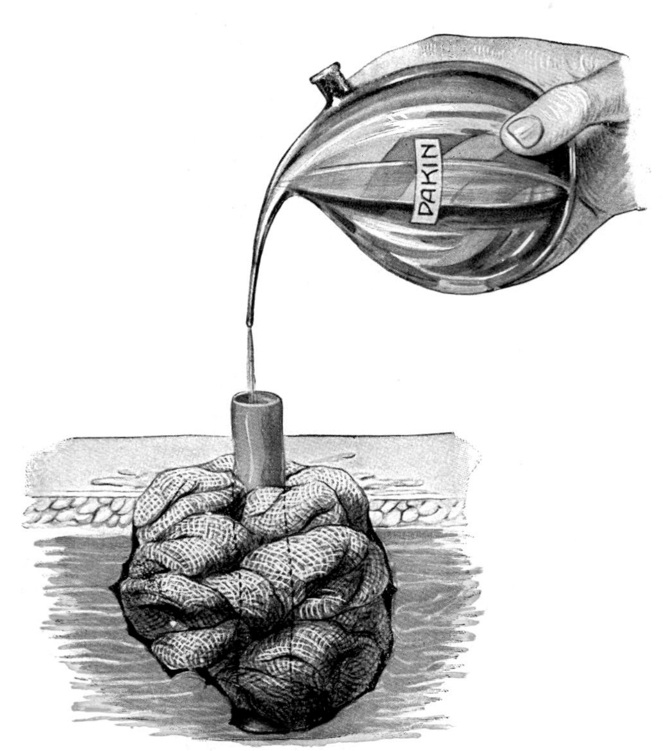

FIG. 294. Chlorinating a wound with Dakin's solution. The tube is passed into the depth of the wound and then loosely surrounded with gauze.

Moisture, or Wet Dressings. Moisture and hyperemia act favorably as a rule upon inflammatory areas. Moisture is applied to the inflamed area in the form of wet dressings. Its specific value is still disputed. I consider it of value when the suppurating focus has been previously drained. I never use an impermeable cover around these dressings since they defeat the purpose of their use. The favorable action exerted by a moist dressing rests mainly in the capillary absorption of the gauze. Due to superficial evaporation a continuous outflow of secretion is engendered. Dressings are moistened with various weak antiseptic fluids, as for example: 60 percent alcohol, boric acid solution, lead acetate, Burow's solution (alum 5.0, lead acetate 25.0, distilled water 500), lead water, potassium permanganate, hydrogen peroxide, etc. These solutions are to an extent deodorant, retard decomposition of wound fluids and growth of bacteria in the dressings, and increase hyperemia. They, however, do not disinfect a wound. Wright's hypertonic saline solution may also be recommended (sodium chloride 50.0, sodium citrate 5.0, water 1000). The osmotic effect of this hypertonic solution is to withdraw fluids from the tissues and thus dilute the concentration of the saline solution. This action results in the outpouring of fluid from the inflamed tissues and brings about a favorable "lymph lavage." Dakin's solution is valuable in severe infections, and in wounds with many sinuses.

To "chlorinate" a wound one should proceed as follows: immediately after the operation the wound is washed thoroughly with Dakin's solution from an irrigator. A Mikulicz tampon of one layer of gauze saturated in the solution is spread over the wound and is pushed in all its cavities and sinuses. One or more specially prepared drainage tubes are inserted into the deepest parts of the wound. The drainage tubes in the wound are then surrounded with layers of cellucotton soaked in Dakin's solution, so that the entire cavity is loosely filled. A few wet layers of cellucotton are placed over the wound surface and are held in place with bandages. The end of the drainage tube projects freely from the dressing (Fig. 294). Dakin's solution is poured into the tube every two hours during the day, so that the dressing is constantly saturated. The patient should not be disturbed at night if he is asleep. The use of a chlorinated soda solution is limited on my service to five days.

A very good method of combating the troublesome pyocyaneus infection often involving granulation surfaces, is a combination of iodoform gauze packing and a moist lead acetate dressing. The use of boracic acid crystals is also often effective. We use few remedies in powder form in the care of wounds.

We recommend the filling of deep wound cavities with balsam of peru. I have also used Granugenol, a wound oil, to stimulate the formation of granulations.

A wound may be kept constantly moist with any one of the aforementioned antiseptic solutions by a constant drip from an irrigator (Fig. 295). The overflow is collected in a basin placed under the area which is being irrigated. Temporary soaking of a wound can be accomplished by using protracted hot baths, preferably of soft soap water. These combine moisture with the hyperemia. It is advisable to use such a bath before changing dressings, since it makes removal of the dressing easier.

On the trunk or portions of the limbs there may be extensive areas of infection such as decubitus or burn wounds which can not be handled efficiently except by continuous baths. The continuous bath, in which the patient may remain for hours or days, should be kept at exactly body temperature; otherwise, too much heat is abstracted from the body or conveyed to it, which in either case is undesirable. The constant temperature of the bath is best maintained by an automatically regulated supply of hot water. Patients are most comfortable in the continuous bath if they are supported in it by a support which can be easily adjusted. A simple continuous bath can be provided by stretching a stout bed sheet in an ordinary bath tub, and by gradually adding hot water as this is needed. Another very simple method of maintaining the heat of the water is to use an electric water heater at the head and foot of the bath tub. The heaters can be removed or inserted as desired. These can also be used for the smaller hand or foot baths. A further advantage of the continuous bath consists in the support which the water gives to the body, so that the entire weight is not on the affected area, especially if this area is over the back or posterior portion of an extremity. These baths further dilute the discharges from wounds and involuntary discharges. By lowering the temperature of the bath, a reduction in febrile reactions can be obtained.

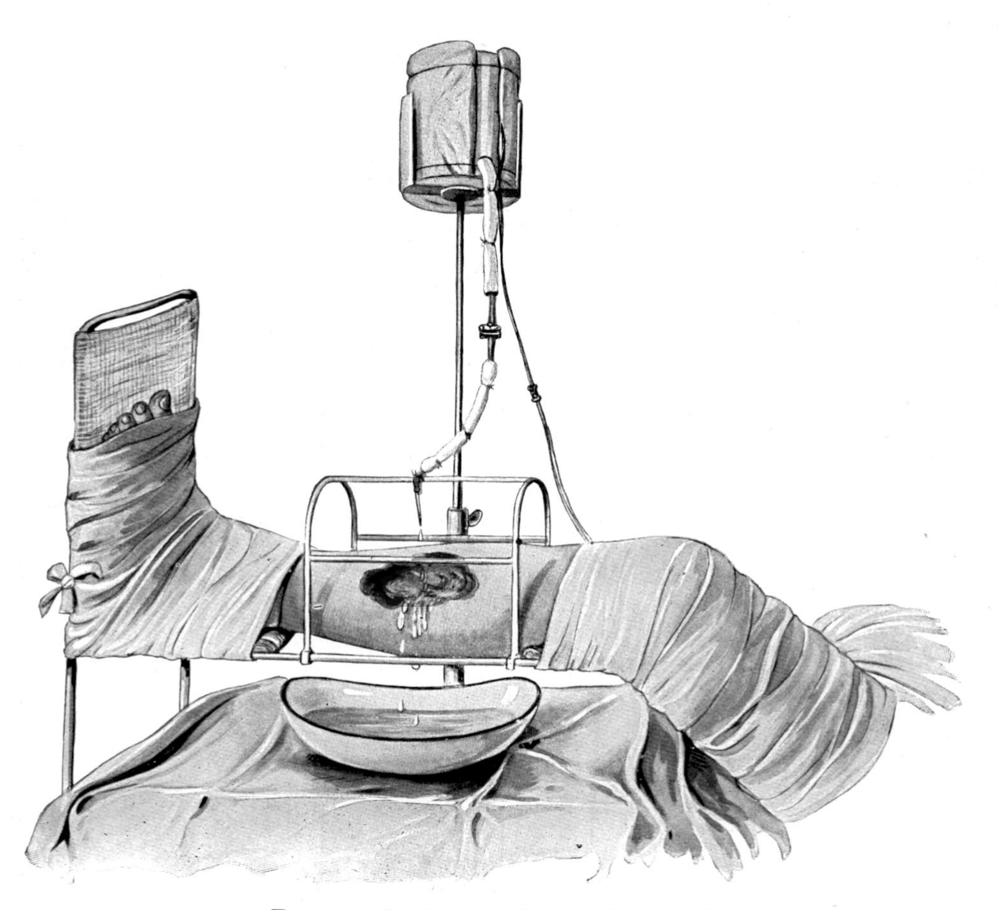

FIG. 295. Continuous irrigation of a wound.

We obtain passive hyperemia of an infected area by lowering the limb, and using elastic bandages (Bier) or by cupping (Klapp). Active hyperemia is obtained by heat (linseed poultices, electric pads, hot-water bags, heaters, natural sunlight, artificial sunlight, warm air, electric light baths). I hesitate to employ Bier's hyperemia in acute suppuration. In my opinion it should be used only when the infected area has been previously treated surgically and when the patient can be constantly watched. The congestion should be induced cautiously with thin rubber bandages, it should not cause pain, and it should not be induced for more than twenty hours a day.

Cupping (Figs. 296 and 297) has the advantage of combining with hyperemia the removal of the suppurative material. It is often used in circumscribed suppurations (furuncles, mammary abscesses, etc.).

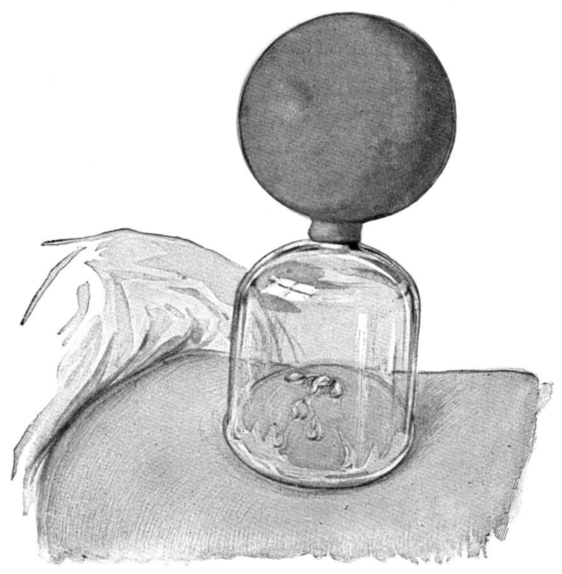

Fig. 296. Cupping-glass with rubber bulb (Klapp).

When the infection has been checked and the wound has begun to heal by granulation, it may occasionally be treated to advantage by the open method. The healing area should be exposed to sunlight and a freely cir-

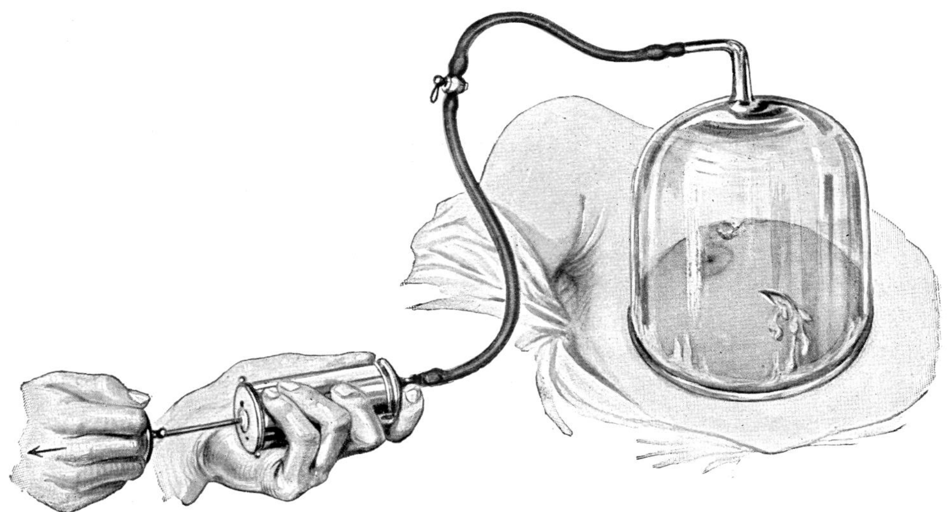

Fig. 297. Suction-bell with pump (Klapp).

culating current of air. The wound should be covered with a layer of gauze fastened around its edges so as to protect it from flies and dust (Fig. 298). Its contact with the wound is prevented by using small rolls, cellucotton rings, or a wire frame. A basin can be placed under the part to catch any tissue discharge. Often a sluggish, odorous wound will lose its odor as soon as the open method of treatment is begun. The method arose from the needs of war and its use has been rather limited in times of peace.

A postoperative infection which fortunately is most rare today is **tetanus.** Muscle spasms, especially of the masseter muscle and the smaller muscles around the mouth, often indicate the onset of this dreaded disease, which demands immediate and strenuous treatment. Catgut stands foremost as the conveyor of this infection during an operation. This is especially true when the non-boilable type of gut is used. If the infection has not obviously

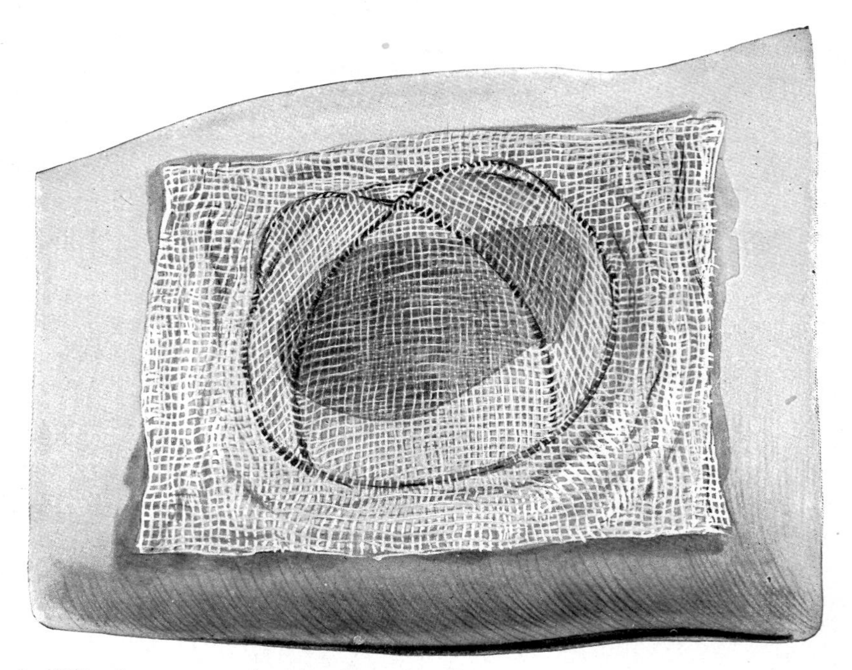

FIG. 298. Wire frame covered with gauze which is fastened to the skin for protection in the open method of wound management.

arisen from another source the supply of catgut should be immediately investigated and a new one used until the old gut has been proved to be uncontaminated. Tetanus may also develop from the penetration into the body of the tetanus bacillus during some previous injury. It may remain quiescent for years (quiescent tetanus infection). As a prophylactic measure 1500 units of antitetanic serum should be injected subcutaneously before a surgical operation in any case where there is any suspicion of latent infection.

CHAPTER IV

THE CONTROL OF HEMORRHAGE

A. ARREST OF BLEEDING

The control of hemorrhage and careful hemostasis are among the most important problems in surgery, whether the hemorrhage is the result of operation, injury, or erosion of a blood vessel during the course of an infection. The prevention and control of hemorrhage is important for several reasons.

A loss of blood exceeding a certain limit is fatal. In healthy adults from 2.5 to 3 liters (2500 to 3000 cc.) is approximately the fatal quantity; this represents about half the total quantity of blood in the individual. The loss of one-fourth of a liter (250 cc.) of blood is usually fatal in a one year old child; while a new born infant may die after losing but relatively few cubic centimeters. Any loss of blood, regardless of the quantity, is deleterious to the patient, the damage being in direct proportion to the quantity of blood lost. The operative field should be carefully examined after every operation and any bleeding should be checked before closing the wound. In this connection one should again emphasize the necessity of thorough anatomical training. A perfectly dry wound is the best insurance against postoperative hemorrhage and hematoma, and one of the most important factors in primary wound healing. Every surgeon should make it a rule never to close a wound, unless it is dry.

The arrest of hemorrhage is either permanent or temporary. The permanent arrest of hemorrhage is accomplished by ligation, by clamping the bleeding vessels with hemostats that are left in place, by tamponing, or by ligating the main vessel at a point of election. The temporary arrest of hemorrhage is accomplished by manual compression of the bleeding vessel at the place of injury, by grasping the bleeding vessel with a hemostat, by manual compression of the main vessel, or by constricting the entire circulation of a portion of the body according to the method of v. Esmarch.

Permanent and dependable hemostasis can only be obtained by ligating the bleeding vessel at the place of injury. All other procedures are inadequate for permanent control.

When operating, the larger visible blood vessels should be ligated before they are divided, so that hemorrhage is minimized. In this way, major operations can be performed with almost no loss of blood. The procedure is as follows: A curved director with handle is passed under the vessel to be incised (we should have on hand a slightly curved and a sharply curved director). With a Deschamp's aneurism needle (Fig. 299), a ligature is passed on the director under the vessel and the latter is ligated at two points in such a manner that the section of the vessel lying between two ligatures is not too short. The vessel is divided between the two ligatures. Instead of ligating the vessel before dividing it, two hemostats may be used and the vessel divided between them (Fig. 300), or when excising a piece of tissue, the vessel on the piece to be excised may be clamped with a hemostat while a ligature is tied on that portion of the vessel which remains.

The first procedure has the great advantage of leaving a clear field of operation, while at the same time the one procedure permanently controls bleeding.

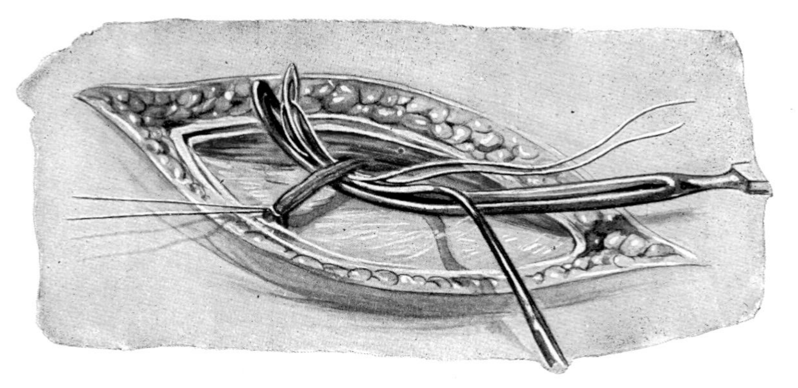

FIG. 299. Double ligature of a blood vessel before it is divided.

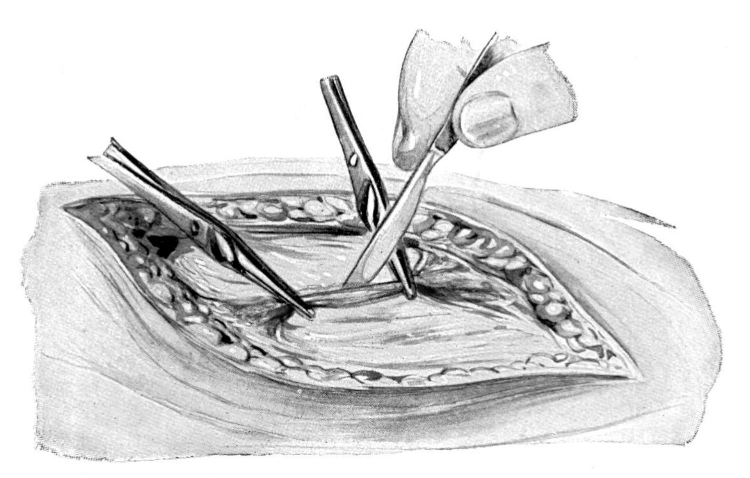

FIG. 300. Dividing a blood vessel between two hemostats.

Mass ligation is done by the same procedure as the ligation of larger vessels. It is practicable when dealing with a large number of very small vessels in a mesentery or a pedicle. Were these to be dissected out, and individually ligated, it would entail an excessive loss of time. In using this method the curved director should be passed so as to include relatively small amounts of tissue and these are doubly ligated or clamped with hemostats so that the tissue may be divided between (Fig. 301). The ligatures should be drawn very tight in the case of slippery tissues, such as the omentum, in order to prevent their slipping off.

Frequently, in operating, the incision is directed across small vessels, which course deep in the tissues, and are so concealed that they are not seen before being incised. Considerable time may be spent in trying to grasp the retracted ends, or the first evidence of injury may be intermediate hemorrhage. If in dividing tissue a sudden severe hemorrhage occurs, the reflex movement of placing the finger over the source of bleeding usually prevents extensive hemorrhage, just as it is used in checking the bleeding of a traumatic wound. This temporary measure must be followed by one which will permanently prevent hemorrhage. Apart from the consideration of sudden severe hemorrhage, any bleeding point arising in the course of an operation should be immediately seized with a hemostat, preferably across the direction of the vessel, with as little surrounding tissue as possible (Fig. 307). I prefer for this the Pean style of hemostat with a plain tip (Fig. 302), while I use

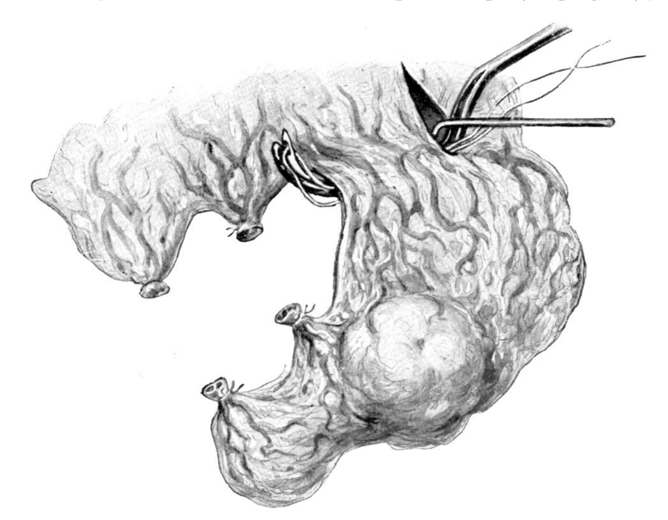

FIG. 301. Ligation en masse of mesenteric vessels; in this illustration, the ligation of the greater omentum.

Kocher's hemostats with toothed tips to grasp vessels in particularly firm tissue (Fig. 303). The Billroth clamp which is especially long is used for grasping deep-lying vessels (Fig. 304). In the United States, the Rochester-Pean hemostat, in both the straight and curved types, is extensively used (Fig. 305).

When the number of hemostats in the wound interferes with the access to, or the view of the field of operation, they should be replaced by ligatures of catgut. It is better technic, as a rule, to ligate as one proceeds. In exceptional instances, or when dealing with large arteries, fine silk thread is to be preferred for ligatures. It is a matter of choice whether the operator or the assistant does the tying and the cutting of ligatures. In my clinic the operator does the tying, the first assistant handles the hemostats, and the second assistant cuts the ligatures. Each hemostat after removal is thrown into an instrument basin and is not used again until it is resterilized (See III. B: "The Asepsis of the Operation").

In ligating vessels caught with a hemostat the surgeon receives the outstretched ligature from the instrument nurse. This he places with both hands near the point of the hemostat. The assistant throws the handle of the hemostat over the ligature and presses its point upward by depressing the handle. The surgeon ties the first knot, being careful that the loop does not include the tip of the hemostat, but only the tissue which is caught by it. The first assistant removes the hemostat, while the surgeon holds the ends of the

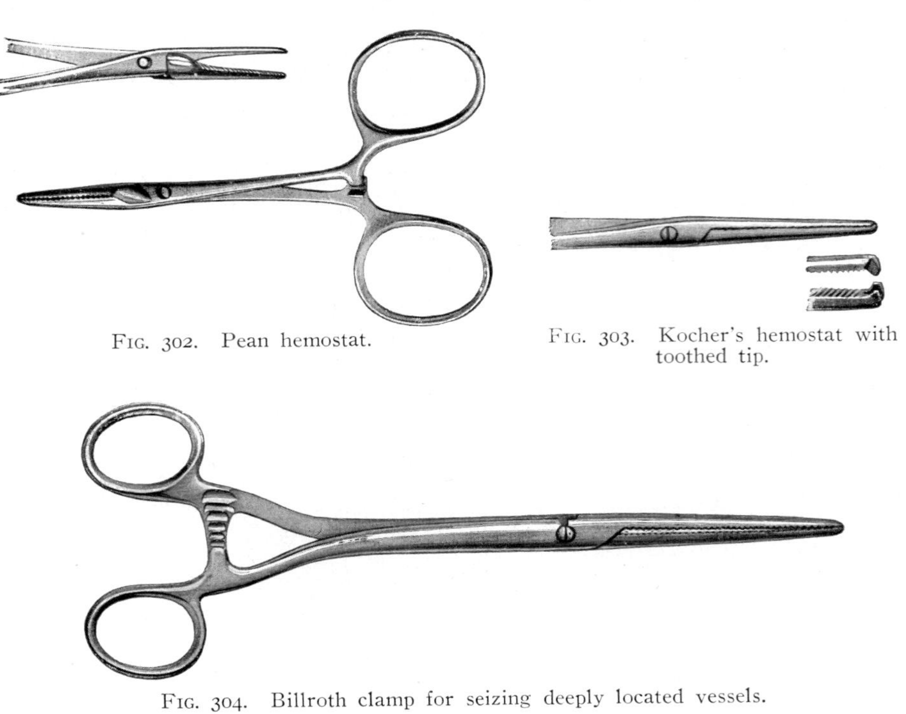

Fig. 302. Pean hemostat.

Fig. 303. Kocher's hemostat with toothed tip.

Fig. 304. Billroth clamp for seizing deeply located vessels.

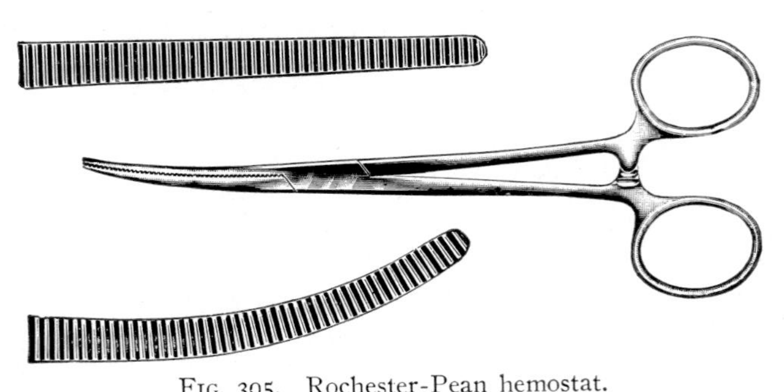

Fig. 305. Rochester-Pean hemostat.

ligature taut (Fig. 307). A second knot is placed over the first, and the second or third assistant cuts the ligature above the knot. Where two or more hemostats have been placed close together, the vessels may be ligated with one ligature (Fig. 308); the hemostats are separated at a large angle, which brings the tips together, thus facilitating the tying of the ligature.

The ligation of vessels and the removal of hemostats should begin at the upper left corner of the wound and follow clockwise along the upper wound margin (Fig. 306). As the ligatures are applied the handle of the hemostat is passed upward out of the wound and toward the opposite wound margin. If this order is followed, ligatures can be placed rapidly, almost automatically, and without a word being spoken. When many ties are to be placed, a "ligature-nut" (Figs. 309 and 310) is a convenience. Time and material are saved in this way and the asepsis is not endangered by passing the ligatures from hand to hand. This simple method of tying suffices for large vessels as well, for example, the femoral artery. All other measures recommended for the increase of safety, such as tying a loop in the end of

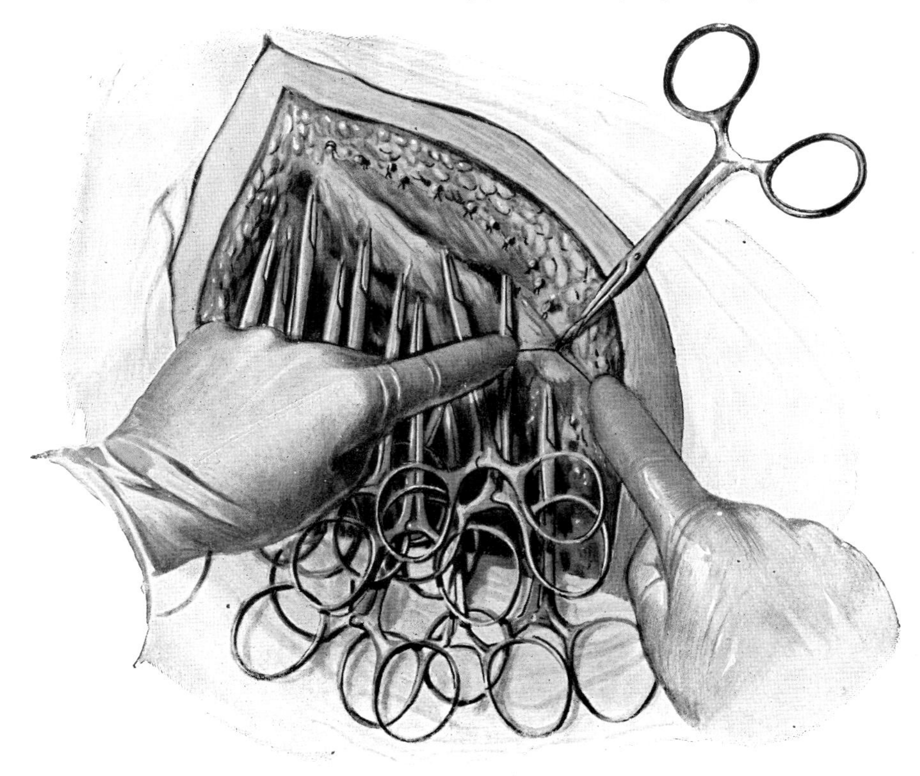

FIG. 306. Tying vessels after they have been clamped with hemostats. The tying starts generally in the upper left corner of the wound and advances clockwise.

a divided vessel, or doubling back the ligated end are artificial and unnecessary.

Every vessel which has been caught by a hemostat should be ligated. There is no exception to this rule. It is a bad practice, resulting in hematomata and secondary hemorrhage, to remove the hemostats after a short time, and to regrasp and ligate only those vessels in which bleeding recurs. The same results occur after the popular method of twisting the hemostat (Fig. 311), in which the vessel is closed by turning the hemostat several times on its long axis. All other substitutes for ligation, such as crushing, and at the same time injuring, the tissue by means of an angiotribe or the popular Blunk clamp, are not reliable. Their use is only justifiable when, due to urgent danger, the operation must be terminated as rapidly as possible.

When the tissue is so firm and dense that it is impossible to separate enough of it with the tip of the hemostat to ligate without danger of the ligature slipping off, the ligature should be carried through the tissue by means of a needle (Fig. 312). A curved needle is used and the ligature is carried through the tissue close to the tip of the hemostat. The ligature is tied on each side of the point of the hemostat.

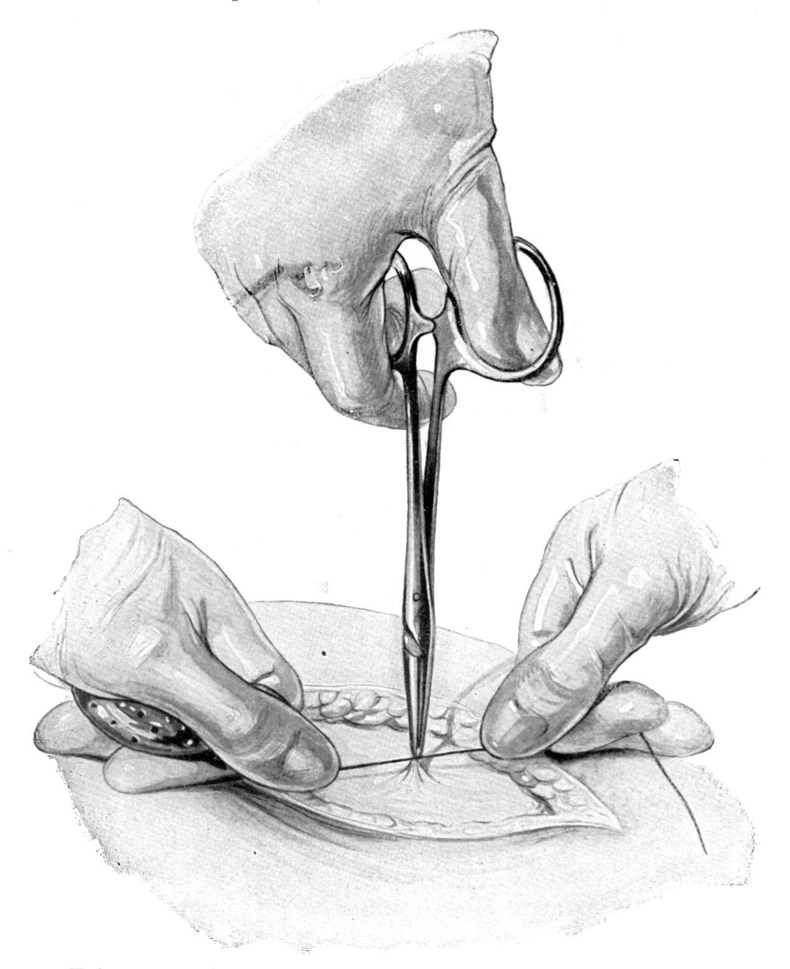

FIG. 307. Tying a vessel under a hemostat. As small an amount of tissue as possible is ligated. The hemostat is raised vertically before it is removed so that the tissue can be easily ligated.

Occasionally it is impossible to ligate a vessel held with a hemostat either by a simple tie or with the help of a needle. It is impossible, for example, to tie the ligature on either side of a hemostat in a very deep and narrow funnel-shaped wound, even with the aid of two tissue forceps to pass and tie the ligature. There are a number of special instruments for such difficult conditions, which from their construction make it possible to carry the thread around the grasped vessel and to hold it in position while the ligature is being tied. The excellent kidney forceps, useful when space permits, is an example. The vessels to be ligated are grasped in a curve and not with the ends of a pointed hemostat; the ligature, passed between the forceps and tissue, slides easily around the tissue along the convexity of the curve of the forceps and does not slip (Fig. 313). Other specially made instruments for similar purposes have not seemed to me so useful (Fig. 314);

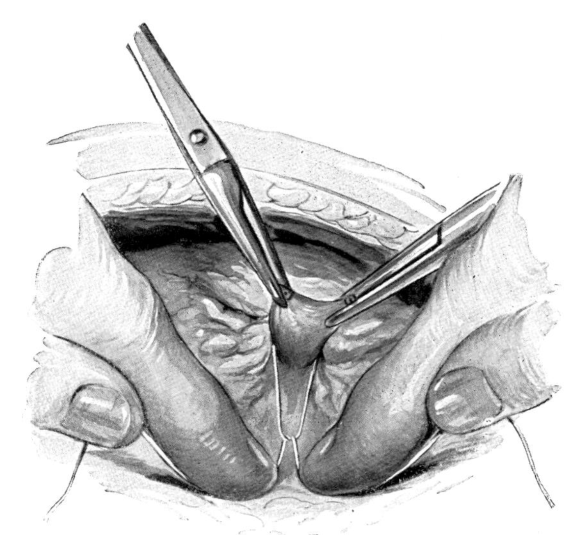

FIG. 308. Tying below two hemostats. The handles of the hemostats are separated so as to approximate the points.

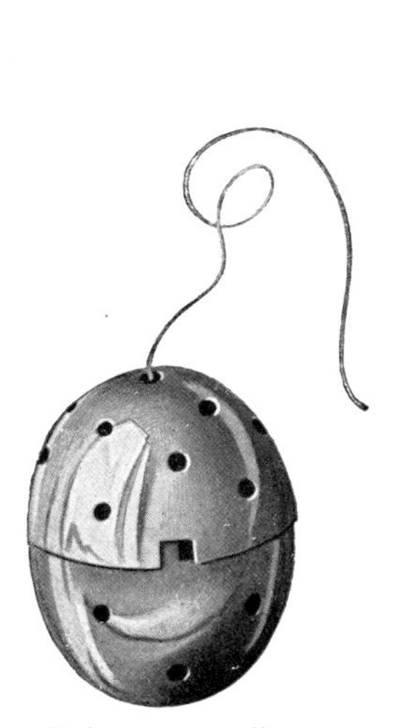

FIG. 309. "Ligature-nut," made of metal. Useful when silk is being used.

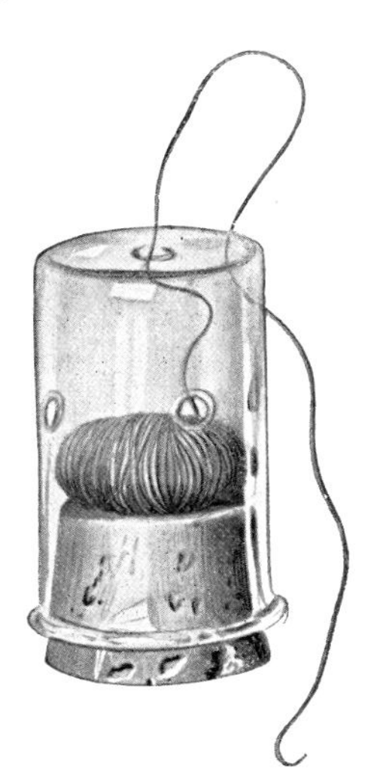

FIG. 310. "Ligature-nut," made of glass with cork stopper.

furthermore they are not at hand when needed because they are used so infrequently. There are other ways of meeting such a difficulty.

If ligation is difficult, a hemostat may be left in place with the handle protruding from the wound for from two to five days, when it may be safely removed because organic closure of the vessel has by that time taken place (Fig. 315). When, for other reasons, the wound is not to be closed primarily, this procedure causes no damage as a rule, and only slight discomfort to the patient. But if the wound is to remain open only because of the presence of one or more hemostats, the benefits of primary closure are sacrificed to this procedure. In any case, this is a measure to be used exceptionally and should never be done unnecessarily because of its ease.

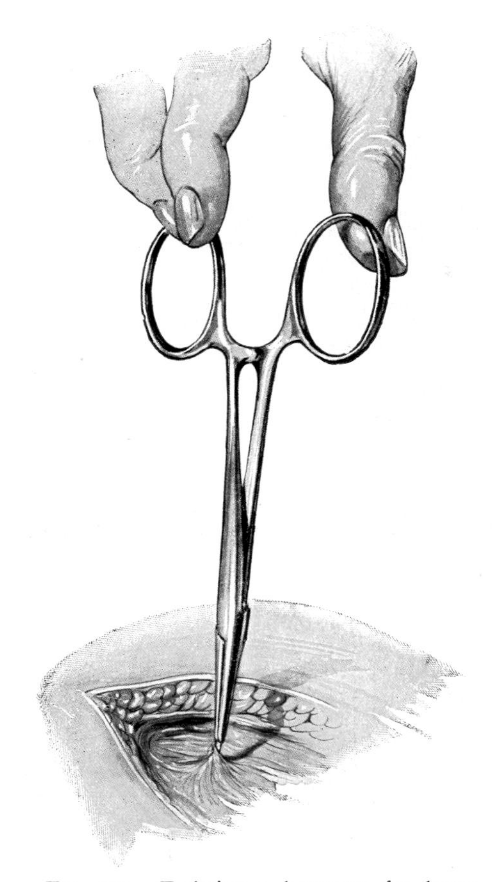

Fig. 311. Twisting a hemostat for hemostasis, permissible only in an emergency.

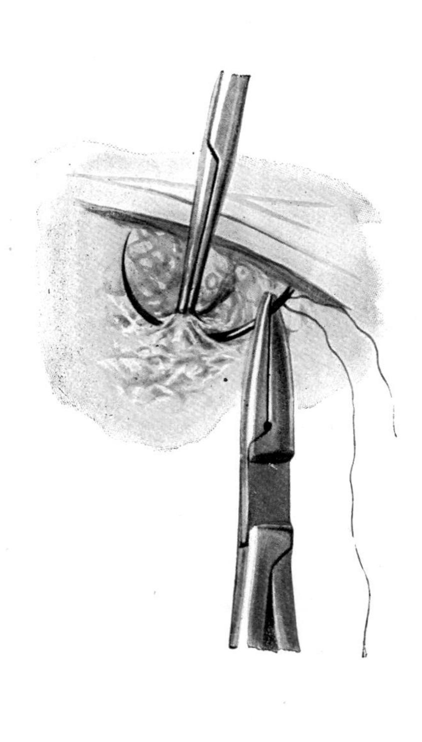

Fig. 312. If the tissue around the clamped vessel is very firm the ligature is carried around it with a needle and then tied on both sides.

Control of hemorrhage by packing (Fig. 316) is a less desirable procedure, that has a possibility of success only in venous or parenchymatous bleeding. A long strip of gauze, if this method is attempted, is impregnated with a chemical styptic, for example: iodoform, adrenalin, 1-1000, horse serum, coagulose, vivokoll, or a 30 percent solution of ferric chloride, is carried with a dressing forceps into the wound and its end pressed firmly against the bleeding area. The gauze is packed layer by layer evenly and firmly until sufficient gauze has been introduced to control the oozing. To retain it and to increase the pressure which the packing exerts, sutures may be used to close the tissues over it. Over the wound, from which the packing protrudes, or which has been sutured over the packing, may be placed a pressure bandage of muslin or rubber, or strips of adhesive plaster. There is a disadvantage to this method also, in that it is impossible to close the wound primarily, and furthermore it may be necessary to open the wound subsequently in order to remove the packing.

In many cases this disadvantage can be overcome by using "buried tampons." These are of two types. Unabsorbable material such as iodoform gauze and sterile gauze, or absorbable material such as a bundle of catgut, animal intestinal wool (Kummel, Jr.), and vivokoll, have been left in the primarily sutured wound, on the assumption that these foreign bodies would become encapsulated or absorbed. However, these materials are not to be recommended except when using unusually small tampons, if even then. Since surgeons have learned to use living tissue as tampons they are finding the foreign materials more and more unsatisfactory. In addition to the purely mechanical pressure which tissue tampons afford, certain of these possess styptic characteristics. The most commonly used living tampons are small pieces of muscle, fascia or fat. They are either free transplants or are adjacent tissue which is turned over the bleeding point on a small pedicle. A free transplant may be taken from the operative wound or from another part of the body, as, for example, when fascia lata is used or muscle from the thigh in operations on the brain. Living tampons are pressed against the bleeding point in the same manner as is gauze, and are secured by catgut or silk sutures (Fig. 317). They are undoubtedly, as far as tamponing is concerned, excellent means of controlling hemorrhage from very soft viscera.

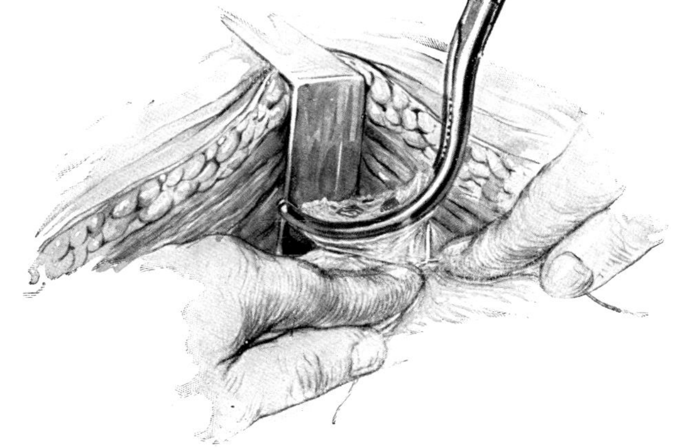

FIG. 313. Ligating a broad pedicle after clamping with a kidney forceps.

The control of bleeding from vessels in bones, where hemostats are obviously of no use, is discussed in Chapter IX: "Operations on the Bones."

To prevent postoperative hematomata in deep wounds, it is important that the wound be closed tightly in layers, even though there has been careful hemostasis. Corresponding layers of the tissues are carefully united to one another with catgut sutures, eliminating dead spaces which may fill with blood and lymph (Fig. 319). In this way also the tissues which were incised at operation are restored to continuity. When a "dead space" results after the excision of tissue, the cavity should not be allowed to remain (Fig. 318), but should be obliterated by mobilizing adjacent tissue (see 1: "The General Principles of Operative Technic").

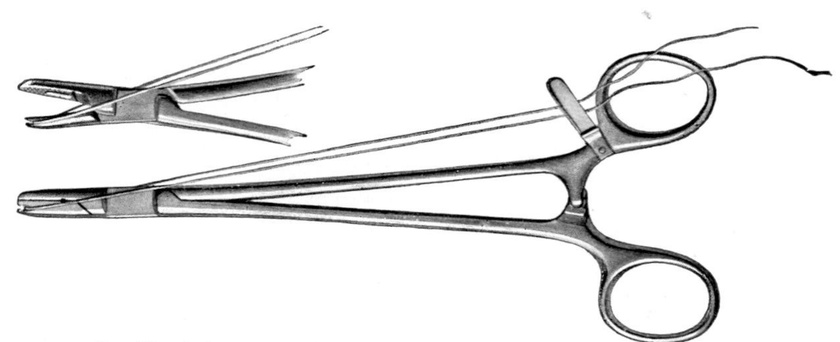

Fig. 314. Combined hemostat and ligature carrier. The hemostat carries the ligature, fastened in a small notch near the point and held taut by the attachment on the handle. As the knot is tied the ligature slips over the tissue grasped by the hemostat and out of the notch.

The danger of hematomata and serum collections is greatest, in spite of careful hemostasis, in the subcutaneous connective tissue. The tissue pressure here is the least, and the skin offers no resistance over an accumulation of fluid. I use large tension sutures to prevent postoperative hematomata in

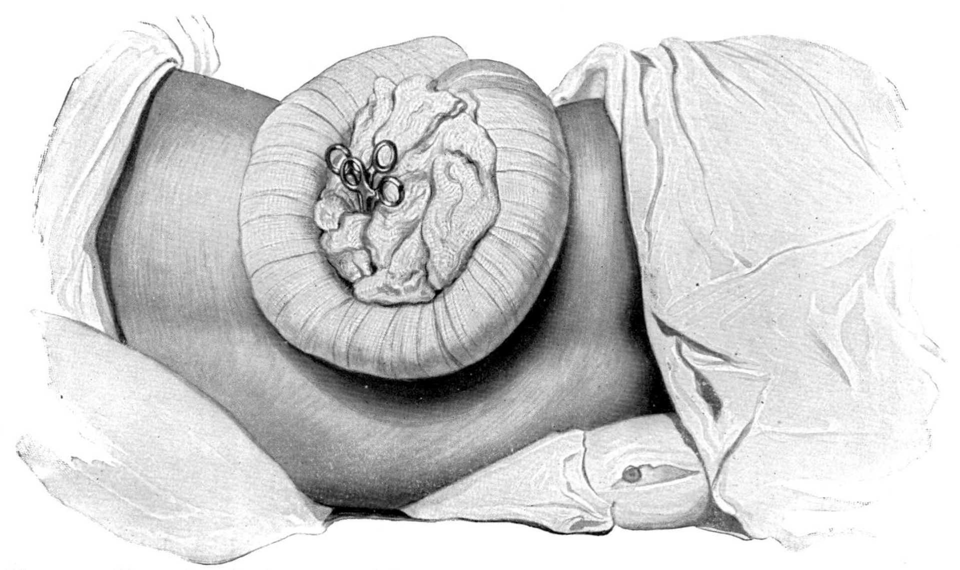

Fig. 315. Protection for hemostats left in the wound, because of inability to ligate the vessels properly. This is a ring fastened to the skin with mastic.

the subcutaneous tissues (Figs. 319 and 320). These have been used routinely for many years, in appendectomies, herniorrhaphies, mastectomies, and wherever postoperative wound collections are apt to occur. They help to support the wound and to obliterate tissue spaces. Before placing the sutures both ends of the wound are grasped by single toothed tenaculi and the wound is drawn lengthwise. Silk sutures of medium thickness on large round cutting edge needles, or on Reverdin needles, are drawn through the wound margins about 4 to 6 cm. apart, the needle entering several centimeters from one margin and coming out on the other side at approximately the same

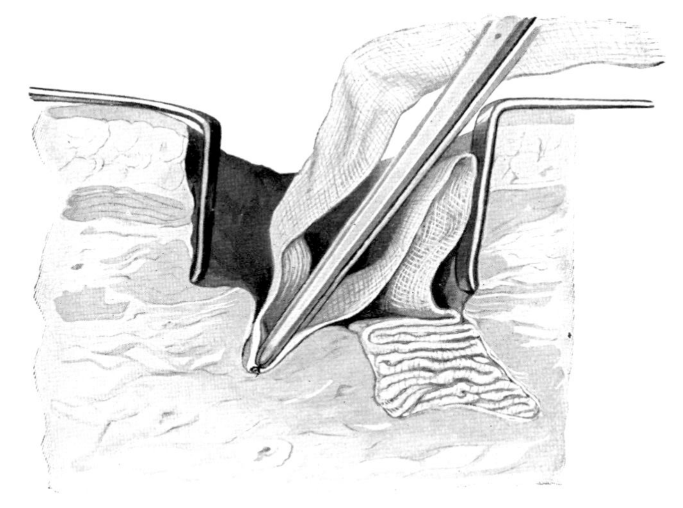

FIG. 316. Gauze packing for arresting hemorrhage in a wound. The layers of gauze should be evenly laid in all parts of the wound and firmly compressed.

distance. These sutures penetrate the whole thickness of the subcutaneous fatty tissue, and catch in the depth of the wound the fascia or even the deeper tissues, so that they can not be seen in the wound. The tension sutures are not tied at once. The ends are held with hemostats. After the

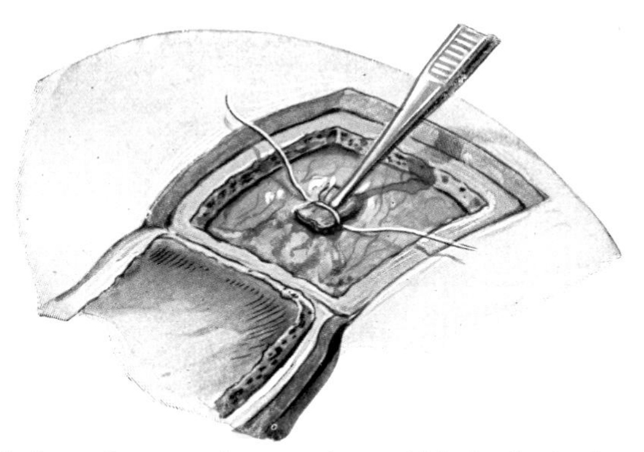

FIG. 317. Hemostasis by a free muscle transplant which is firmly fastened to the bleeding point.

entire wound, including the skin, is closed in the usual way, the deep tension sutures are tied firmly over a gauze roll (Figs. 319, 320 and 321). These sutures are removed in my clinic at the same time that the skin sutures are removed, although some surgeons permit them to remain for a longer period. With the use of tension sutures hematomata in all parts of the wound are less likely to form. Wire sutures and wire plate sutures which are used for closing wounds under excessive tension also prevent to a considerable degree the formation of serum collections and hematomata.

The procedure seems to me to be better than the extensive, expensive compression bandage which so easily becomes loosened, or, the use of heavy sand bags over the wound, which cause the patient discomfort and pain. If inadvertently the sand bags should come in contact with secretion from the wound, they form an excellent harbor for bacteria. When sand bags are used care should be taken to see that they are not too full, that no sand can escape from them, that they cover the wound fully, and that they do not lie on as rigid blocks.

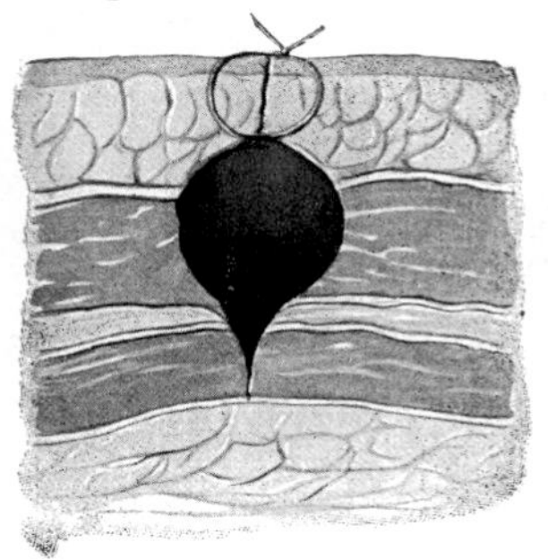

FIG. 318. Postoperative fluid collection in a wound, which was not sutured in layers, as it should have been.

Local styptics are of little use in severe hemorrhage, but are occasionally useful in slow venous hemorrhage or parenchymatous oozing. Those most commonly used are adrenalin, 1 to 1000, a 30 percent solution of ferric chloride, hydrogen peroxide, normal saline solution, heated to 50° C., the cautery, vivokoll, coagulen, stypticin, etc. There is no question but that every hemorrhage must be checked. Liquor ferri sesquichloride in a 30 percent solution has given us the best results. I have used it for many years in a large number of aseptic operations, such as goiter and hernia, and never found it injurious or detrimental to primary healing.

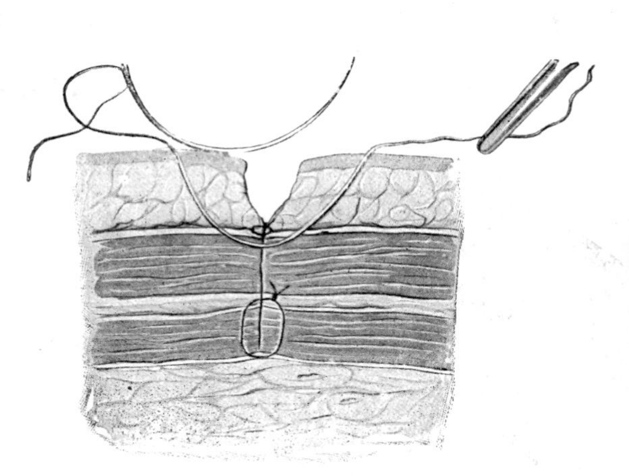

FIG. 319. Wound closure by layers and deep tension suture.

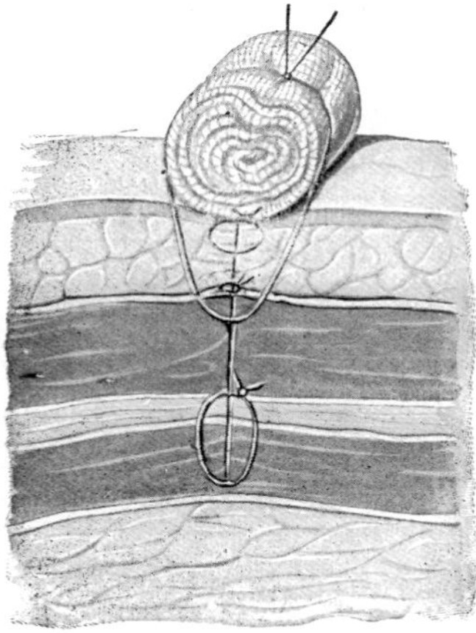

FIG. 320. Wound closure by layers and deep tension suture knotted over a roll of gauze.

Besides the local styptics, there are preparations for injection into the blood stream for the control of bleeding. They are supposed to be very effective in patients with hemorrhagic tendencies, as in hemophilia or jaundice, and they are used not only preventively, but also after operation. Although a variety of substances have been recommended for intravenous use in hemorrhage, especially if this is associated with a hemorrhagic diathesis, very few, if any of these are effectual in actual practices. Calcium salts have been used by mouth or by rectum as well as intravenously. Since the extent of calcium absorption from the bowel is not definitely known, the salt should be used intravenously, if at all. Five cc. of a 10 percent solution of calcium chloride can be given daily. Five cc. of normal horse serum has also been very

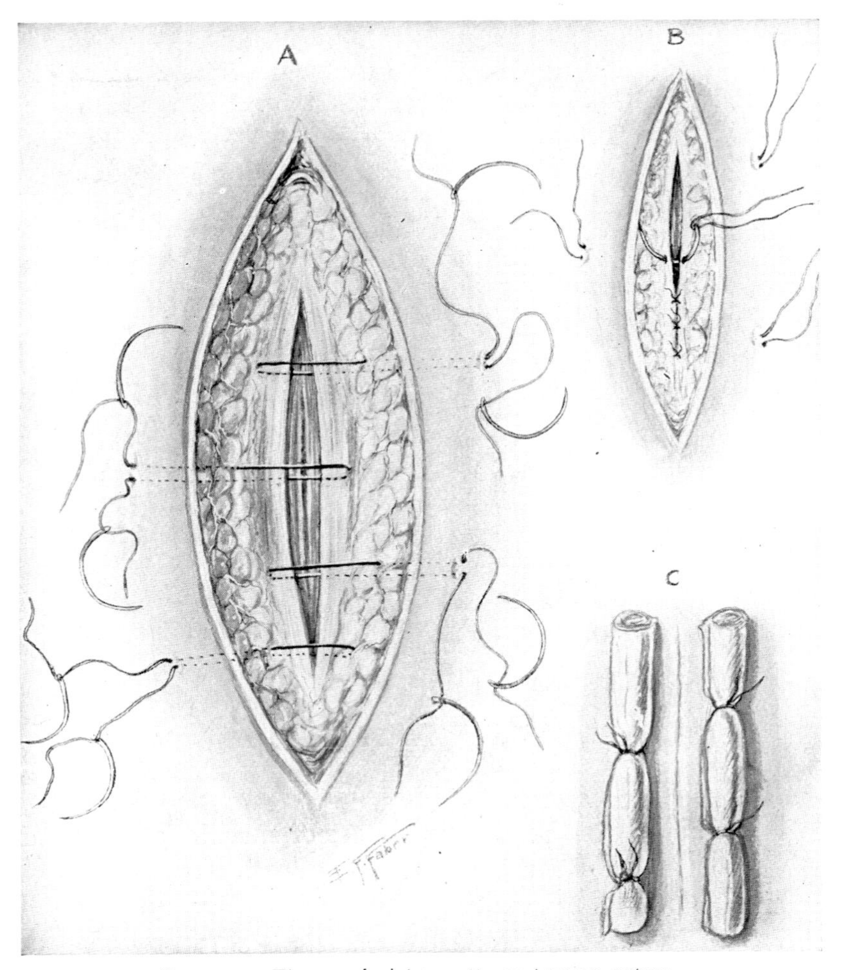

FIG. 321. Figure of eight mattress tension suture.

widely used, but here again the likelihood of any definite results are open to serious question.

The Spanish preparation, Nateina, for controlling hemorrhage in hemophilia is of great value. Its use has been discussed in a previous chapter. There is one reliable measure for rapidly checking repeated bleeding in patients threatened with extensive hemorrhage. This method is the transfusion of blood. (See Kirschner; German Surgical Congress, 1924.) When transfusion is used to prevent bleeding it may be done on the day preceding the operation or during the operation. I give, as a rule, 500 cc. of blood for this purpose. The transfused blood supplies the patient with those components of the blood which are necessary for coagulation. It is the best means of combating the sequelæ of blood loss from injury or operation.

In my experience rœntgen ray exposure of the spleen has been of no benefit in postoperative hemorrhage, even in the hemorrhagic diathesis. On the other hand it would seem that Seifert's recent suggestion of the prolonged use of irradiation by direct sunlight of the entire body is useful in preventing the hemorrhagic tendency associated with jaundice. Seifert states that in jaundice the bleeding time, which is a function of vessels, is not disturbed, but the coagulation time, which depends on the constituents of the blood, is at fault. The prolonged exclusion of bile from the duodenum results in a depletion of the fat soluble vitamin D, and an associated disturbance in

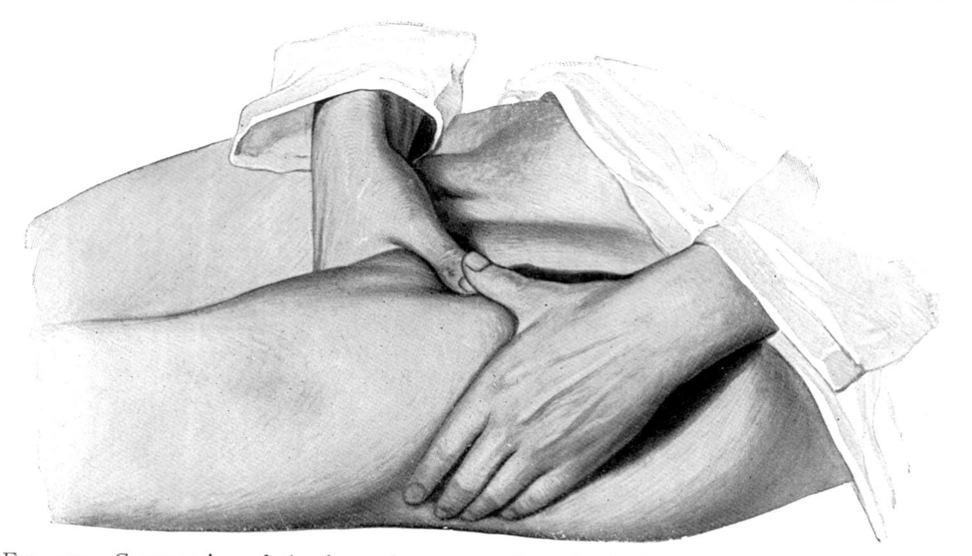

FIG. 322. Compression of the femoral artery against the horizontal ramus of the os pubis.

intermediary calcium metabolism. Just as in rickets where this deficiency of vitamin D can be compensated for by the use of sunlight, so also in obstructive jaundice light therapy seems to play an important role. Seifert reports a reduction in the coagulation time of the blood of jaundiced patients from an average of 12.5 minutes to 3.5 minutes after 10 to 14 days of sunlight therapy.*

The use of adrenalin with the local anæsthetic will reduce the bleeding from smaller vessels during the division of tissues. I frequently use a novocain-adrenalin mixture to prevent oozing even though the operation is done under general anæsthesia. This is especially true in oral and nasal operations, where small quantities of blood may obstruct the view, and subject the patient to the danger of aspiration. It is also used in operations on the head, spine, breast and prostate. A 0.5 to 1 percent novocain-adrenalin solution is used. As a result of the anæsthetic effect of the novocain, the

* Too much emphasis should not be placed on this observation since coincidental therapy, as for instance the intravenous use of glucose, may be an important factor in the reduction of the coagulation time. I.S.R.

general anæsthesia need not be induced early in the operation. Since the vaso-constrictor action of suprarenal extracts is evanescent secondary hemorrhage must be guarded against by careful hemostasis. Every bleeding point must be ligated as well as the visible vessels which do not bleed when incised. My assistant, Borchers, has developed a method for the use of suprarenal extracts previous to operation. He uses 10 minims in 100 cc. of distilled water. More than 200 cc. of such a solution should not be used in any operation. The solution is injected around the operative site and 10 minutes should elapse from the completion of the injection until the incision is made.

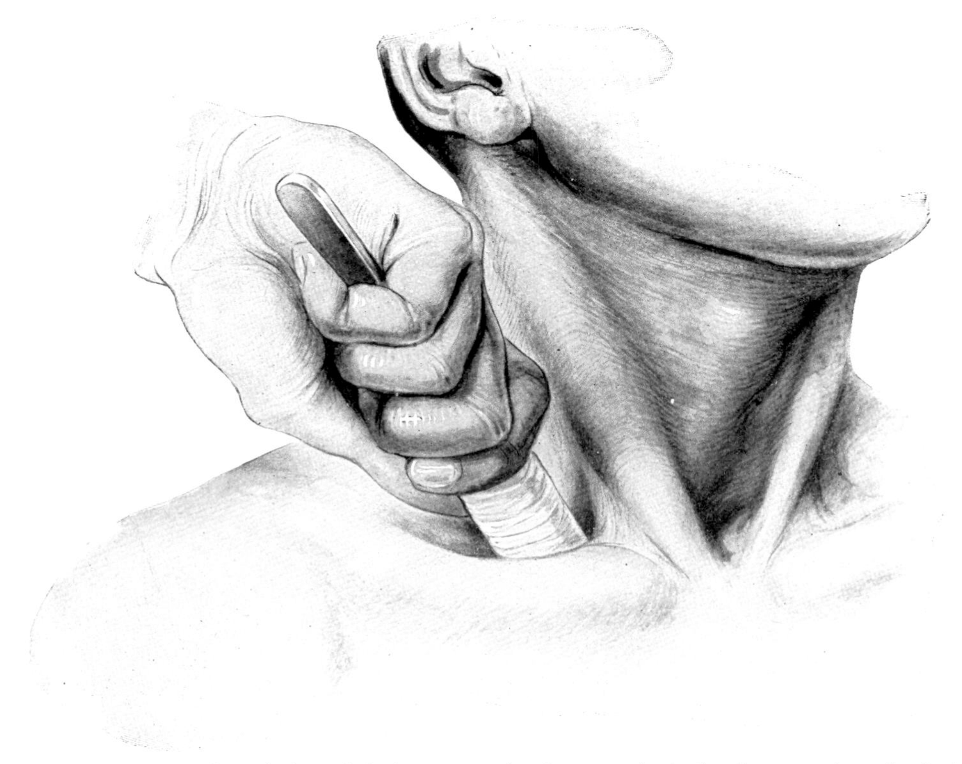

FIG. 323. Compression of the subclavian artery in the supraclavicular fossa against the first rib. A padded handle is used.

Another method for reducing operative hemorrhage is the permanent or temporary ligation of the major vessel supplying the area of operation, at the point of election. We use this preventive method occasionally, as when in operations on the maxilla the external carotid artery is ligated; or when in operations on the tongue the lingual artery is ligated; the hypogastric artery before the extirpation of the rectum; the subclavian artery before exarticulation of the arm at the shoulder; the femoral artery before exarticulation at the hip. Ligation of the main vessels alone as a hemostatic in severe hemorrhage is not always sufficient, because of the very extensive collateral circulation which may exist between adjacent vessels having a separate origin. This is therefore not a permanent hemostatic measure. The same applies to manual compression of large vessels, which is resorted to in sudden, large hemorrhage as the first and quickest way of controlling the bleeding. Compression may be used as a temporary measure when the walls of large arterial trunks are so sclerotic that they might be damaged by a ligature.

To compress the femoral artery an assistant places both hands around the patient's thigh near the inguinal ring and with one thumb over the other presses the pulsating femoral artery firmly against the horizontal ramus of the os pubis (Fig. 322).

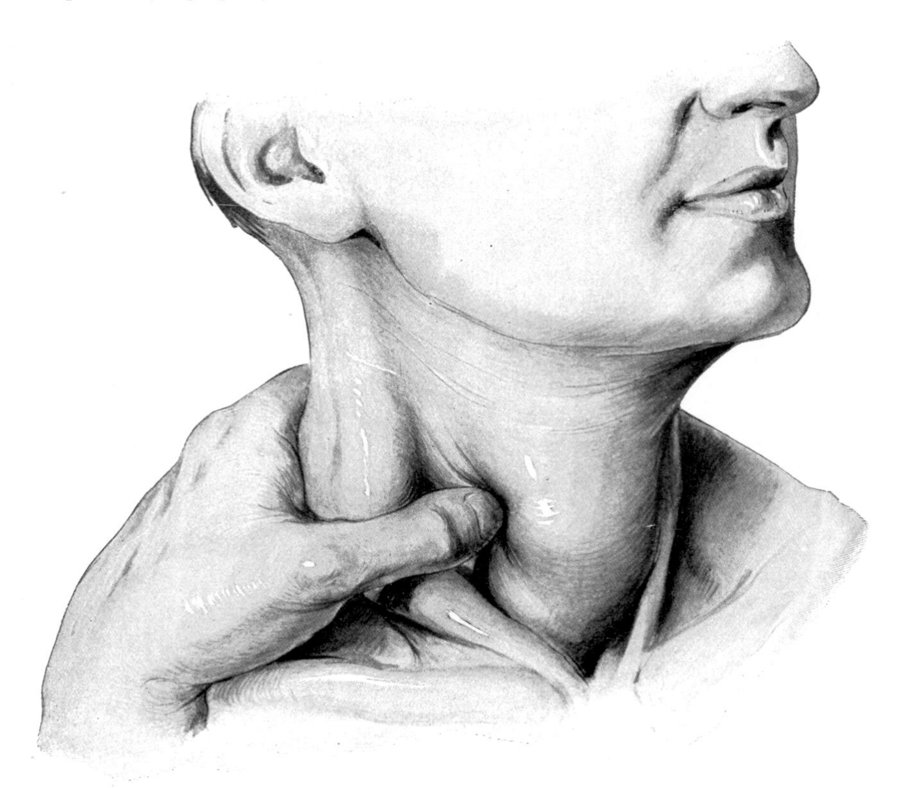

Fig. 324. Compression of the common carotid artery against the carotid tubercle on the transverse process of the sixth cervical vertebra.

Hemorrhage from the forearm or just above the elbow can be controlled by pressure on the main artery, easily recognized by its pulsation, either in the medial bicipital sulcus, against the humerus, or if the bleeding is from a higher point, just over the clavicle against the first rib and lateral to the sternocleidomastoid muscle (Fig. 323). Because the finger soon becomes fatigued, it is better to make pressure on the artery at this point with the handle of an instrument, an elevator or spatula, which has been padded with cotton or gauze. Critical hemorrhages of the head and upper part of the neck can be controlled for a short period of time by pressing the common carotid artery against the carotid tubercle on the transverse process of the sixth cervical vertebra (Fig. 324). If pressure is made on both common carotid arteries, it must be released for short periods of time.

Pads and many of the special types of tourniquets for controlling bleeding have fallen into disuse, as have the many hemostatic contrivances developed during the war, for example, the much reputed Sehrt clamp. These are poor substitutes for the rubber bandage.

The Esmarch rubber bandage is the best method for hemostasis during operations on the extremities. It should be used according to Esmarch's original description. A rubber bandage is tightly wrapped around the extremity from the distal end to the place of operation, thus forcing blood from the limb. Proximal to the operative site a rubber tourniquet is drawn tightly around the extremity and the rubber bandage is then removed (Fig. 325).

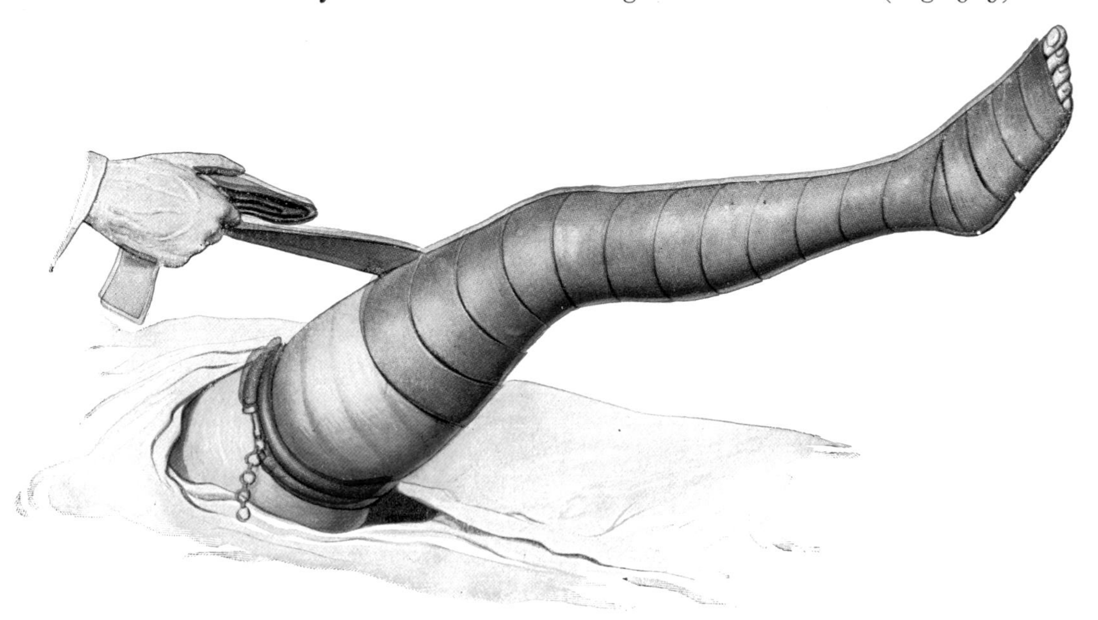

FIG. 325. Classic application of the Esmarch bandage. The limb is spirally wrapped in the proximal direction with a rubber bandage. A tourniquet is then applied at the base and the bandage removed.

A practical procedure, and one that is especially indicated where there is an open wound which prevents the use of the rubber bandage, is simply to elevate the extremity for a few moments and then constrict it above the level of operation with a rubber tourniquet.

In the Esmarch method of hemostasis the tourniquet may be a rubber tube, a rubber bandage, or a pneumatic cuff.

The rubber bandages are usually 6 cm. wide and are made of different thicknesses, according to their intended use: arm or leg, adult or child. The tourniquet tubings also are of different thicknesses from 1.5 cm. for the Momburg hemostatic belt, to 2 or 3 mm. for the fingers and toes.

Perthes has suggested a pneumatic tourniquet consisting of an inflatable cuff surrounded by an adjustable metal band. The cuff is inflated by means of a pump until the circulation is obstructed. The pressure necessary can be read on a manometer (Fig. 326). Kirschner, following Perthes' principle, has introduced a much simpler apparatus for use on the extremities. The apparatus, made in two sizes, consists of a pneumatic cuff covered with cloth, that is held in place by a bandage or by straps. The cuff can be inflated with a bulb or an ordinary bicycle pump until it constricts the circulation. A manometer attached to the side indicates the height of the pressure. When the peripheral pulse is obliterated the valve on the tube is closed, maintaining the pressure. The pressure can be controlled by opening the valve from time to time for further inflation.

The pneumatic cuff with my modifications possesses a great many advantages over the rubber tourniquet. The apparatus can be applied quickly and easily, since it need only be slipped around the extremity. To apply the apparatus it is not necessary to change the position of the limb. It can be applied even if the sterile covers have been put on the extremity. The apparatus can be applied previous to operation and inflated when needed. The constriction of the vessels can be diminished promptly during an operation without endangering the asep-

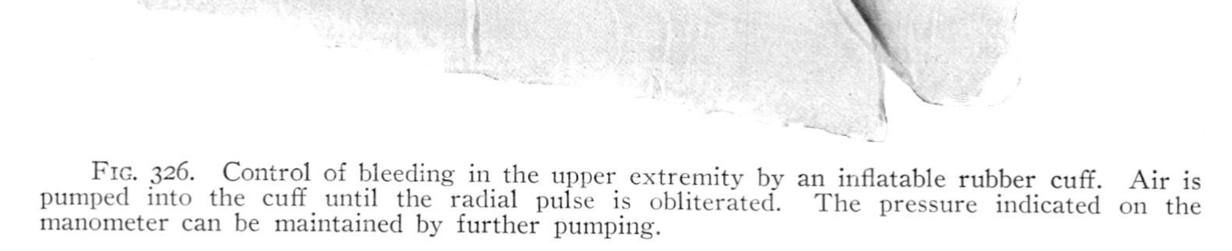

FIG. 326. Control of bleeding in the upper extremity by an inflatable rubber cuff. Air is pumped into the cuff until the radial pulse is obliterated. The pressure indicated on the manometer can be maintained by further pumping.

sis, by the simple procedure of opening the valve; it can then be restored within a few seconds by inflation. The pressure can be carefully regulated so that hemorrhage can be controlled without undue pressure on the nerves or on sclerosed vessels. These advantages can not be obtained with the rubber tourniquet. The only advantage of the tubing is that it takes less space than the pneumatic cuff. I routinely use the pneumatic cuff for controlling hemorrhage except where there is not room to apply it, as in high amputation of the arm or leg, when we use Esmarch's rubber tourniquet.

The technic for the use of the pneumatic cuff is as follows: the cuff, uninflated, is placed around the extremity at the place desired and fastened snugly. The pneumatic cuff is placed (Fig. 328) at the highest possible level of the thigh, around the thickest section of the forearm, just below the elbow joint, or as high as possible on the arm. After opening the valve the cuff is inflated until the arterial pulse disappears at the periphery, or until the blood stops flowing in operations which have already begun. The pressure required for the arm is about 120 mm. Hg. and for the thigh 125 mm. Hg., but the exact pressure must depend on the blood pressure of the patient. The pressure should at no time be carried beyond the height necessary to check the flow of blood, so that the nerves and the walls of the arteries may not be subjected to injury. After the cuff is inflated to the required pressure the

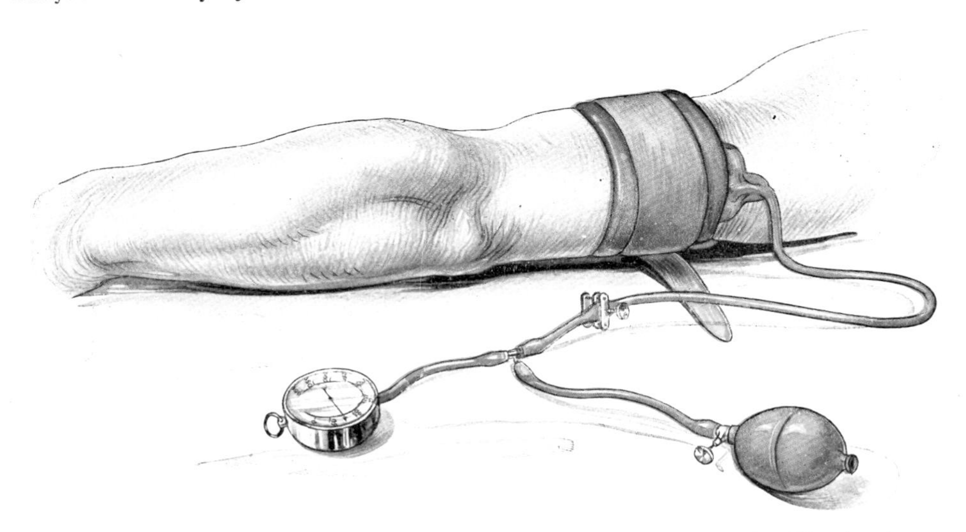

FIG. 327. Pneumatic cuff for control of the blood supply to a limb (Kirschner).

valve is closed. From time to time during the operation, or if a drop in pressure is indicated by beginning hemorrhage, the valve is opened and the cuff is again inflated. It is only necessary to open the valve to remove all constriction from the extremity. This is of great value in testing hemostasis, for example, in an amputation stump, for it is very easy to reapply the constriction by inflation of the cuff. The apparatus is removed after the air is released.

The technic for constricting an extremity with an elastic tourniquet, such as a rubber tube, is as follows: the tube is placed around the side of the extremity on which the large vessels run, one end of the tube is held firmly on the limb with the left hand, the other end is pulled vigorously with the right hand and carried once around the limb (Fig. 329), in such a way that it crosses and fastens the extremity held by the left hand. The first end need no longer be held since it will not become loose, and the tube is again carried around the limb stretching it moderately with both hands. The end of the tube is fastened by hooking, tying, by pushing it under another part of the tubing, by clamping with a hemostat, or by tying the ends together with a cord. Still better is the use of a hard rubber block (Fig. 330) in which the end of the tube is fastened by its own contraction when tension is released, and from which it can be removed by one motion.

In high amputation of the thigh and arm care should be taken that the tourniquet does not slip off the resulting short stump. If the tubing is long enough, it may be carried in a figure-of-eight around the body, that is, around the thorax and under the opposite axilla. The tubing can also be held in place by Wyeth's pins inserted either on the lateral or medial side of the thigh or on both sides. The ends of the pins are protected by a shield or cork. The tubing is placed just proximal to the pin (Fig. 331). The simplest and most dependable way is to apply the tubing and then stitch it securely to the skin (Fig. 332).

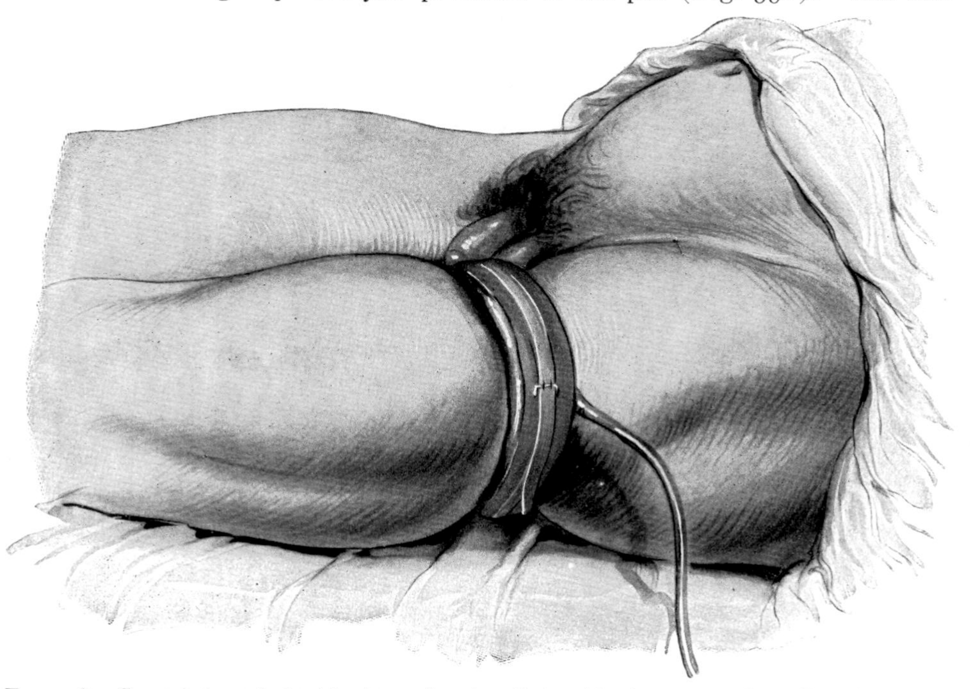

FIG. 328. Constriction of the blood supply of a limb with the pneumatic cuff. The cuff is inflated until the peripheral arterial pulse disappears.

In high amputation of the thigh the tubing may also be carried over a bandage placed on the lateral side of the thigh, and the ends of the bandage tied around the waist. In high amputation of the arm, the tubing is placed over a bandage which is carried around the neck to be tied in the opposite axilla (Fig. 333).

Compressing the abdominal aorta (Momburg) makes possible operations above the groin with insignificant loss of blood, for example, exarticulation of the hip, pelvic operations, obstetrical operations. While temporary constriction of a single limb does no harm to a patient, constriction of the abdominal aorta places a tremendous burden on the patient's circulatory system, which may cause serious, even fatal results. The intestine may be injured by the pressure. Because of these dangers this procedure should be avoided as much as possible, but if used it should be used for very brief periods and with the greatest care.

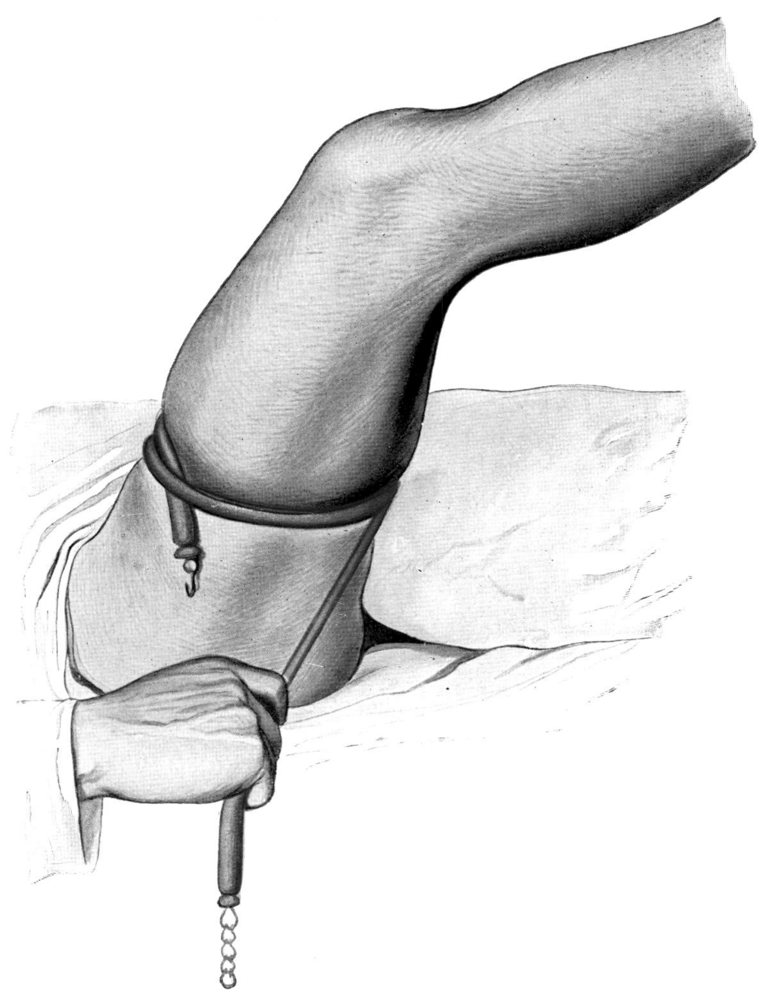

Fig. 329. Method of applying the Esmarch tourniquet. The first end of the tube is fastened by the first turn around the thigh.

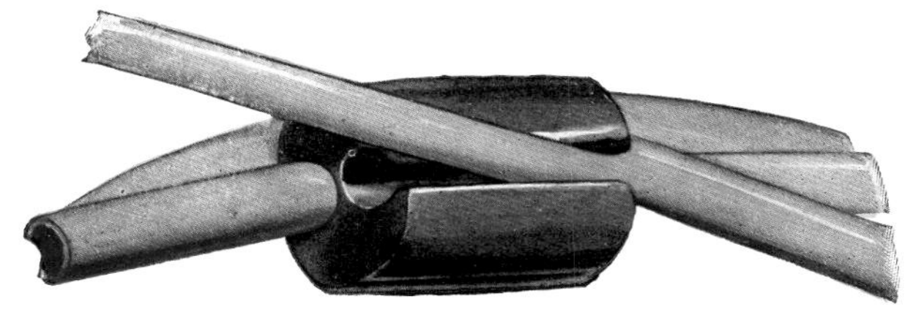

Fig. 330. Hard-rubber block for fastening Esmarch's tourniquet if it is not fastened by the links.

If a rubber tube is used for compression of the aorta, it should be about 1.5 cm. in diameter, at least 1.5 m. long, and made of the best material.

The patient is placed so that we can reach freely under the lumbar region of the vertebral column. The tubing is wrapped over a felt pad around the waist, one turn of the tubing fastening the first end. While an assistant

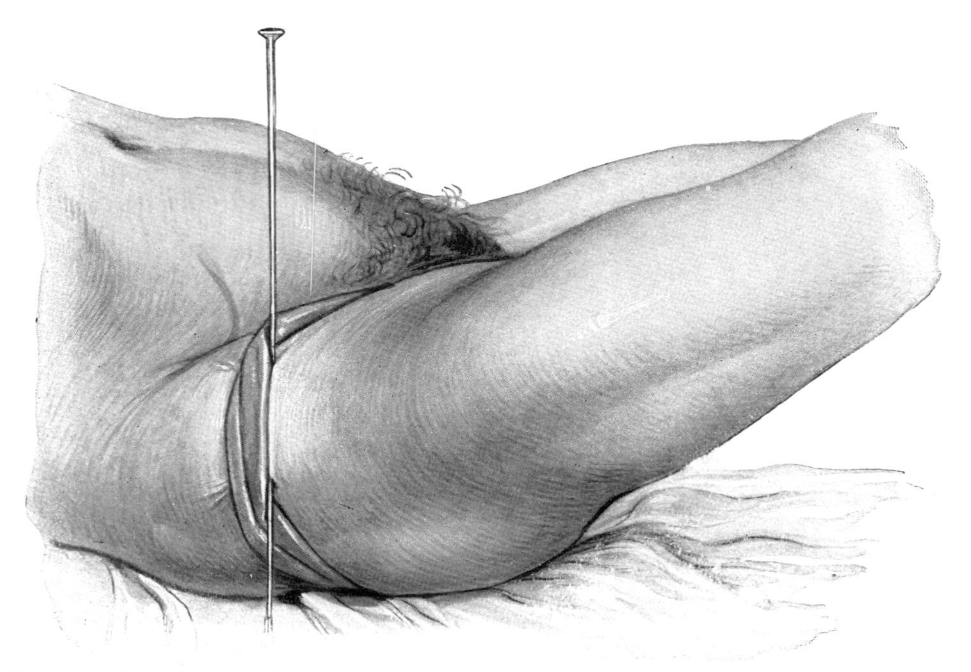

FIG. 331. Skin pin to maintain the position of Esmarch's tourniquet in high amputations of the thigh.

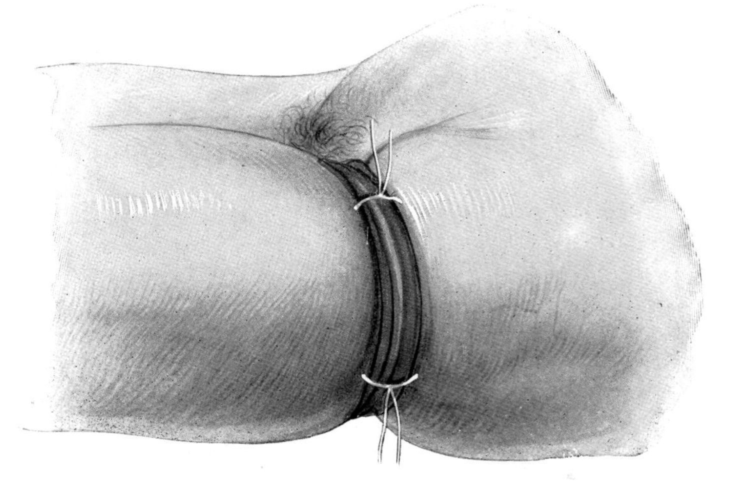

FIG. 332. The use of sutures to maintain the position of Esmarch's tourniquet.

watches the femoral pulse, the tubing is wrapped tightly around the waist. As soon as the pulse can no longer be felt the end of the tubing is fastened. Two to four turns of the tubing are usually sufficient (Fig. 334). Tourniquets are placed on both legs, below the hips and below the knees, if this

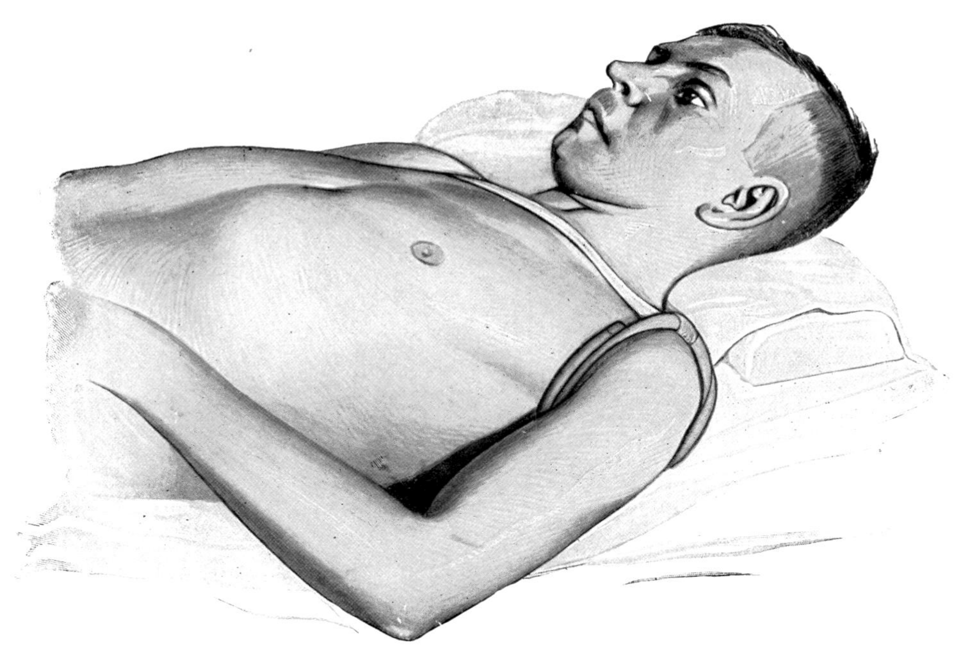

FIG. 333. Maintaining the position of Esmarch's tourniquet with a bandage carried through the opposite axillary space, in an amputation of the upper extremity.

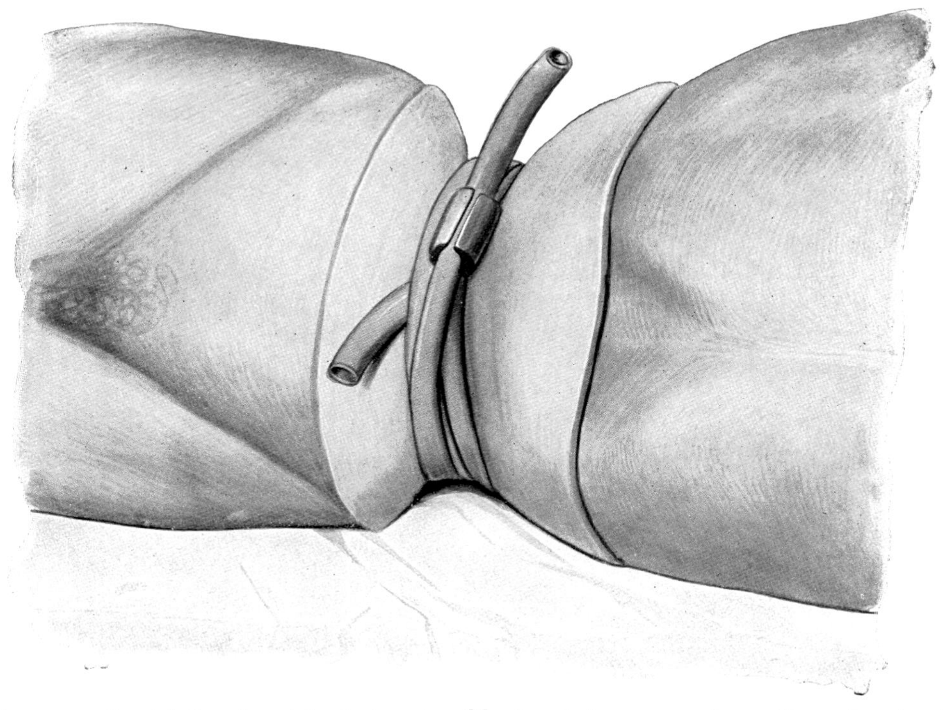

FIG. 334. Constricting the abdominal aorta (Momburg) by means of a rubber tube placed around the waist over a strip of felt.

does not interfere with the operation. After the Momburg belt is removed, the tourniquets are removed one at a time at short intervals, in order to return the blood gradually to the general circulation, and so prevent a sudden over-burdening of the heart. It is better to place these four constrictors before applying the Momburg belt, thus making the effect of aortic constriction less abrupt.

The abdominal aorta may also be compressed by means of a lever, as described by Hans. Aside from being an effective device for aortic compression, it has the added advantage that the degree of pressure can be altered instantly and that the compression need not be maintained unnecessarily throughout the operation. It seems to cause less injury to the intestines. I prefer this method of aortic constriction if one must be used (Fig. 335).

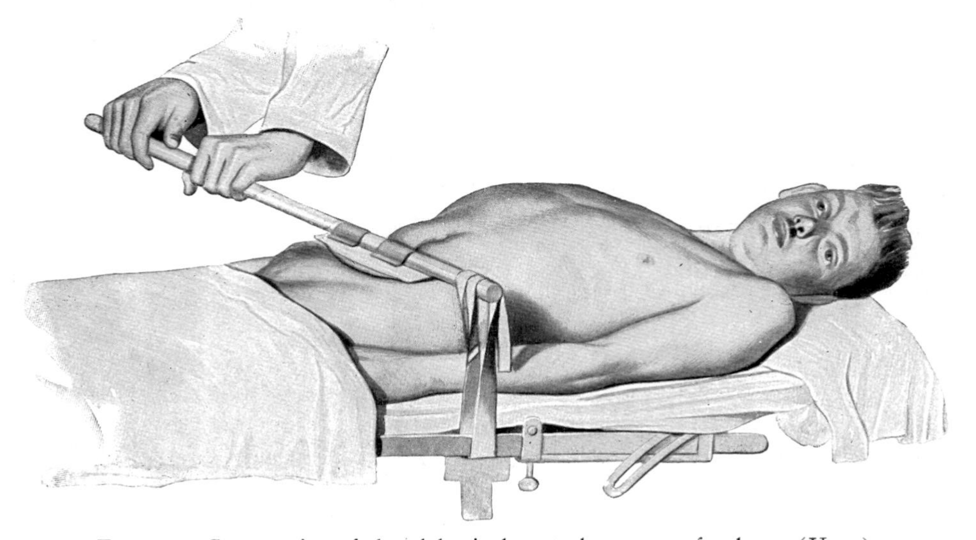

FIG. 335. Compression of the abdominal aorta by means of a lever (Hans).

The end of a strong wooden rod is passed through the loop of a chrome leather belt of suitable length which is fastened to the edge of the operating table, at the level of the patient's waist. The rod is placed across the patient's abdomen over a pad of sponge rubber, or a folded sheet. The free end of the rod acts as a lever which is depressed by an assistant with just enough force to control the bleeding or to obliterate the pulse before the hemorrhage occurs. The assistant may regulate the pressure by shifting a sliding weight on the wooden rod. The contrivance should be tested before the operation, observing the pulse in the femoral artery.

While a rubber tourniquet does not endanger the nerves of the lower limbs, which are well protected by thick muscles, the nerves of the arm may be so injured by pressure that complete or partial paralysis results. Even though the prognosis of such paralysis is favorable, it may cause disability and discomfort for weeks. In spite of the most careful precautions, paralysis can not always be avoided. The following precautionary measures should be observed when constricting the arm (Fig. 336). Never use tubing or a thick rubber bandage, but always a wide soft rubber bandage. The bandage should be wrapped several times around the arm, each layer only partly overlapping the previous one. It should be under just enough tension to obliterate the radial pulse. While the pneumatic cuff is the best method for constriction of the arm, even with this, there may be nerve injury. There is no danger of injuring the nerves in constriction of the muscle-padded forearm; for this reason, it is always preferable to constrict the circulation just below the elbow in operations on the lower forearm or hand.

For severe traumatic hemorrhage from an extremity an Esmarch tourniquet is the best means of controlling the bleeding, because its action is both rapid and sure. The constriction should never last longer than three hours, because of the danger of tissue changes or even gangrene. In view of this danger, the surgeon himself should make it a rule to remove the tourniquet. It is easy to forget to remove the tourniquet after the operation, and this neglect may lead to serious consequences. The patient may still be under the influence of the anæsthetic and unable to express clearly his suffering, or

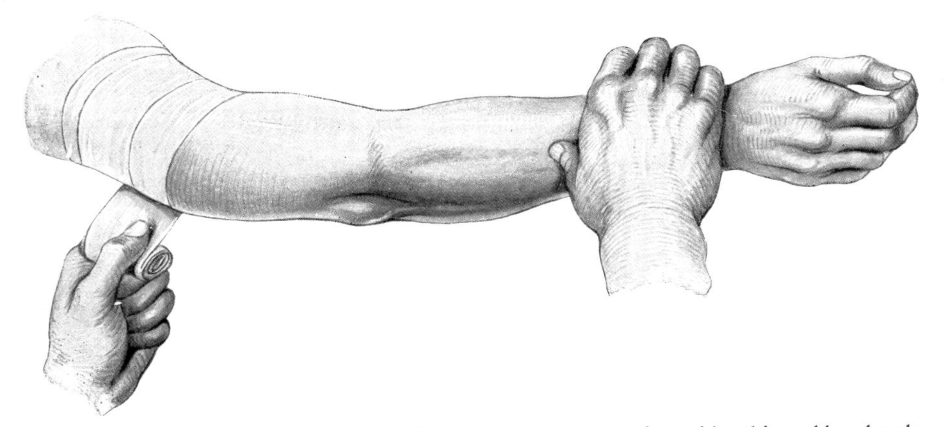

FIG. 336. Local anemia of the forearm (Esmarch) by means of a wide, thin rubber bandage, applied until the radial pulse disappears.

his complaints may be interpreted falsely as "wound pain" and morphine be given.

A reactive hyperemia usually follows the removal of the tourniquet after an operation, which may result in an increase in the escape of blood from the incised vessels and a greater tendency toward hematomata. This danger is even greater because a vessel may be cut during operation but not bleed if the tourniquet is tight, and so not be seen and not ligated. It is a good practice, when there is a possibility that a vessel may have been injured during operation, as in plastic operations on tendons, to remove the tourniquet before closing the wound and to ligate any visible bleeding points.

It should be kept in mind that if an operation is to be performed without a tourniquet, the amount of blood at the site of operation depends to a great extent on its position in relation to the rest of the body. The patient should be placed so that the area of operation is at a higher level than the rest of the body, that there is an incline from it to the heart, and that there are no compressing bands, such as garters, or tight clothing, which prevent a free venous return toward the heart. For operations on the head and neck, the head is usually raised; for operations on the hand and arm, the arm should be raised above the axilla; and for operations on the leg, the leg should be elevated well above the level of the hip. (See Chapter I, C. "Position of the Patient".) These rules are too often not observed.

A method for diminishing the amount of blood lost in operations on the head, neck, and body has been developed by Klapp. He suggested that the extremities be used as reservoirs of blood, a condition just opposite to that produced by the Esmarch bandage, by placing tourniquets around them while they are plethoric. The blood remains in the extremities during the course of the operation but when it is completed the tourniquets are removed and the blood returns to the general circulation. It was hoped that in catastrophes from an anæsthetic the unaffected blood in these reservoirs could be released into the general circulation to dilute that which carried the anæsthetic. In effect this procedure amounts to an autotransfusion. In Klapp's experiments both lower extremities were constricted high in the thigh. The procedure has as yet no definite practical significance. In other experiments along this line an attempt has been made to apply increased air pressure at the site of operation, as well as to subject the entire body to a subatmospheric pressure except at the operative site so that the blood might be drawn away. The complicated apparatus necessary and the danger of air-embolism offer difficulties to the use of such procedures.

B. TREATMENT AFTER HEMORRHAGE

Profuse hemorrhage from operation or injury with resulting acute anemia, and its sequelæ, requires energetic and immediate treatment to save the life of the patient.

1. Principles of Treatment

One must first be sure that the bleeding has actually stopped and that precautions have been taken to prevent its recurrence. If these conditions have not been fulfilled it is important to follow immediately the previously discussed methods for the control of hemorrhage. Only when this task has been accomplished has the management of hemorrhage been started along the proper line.

It is of vital importance in these cases to direct any blood remaining in the patient to the heart and to the medullary centers, which may be attempted by lowering the upper portion of the trunk and the head (Fig. 337) and elevating the lower portion of the trunk and the extremities. This may be further assisted by applying Esmarch bandages to the extremities in order to drive the residual blood in these to more important structures. External heat in the form of hot water bottles, electric pads, or an electric cabinet should be supplied to overcome the subnormal temperature. In an attempt to whip into action the depressed vasomotor system, 1 cc. of a 1:1000 solution of adrenalin may be given intravenously. For existing "cardiac weakness" many of the remedies used for cardiac stimulation (strophantin, digalen, caffein) are recommended for intravenous use. (Though the use of these remedies is widespread their value is indeed questionable. There has been no verification of the belief that digitalis, even intravenously, acts instantaneously, or that it is of use in the heart whose main need is merely more blood. I.S.R.) Ten to 50 cc. of a 20 to 40 percent solution of glucose have been found efficacious in many of these cases. The action of this may be due to the fact that the hypertonic solution increases the blood volume by its osmotic effect.

However, these measures do not strike at the root of the evil. The important point is to refill the empty vascular system with fluid, and if necessary to provide oxygen carriers, in the form of red blood corpuscles. The first can be supplied by the introduction of an isotonic solution, the second, only through a transfusion of blood. It must be remembered, that

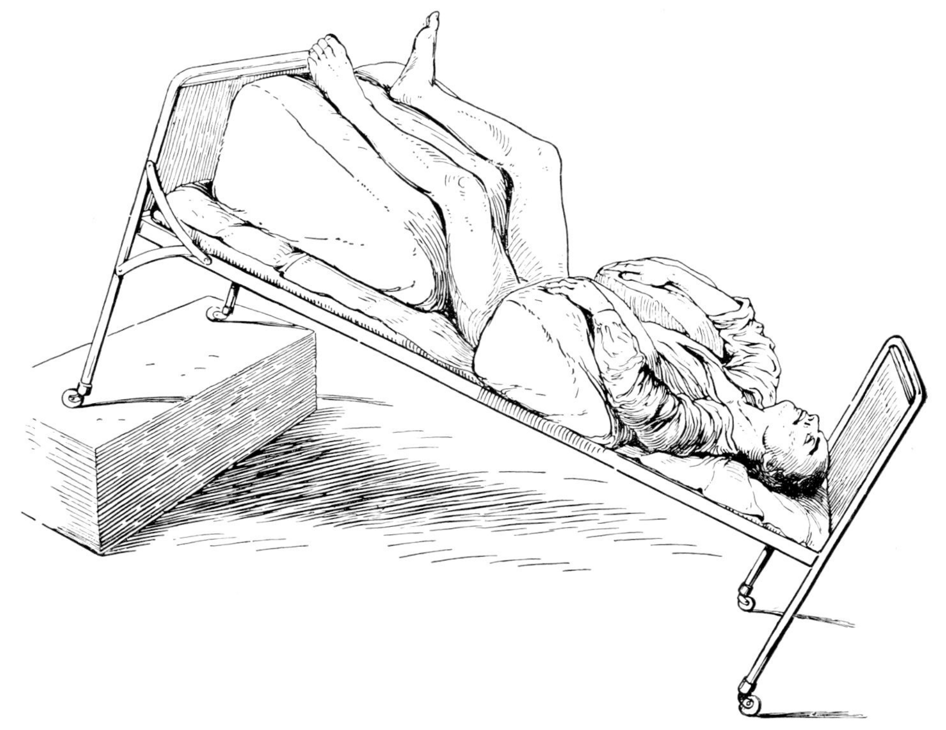

FIG. 337. Position after severe hemorrhage. The limbs are elevated, the head lowered as much as possible, and the foot of the bed is raised on blocks.

animals, which have been exsanguinated to a point incompatible with life, can not be saved by saline injections, but only by blood transfusion.

If patients are able to drink, they may be given hot liquids by mouth, but fluids by mouth can not be relied upon in patients who have had extensive hemorrhage. They may be unconscious and unable to swallow the liquids, they may vomit, or the fluid ingested may remain in the stomach for an indefinite time. For these reasons, the burden of treatment rests upon the rapid introduction of large amounts of fluid into the body by other routes.

The technic of the various procedures for the introduction of fluid will be discussed since there are many other indications for this type of therapy. The body must be provided with fluid, nourishment, blood or medicinal agents, when the introduction and the absorption of these substances can not be carried out in the natural way, in sufficient quantity, with sufficient rapidity, in an unchanged form, or when we fail to obtain cooperation from the patient. The rectal, subcutaneous, intramuscular and intravenous routes are commonly employed.

The rapid introduction of fluids into the body with a syringe is called an injection. When the procedure is prolonged and the fluid is given more slowly by gravity, it is called an infusion.

Regardless of the method of introducing fluid, it must be remembered that an excess quantity is a burden and thus injurious to the body, for this superfluous fluid must be pumped by the heart through the blood vessels, and must be excreted by the kidneys. It is, therefore, improper and injurious to force an arbitrary amount of fluid into the body without considering the needs or the capacity for handling it. Disturbance of the water balance from too much water is as injurious as from too little water. While the body can protect itself against overloading the blood with water introduced rectally or subcutaneously, by reducing absorption and by adequate storing of the water in the body tissues (liver, muscles, and other tissues), it is defenseless in the presence of an overload rapidly given intravenously. For that reason, care must be exercised as to the exact quantity of fluid introduced. The 24 hour urine output and the blood pressure offer assistance in determining the necessary amount. (Hemoglobin estimations, hematocrit readings, and estimation of the serum protein are also helpful. I.S.R.)

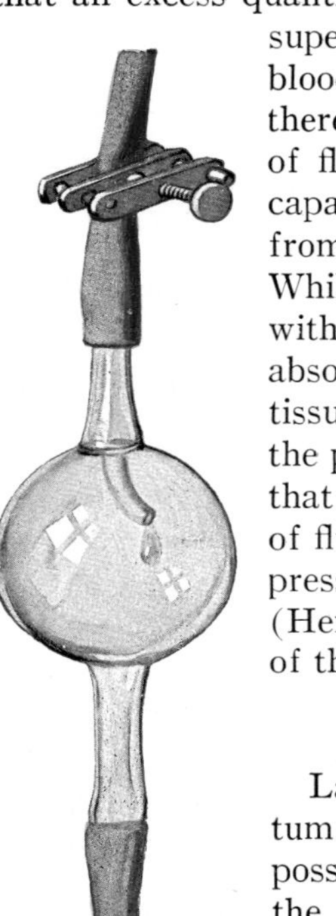

FIG. 338. Drop bulb (Martin) for observing rate of flow. The rate can be controlled by a screw clamp on the rubber tube.

2. THE INTRODUCTION OF FLUIDS BY RECTUM

Large quantities of fluid can be absorbed from the rectum and colon. A preliminary cleansing enema is given if possible. Because large quantities of water introduced into the rectum incite peristalsis, not more than 150 to 200 cc. should be introduced at one time for absorption. To prevent peristalsis it will be found useful to add to the solution a little opium (20 drops of the tincture). A Nelaton catheter is inserted into the rectum and a syringe containing the fluid at body temperature is attached to it. The fluid is then slowly injected into the intestine. Drugs may be introduced by this form of injection. The popular nutrient enemata consisting of milk, eggs, wine, etc., should never be used since the rectum does not absorb albumin and fats, which are the constituents of these enemata. It is also likely that glucose is not absorbed from the large intestine. These substances disappear by decomposition, not by absorption.

When large quantities of fluid are to be given by rectum, the drop method should be used. A soft, thin Nelaton catheter is introduced into the rectum for a distance of about 15 cm., and is connected with an irrigating jar or funnel, placed about 1 meter above the anal orifice. A Martin dropball is inserted in the tubing (Fig. 338), through which the rapidity of the drops can be observed. A regulating tube clamp is placed between the drop-ball and reservoir and adjusted so that a drop falls every 1 to 3 seconds. If fluid accumulates in the drop-ball, the clamp must be adjusted to retard or inter-

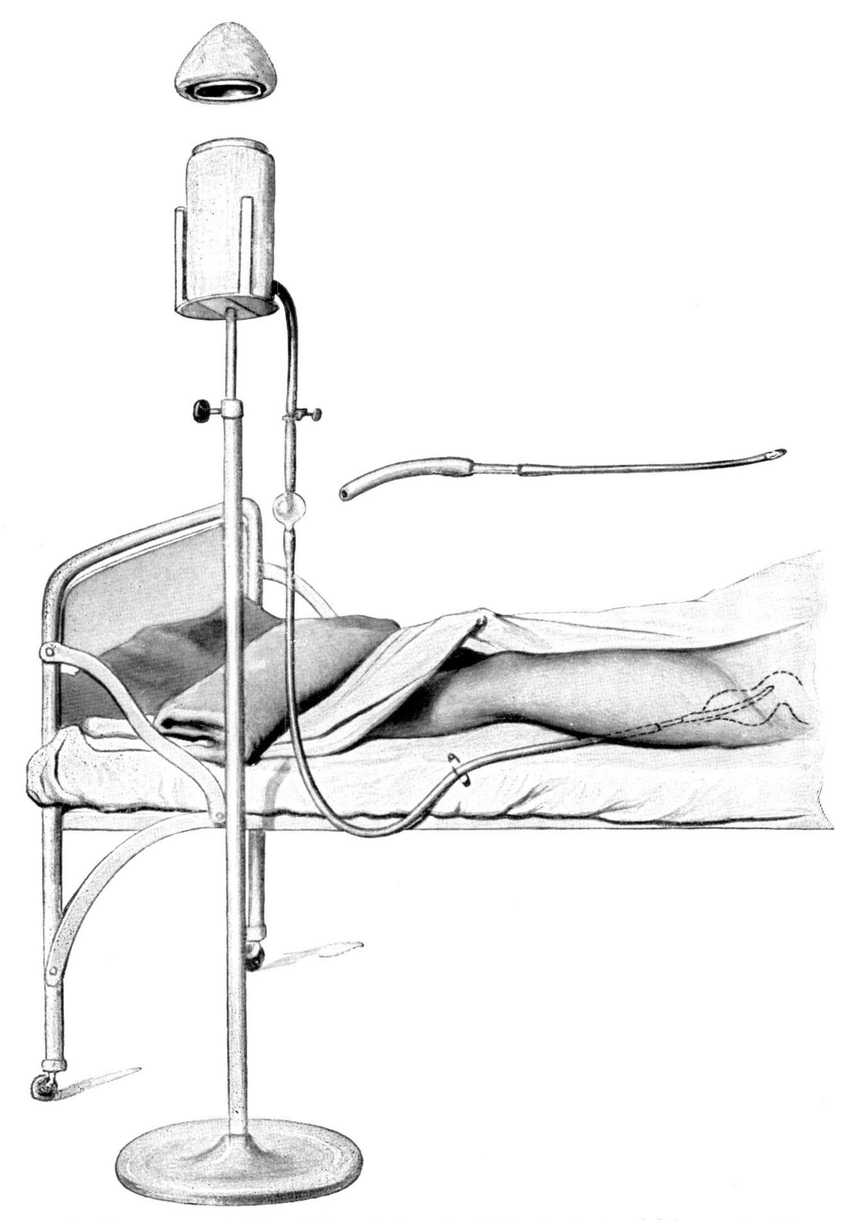

FIG. 339. Continuous rectal drip. The solution should be kept at a fairly constant temperature by an electric heater or by using a vacuum bottle.

rupt the flow. The reservoir and tubing are wrapped with cotton, so that the fluid will reach the intestine still warm (Fig. 339). The fluid may be kept warm by placing an electric heating pad around the reservoir or by the use of hot water bottles. In this way the patient can be given as much as 5 liters of fluid a day, and usually tolerate it for several consecutive days. To prevent rectal irritation, it is advisable to remove the catheter from the rectum for several hours at a time. The quantity of fluid given should depend upon the output of urine, which should amount to about 1500 cc. in 24 hours. In considering output one should also take into account the loss of fluids by vomiting and by drainage from fistulæ.

By this drop-method fluid alone, or fluid with the addition of various substances can be introduced. The fluids usually given are physiologic salt solution; Ringer's solution (sodium chloride 9.0, potassium chloride 0.2, sodium bicarbonate 0.1, distilled water 1000.0), or tap water. The following substances have been added to fluids given by rectum, for their possible caloric value: glucose 7.5 percent, 1 liter of which contains 220 calories; Kalorose 4.5 percent; dextrin 10 percent; alcohol 3 percent; the egg albumin preparation, Riba, 20 percent, and peptone. Any medicament that does not irritate the intestine can be added to any of these solutions. (However from the investigations of Carpenter it is highly probable that of these alcohol only is absorbed to any extent. I.S.R.)

3. The Subcutaneous and Intramuscular Administration of Fluids

Isotonic fluids can be absorbed when injected into the subcutaneous connective tissue. The fluid should be given in an area abundant in loose subcutaneous tissue, but one which does not interfere with the comfort of the patient's position, and also one in which a possible infection might easily be controlled. Such areas are beneath or above the breasts; the dependent sides of the abdomen; the medial side of the thigh and the flexor surface of the arm. It is not practical to inject fluid where the skin is attached to the muscles by fibrous bands, as on the lateral side of the thigh. The fear of injuring large vessels in using the flexor side of the limbs appears to me unwarranted.

The syringes and needles should always be sterilized by boiling; alcohol sterilization is not efficient. Glass syringes holding 1, 5, 10 and 20 cc., are the best to use. The hands need not be sterilized before an injection, but they should be dry, so that the point of insertion of the needle does not become contaminated from drops of water off contaminated hands.

When a large quantity of fluid is to be given it should be warmed to body temperature before injection. Although air introduced under the subcutaneous connective tissue does no harm in itself, it is advisable before injection to turn the syringe with the point up, and gently push in the piston to remove all air bubbles from the fluid. The needle should not be large, but of such a gauge as to permit the free flow of the fluid. For oil, the finest needle may be used. The place of injection should be disinfected by wiping the skin with alcohol, ether, or ether-alcohol. A fold of skin is picked up with the left hand, and with the right hand the needle, tightly attached to the syringe, is pushed sharply into the subcutaneous connective tissue, at a place in the skin which the finger has not touched (Fig. 340). The fluid is emptied by pushing the piston slowly forward. The needle is then quickly withdrawn. Too large an amount of fluid should not be injected at any one place, because there is danger of necrosis of the overlying skin from prolonged tension, with its accompanying ischemia.

The mistake is often made of not inserting the needle through the entire thickness of the skin. The result will then be a somewhat painful intracutaneous injection.

It is not necessary to seal in the injected fluid. The needle hole need only be closed if, after a large quantity has been injected, there is some leaking, or if large cannulæ are used. A collodion patch is sufficient.

Intramuscular injections of fluid are done in the same way as the subcutaneous injections. The needles must be sufficiently long, and they should be plunged vertically into the depth of the muscle. The proximal lateral quadrant of the thick gluteal muscles is usually the site chosen. If it is necessary to make several injections, as, for example, in the treatment of tetanus

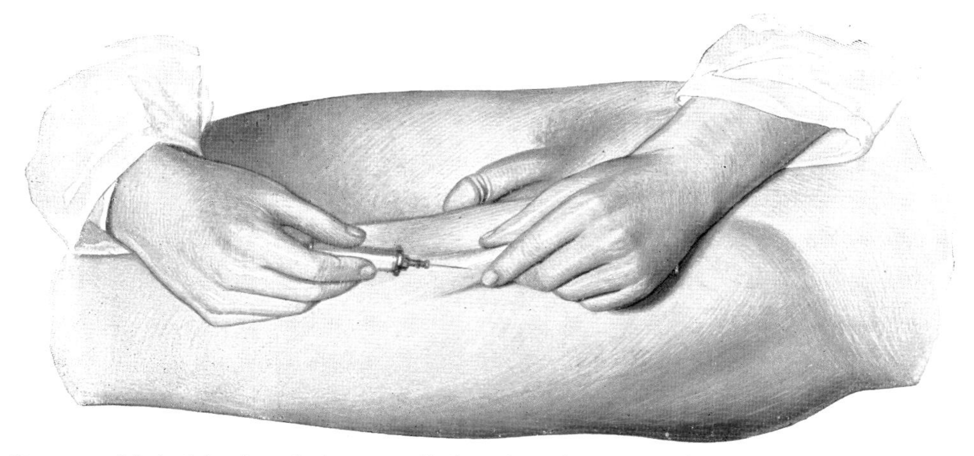

FIG. 340. Method for introducing a needle into the subcutaneous tissues. The skin is pinched into a fold.

with intramuscular injections of magnesium, any other accessible muscle may be chosen. The vicinity of large nerves and blood vessels should always be avoided. Before injecting any fluid, it should be carefully determined that the point of the needle is not in a blood vessel. To determine this, either the syringe is detached, or it is left on and slight suction is made with it. If blood appears, the point of the needle must be shifted or reinserted at another point.

Rapid injection of large quantities of fluid, 50 cc. or more, with a syringe into the subcutaneous connective tissue is difficult because of the resistance of the tissues and produces pain from tension. For these reasons, the slow introduction of the fluid by gravity from a high reservoir, a funnel or irrigating jar, is preferable. The needles, tubing, and reservoir should be sterilized by boiling. A Y tube with two needles may be used (Fig. 341). The diameter of the needles should be about ¾ mm. The rapidity of the flow is regulated by raising or lowering the reservoir. By inserting the needles in several places, more than a liter of salt solution can be introduced within an hour. After removal of the needles the points of insertion are closed with collodion patches. The Martin drop-ball may be used in the hypodermoclysis set-up, in order to visualize the rapidity with which fluid is being introduced.

I do not, however, recommend the drop method for prolonged subcutaneous injections of normal salt solution or Ringer's solution. It prolongs the

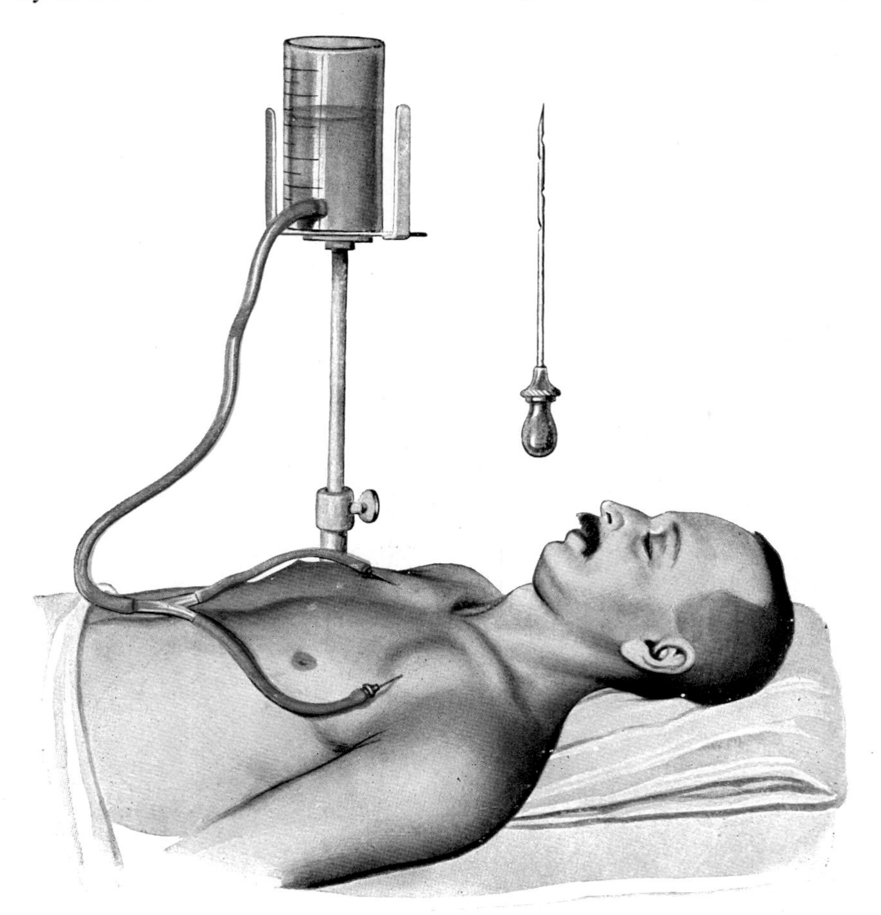

Fig. 341. Subcutaneous injection of large quantities of fluid in the intraclavicular fossa. The needle illustrated has a series of holes.

discomfort and, because of the length of time the needle is in the skin, it predisposes to infection. I prefer the continuous intravenous infusion.

4. The Intravenous Introduction of Fluids

Small quantities of fluid are introduced into the veins by direct puncture of a vein with a sharp needle through the skin; large quantities of fluid are introduced by tying a blunt cannula in an exposed vein. A superficial vein is usually chosen, as a rule, the median vein in the antecubital fossa of the left arm. In order to avoid injury to the artery if the vein is missed, or if fluid is injected around instead of into the vein, a vein lying directly over the course of the artery should not be chosen. In special cases any other accessible vein may be used, for example, a vein on the hand, in the forearm, the basilic vein of the arm, the external jugular vein, the saphenous vein, or, in case of necessity, even a deep vein, as in infants, the longitudinal sinus.

Before beginning an intravenous injection at the bend of the elbow, the arm should be allowed to hang down for a time to fill the veins, and then a tourniquet applied snugly around the arm, without, however, obliterating the

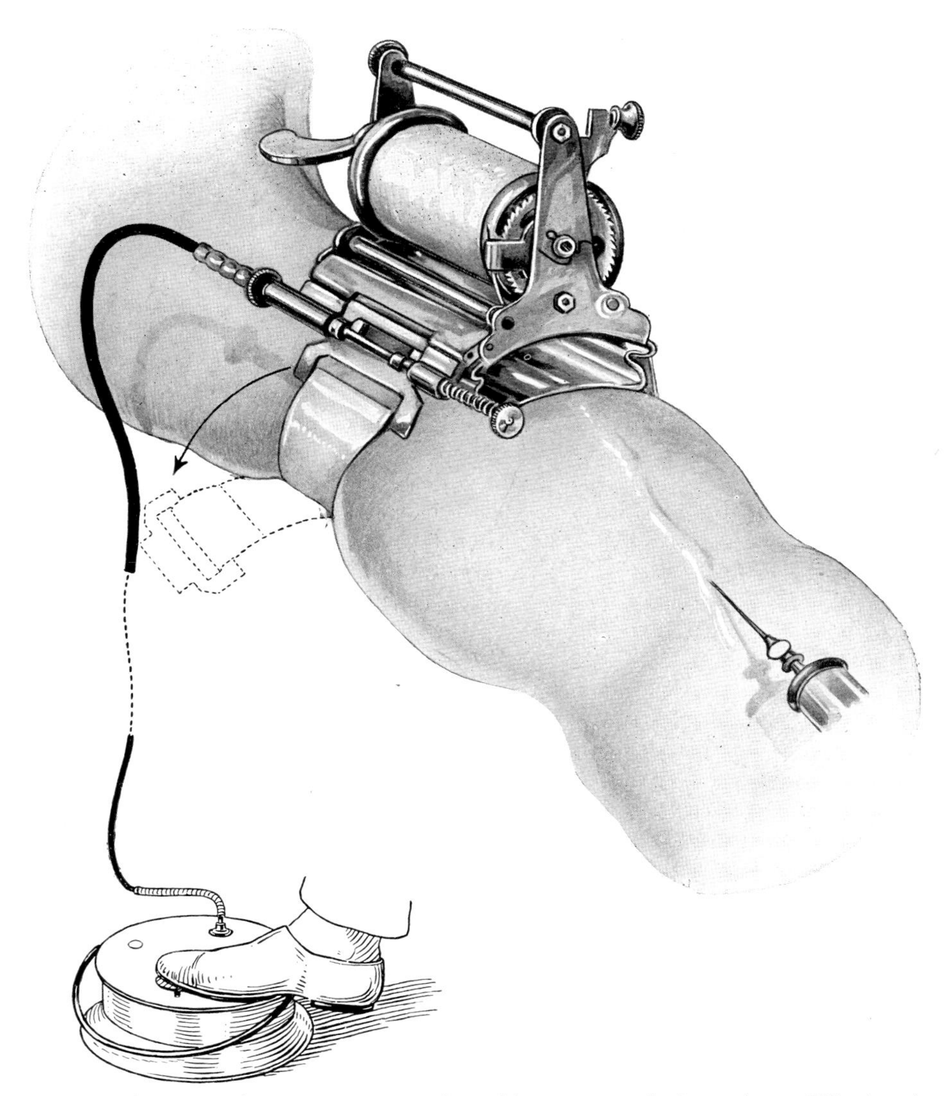

FIG. 342. Apparatus for venous compression with an automatic foot release (Kirschner).

radial pulse (Fig. 343). If an assistant is not present to apply or release the tourniquet, a device is available which has an automatic foot release (Fig. 342). The extended elbow is grasped from behind with the left hand and the skin drawn tight. A fine needle, securely connected to the syringe, is inserted into the vein in a proximal direction and parallel with it, until the needle point has penetrated the lumen of the vein. The syringe should not be entirely filled with the solution to be injected, so that the piston can be further withdrawn to determine whether blood flows readily into the syringe. If it does not flow, the needle must either be shifted or reinserted. When blood flows freely into the syringe, the tourniquet is loosened, the arm and syringe are raised so that the piston end of the syringe is higher than the needle and any air present collects in the upper end. The contents of the syringe are then slowly injected. During the injection the patient is carefully watched and if any untoward symptoms develop, the injection is immediately stopped, the arm is lowered and the tourniquet reapplied to prevent any more of the solution reaching the general circulation. When the injection is completed, the needle is withdrawn quickly, pressure is made over the point of injection for a few seconds, the arm is elevated and a small dressing applied.

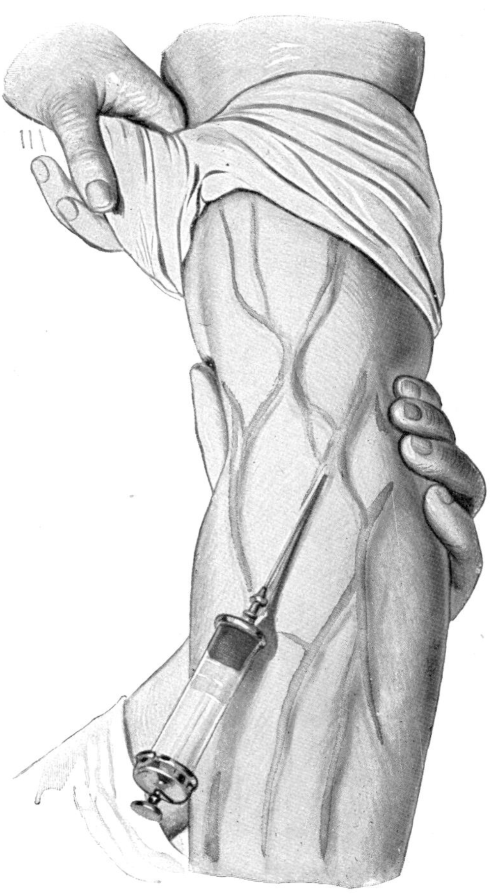

Fig. 343. Inserting a needle into a superficial vein at the bend of the elbow.

Blood can be removed from a vein by the same method, except that the piston is all the way in the syringe when the needle is inserted and a larger needle is advisable. The tourniquet should not be released while blood is being withdrawn. To prevent clotting, the syringe should be emptied immediately and, because of the difficulty of removing clotted blood from a syringe, the barrel should be promptly rinsed with water. It is not necessary to insert the needle in the distal direction when withdrawing a small quantity of blood, for it can be obtained from an insertion in the proximal direction.

Since the venous blood pressure in a greatly congested venous system rises considerably, it is not always necessary to use a syringe for withdrawing blood, for blood will flow freely from a well distended vein. The flow can be increased by movements of the hand. The patient may be instructed to open and close the hand over a rod. Thus, in venesection a large needle can be inserted into a distended vein at the elbow, and the blood allowed to flow into a basin, or flask, if the blood is to be used again. Venesection may also be performed in the classic way by slitting the vein wall with a knife. This form of venesection is preferable for rapid relief of a congested venous system. The old practitioners strictly observed the custom of slightly bending the elbow-joint before incising the vein, in order to separate the vein from the brachial artery by stretching the bicipital fascia and thus lessening the danger of injuring the artery. This precaution is hardly necessary today, since a knife is used under the guidance of the eye, instead of the poorly protected spring lancet phlebotome, so difficult to control. With the point of a knife placed at an angle of 45 degrees, the skin, anæsthetized if necessary, and the anterior wall of the vein are incised, so that the vein is opened for about 1 cm. (Fig. 344). The skin edges are retracted to remove any obstruction to the flow of blood. From 200 to 500 cc. of blood are usually removed, though as much as 1500 cc. may at times be withdrawn. The bleeding stops as soon as the tourniquet is removed and the arm elevated. The wound is closed with a pad, over which is placed a firm bandage.

When there is no vein at the elbow, or in another part of the body that can be seen or felt distinctly enough for the insertion of a needle, or when

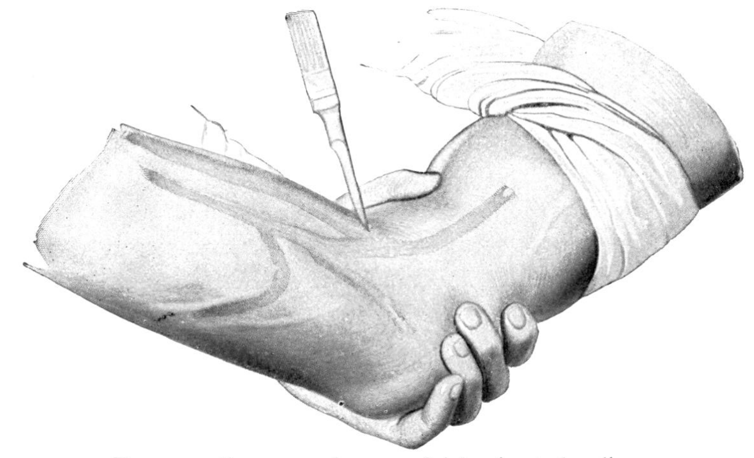

FIG. 344. Exposure of a superficial vein at the elbow.

a cannula is to be placed in the vein for continuous intravenous injection, an incision must be made to expose a vein. This is done under local anæsthesia but, in order to prevent contraction of the vein, no adrenalin is added to the 1 percent novocain solution. A tourniquet is applied with the arm dependent so that a suitable vein may be found. The skin over the vein selected is marked with a blue dye, and the tourniquet removed. To expose a visible vein a longitudinal incision is made directly over it, or when the vein can not be seen a transverse incision across the bend of the elbow is made and a suitable vein can then be found.

If a specially shaped cannula is to be tied in a vein, the vein is exposed on all sides for a few centimeters and any branches entering it at this point are ligated. Three silk ligatures are carried under the vein with an aneurism needle. One ligature is tied as far distally as possible, so that the flow of blood from the forearm to this vein is obstructed. The ends of the middle ligature are then loosely looped once, but without compressing the vein. The ends of the proximal ligature are caught in a hemostat and are used by an assistant to make upward traction on the vein until the lumen is occluded and the flow of blood from the proximal end of the vein controlled. The exposed segment of vein is now shut off from all blood supply. The surgeon can open the vein and introduce the cannula without being disturbed by any bleeding. He grasps the vein with a forceps close to the distal ligature, and with knife or scissors makes an oblique opening along its anterior wall (Fig. 345), inserts the cannula into this opening, without releasing the proximal ligature, and ties the middle ligature securely so as to hold the cannula in position. The cannula, which has a shoulder just back of its tip, is thus fastened in the vein securely so that there can be no leakage around it. No air should be allowed to enter the vein while introducing the cannula. The container, which may be an irrigating jar or funnel, but preferably a graduated

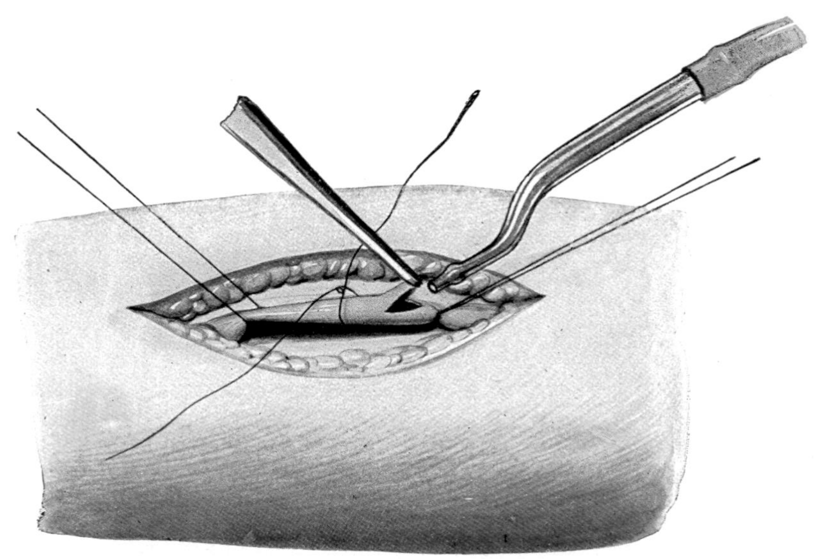

FIG. 345. Tying a cannula in a vein.

cylinder, the tubing, and the needle must be free from air. By holding the filled container low at first, then raising it gradually, the tubing fills and its end is clamped. While introducing the cannula into the vein, a little of the fluid is allowed to run out.

As soon as the cannula is tied in place, the proximal ligature is loosened, but not withdrawn, the pinch-cock on the tube is opened and the arm laid horizontal to the body. The fluid flows into the vein, the rapidity of the flow being regulated by the screw adjustment of the pinch-cock or through changing the level of the fluid container. A Martin drop-ball (Fig. 338) may be used to permit observation of the rate of flow.

At the end of the infusion, the proximal ligature is tied and the cannula removed, after cutting the middle ligature. The small skin wound is closed by sutures or wound clips.

This method of intravenous infusion is particularly adapted for the introduction of physiologic solutions of sodium chloride, glucose, or blood. Drugs in the customary dosage (adrenalin, strophanthin, digalen, pituitrin, etc.) may be added to the solutions.

This method is particularly suited for the reintroduction of sterile blood found in a body cavity, thorax or abdomen (autotransfusion) (Fig. 346). It is best to use a glass funnel or cylinder as a reservoir for the blood. The top of either should be covered with four layers of gauze, and attached to a vein cannula by means of a short rubber tube. The blood removed from the body cavity by suction or with sponges is poured through the gauze filter and runs

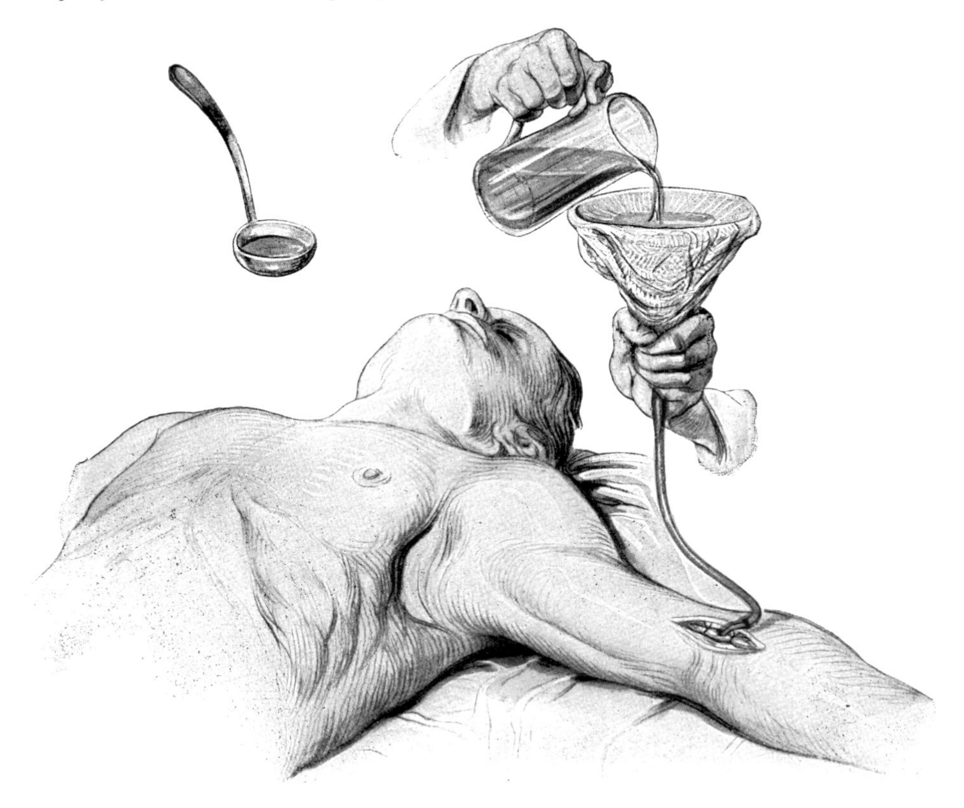

Fig. 346. Autotransfusion of blood. Blood is removed from the abdomen with aseptic precautions and reinjected into a vein, after being passed through several layers of gauze to remove possible clots.

directly into the vein. It can be diluted with normal salt solution or it may be citrated.

When it is desired to introduce fluids intravenously over a long period, the intravenous injection should be given by the drop method. The apparatus can be left attached to the vein for several days; the fluid can be given continuously or the flow can be interrupted every hour. The fluid should, as a rule, run in very slowly. The container is kept warm during this time with an electric heating pad. The arm which is used is fixed in an almost extended position to a wire splint and the tubing is fastened securely to the bandage. In order not to overburden the heart, the quantity of fluid conveyed should be gauged by the quantity of the 24 hour output of fluid.

5. Blood Transfusion

General Principles

Human blood alone can be used in the transfusion of humans. The use of heterogenic blood is not only useless, but fraught with the gravest danger. The blood can be transfused by the indirect method, in which case the blood of the donor is collected first in a vessel and is then conveyed from this to the recipient; or, it may be transfused by the direct method, in which case the blood from the donor is transfused directly into that of the recipient. The direct transfusion may be accomplished in one of several ways: by connecting an artery of the donor and a vein of the recipient (arteriovenous transfusion); by connecting a vein of the donor with a vein of the recipient (venovenous transfusion). For these, the blood from the vessel of the donor can be conveyed to that of the recipient either through an intermediate tube, or through direct vascular continuity as by vessel suture. A pump may be inserted in the line between the donor and recipient to act both as a means for measuring quantity, and also to provide suction and pressure for the removal and introduction of the blood. Most of these procedures have but a historical value at the present time. I use almost exclusively vein to vein transfusion, with the aid of Oehlecker's apparatus, which is similar to many of the direct apparatus used in the United States. Occasionally I use the indirect method. There are many types of transfusion apparatus but few possess any distinct advantage over the others. The surgeon should become familiar with one and use only it.

Blood transfusion is not only the most effective, but probably the only available procedure by which inevitable death from exsanguination can be prevented. It is also the most valuable non-mechanical hemostatic that can be used prophylactically. Transfusion is the best means of preparing debilitated and anemic patients for operation. It is also the best and most rapid means of restoring strength to a patient who has collapsed from acute disease or from an operation.

The transfusion of blood entails numerous dangers to the donor and recipient. To avoid these demands special precautions. We must particularly watch (a) that no diseases are transmitted; (b) that in bringing together the blood of the donor and of the recipient, neither hemolysis nor agglutination of the red blood corpuscles occurs; (c) that the blood does not coagulate, and (d) that air embolism does not take place.

(a) An accurate record of the previous medical history, and a minute examination of the donor and the recipient in regard to acute and chronic infectious diseases (tuberculosis, syphilis, malaria) is essential. If there is time, the results of the Wassermann reaction should be awaited. The family background, age, sex, and occupation of the individual should be considered, but these are not absolute criteria. Young healthy adults are preferable as donors. Sailors and others who have traveled in tropical countries should be avoided as donors unless there is time for a thorough study of them. If there is any question of infectious disease of the recipient the indirect method of transfusion should be used to protect the donor.

Although I very frequently transfuse patients, I have never lacked for willing and suitable donors. I rarely experience the need of using professional donors or "blood cows" as we are wont to call them in Germany. When relatives or friends can not be used there are usually volunteers who can be found. (In the United States professional donors are widely used. I.S.R.)

(b) The blood serum of certain individuals agglutinates the blood corpuscles of other individuals in a very definite order. Based upon this, Landsteiner and Moss have divided individuals into four groups, corresponding to the reaction of their blood corpuscles to the blood serum of the other groups.

Group I. The serum of this group agglutinates the red blood corpuscles of no other group. The red blood corpuscles however are agglutinated by the serum of every other group.

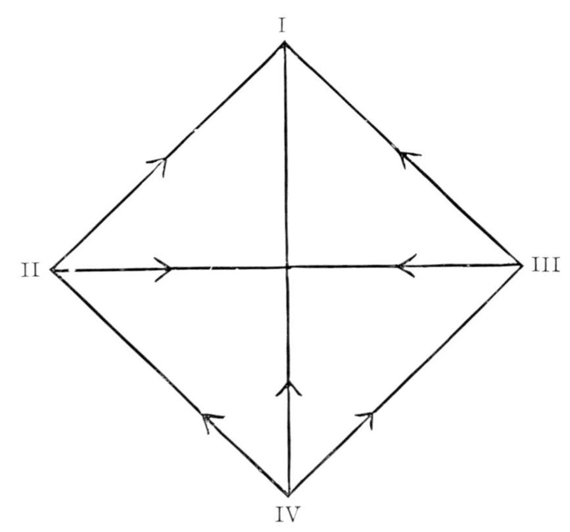

Schematic representation of cross-agglutination. The arrows show which group sera agglutinate the corpuscles of other groups. (Landsteiner and Moss Classification.)

Individuals in this group are known as **universal recipients,** since they can receive blood from any group, including their own. Individuals of Group I, however, are donors for their own group only.

Group II. The serum of this group agglutinates the red blood corpuscles of Groups I and III. The red blood corpuscles of this group are agglutinated by the serum of Groups III and IV.

Individuals of this group are recipients for blood from Groups II and IV, and donors for individuals of Groups I and II.

Group III. The serum of this group agglutinates the red blood corpuscles of Groups I and II. The red blood corpuscles, however, are agglutinated by the serum of Groups II and IV.

Individuals in this group are recipients for blood from Groups III and IV, and donors for Groups I and III.

Group IV. The serum of this group agglutinates the red blood corpuscles of all other groups. The red blood corpuscles of this group are not agglutinated by the serum of any other group.

Individuals in this group can receive blood only from those belonging to the same group and are donors for members of all other groups. They are therefore known as **universal donors.**

The serum reaction (agglutination) can also be interpreted from the drawing above, in which the arrows indicate that the serum of the group from which the arrows emerge agglutinates the blood corpuscles of the group against which they point. (The classification which Kirschner gives is known in the United States as the Landsteiner and Moss classification. The American Association of Clinical Pathologists has recently adopted the Jansky classification. In the latter Groups I and IV are reversed, while Groups II and III remain the same, thus Group I is the universal donor group, while Group IV is the universal recipient group. I.S.R.)

According to Moss, the percentage of individuals in each of the four groups is: Group I 5 percent, Group II 40 percent, Group III 10 percent, Group IV 45 percent. Once the group is established a change in the grouping of an individual does not occur. The group is established during the first year of life. Members of the same family and of the same sex do not necessarily belong to the same group.

In blood transfusion the serum of the recipient should never agglutinate the red blood corpuscles of the donor. No particular harm, beyond an occasional slight chill, will result if the donor's serum agglutinates the cells of the recipient, since the donor's serum is quickly diluted by the large volume of the recipient's blood. Though it is preferable to have both donor and recipient from the same group, it is permissible to use a donor whose serum agglutinates the recipient's cells. It is absolutely necessary to establish whether the blood serum of the recipient agglutinates the red blood corpuscles of the donor. Hemolysis does not occur without agglutination, so that a separate test for hemolysis is unnecessary.

The agglutination test is done by the hanging drop: a drop of a serum of known type is mixed thoroughly with a drop of the blood to be examined. The result appears immediately and is interpreted macroscopically or under the microscope. Chemically clean instruments are required for satisfactory results.

VARIOUS BLOOD AGGLUTINATION TESTS EMPLOYED

The recipient's serum is mixed with the donor's blood. From 4 to 5 cc. of blood are removed by vein puncture from the recipient and are allowed to settle until the serum separates. To expedite matters, the blood can be centrifuged. A trace of blood only, obtained by a needle-prick from a finger tip of the donor is placed in a drop of the recipient's serum. Transfusion is possible when agglutination fails to appear. From this test information is obtained as to whether or not the recipient's serum will agglutinate the donor's blood corpuscles, but not whether the donor's serum agglutinates the recipient's blood corpuscles. As stated previously, the latter reaction, however, is not essential in choosing a donor.

The recipient's blood is mixed with the donor's blood in a 10 percent solution of sodium citrate. A drop of blood from the recipient and one from the donor are mixed with a drop of a 10 percent sodium citrate solution to prevent coagulation. After standing for a few moments the mixture is examined under the microscope for agglutination. A positive agglutination excludes the donor being used for that particular recipient. This test can be carried out rapidly, but it is impossible to tell whether the donor's or the recipient's serum has caused the agglutination. A useful donor might be rejected by the agglutination of the recipient's blood corpuscles through the donor's serum, because the agglutinating serum is unknown, and precious time may be lost searching for another donor.

The first method of examination is used for cross-agglutination by mixing a drop of the recipient's serum with a drop of the donor's blood and a drop of the donor's serum with a drop of the recipient's blood. If after standing a few moments no agglutination takes place in either test we have the proper recipient and donor. The examination takes about twice as long as method 1, but is somewhat more sure.

The American method of group determination of recipient and donor. For this are required sera from individuals in Groups II and III. A drop of serum of Group II with a similar quantity of blood from the individual being tested are mixed on a glass slide. If agglutination of the red cells takes place, the blood examined belongs to Group I or III. If the same blood is mixed with Group III serum and agglutination again takes place, the individual belongs to Group I or II. Both tests taken together demonstrate that he must belong to Group I. The group can be established rapidly from the following table:

		Serum:			
		I.	II.	III.	IV.
Blood corpuscles:	I.	—	+	+	+
	II.	—	—	+	+
	III.	—	+	—	+
	IV.	—	—	—	—

I have for years used the first method of testing for agglutination with very satisfactory results. It is carried out in a few minutes, is dependable and a criterion for all suitable donors.

Agglutination, as observed under the microscope, consists in clumping of the red blood corpuscles. Macroscopically, the occurrence is distinguished by the appearance of small, brick-red clumps. When the red blood corpuscles under the microscope remain unchanged, and when the drops appear uniform to the naked eye, agglutination has not occurred and the transfusion may be performed.

(In the United States the feeling is becoming more general that a Group IV donor should be used whenever possible. However, in the very sick patient I prefer to use a donor from the same group as the recipient after performing the cross-agglutination test. I.S.R.)

(c) In order to perform a **transfusion by the indirect method** coagulation is prevented by the use of anticoagulants. The former method of defibrination by beating with a glass rod, with a fork, with a small forceps, by shaking with glass beads, etc., has been discarded, because, on the one hand, many constituents of value in coagulation and for nutrition are extracted from the blood, and, on the other hand, toxins develop during defibrination, from destruction of the corpuscles. As a rule, coagulation is prevented by mixing the blood with sodium citrate, which does not, apparently, affect the hemostatic efficacy of the transfused blood within the recipient. A 2.5 percent solution of sodium citrate is used. Twenty cc. of the sodium citrate solution are placed in the blood collecting receptacle, the blood is allowed to flow into the container, which should be kept in constant motion, and sodium citrate solution is gradually added until the citrate solution is in the proportion of 1 part to 10 parts of blood. This 0.25 percent citrated blood mixture can be

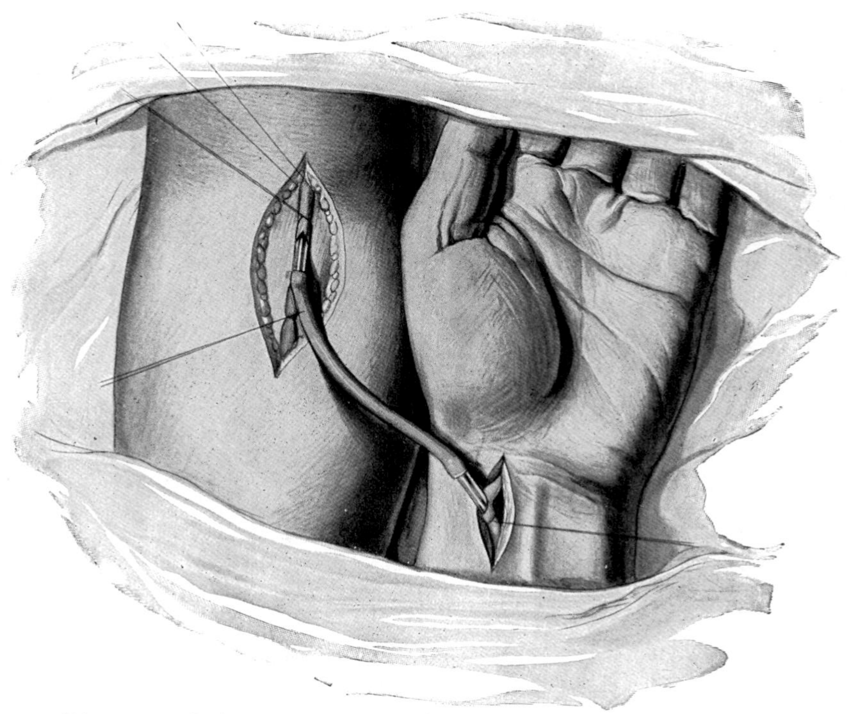

FIG. 347. Direct transfusion of blood by connecting the donor's radial artery with the recipient's cubital vein by means of rubber tube. This method is rarely ever used.

kept on ice for a long time without the blood coagulating. The use of glass cannulæ decreases the danger of coagulation.

Before every transfusion, the containers, cannulæ, and tubing coming in contact with the blood, are rinsed out with a 2.5 percent sodium citrate solution, and a little of the solution is allowed to remain in them.

THE TECHNIC

The simplest form of transfusion is the withdrawal of blood from a vein of the donor with a syringe and needle and the immediate injection of the blood into a vein of the recipient. Even when the needles remain in both veins, but little blood can be conveyed in this manner, which is of no value in massive replacement of blood, even though it may have a biological effect. (The editor must take exception to this statement since in this country large amounts of blood are rapidly transfused by the syringe-cannula method. I.S.R.)

To transfuse larger quantities of blood indirectly, the blood is collected by puncture or by venesection in a graduated cylinder containing a few cubic centimeters of sodium citrate solution; the blood is then mixed with the necessary quantity of sodium citrate solution as it is collected, and conveyed to the vein of the recipient by means of a glass cylinder covered with four layers of gauze, connected by rubber tubing to a needle in the vein. We see no advantage over this simple procedure in the apparatus of Kimpton-Brown or Percy, which we have used many times.

The old method of direct transfusion, connecting a donor's artery with the recipient's vein by vessel suture or tubing (Fig. 347), is no longer practised.

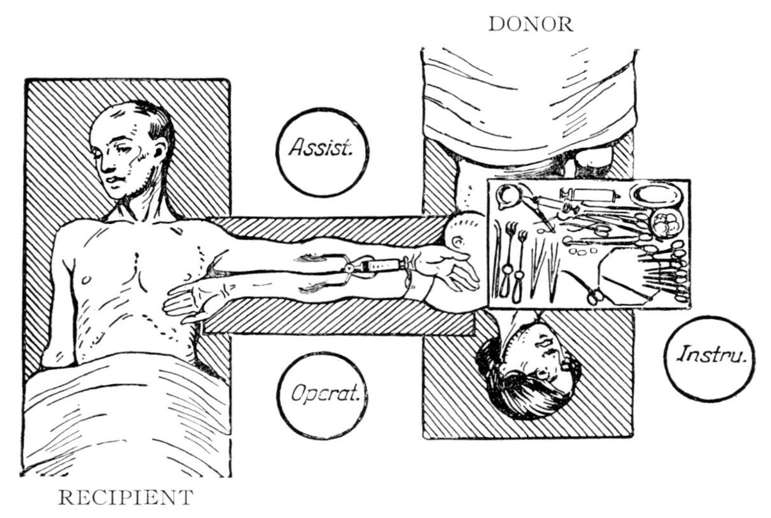

Fig. 348. Usual position of the donor and recipient, and of the operator and assistants, in an unmodified transfusion of blood.

Transfusion with Oehlecker's apparatus is, in my opinion, more satisfactory than with any other method. It is simple, dependable, the amount of blood given may be measured, and the blood may be given rapidly, slowly, or the flow interrupted. It lies between indirect and direct transfusion methods, since there is a direct connection between a vein of the donor and a vein of the recipient, but the blood deviates from the direct path to go through an interposed glass syringe, which acts both as a pump and as a measuring device. It should properly be called the unmodified method. Since this method requires direct connection between the veins of the donor and recipient and the individuals are in such close proximity, there is danger of infection of the donor by the recipient. For this reason Oehlecker's method, or methods similar to it, should only be used when the recipient is unquestionably non-infectious. Since this is the method of choice, it will be described in detail.

Oehlecker's apparatus (Fig. 349) consists of a three-way stop-cock, one outlet of which is for the attachment of a glass syringe provided with a ground glass piston, and two curved outlets for the attachment of rubber tubing from the cannulæ in the veins of the donor and recipient. In the first position of the stop-cock, all three outlets are closed; in the second position the syringe is in connection with one of the cannulæ, while in the third position it is in connection with the other.

The sterile three-way stop-cock, connected with the two vein cannulæ and syringe, is filled with 2.5 percent sodium citrate solution to force out the air, and turned to the first position. Two sterile glass syringes are lubricated with citrate ointment and filled with a few cubic centimeters of sodium citrate solution.

℞	Sodium citrate.		
	Lanolin.		
	Distilled water	aa	10.00
	Liquid petrolatum		70.0
	M.ft. Ung.		
Sig.	Warm and mix thoroughly before using.		

The donor and the recipient are placed in opposite directions upon two operating tables or beds of equal height, lying, if possible, on their backs, so that the left side of the recipient is adjacent to the left side of the donor (Fig. 348). They lie parallel so that the head of one is at a level with the feet of the other, thus bringing the left arms adjacent to each other. The operating tables are so arranged, that when the left arms are abducted at a right angle, and extended at the elbow they will be at the same height. The space between the two operating tables, which is just enough to allow room for one person, is bridged with a board, about 35 cm. wide and padded, at the level of the shoulders of the two subjects. The operating tables should be tied together. The arm of the donor is constricted, and in order to locate a suitable vein, the arm of the recipient is also temporarily constricted. The radial pulse of the donor must remain perceptible throughout the operation. The pneumatic cuff may be used as a tourniquet and the pressure regulated by the pressure gauge. The veins to be used are marked with a blue dye. After disinfection with a tannin-alcohol solution the arms of the donor and recipient are fastened together with bandage or adhesive tape, so that the two veins are directly side by side on the board. After the sterile covers are in place the operator seats himself on a revolving chair, to the right of the donor; the assistant sits opposite the operator. The instrument nurse stands on the free side of the donor. An anæsthetist or nurse stands on the free side of the recipient.

During the operation the recipient is always handled first. If any obstruction should occur to the passage of blood from delay, it may be overcome by aspiration.

After injecting novocain, which does not contain adrenalin, the veins are freely exposed for several centimeters, or needles inserted directly into them in the same direction as the cannulæ are to be inserted. Three ligatures are passed under each vein, if the veins are exposed. The distal ligature in the recipient is immediately tied, as is the proximal ligature in the donor. The proximal untied ligatures in the recipient are drawn taut, so that the blood can not escape when the vein is incised. The vein is incised close to the distal ligature and the recipient's cannula, connected to the three-way stop-cock is introduced in a proximal direction and tied with the middle liga-

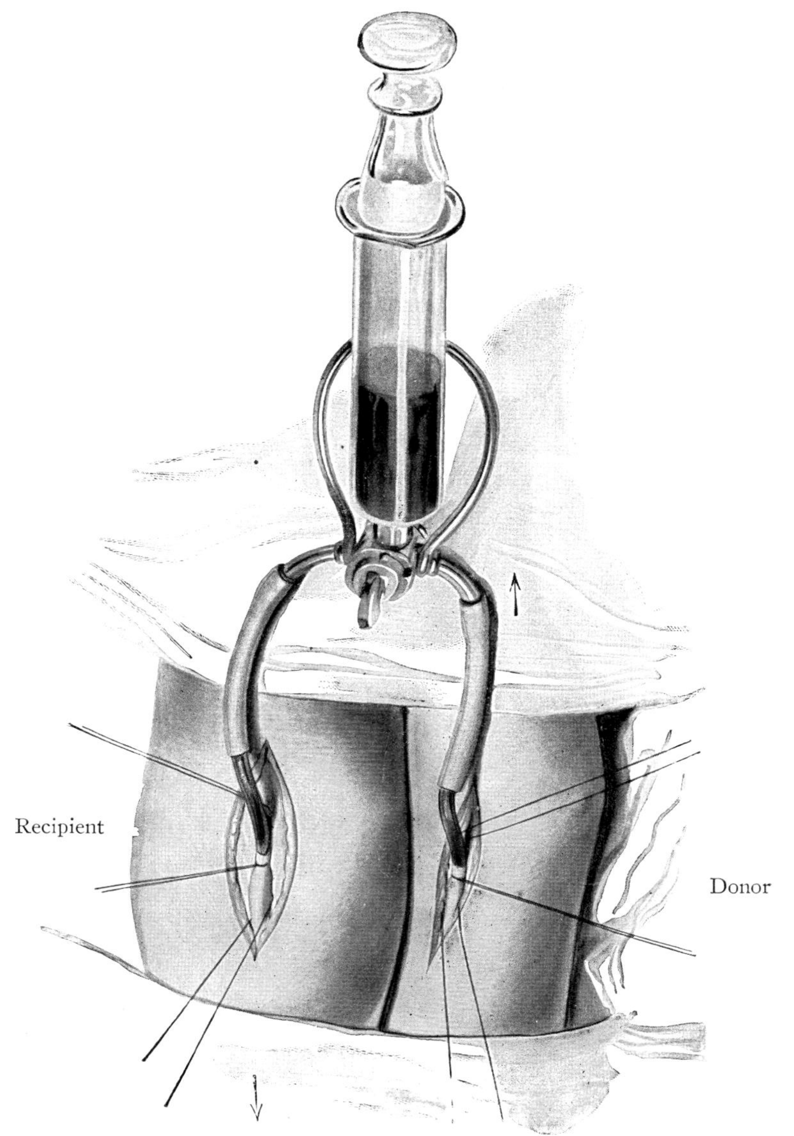

Fig. 349. Blood transfusion with Oehlecker's apparatus. A three-way stop-cock controls the direction of the blood flow.

ture. In a similar manner the other cannula is tied in the vein of the donor, however in the opposite, or distal, direction.

After a glass syringe moistened with a few cubic centimeters of sodium citrate solution is attached the three-way stop-cock is opened by turning the stop-cock towards the donor, and the connection is established between the syringe and the donor's vein. If the tourniquet is properly adjusted, blood will immediately flow into the syringe and drive out the piston with its own force. If this does not occur, it may be necessary to loosen the tourniquet slightly, or to shift the position of the cannula in the vein, rather than to try to withdraw the blood with the syringe. As soon as the piston is at 50 cc.,

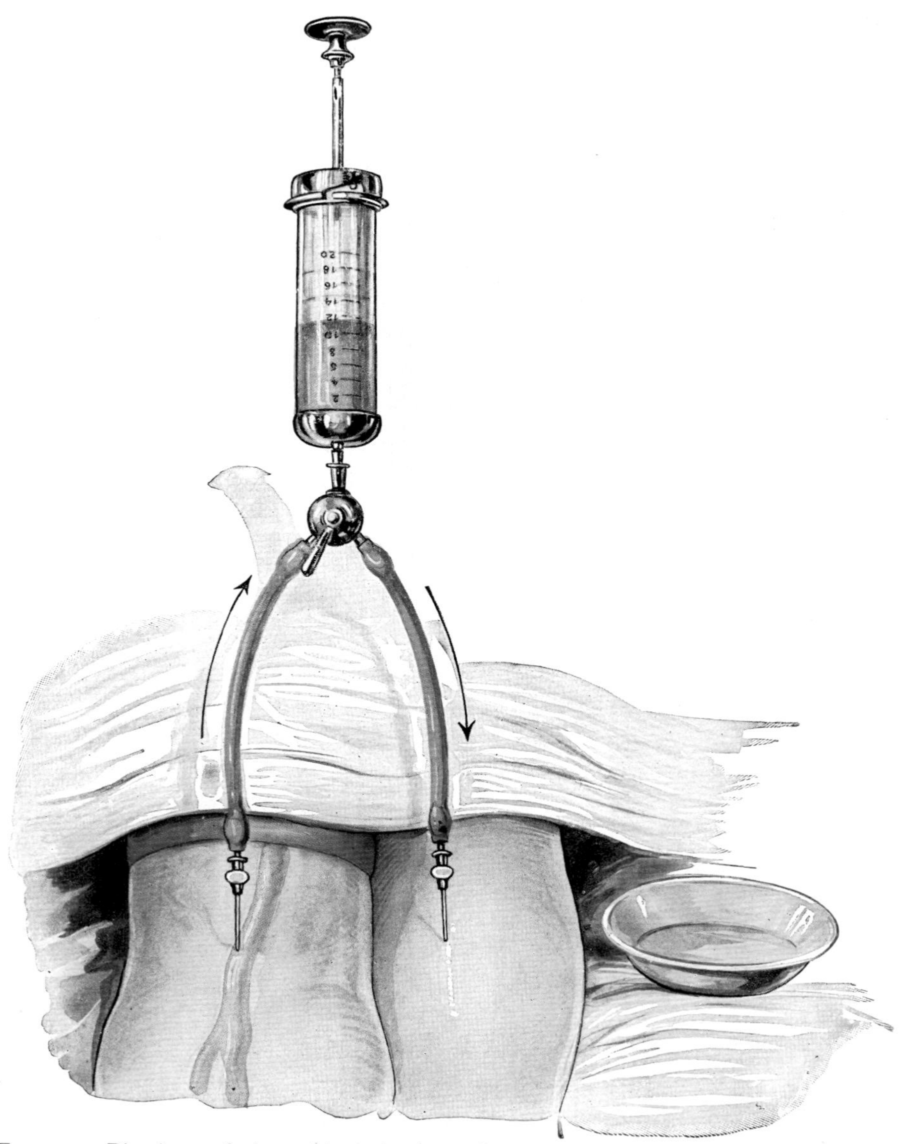

FIG. 350. Blood transfusion with a simple syringe, two-way stop-cock and two needles.

the stop-cock is turned towards the recipient, thus opening the circuit between the syringe and the recipient's vein and the blood is injected into this vein by pushing in the piston. The recipient is watched closely for a few minutes. If any untoward symptoms appear, pallor, dyspnea, cramps, excitation, collapse, etc., the transfusion is immediately stopped. If the symptoms are mild and disappear rapidly, more blood may be cautiously injected, but the injection must be discontinued if serious disturbances again occur, because it is evident that the recipient does not tolerate the donor's blood. Because of the possibility of such disturbances, the recipient is closely observed for several moments after the contents of the first syringe are injected, and the transfusion is continued only when no threatening symptoms occur (biological test). To continue the transfusion, the following manipulations are made: the stop-cock is turned toward the donor's vein, the syringe is filled, the stop-cock turned toward the recipient's vein, the blood injected, the stop-cock reversed toward the donor's vein, etc. Should the piston not slide freely, the stop-cock is closed, the syringe discarded and replaced by a new one moistened with a few cubic centimeters of sodium citrate solution and lubricated with sodium citrate ointment. The first syringe is cleansed with sodium citrate solution and made ready for use again by the instrument nurse. When a cannula becomes clogged, sodium citrate solution can be forced through it with the syringe.

The amount of blood transfused depends upon the purpose of the transfusion and upon the condition of the recipient and donor during transfusion. From 100 to 1000 cc. of blood may be transfused. When the transfusion is to be terminated, the stop-cock is closed, the glass syringe is taken off, and the tourniquet around the donor's arm removed. The proximal ligature on the vein of the recipient and the distal ligature on the vein of the donor are tied. After cutting the ligatures holding the cannulæ in place, the cannulæ are removed and the skin wounds closed.

The donor may lose 500 to 1000 cc. of blood without disturbance, although he occasionally complains of weakness. A substantial meal with a bottle of beer or a glass of wine will help overcome such after effects.

It is not absolutely necessary in direct transfusion, with or without Oehlecker's apparatus, to expose the vein and tie in a cannula. A needle may be inserted through the skin directly into the vein. Needles, inserted through the skin, are more apt to become clogged, in our experience, even though very large ones are used. Therefore when large amounts of blood are to be transfused I prefer a cannula tied into the exposed vein. Instead of the Oehlecker apparatus, a simple two-way stop-cock and an ordinary record syringe may be used (Fig. 350).

CHAPTER V

OPERATIONS ON THE SKIN AND SUBCUTANEOUS CONNECTIVE TISSUE

A. INCISION, UNION AND TRANSPLANTATION OF SKIN

1. Skin Incision and Suture

Most operations are begun by dividing the skin and the subcutaneous connective tissue, the skin incision. It is important to use the greatest possi-

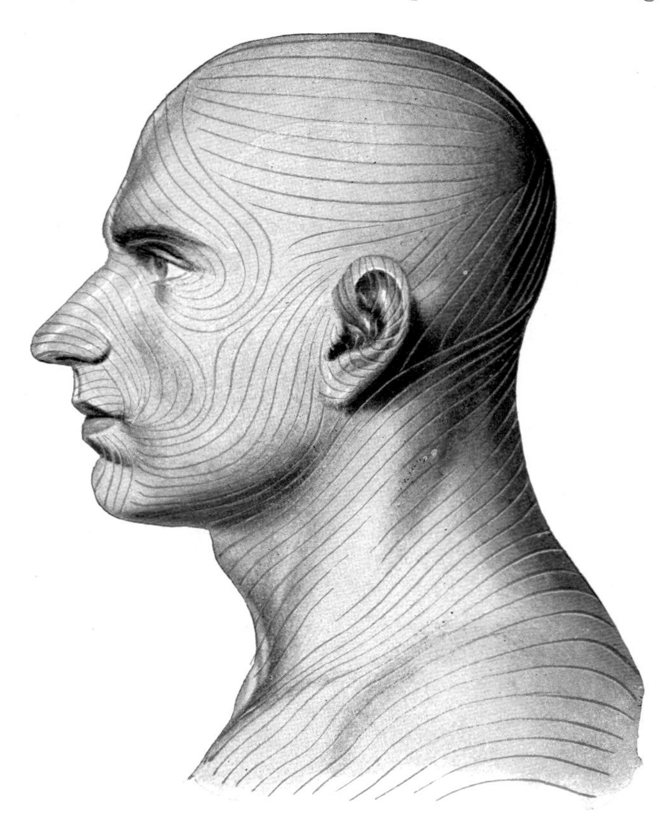

Fig. 351. Tension lines of the skin on the head and on the neck.

ble precision in making the incision, so I always mark the line for the skin incision in advance (Chap. III. "The Asepsis of the Operation"). The scar which remains after healing of the wound is a permanent, visible reminder of the surgeon's activity, which is reason enough to use every precaution so that it results in the least possible functional and cosmetic disturbances. The skin incision should not be unnecessarily large, but must be long enough to expose fully the field of operation. However, deference to cosmetic results should never mislead one into making a smaller skin incision than is required for free access to the area of operation.

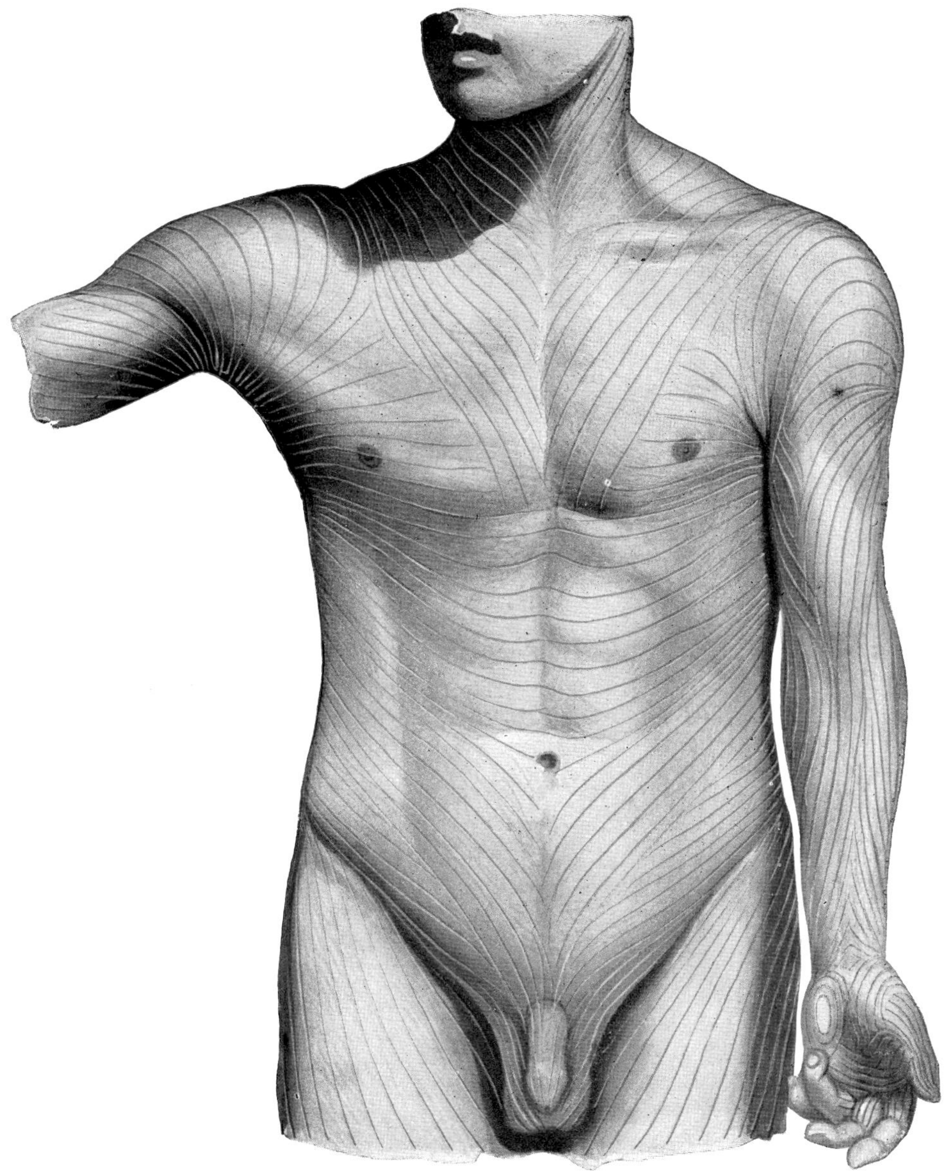

FIG. 352. Tension lines of the skin on the anterior surface of the trunk and upper extremity.

The direction in which the skin is incised is of importance (Kocher) in considering the ultimate appearance of the skin cicatrix. If the skin is divided in the direction of the skin folds, a narrow, delicate, often invisible scar is apt to result, while an incision perpendicular or diagonal to the direction of tension often results in a scar that in time widens, and may become depressed or elevated. Constitutional factors play an important role in this, since in many individuals there is a tendency toward the formation of simple scars, while in others there is a tendency towards keloid formation. I always make the skin incision in the line of tension direction, unless it is necessary, in order to obtain access to the zone of operation, to use a different line of incision. The direction of tension lines, which is the same in all

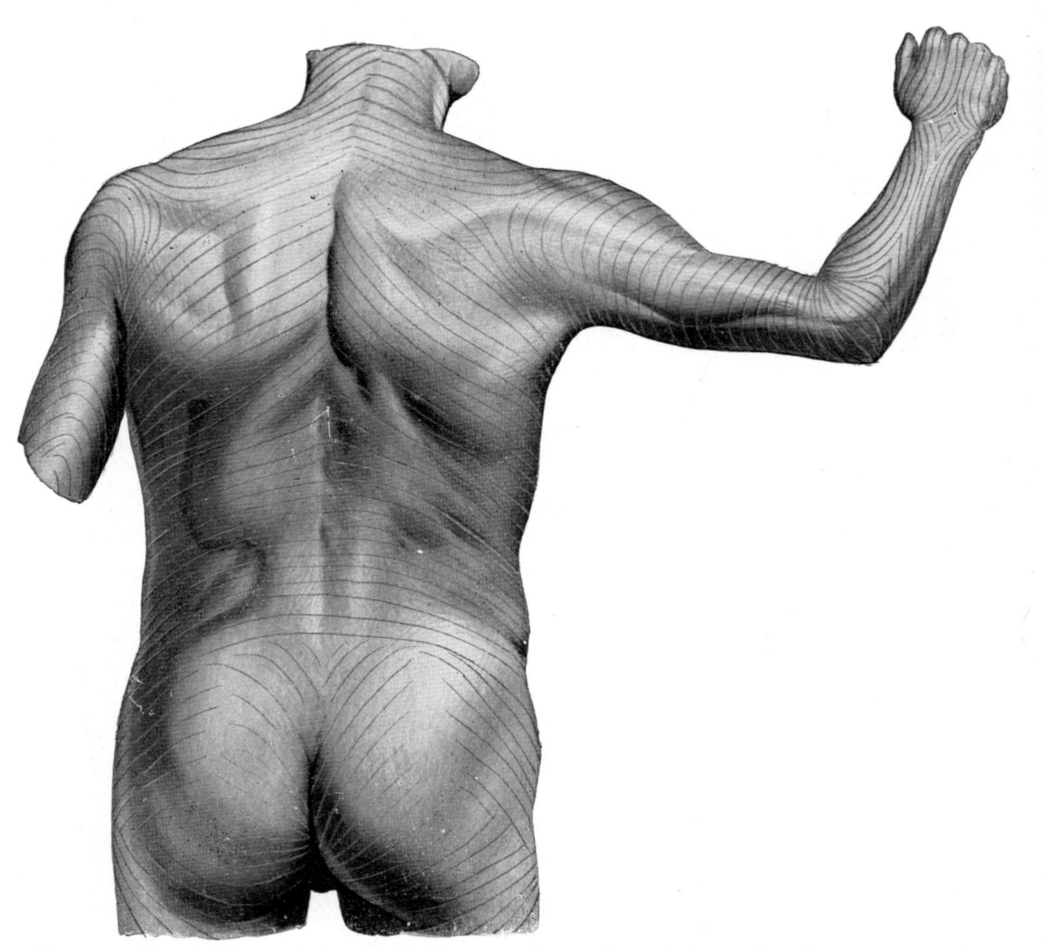

FIG. 353. Tension lines of the skin on the posterior surface of the trunk and upper extremity.

individuals, is recognized by the direction of the folds of skin and hairs, that lie in the same way. These lines are shown in Figures 351-354. The line of incisions on the face should be directed toward the ear because of the position of the facial nerve. The skin should be incised evenly with a sharp knife, perpendicular to its surface. A slanting incision through the skin, which is sometimes recommended, results in no better scar (Fig. 355).

The removal of cicatricial keloids, which may even develop in a stitch wound, and which may assume grotesque forms, is not possible by excision and suture, because the new cicatrix will degenerate in the same manner within a short time. Fair results may be obtained occasionally by injecting a chemical substance over a period of months, as will be described later, under the treatment of cicatrical contractions of the skin. I have obtained moderately good results, at times, by excising the scar and treating the unsutured wound with radium irradiation, the wound being allowed to heal by granulation.

The skin wound is closed by suture at the end of an aseptic operation; in septic operations or, if the asepsis is questionable, it is left more or less open. In suturing a long incision that was made across the lines of tension, the displaced margins of the wound must be carefully sutured in their correct relation to each other. To do this, the incision is stretched lengthwise by means of two pointed hooks placed in its corners (Fig. 356). A suture is then placed at the center, the skin is stretched between this suture and one of the hooks, another suture is placed at the center of this section, and this is continued until the sections between the sutures thus placed become sufficiently small to permit the remaining sutures to be placed without difficulty. If very large or irregular skin incisions are necessary, I mark the skin with a dye, before making the incision, with several lines perpendicular to the line of incision. When the sutures are to be placed, these lines indicate corresponding points on the opposite skin margins.

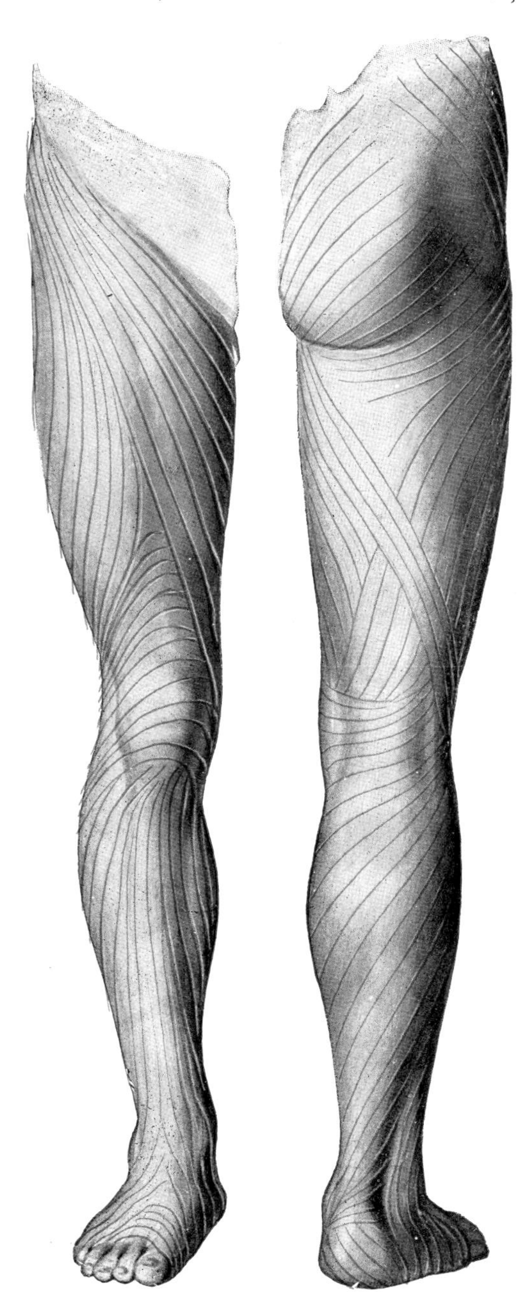

FIG. 354. Tension lines of the skin of the lower limb.

The skin incision may be closed with interrupted or continuous sutures of silk, linen, catgut, horse-hair, or wire, or by skin clips (Fig. 357 and 358). The finer the suturing material is, the less apt is it to lead to infiltration or to infection of the stitch holes, and thus the less visible is the cicatrice as a rule. For sutures on the face, it is preferable to use fine silk, or still better, horse-hair or very fine wire. Horse-hair can be boiled.

For skin sutures either curved, cutting point needles (Fig. 356), or straight needles with lancet points are used (Figs. 67 and 72).

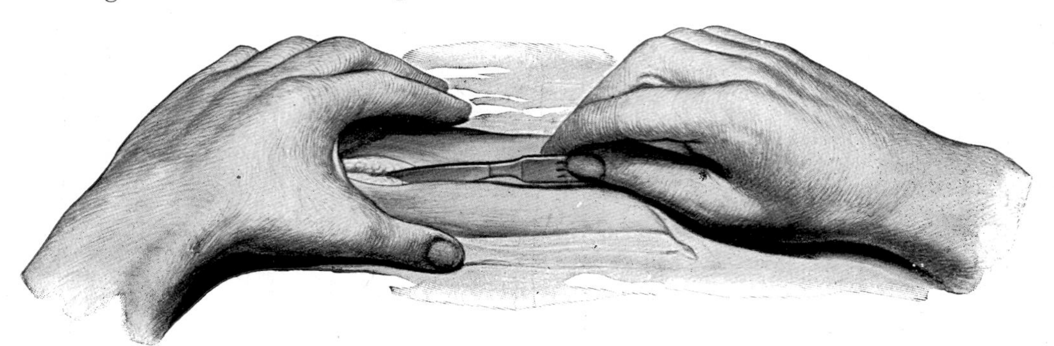

Fig. 355. Skin incision. The skin is stretched with the left hand. The knife is held like a violin-bow.

The interrupted suture has an advantage over the continuous suture in the presence of hematomata or serum collections in the wound, since one or two sutures may be removed without fear of opening the entire wound. The knot of the interrupted suture should not be placed over the line of incision, but beside it (Fig. 65). In continuous suture the stitches are placed

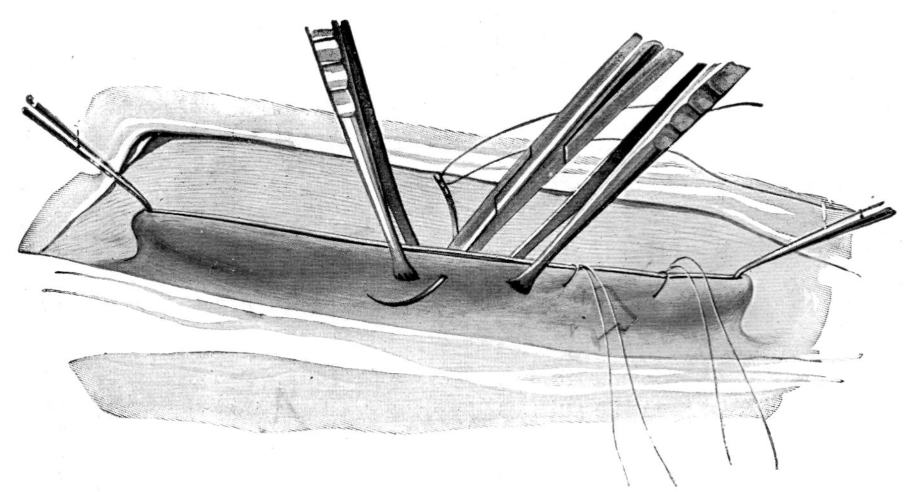

Fig. 356. Closing a skin wound by interrupted sutures. The skin is stretched by hooks put in at both ends of the skin incision, it is pressed together with tissue forceps, and interrupted sutures are inserted and tied.

one after another, an assistant holding the suture taut between each stitch so that the wound margins are drawn together by the previous stitch (Fig. 66). Complicated sutures, such as the interlaced or the mattress suture (Fig. 67), possess no particular advantages over the simple sutures.

Catgut sutures need not be removed, since they fall off by themselves after a short time, which is of advantage in children and nervous patients, or

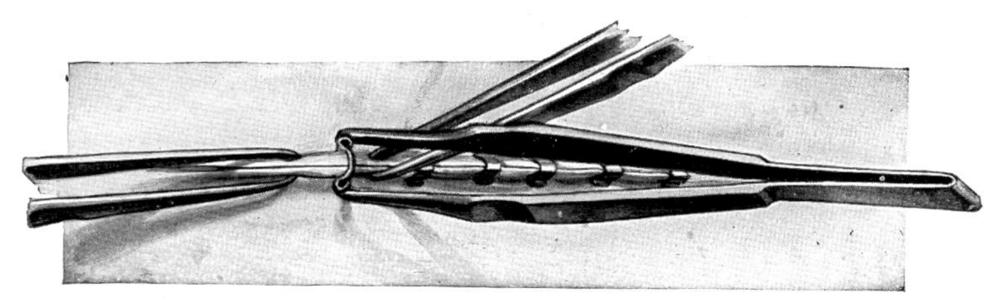

FIG. 357. Closing skin incision with Michel's clips.

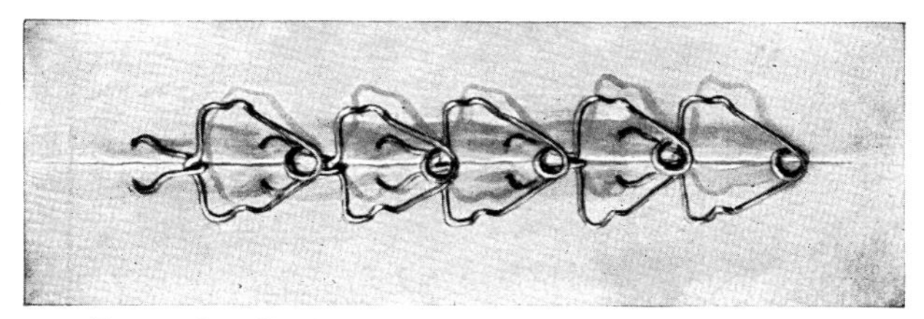

FIG. 358. Closing skin incision with Herff's clips.

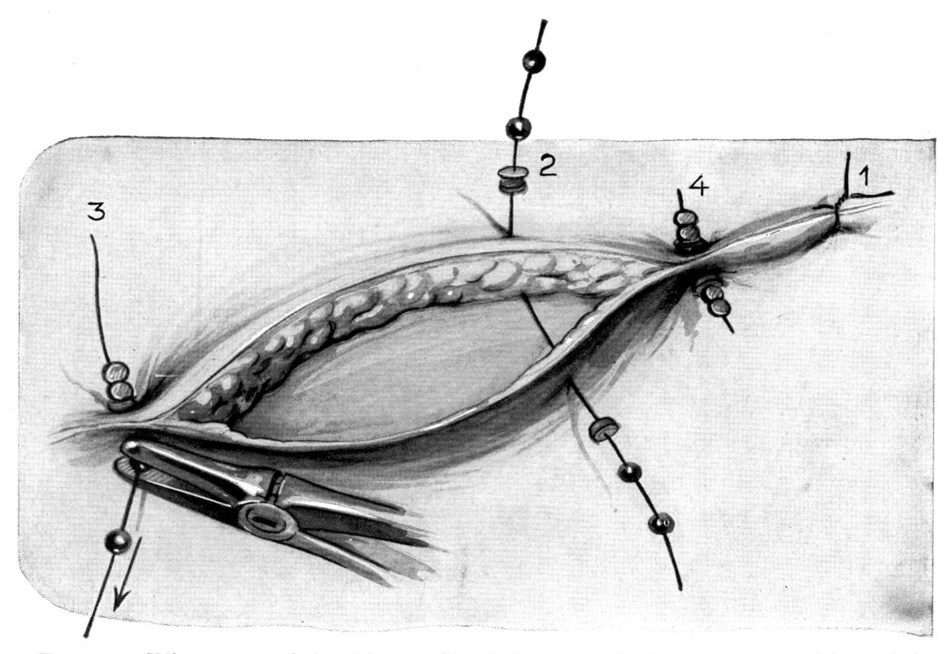

FIG. 359. Wire suture of the skin. 1. Simple interrupted wire suture, closed by twisting. 2. Individual components of wire and shot suture before closing. 3. Wire and shot suture being applied. 4. Completed wire suture.

when a wound is to remain tightly bandaged for a longer period of time than usual. Catgut should not be used if the skin is to be subjected to considerable tension.

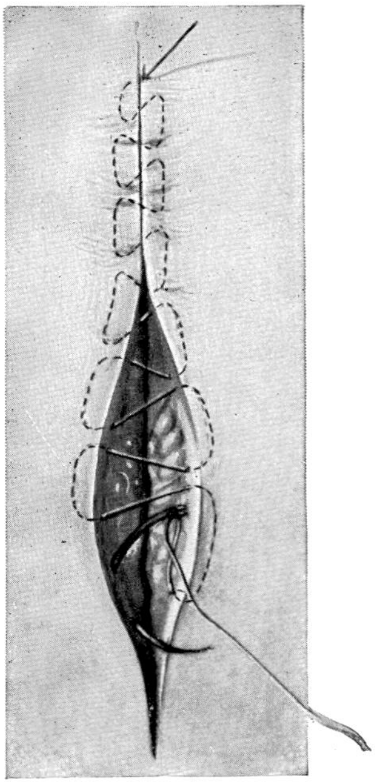

Skin wounds may also be closed with metal clips, Michel's clips being more dependable than Herff's clips (Fig. 358). Both may be used more than once. They have the advantage of piercing only the outer layer of the skin and do not carry superficial infection into the deeper tissues. Michel's clips are applied by simply pressing them together with a special forceps. The removal of the Michel clip is sometimes a little difficult and requires a special instrument. The new clip of Wachenfeld-Kifa (Fig. 364) is easily applied and very easily removed by the same instrument.

To fasten a wire suture (Fig. 359), the ends of the wire are either twisted or secured by shots clamped firmly onto the wire, under which one can put lead or rubber plates.

Fig. 360. Subcuticular suture (Halsted). The first end is fastened with a knot and then the suture is carried from side to side just beneath the skin.

Halsted's subcuticular suture (Fig. 360) has the advantage of not making any visible stitch holes. A fine curved needle threaded with fine silk or catgut, knotted at one end, carries the suture from side to side just beneath the surface of the skin. The needle, carried parallel and as close as possible to the skin surface, catches alternately a small section of the corium of each side of the wound, so that the stitches are placed as close together as possible. The thread is drawn taut

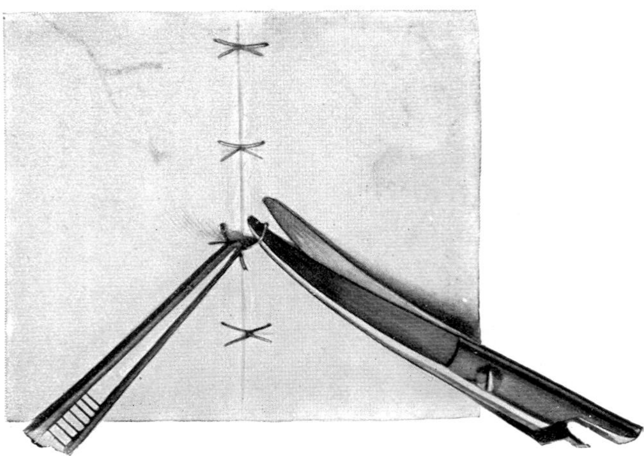

Fig. 361. Removal of a skin suture. The stitch should be cut close to the skin at one side and then pulled out.

after every stitch. The suture is fastened at the end of the wound, either by leaving the end long and fastening it to the skin under light tension with adhesive plaster or a collodion patch, or by tying it. When linen or silk is used, the suture must be removed later. This is unnecessary when catgut is used.

The skin margins should not be allowed to become inverted when they are sutured. An assistant must "adapt" the skin margins. To do this, the assistant holds the edges of the skin together with two toothed forceps (Fig. 356) so that the edges are pressed against each other and elevated, while the operator is placing and tying the sutures between the points held by the two forceps. When the skin is released, the wound margins lie evenly together. If it is impossible to hold the skin margins together because of their rigidity, thickness, or tension, then the assistant must evert each edge separately while the surgeon ties the suture. Again the margins will fall evenly together when released. The distance between sutures and the amount of skin caught in each suture depend upon the thickness of the skin and the amount of tension on the suture.

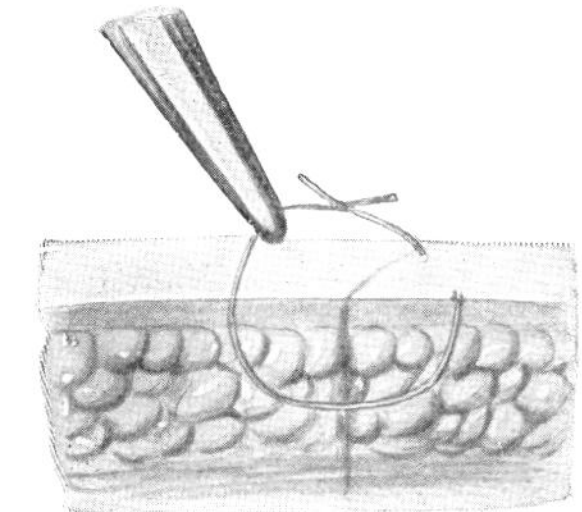

FIG. 362. Removal of a skin suture after cutting the thread close to its exit from the skin.

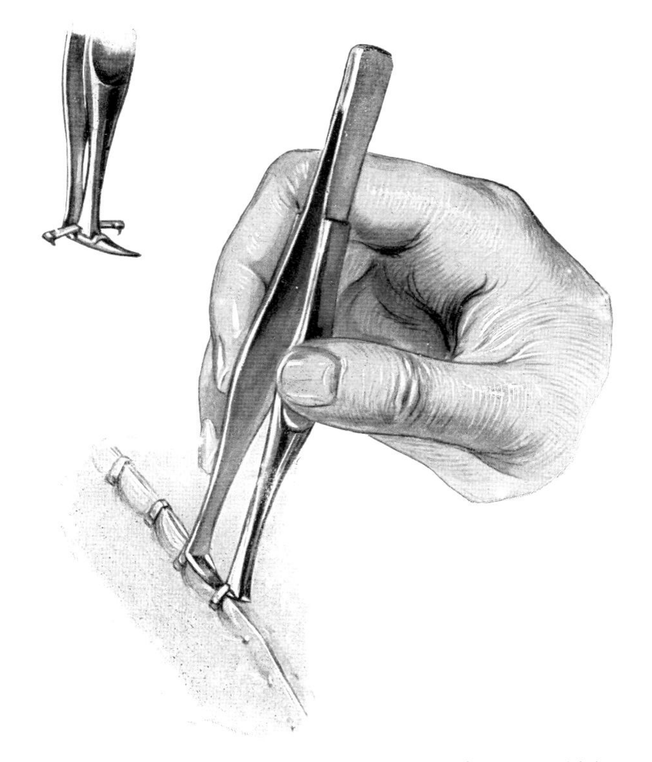

FIG. 363. Removing a Michel clip with a special forceps, which spreads it.

Tension on the skin sutures should be reduced as much as possible if narrow scars are desired. Therefore, when a good cosmetic scar is the object, the subcutaneous fascia and any superficial muscle fibers, such as the platysma, are united previously by buried catgut sutures, and if possible, so intimately that the edges of the skin are pectinated. When the skin is under great tension, the subcutaneous sutures should be placed carefully and plentifully, so that they will take up as much of the tension as possible. When the tension can not be relieved in this manner, the wound is drawn together by a few tension sutures, which are wide interrupted sutures of silk, wire, or silk worm gut, and the wound margins then sutured in the usual manner.

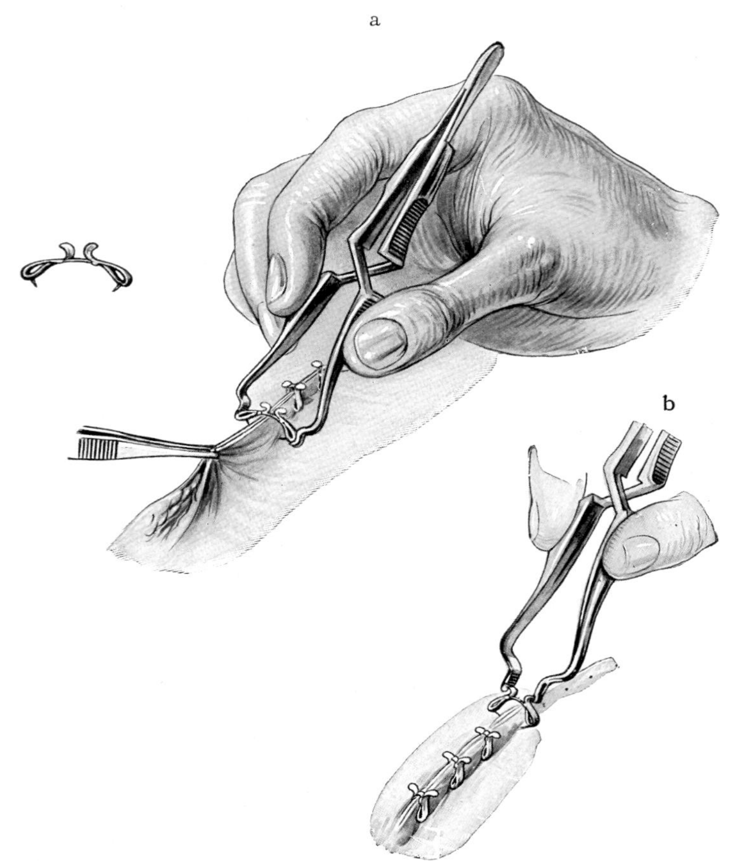

Fig. 364. a. Inserting the skin clips of Wachenfeld-Kifa. b. Removing the skin clips of Wachenfeld-Kifa.

I remove sutures and clips on the eighth day. Apparently, earlier removal does not result in any finer cicatrices. When a stitch is to be removed, it is grasped with a tissue forceps and is cut close to its point of entrance (Figs. 361 and 362) into the skin. The long end is pulled on, thus removing the suture without carrying any of it which lay outside the skin through the tissues.

If the wound has not entirely healed, alternate skin sutures are left in, to be removed later. The old Michel clips must be removed with a special instrument (Fig. 363), while the Wachenfeld-Kifa modification of these can be removed with anatomical forceps.

2. Closure of Defects by Direct Union of Wound Margins

The elasticity of the skin often permits the uninterrupted union of two wound margins, though they are of different shapes or lengths. Where there is too much skin present the stitches are placed further apart, while where

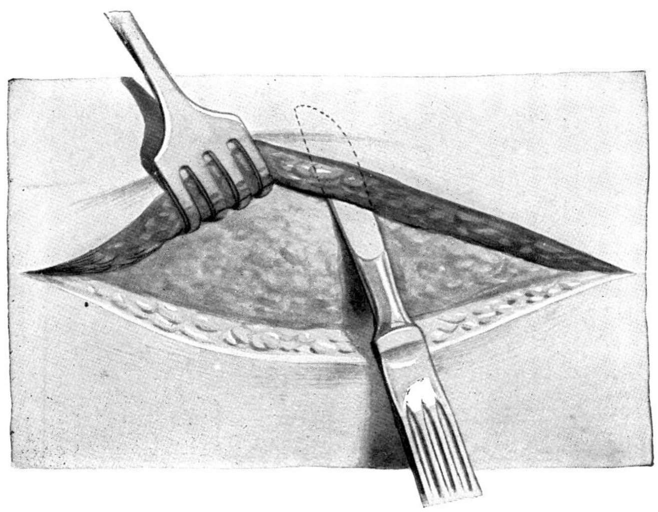

Fig. 365. Mobilizing the edges of a wound so that they may be drawn together over a defect. The skin and subcutaneous tissue are elevated with sharp hook retractors and the edges are freed by extensive undercutting.

there is too little skin the stitches are placed closer together. It is also possible because of the elasticity of the skin to cover fair sized defects by pulling together the margins of the wound with wire sutures, retained with lead plates and shot.

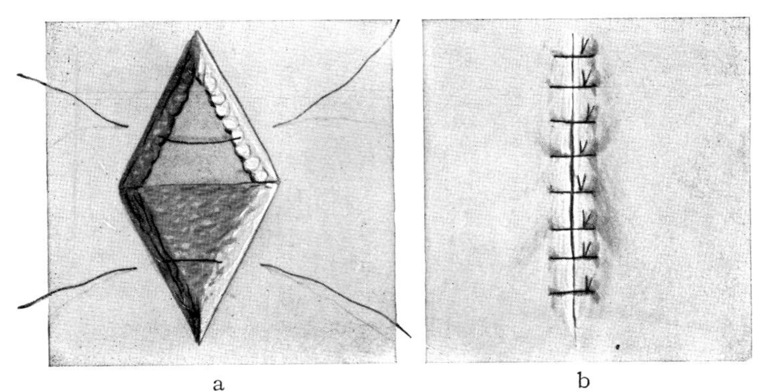

Fig. 366 a and b. Closing a diamond shaped defect by drawing the margins together with sutures.

The elasticity of the skin and the ease with which the skin can be mobilized from the subcutaneous tissues vary considerably in different parts of the body. These are greatest about the scrotum, the labii pudendi, the neck, the abdomen, and the female breast, but limited on the palmar surface of the hand, the plantar surface of the foot, and over the skull. Large defects can be closed occasionally by undercutting the skin margins (Fig. 365), especially where the skin is naturally adherent to the underlying tissues,

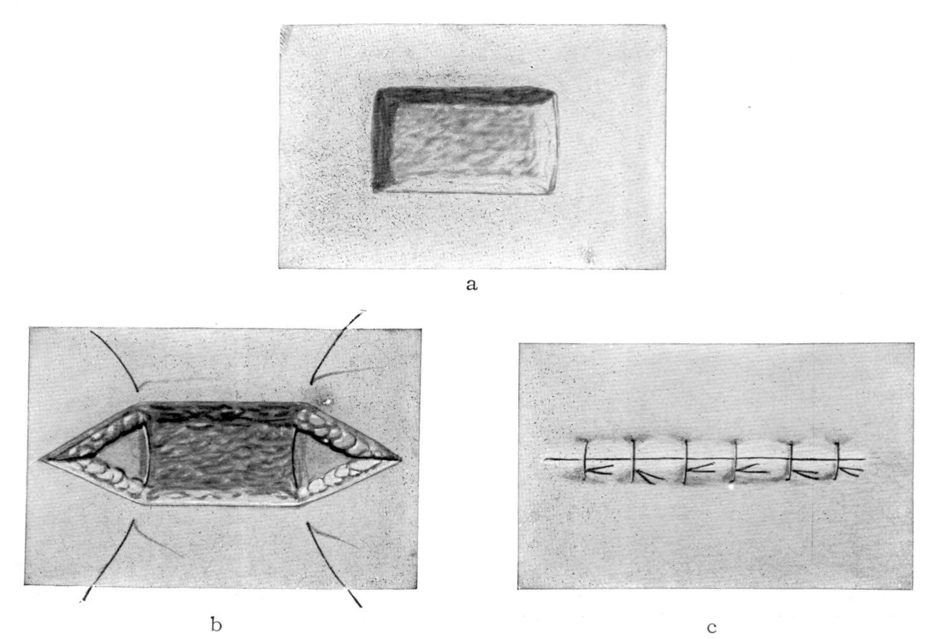

a b c

FIG. 367 a-c. Closure of a rectangular gap. Triangles of skin are cut from each end and the wound closed lengthwise.

as on the chin, over the spinous processes, over the crest of the ilium, and over the tibia. In large wounds the undercutting may be 10, 20 or more centimeters in width.

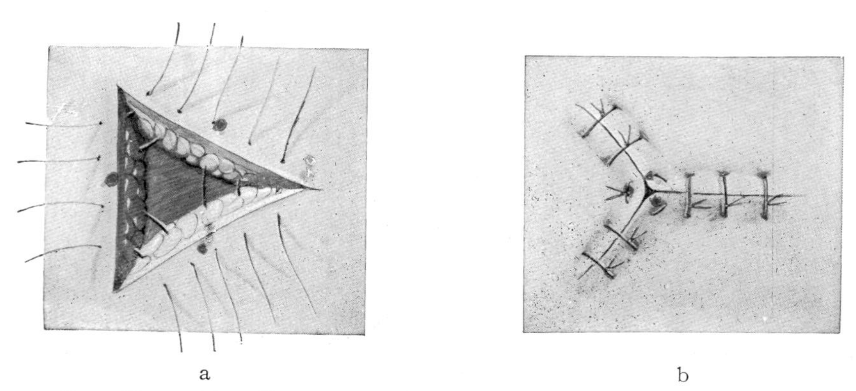

a b

FIG. 368 a and b. Closure of a triangular defect by suturing each angle.

Variously shaped skin defects can be closed easily, regardless of their diverse size. The treatment of these variously shaped defects, the closing of which can be done easily is well standardized. Therefore in closing defects

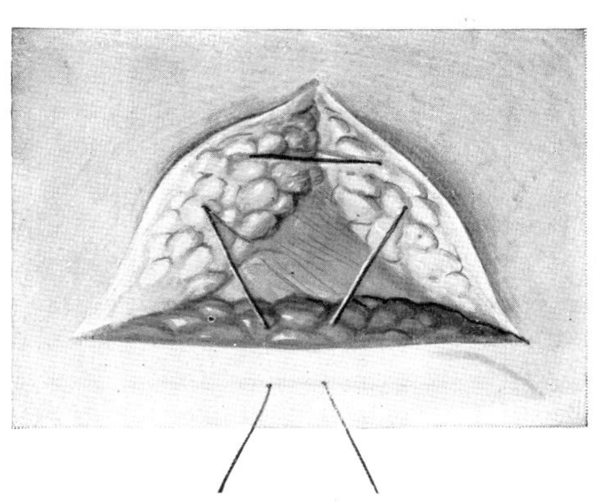

FIG. 369. Closure of a triangular defect by approximating the three sides with a subcutaneous suture.

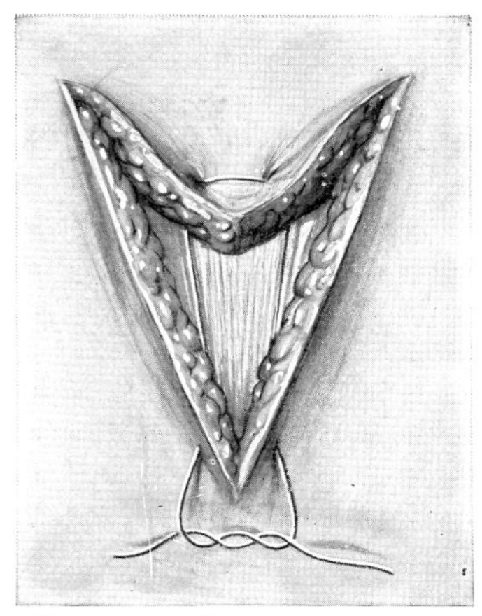

FIG. 370. Corner suture. Approximating an angle and a side in a triangular gap.

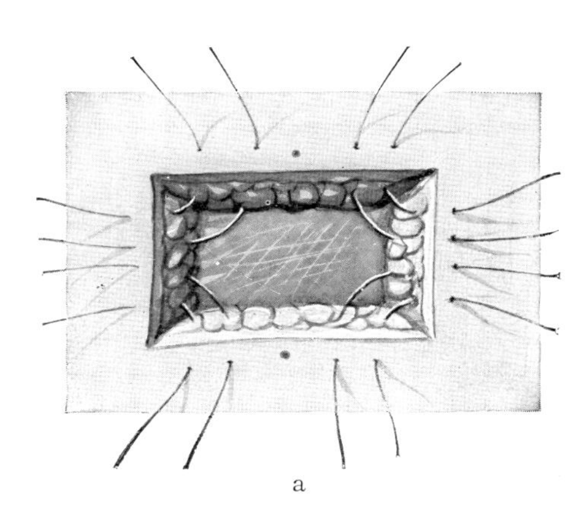

a

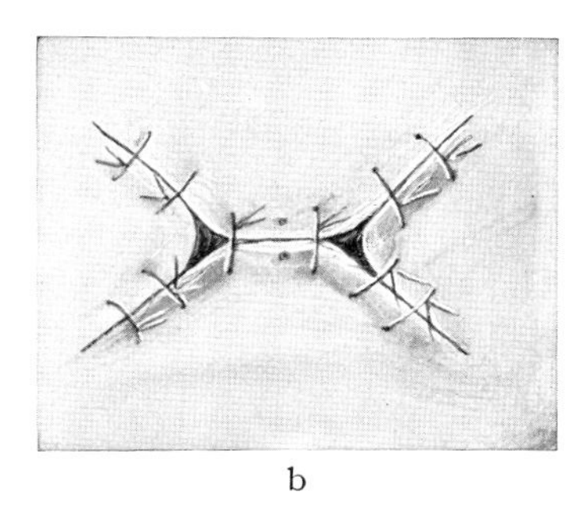

b

FIG. 371 a and b. Closure of a rectangular defect by suturing the four corners and the centers of the long sides.

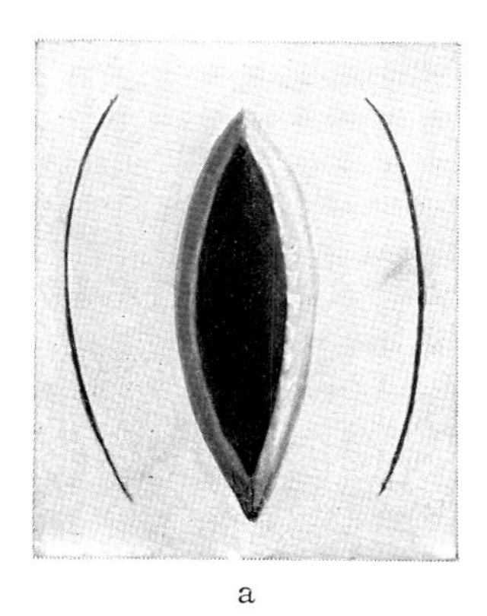

a

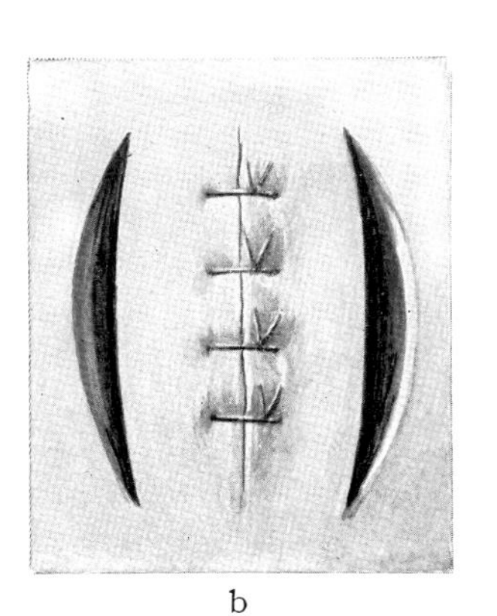

b

FIG. 372 a and b. Closure of an oval defect with lateral incisions to relieve tension.

immediately, or subsequently, certain typical shapes such as an oval, a triangle, or a square are outlined.

An oval or a rectangle is sutured transversely (Fig. 366), after being drawn lengthwise by two one-pronged hooks placed in the ends. The wound

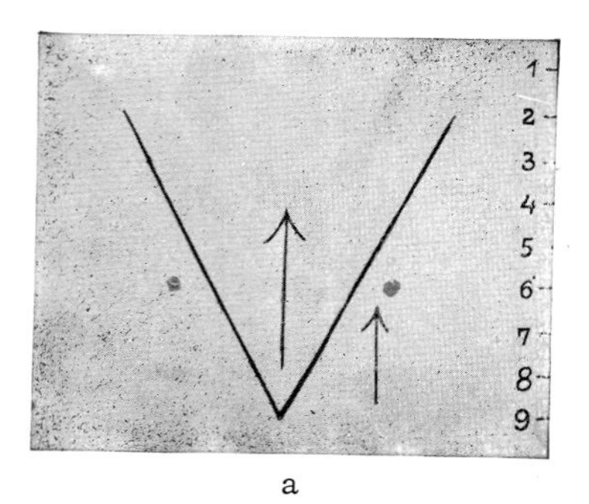

a

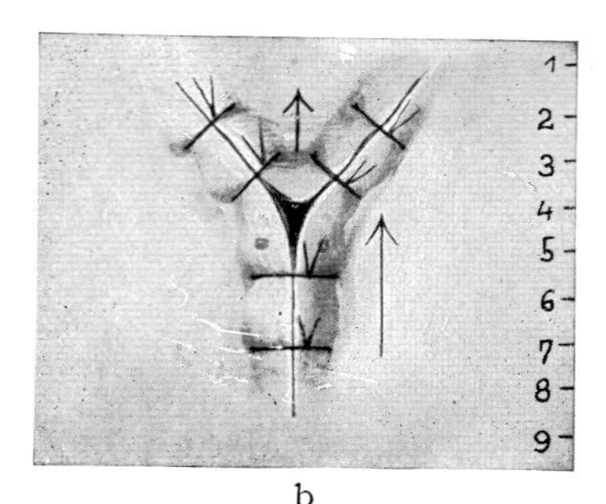

b

FIG. 373 a and b. Plastic operation by sliding V shaped flap, sutured as a Y.

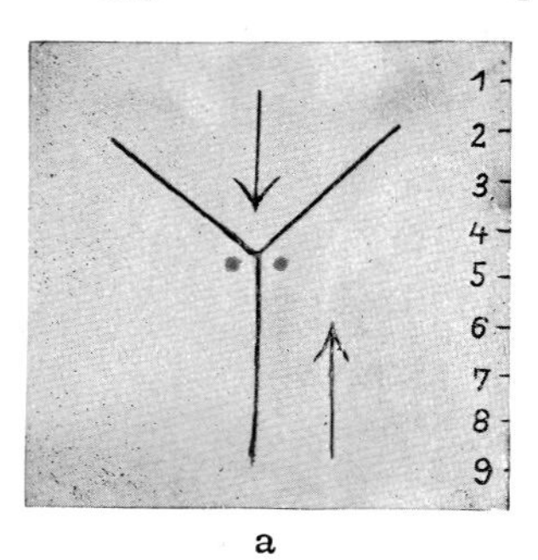

a

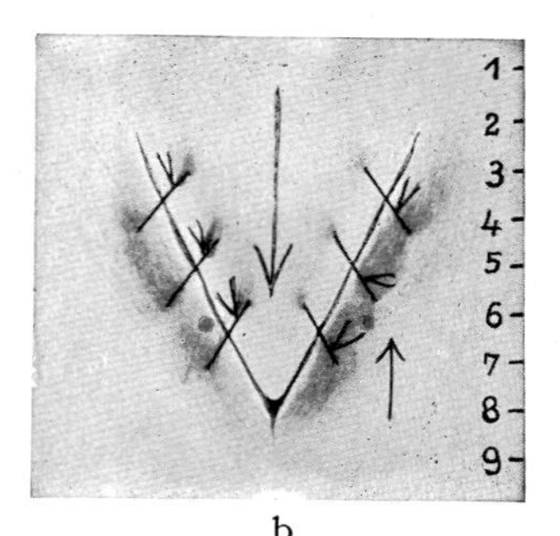

b

FIG. 374 a and b. Plastic operation where Y shaped incision is sutured as a V.

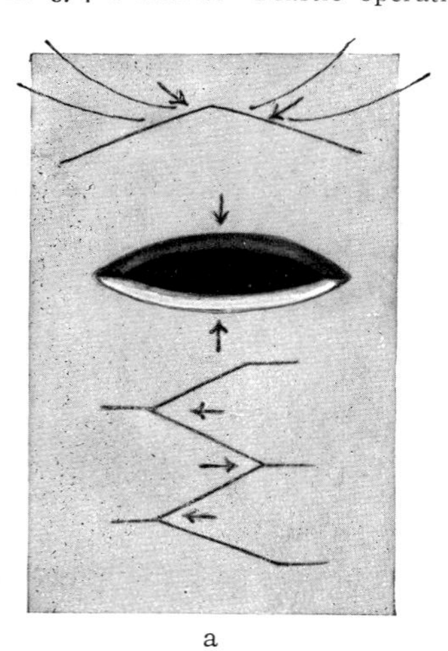

a

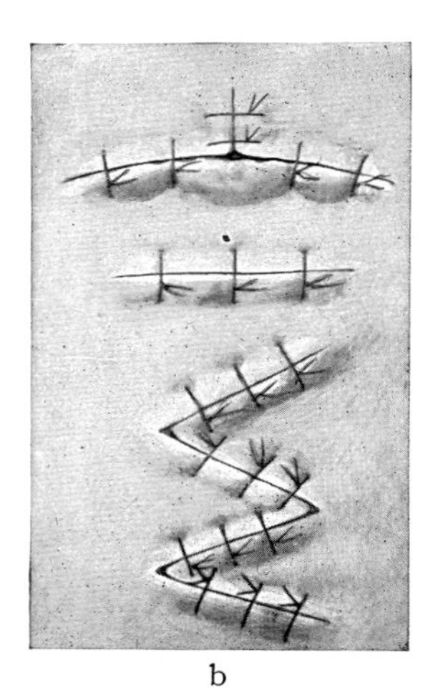

b

FIG. 375 a and b. Sliding the skin after several Y shaped incisions which are sutured as V's.

margins may be separated from the underlying tissues if necessary. The procedure is so simple, that rectangular defects may be made to assume an oval shape subsequently, by cutting out pointed sections from the narrow sides

(Fig. 367). We meet here for the first time with the remarkable fact, that a further loss of skin facilitates the covering of an existent skin defect.

Triangular defects are closed by suturing the angles as shown in figure 368. The suture begins at the angles and is carried inward. When this

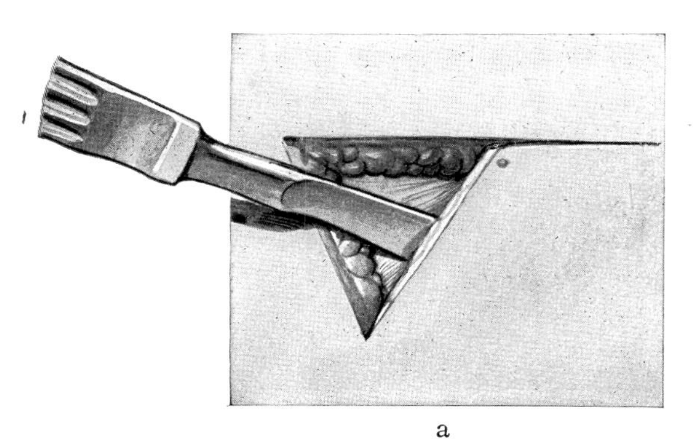

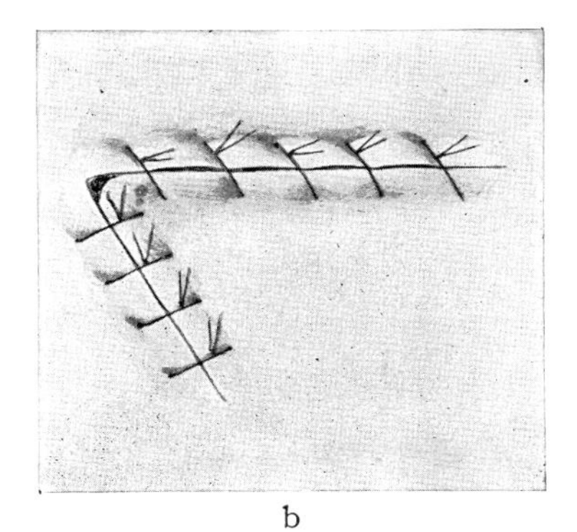

a b

FIG. 376 a and b. Covering a triangular defect by extending one wound margin in a straight incision. Undercutting the edges, and the finished suture.

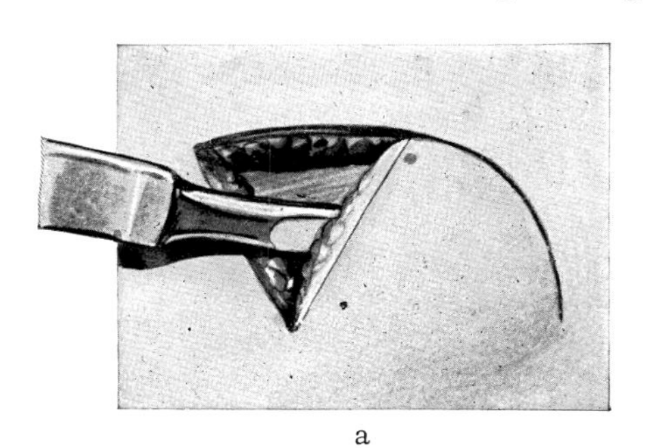

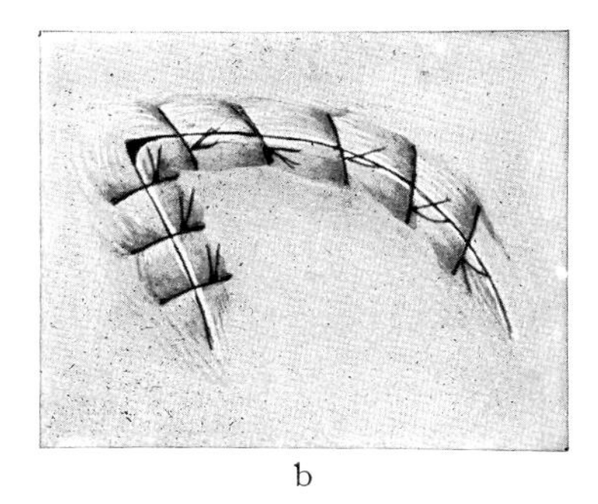

a b

FIG. 377 a and b. Covering a triangular defect by an extension of a wound margin laterally in an arc. Undercutting the edges, and the completed suture.

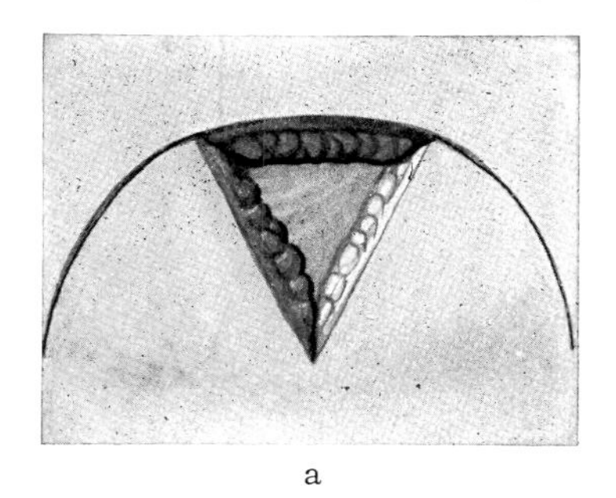

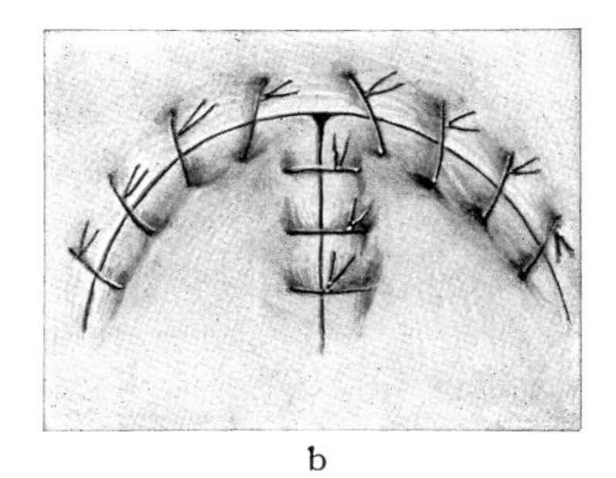

a b

FIG. 378 a and b. Covering a triangular defect by extension of a wound margin in an arc at each side. The edges are undercut and then sutured.

type of suture is used tension on the suture lines is lessened by the insertion of either a cuticular or subcuticular suture which passes through the center of two sides and both ends of which are carried through the center of the third side to be tied there (Fig. 369).

In a similar manner the base of a triangle can be caught by a suture which is then passed through the sides of the angle opposite it (tip-suture Fig. 370). A rectangle can be closed by suturing first the four corners, as

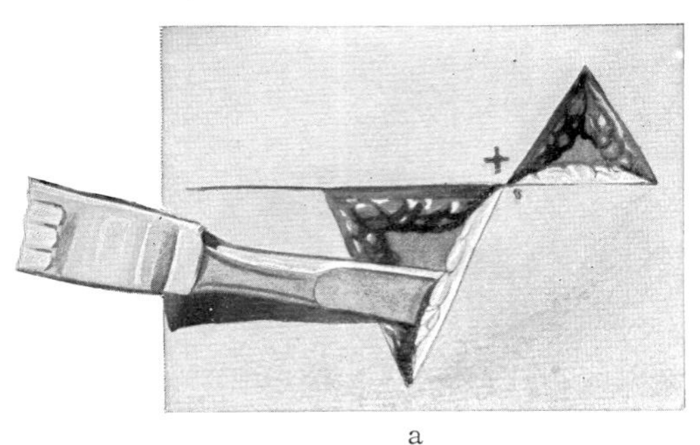

a

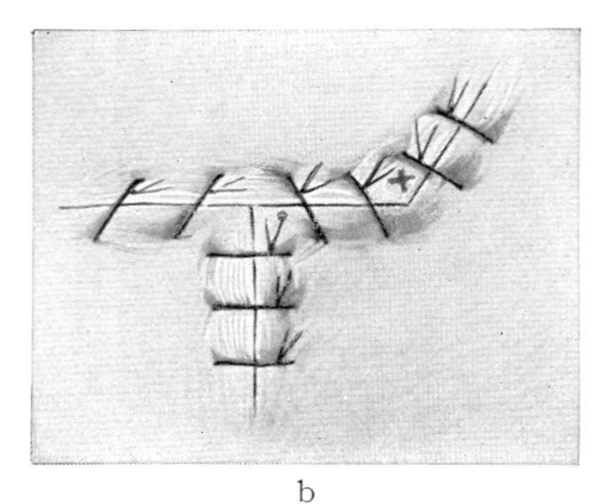

b

Fig. 379 a and b. Repairing a triangular defect by a direct extension of the wound margin to one side. A triangle is cut from the opposite side and the wound is sutured after mobilization of the flaps.

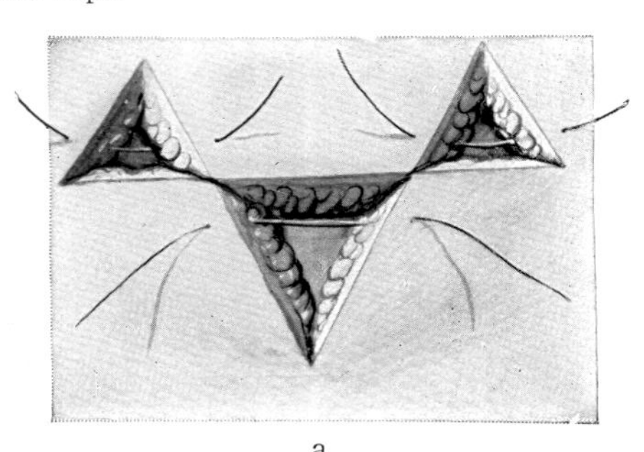

a

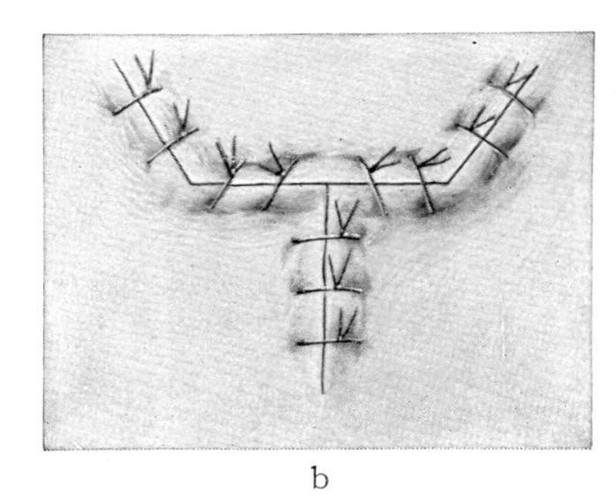

b

Fig. 380 a and b. Repairing a triangular defect by direct extensions of a wound margin toward both sides. A triangle is cut from each side and the wound sutured after mobilization of the edges.

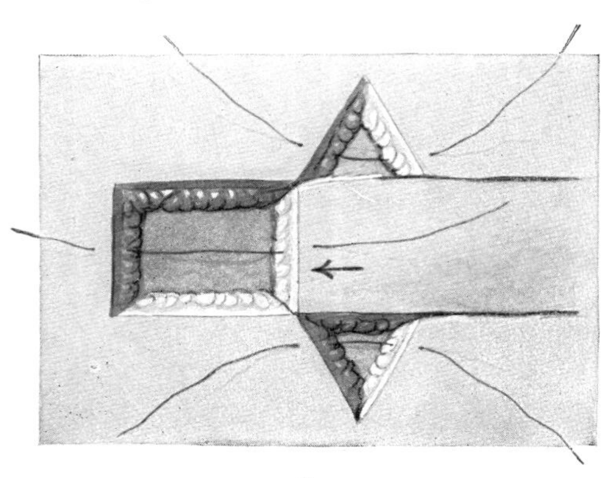

a

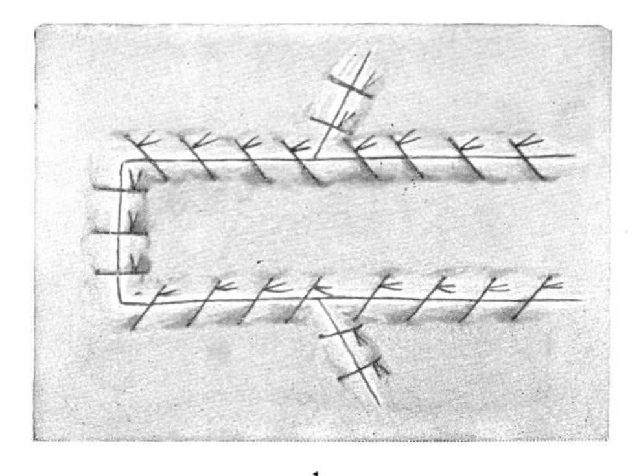

b

Fig. 381 a and b. Repairing a rectangular defect by lateral extension of two parallel wound margins. Two triangles are excised and the wound sutured after extensive freeing of the wound margins.

in suturing the adjacent sides of a triangle, and then by suturing the two approximated long sides with interrupted sutures (Fig. 371).

Lateral incisions provide a method for relieving the tension on the margins of a cutaneous defect which are to be drawn together by suture (Fig. 372). The resulting defects are either not sutured, or when closed the suturing is done in such a way as to bring the tissues together in the desired direction under the least tension. In the latter case the incisions to relieve tension must necessarily be made in a suitable shape. Thus, for this purpose, a V shaped incision may be sutured as a Y (Fig. 373), or a Y incision closed as a V (Fig. 374).

By making several adjacent Y shaped incisions and suturing them in the form of V's, a surplus of skin can be produced which will permit the closure of a defect without tension (Fig. 375).

If the edges of the incisions made to relieve tension are undercut, a much greater degree of mobility can be obtained from the loose flaps of skin. In this way triangular defects may often be closed by means of straight (Fig. 376) or curved (Fig. 377) extensions of the wound margin from one or both sides (Fig. 378), and by undercutting the edges. This principle is applied in the operation for "rotation of the cheek" (Esser). Rectangular

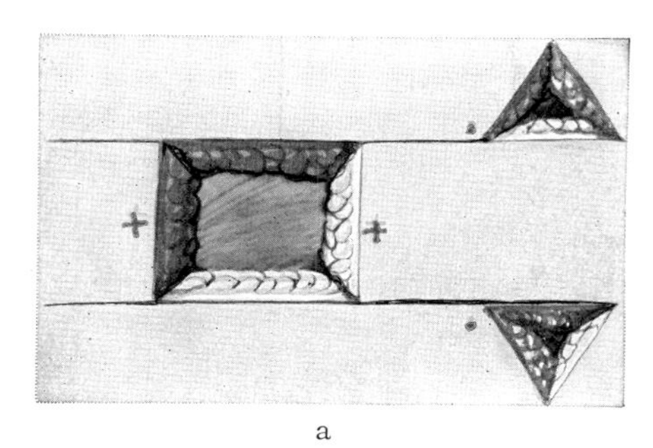

a

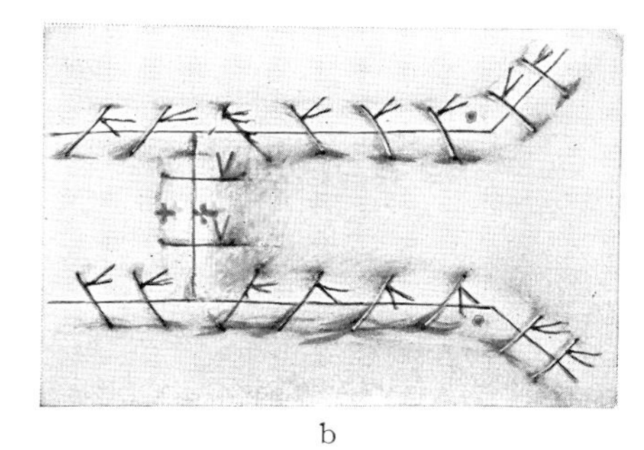

b

FIG. 382 a and b. Repairing a rectangular defect by extension of two parallel wound margins toward each side. Two triangles are cut as illustrated and the wound sutured after undercutting the edges.

defects may be repaired by lateral extension of two parallel wound margins to one (Fig. 381) or both (Fig. 382) sides, and mobilizing the rectangular flap, or flaps, and their margins by undercutting.

Frequently when the skin is drawn over the defect there is considerable strain at certain points, and the burden of this tension rests on a few sutures. If triangles of skin are excised at the points of strain, the tension will be relieved, and, at the same time, distributed over a larger number of sutures. In closing a triangular or a rectangular defect, therefore, triangles may be cut to the outer side of the parallel extensions of the wound margins, as previously described (Figs. 379-382).

3. Repair of Skin Defects by Pedunculated Skin Flaps from the Vicinity

The procedures just described of extending and undercutting the wound margins form a transition to the pedunculated skin flap. One side of the skin flap is continuous with one side of the defect (as in Fig. 388), the skin flap from directly adjacent tissue, or the margins are separated by intact skin (as n Fig. 386), the skin flap from the vicinity. The important point of every flap is its nutrition.

There are a number of general rules to be observed in this connection. It is of the greatest importance for the nutrition and the cosmetic results in many plastic operations that the incision be accurately made. I, therefore, outline on the skin with a dye the exact line of incision before beginning, or at least during the course of a plastic operation. A tape measure, compass, pieces of rubber bandage for models of defects and flaps are indispensable (Figs. 400 and 431). The models cut from old rubber bandages are better than those from the customary Billroth cambric. The flaps should always be cut slightly larger than the defect, because they shrink when detached and they must not be stretched in their new location.

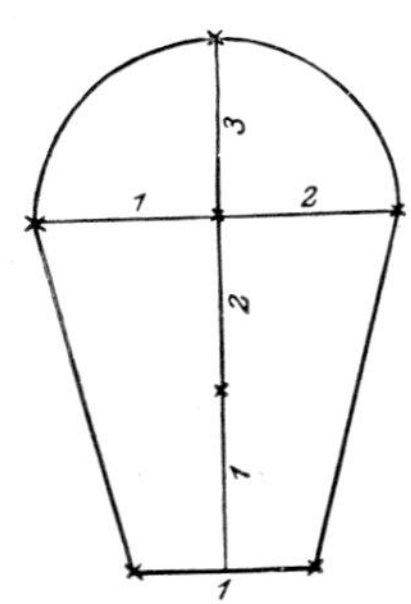

FIG. 383. Correct proportions of a pedunculated skin flap. The width of the pedicle of the flap should not be less than half the greatest width of the flap; the flap should not be longer than three times the width of the base of the pedicle.

I use local anæsthesia without hesitation, for I do not believe that it lowers the vitality of the flaps. The pedicle of the flap should be as wide as possible, as a rule not smaller than half the greatest width of the flap. The flap itself should be as short as possible, as a rule not longer than three times the narrowest part of the pedicle (Fig. 383). Since the arteries supplying the skin run in the subcutaneous connective tissue directly upon the superficial fascia, they are preserved only when this fascia is included in the flap. As far as nutrition is concerned it makes no difference whether a flap on the body and on the extremities is pedunculated proximally or distally (Fig. 396).

The rules for laying out a flap are only general and can be partially infringed upon with impunity, if certain precautions are taken. These depend upon the fact that the flap to be transplanted will become gradually accustomed to a lessening of nutrition or, that by gradually reducing other nutritional channels, the flap will be thrown more and more upon the only remaining source of subsistence, the flap pedicle. With this in mind, the following measures are applicable:

An incision is made around the flap, leaving the site of the pedicle intact, the flap is then sutured in situ, either without being undercut or, in some cases, after being freed from its bed. It is allowed to heal and at a later operation it is pedunculated. A second procedure is to raise either a part of or the entire flap from its bed, insert a layer of gauze, Billroth cambric, or rubber tissue under it, to prevent the flap from adhering, and over this to replace the flap, suturing the edges to avoid shrinking (Fig. 384). The flap is released and pedunculated in several stages. The newly released portions are prevented from reuniting by inserting larger pieces of material or by suturing the edges in tubular form for the pedicle (Fig. 401). Or a third procedure is to begin with the formation of the pedicle of the flap, preventing re-adherence of the pedicle by tubular suture (Fig. 419) or by means of suitable inlays. The pedunculation is carried out in several stages, and the flap released as the last step. It is possible to obtain by this method flaps and pedicles of amazing length.

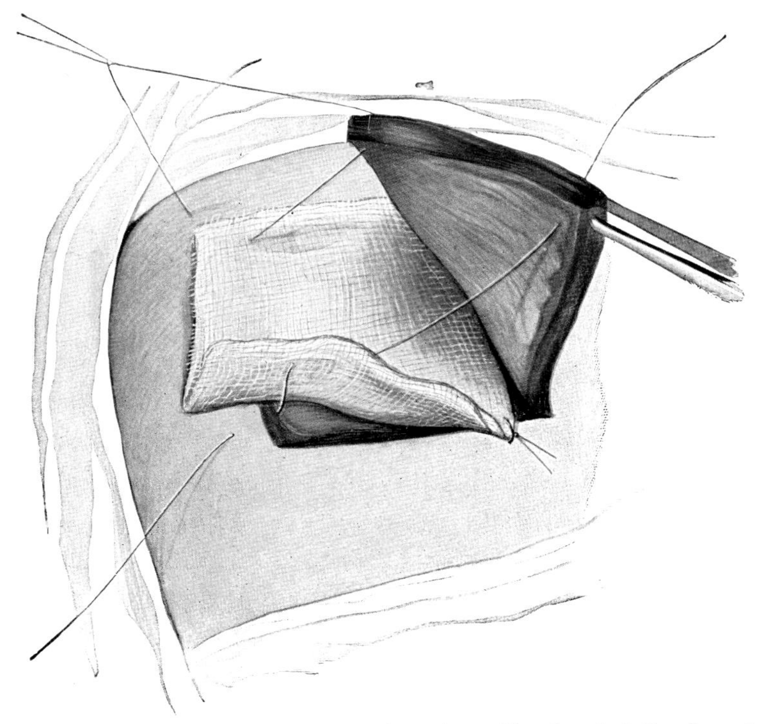

Fig. 384. Preparing a skin flap for transplantation. The detached flap is replaced in its wound-bed, where union is prevented by inserting a layer of gauze. Its entire circulation is received through the pedicle.

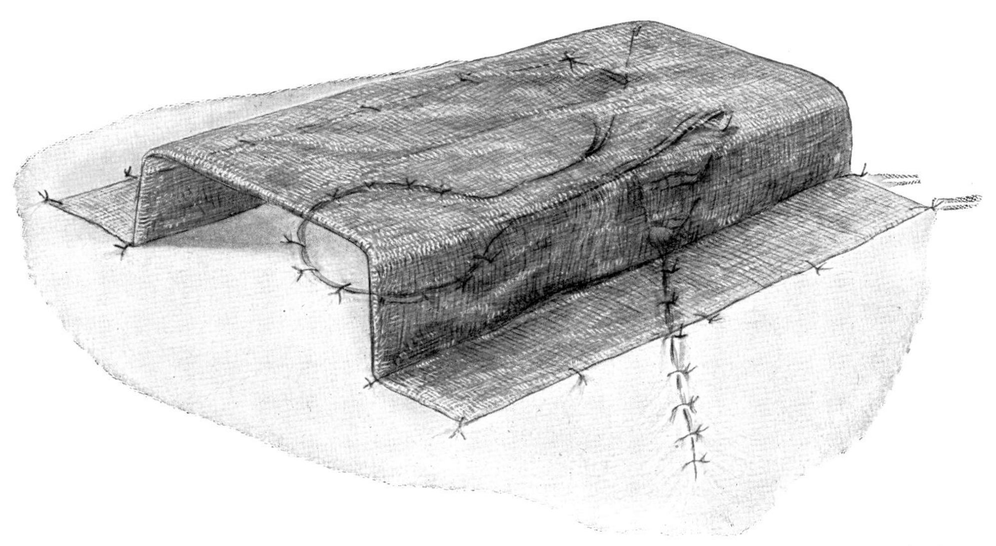

Fig. 385. Wire netting used as a protective dressing in plastic surgery, to prevent injurious pressure and to allow observation and exposure to the air.

The pedicle of a skin flap should be twisted or bent as little as possible, so that there will be no interference with the exchange of tissue fluids. When the pedicle is included in a dressing, it must be protected from pressure. This can be done by a frame of cardboard, wood, or wire netting fastened in place

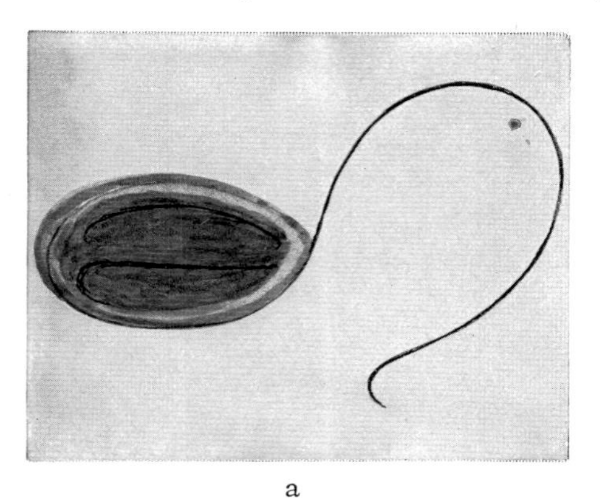

a

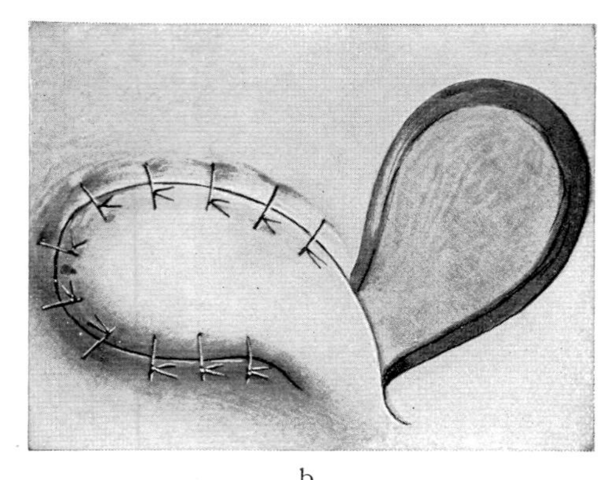

b

FIG. 386 a and b. Formation of an adjacent pedunculated flap that is placed in the primary defect by rotating the pedicle.

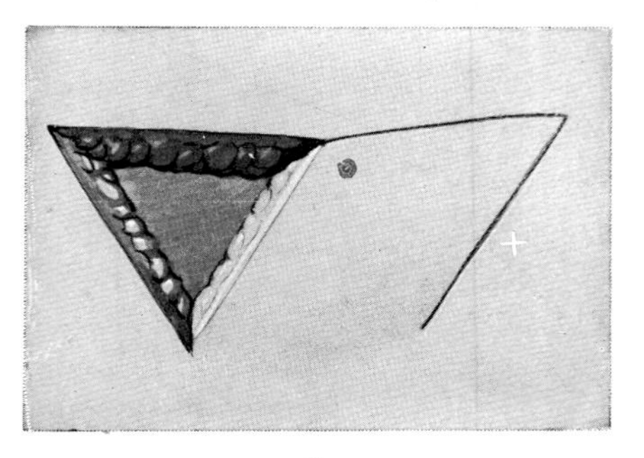

a

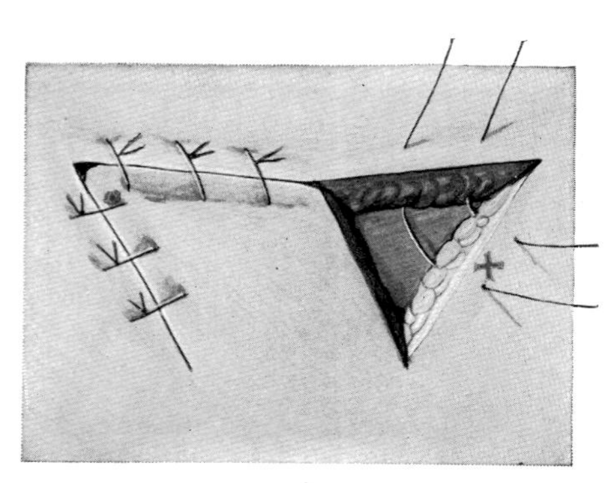

b

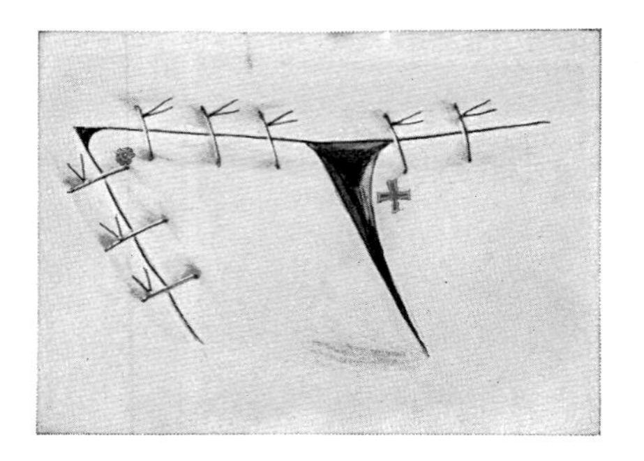

c

FIG. 387 a to c. Unilateral rhomboidal flap for closing a triangular defect. The newly formed triangular gap is closed by direct suture after mobilization of its margins.

over it (Fig. 385). It is better to leave the pedicle entirely free, so that its condition can be watched at all times.

The flap should fit freely in its new bed. It must not be forcibly stretched because of the danger of impeding the ebb and flow of tissue fluids.

Like all tissue grafts, skin flaps that are to be transplanted should be handled with the greatest care. The margins of the flap should preferably be straight or rounded, for angles and corners endanger nutrition. All these rules are

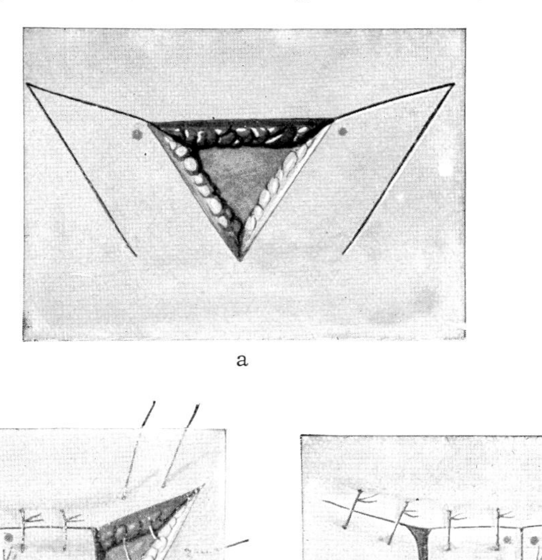

a

b c

Fig. 388 a to c. Bilateral rhomboidal flaps for closing a triangular defect. The newly formed triangular gaps are closed by direct suture.

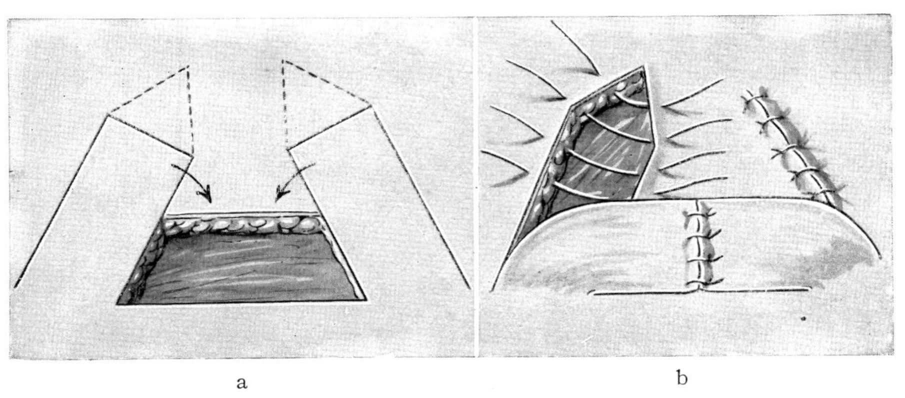

a b

Fig. 389 a and b. Bilateral rhomboidal flaps for closing a rectangular defect. The newly formed four-cornered gaps are closed by direct suture, after the ends are pointed by cutting out a triangle. The suture of the secondary gaps relieves the tension on the suture line of the flaps.

but general principles and should be influenced by the differences in the nutrition of the skin in various parts of the body, as well as in different individuals. The scalp, for instance, is particularly well nourished.

In those regions where arteries run for long distances in the subcutaneous tissues parallel to the skin, flaps receiving their nutrition from these arteries may be especially long and their pedicles especially small. The arteries

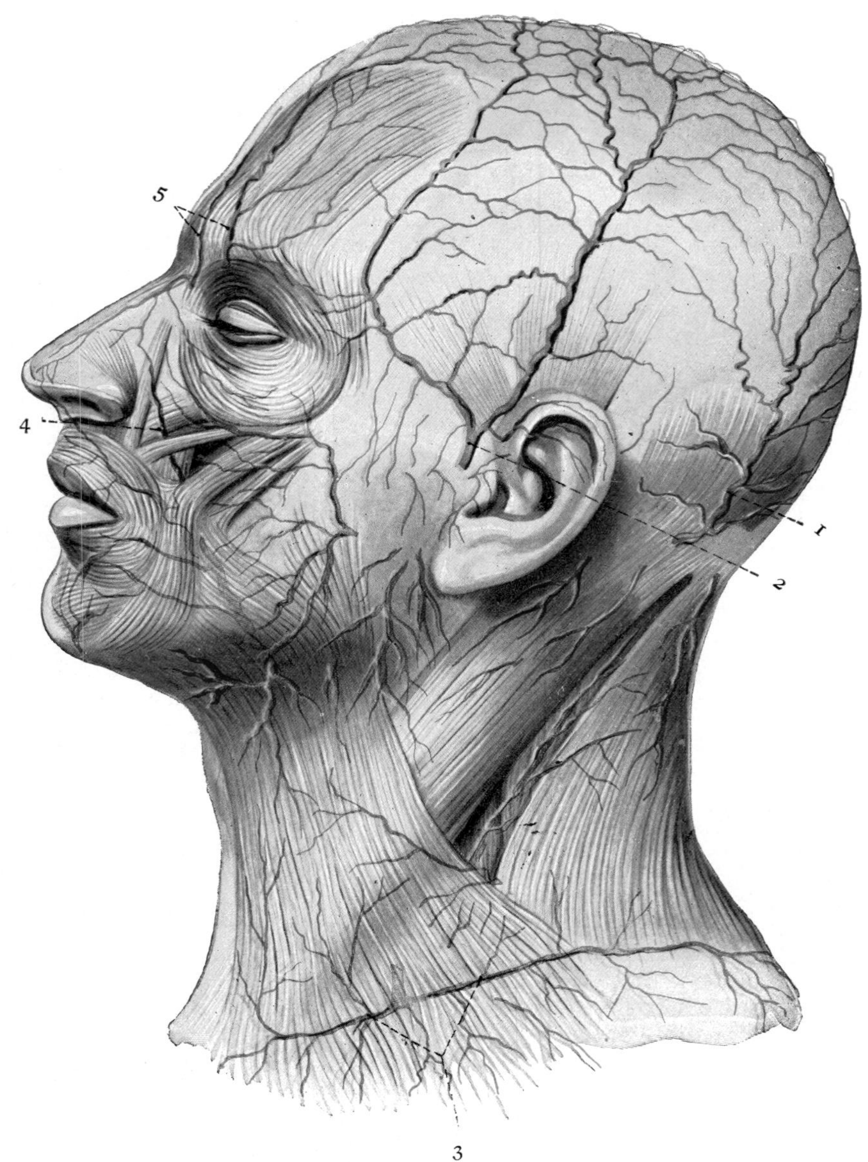

FIG. 390. Superficial arteries of the head and neck which are important in the formation of skin flaps (Manehot). 1. Occipital artery. 2. Temporal artery. 3. Anterior and posterior supraclavicular arteries. 4. Angular artery. 5. Frontal artery.

adapted to the formation of such flaps (Figs. 390, 391) are: 1. the temporal artery (Lexer's pistol-flap), running up directly in front of the ear (Figs. 397, 398); 2. the transverse facial artery, that runs from the temporo-maxillary articulation to the ala nasi; 3. the external maxillary artery and its

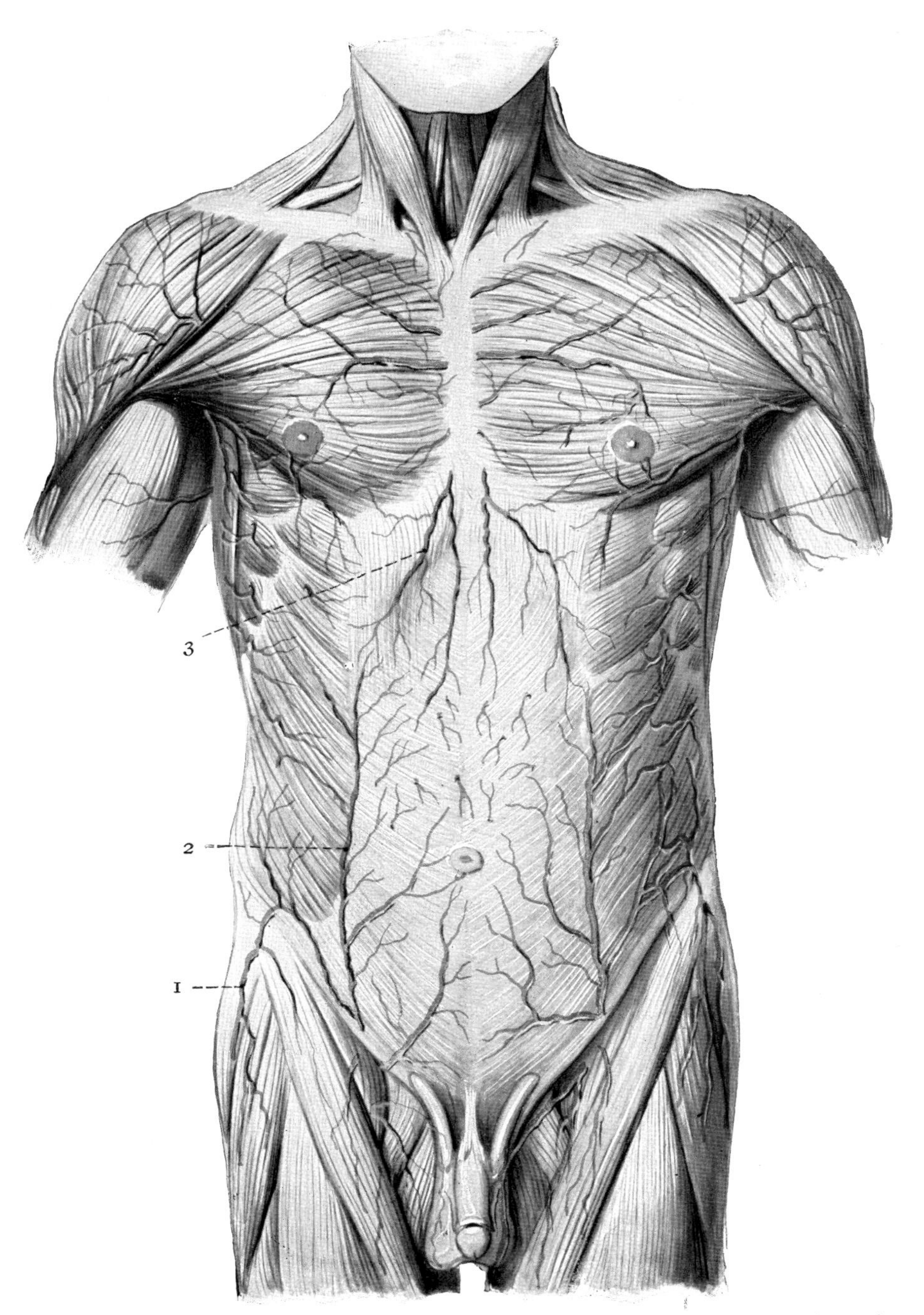

Fig. 391. Superficial arteries of the trunk which must be considered in the formation of skin flaps (Manehot). 1. External femoral artery. 2. Superficial epigastric artery. 3. Superior epigastric artery.

continuation, the angular artery, the former appearing on the face over the anterior border of the masseter muscle and passing from here to the angle of the mouth, thence along the border of the ala nasi to become the angular

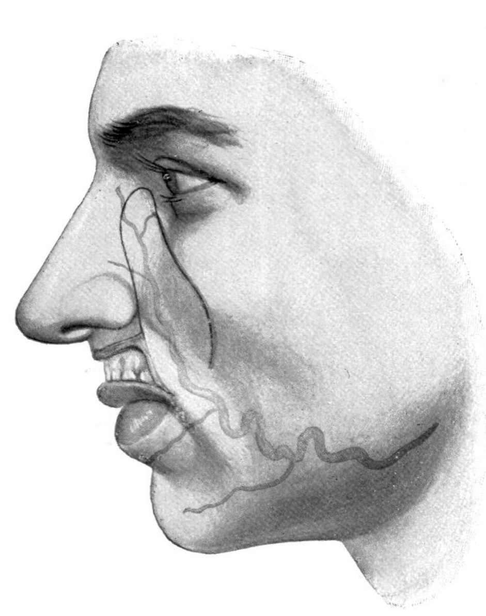

FIG. 392. Skin flap located in the nasolabial fold and supplied by the angular artery.

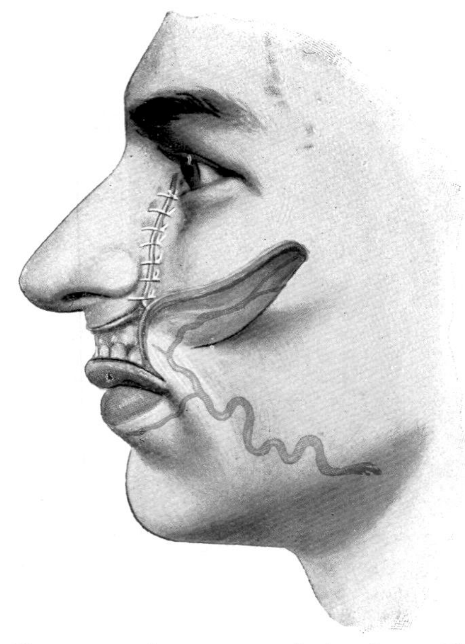

FIG. 393. Appearance of the flap. The flap of the former illustration has been mobilized and the resulting gap closed by suture.

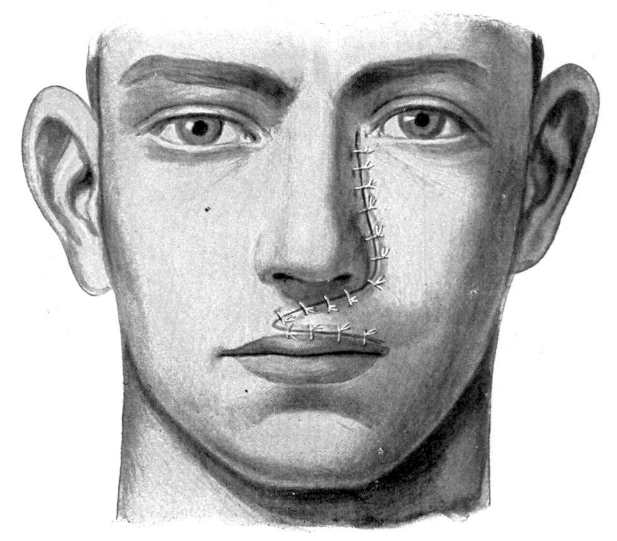

FIG. 394. Flap sutured in position in the defect on the upper lip.

artery, which passes to the inner canthus (Figs. 392, 393, 402); 4. the frontal arteries, which are in part a continuation of the latter, and in part, frontal branches of the superficial temporal and supra-orbital arteries, and which run from the inner canthus towards the forehead, and finally, 5. the occipital artery, which appears behind the mastoid process and is directed somewhat backward as it ascends on the cranium. If these vessels can be palpated

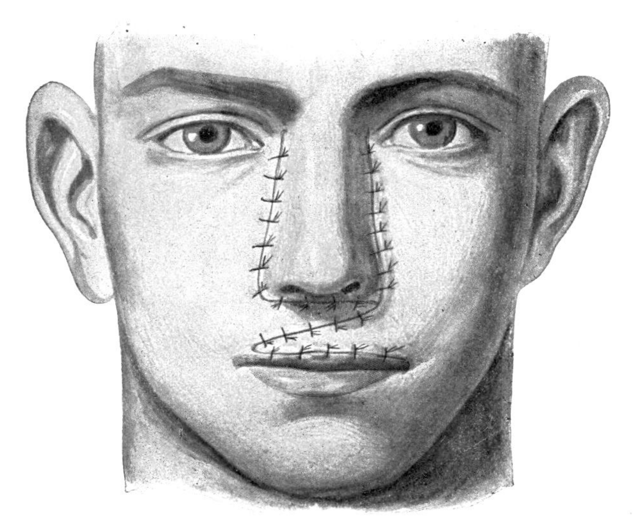

FIG. 395. The entire upper lip is reconstructed by two skin flaps taken from the nasolabial fold of each side, each flap supplied by the angular artery.

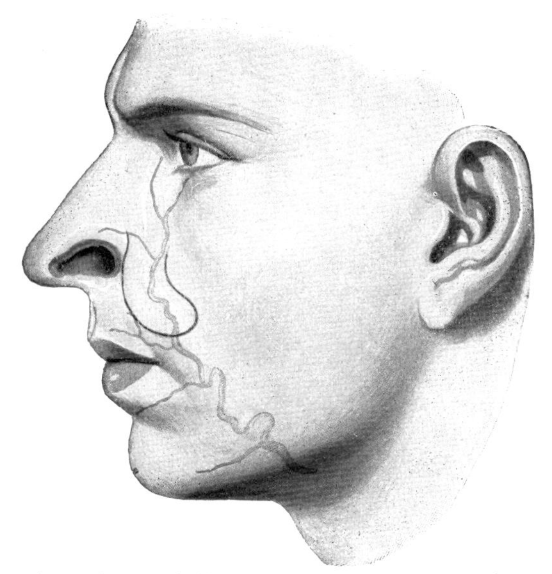

FIG. 396. Flap taken from the nasolabial fold to repair a nasal defect. The direction of the flap is opposite to the course of the angular artery.

under the skin, which is possible, for example, in the temporal artery as far as its ramifications on the forehead, I outline the course of these with a colored solution, adding the approximate course of the smaller vessels so that they can be visualized in outlining the flap.

It is possible to utilize as a pedicle for a flap a cutaneous bridge which

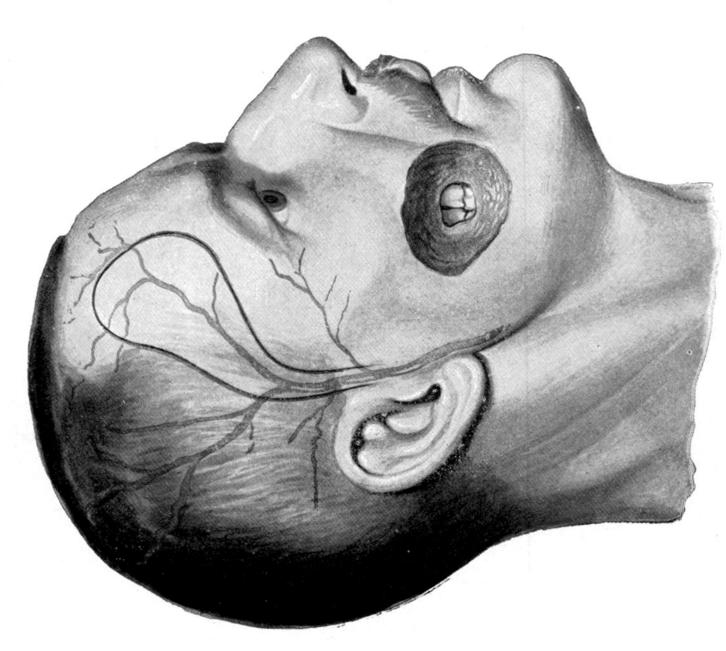

Fig. 397. Outlining a flap where the major portion of an artery is included in the flap. The base of the pedicle in this case can be very narrow and the flap can be very long. This is known as a bridge flap.

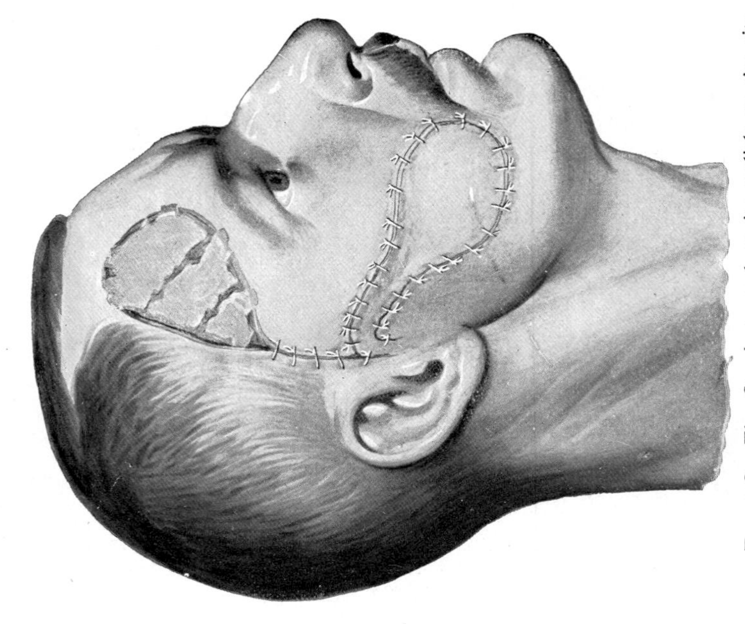

Fig. 398. The flap is turned on its pedicle to the site of the defect and sutured in place. In order to do this it is necessary to divide the skin between the defect and the base of the pedicle.

may be only a few millimeters wide but which will include the major artery supplying the area from which the flap is to be taken. The flap itself under these circumstances may be surprisingly large (Fig. 397). I have given up the use of any flap which does not contain a supporting artery (Fig. 402).

Bilateral pedunculated skin flaps may be used to cover a large defect. In these bilateral flaps the vascularization so obtained is much more efficient than that obtained from two individually nourished flaps. It is wise, how-

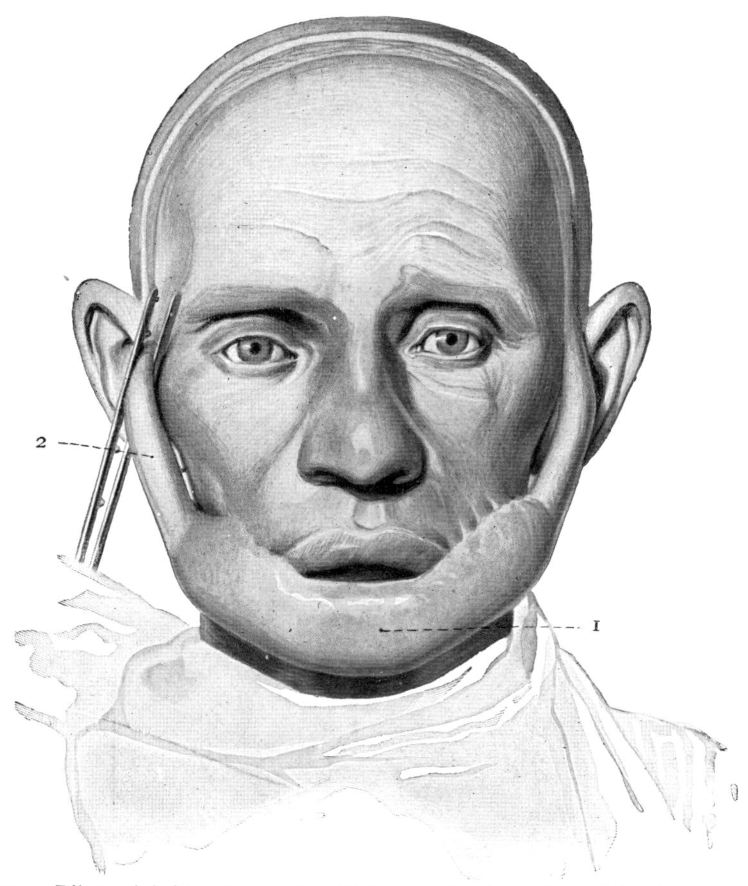

FIG. 399. Bilateral bridge flap (1), which contains in each pedicle the temporal artery. The pedicles are sutured in the form of a tube. The blood supply of one flap (2) is partially restricted for short periods in order to promote vascularization of the flap in its new bed.

ever, to shape the pedicles so that each pedicle can supply half of the flap. Such visor flaps are used very often to cover skin defects on the face. One may use for this purpose flaps from the neck, outlined as a collar incision, or flaps from the forehead or from the sinciput (Fig. 399), supplied by both temporal arteries. Bridge flaps may also be used for covering ulcers on amputation stumps (Samter) (Fig. 732).

In plastic operations, where the flap intended for use does not adjoin the defect directly, the pedicle of the flap must be carried over an area of intact skin. To protect the deeper surface of the pedicle from drying and from

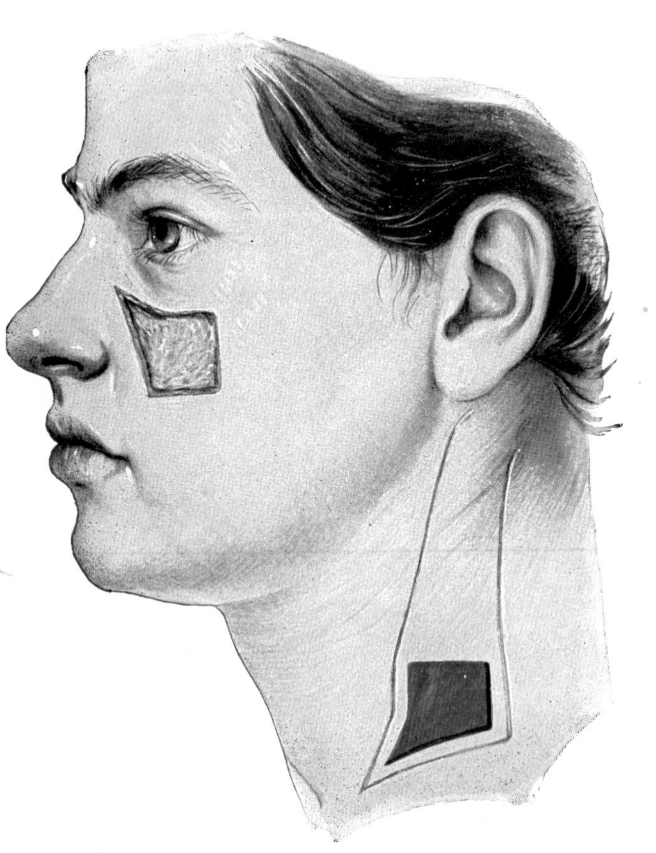

Fig. 400. Outlining a skin flap around a model of the defect to be covered.

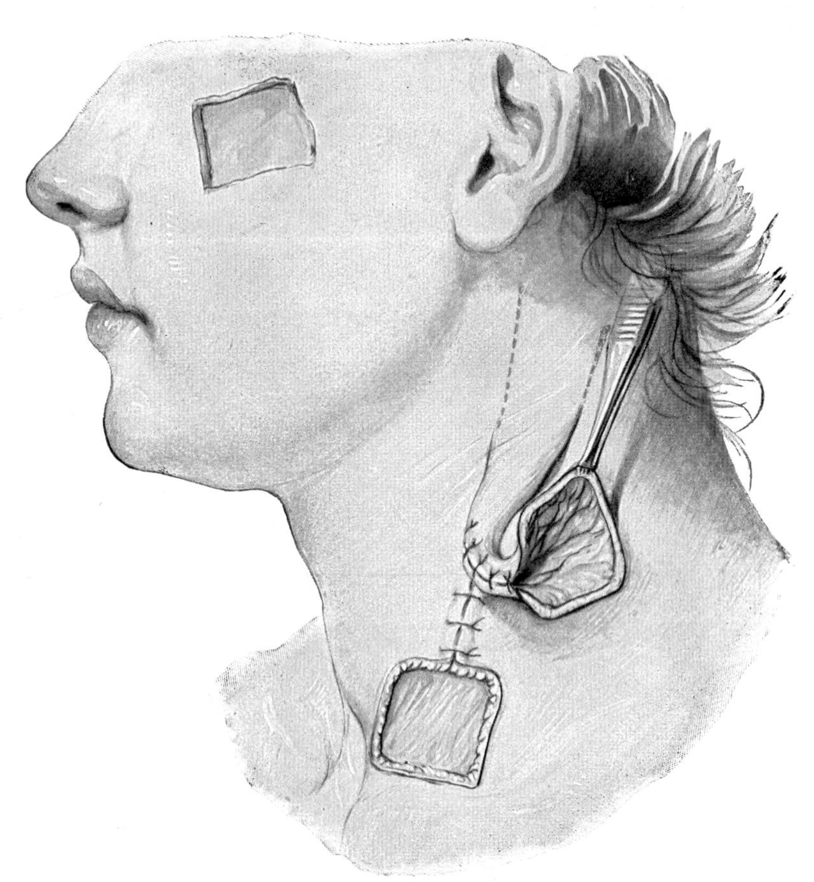

Fig. 401. Tube pedicle flap (Filatow). Intermediate stage.

infection while preparing the flap, it is advisable to sew it together in the form of a tube with the skin on the outside (tube plastic after Filatow, Figs. 399, 401, 419 and 425). If it is desired to avoid carrying the pedicle over the skin, and if the pedicle is not to be used later, it is possible to divide the skin under the pedicle, after transplantation of the flap and to suture the pedicle into the new wound (Fig. 398). When the pedicle of an arterial flap is not covered with skin, it must be entirely buried in the subcutaneous tissue, either by dividing the detached bridge of skin, imbedding the pedicle

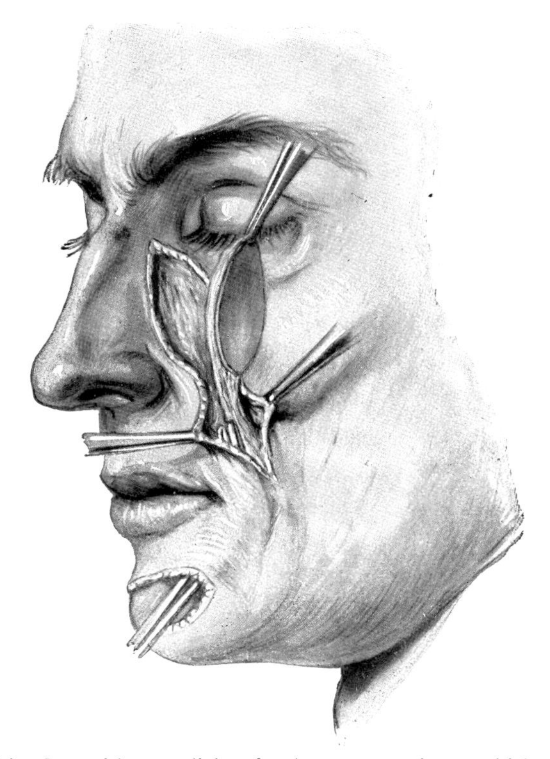

FIG. 402. A skin flap with a pedicle of subcutaneous tissue which contains the angular artery. The flap is drawn to the site to be filled in through a subcutaneous tunnel in which the pedicle remains (Esser).

and suturing the skin over it, or by tunneling under the skin and pulling the flap and pedicle under the skin bridge (Fig. 402).

The factors concerned in the division of a pedicle which lies over a bridge of skin are discussed on page 384. A skin flap which has been separated subsequently from its nutrient pedicle differs more from the surrounding skin in color and consistency, as a rule, than one whose pedicle remains attached to the original parent tissue.

The defect resulting from the removal of a flap is taken care of according to the general rules covering plastic procedures. It may be closed by drawing the edges of the wound together, or by free grafts (Thiersch). In shaping the primary flaps, one should carefully consider the feasibility of closing the secondary defect. This is well illustrated in the formation of the Gersuny type of sliding flaps (Figs. 403, 404). Gersuny attains this object by cutting the flap so that one or more corners are pointed. The point of the flap can be used to cover the secondary skin defect resulting from the removal of the

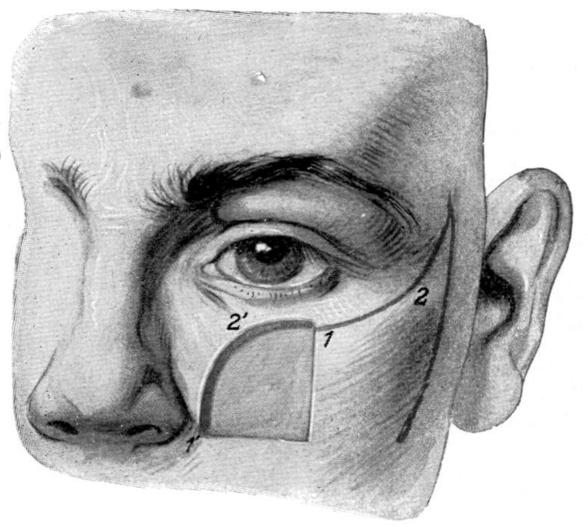

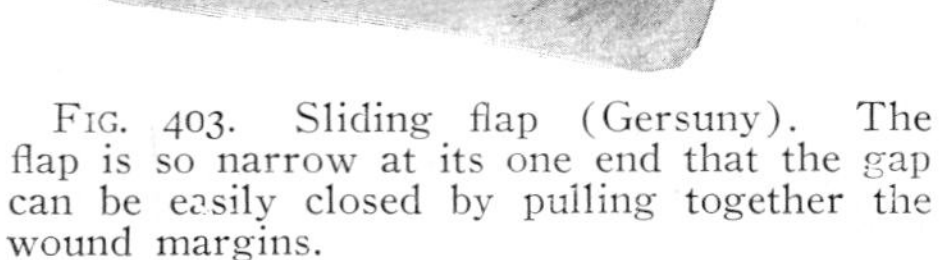
Fig. 403. Sliding flap (Gersuny). The flap is so narrow at its one end that the gap can be easily closed by pulling together the wound margins.

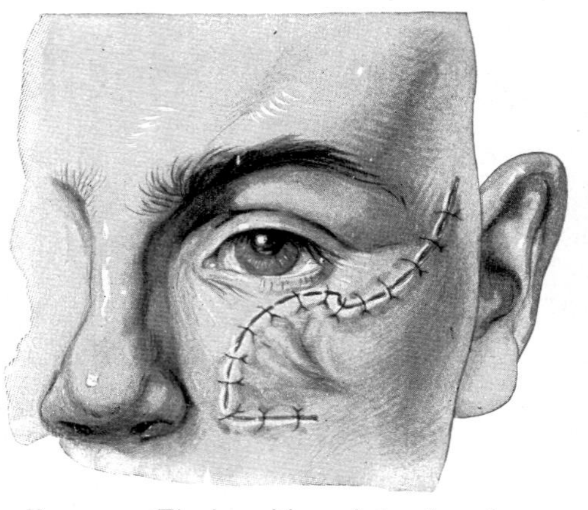

Fig. 404. Final position of the flap shown in the previous illustration and suture of the secondary gap.

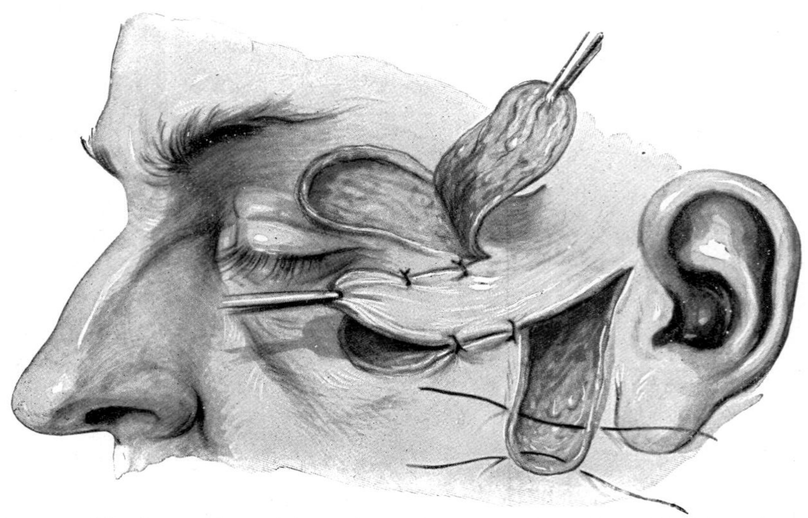

Fig. 405. Plastic to close defect above the external canthus (Esser). A two point flap is made. One flap serves to close the primary skin defect, and the second flap covers the bed left by elevation of the first flap. The remaining defect is closed by suture or by a Thiersch graft.

primary flap, while the pointed corner of this defect can be drawn together with relative ease.

The closure of the secondary defect is sometimes as serious a matter as the closure of the primary one. In such cases the use of a two point flap (Esser) may be of advantage (Fig. 405). The procedure consists in shaping a two point flap in such way that the first point can be drawn into the primary defect, the second point, into the defect left by removal of the first point. The less important defect left by the removal of the second point can be closed in one of the usual ways. Naturally, the procedure is only of advantage if the second point can not be used to close the primary defect. This procedure might well be called a "spoke-plastic."

4. Repair of Skin Defects by Pedunculated Flaps from a Distance

Since the skin of widely separated parts of the body, especially of the extremities, can be brought into contact by posture, it is possible to use pe-

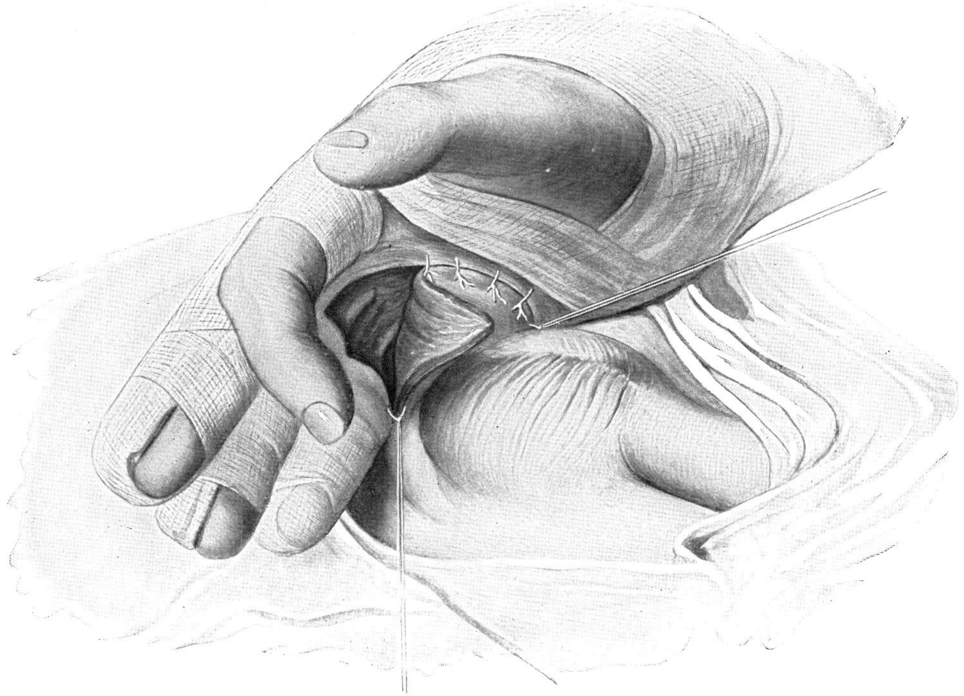

Fig. 406. Skin graft of the hand from the scrotum. The pedicle will be cut when the graft becomes adherent.

dunculated skin flaps from an entirely different area to repair a defect, if the area of the defect and of the flap can be brought together by posture. The defect left by the removal of the flap can be closed primarily, secondarily, or by Thiersch grafts. Skin losses on the fingers, hand, and forearm can thus be replaced with skin from the scrotum (Figs. 406, 407 and 412), the abdomen (Figs. 408 and 410), the breast, the back, and the thigh, and, on the other hand, skin losses on these parts of the body can be covered with pedunculated flaps from the forearm. For facial repair we may use skin from the hand, the forearm, and the arm (Fig. 411). It is possible to transfer skin flaps with temporary pedicles from one leg to the other (Fig. 409), or to bring a foot in contact with the opposite leg, or with a hand for a skin graft. The breast on the same side has been used to cover a thigh stump.

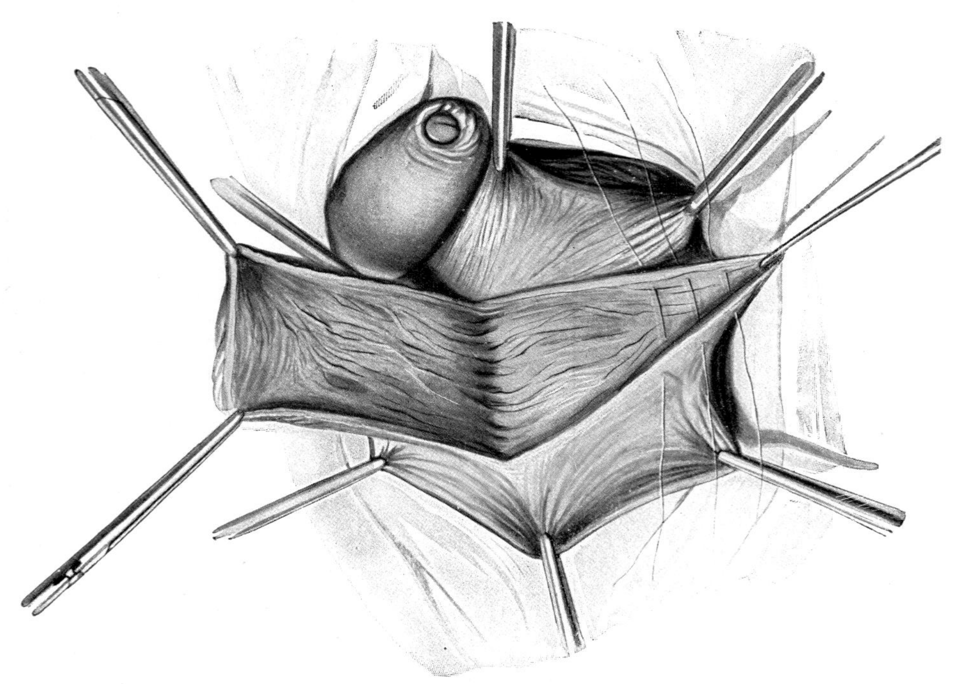

FIG. 407. Flap formation from the skin of the scrotum with a temporary pedicle. The resulting skin defect is closed by direct suture.

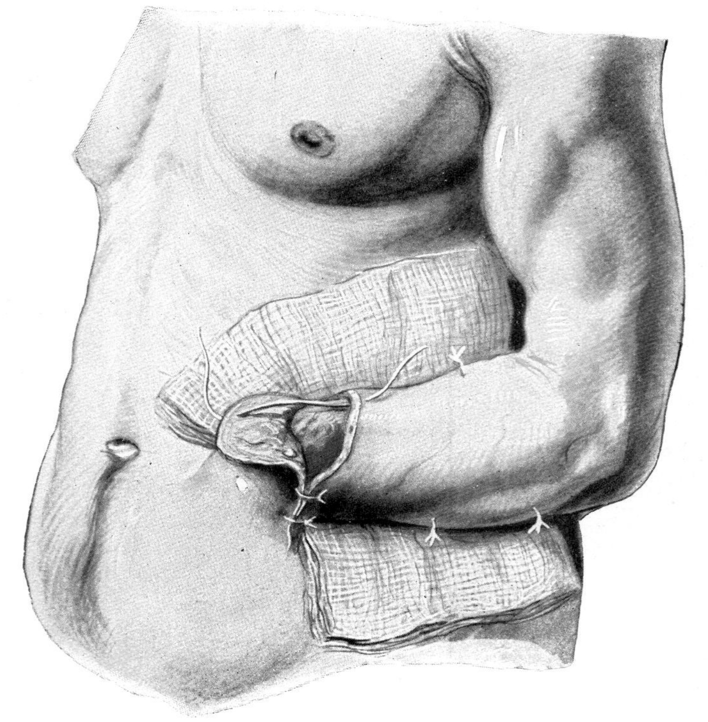

FIG. 408. A flap from the abdomen is used to cover a defect on an amputation stump of the forearm. The pedicle will be cut when the graft becomes adherent.

When a defect of an extremity is corrected by inserting it under a raised bridge flap, it is called a "muff plastic" (Fig. 410).

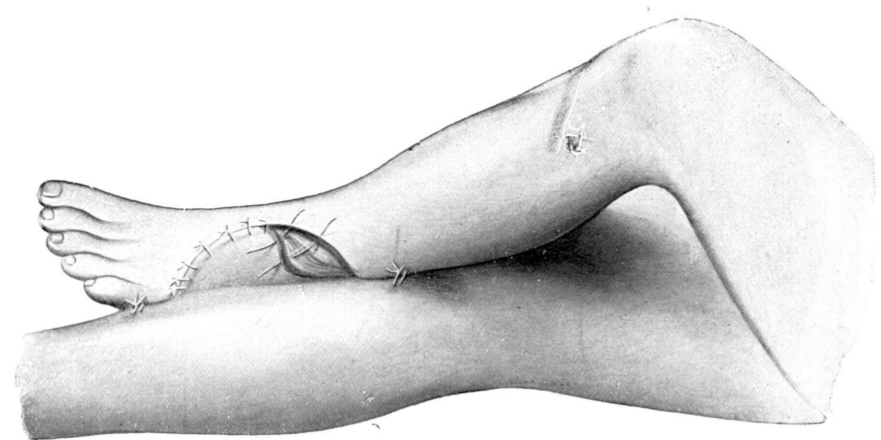

FIG. 409. Pedunculated skin graft from one leg to the other.

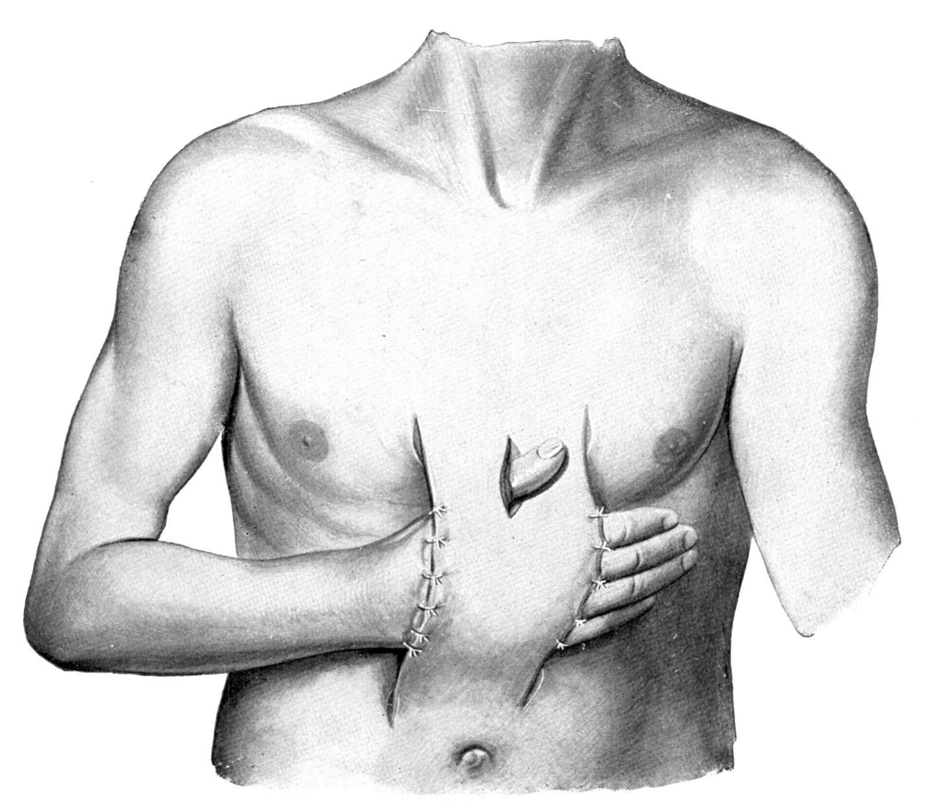

FIG. 410. Pedunculated graft from the abdomen to the back of the hand.

When two distant parts are brought in contact for transplantation of a pedunculated flap, they must be carefully immobilized so that there will be no tension nor pressure on the pedicle. When an extremity must be held in

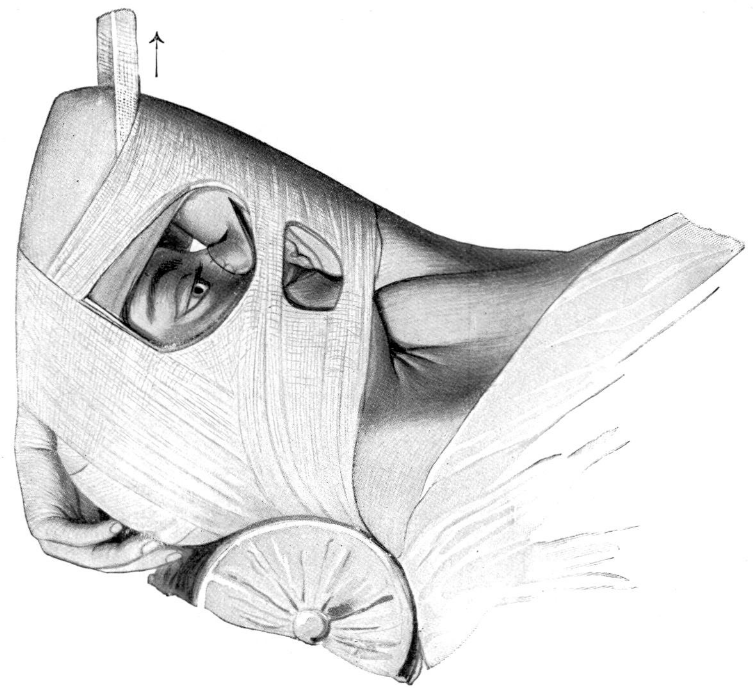

FIG. 411. Method of holding upper extremity to the face after a pedicle graft to the nose (Italian Method). This method permits the graft to be seen freely. The band under the elbow which is provided with a weight compensates for any change of position of the arm.

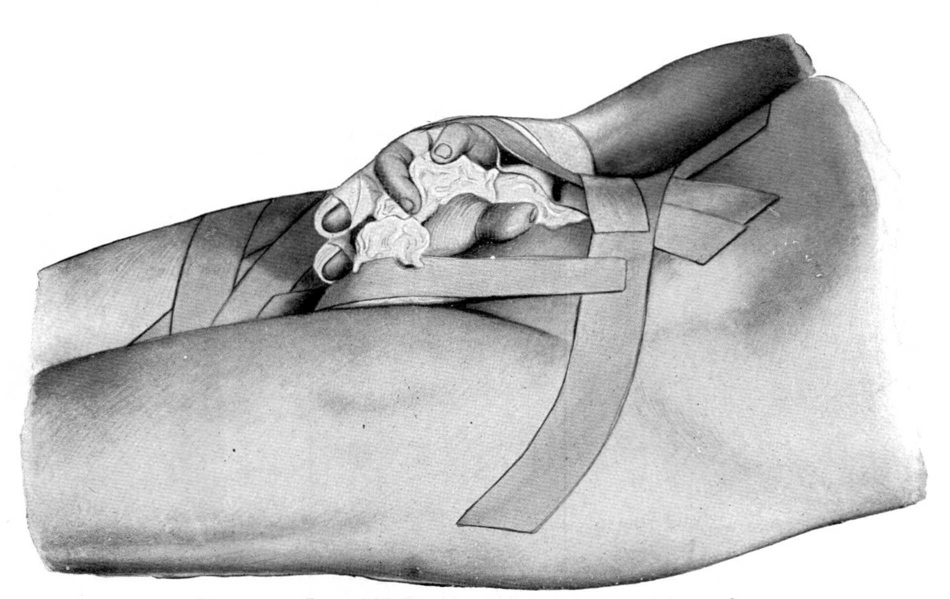

FIG. 412. Immobilizing the parts after a pedicle graft.

a constant position, often an uncomfortable one, for from ten to fourteen days, some type of restraint must be used. A plastic of the face during warm weather frequently taxes a patient almost beyond his endurance. The patient should be given narcotics, morphine or bromides, or hypnotics, to help him through this period. Before the flap is raised and the extremity fixed in place, the position most tolerable for the patient should be determined. In planning the flap, the extremity is placed in contact with the defect in the

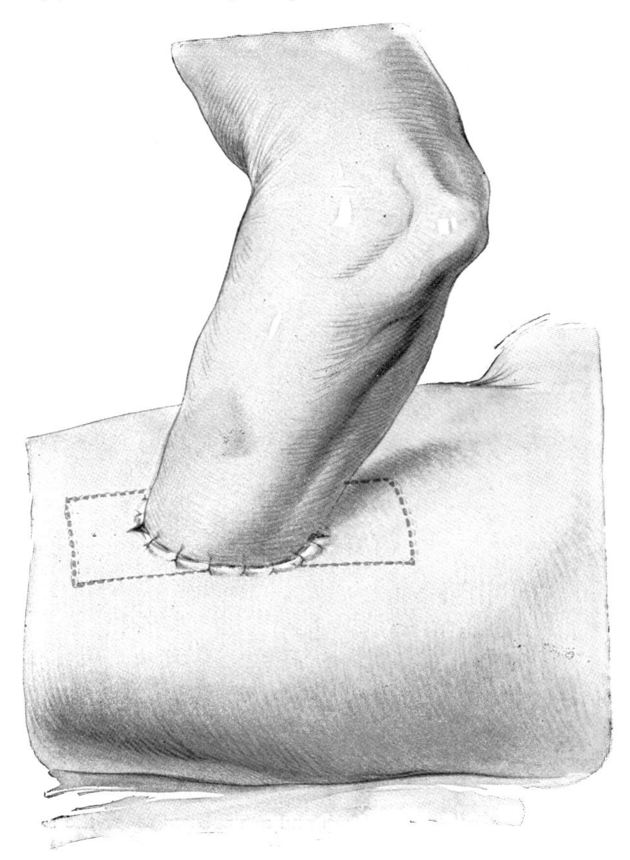

FIG. 413. Temporary implantation of amputation stump, first stage. The amputated surface of the forearm is sewed in a specially prepared site in the thigh.

most favorable position, and the outline of the flap is marked with a colored solution. The entire flap should be cut with the aid of a model, if possible. After the flap is cut the resulting defect is closed by suture or by Thiersch grafts, the limb is brought to the proper position and the flap sutured in place.

To immobilize the parts (Figs. 411 and 412) adjacent skin areas may be fastened together with mastic, strips of adhesive plaster, or frequently skin sutures are used. However, plaster casts are absolutely essential in many cases. Often it is possible to allow some motion, limited by the length of the pedicle, so that the weight of the extremity may rest upon the other part, or sometimes adjustable weights may be used to raise the part and thus counterbalance its weight (Fig. 411). In any type of dressing, it must be possible to observe the pedicle freely, in order to be sure that it is always in the proper position.

Local anæsthesia is of special value in distant plastic operations. It prevents tearing out of the flap pedicle and vomiting, that so frequently occur during the recovery from a general anæsthetic. Postanæsthetic vomiting may result in dangerous suffocation in a patient who has had the "Italian" type of plastic, in which the arm is fastened over the mouth.

A special form of plastic operation which is used particularly to cover stumps, consists in implanting the surface to be covered into the area from which skin is to be removed, through a skin incision. After healing, the two

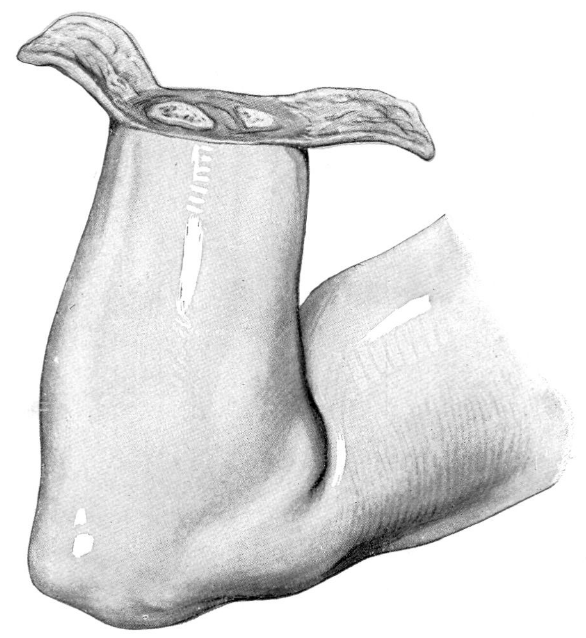

FIG. 414. Temporary implantation, second stage. The flaps outlined in the previous illustration are elevated with the amputation stump and are used to cover the stump surface.

parts are united, like Siamese twins (Fig. 413). When they are to be separated, flaps of skin around the implanted extremity are removed with it, and these flaps are then used to cover the denuded area (Fig. 414).

In the ordinary flap operation from 10 to 14 days should be sufficient time for the pedunculated flap to become physiologically united to its new bed. The flap can be gradually made independent of its pedicle by constricting the pedicle for prolonged periods (Figs. 399, 415 and 418) with an elastic clamp, a rubber tube, or through frequent injections of adrenalin, thus forcing it to depend upon its new bed for its blood supply. When the nutrition from the new base is uncertain, the pedicle should be separated after a longer period. To determine how much nourishment a newly transplanted flap is receiving from its new bed, one should observe to what extent the flap retains its healthy color after temporary constriction of the pedicle, or pedi-

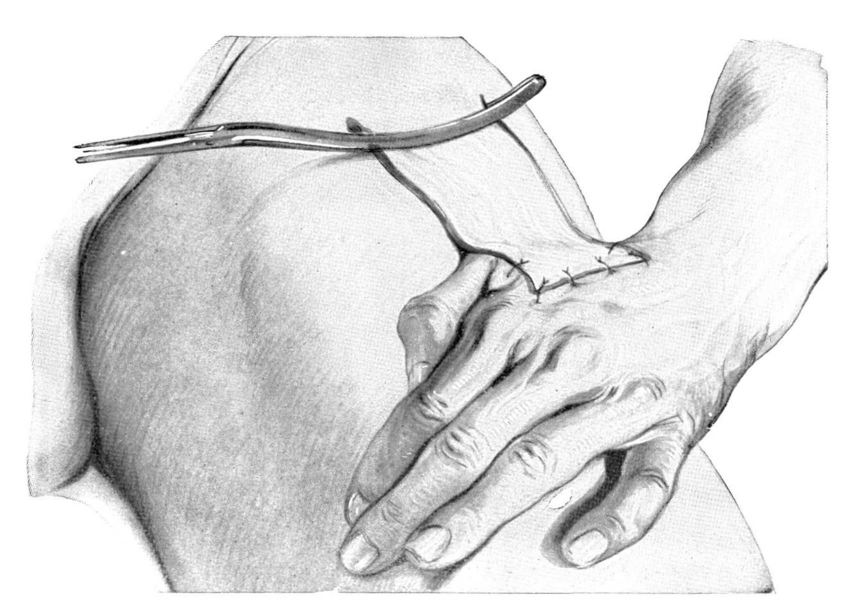

FIG. 415. Migratory flap, first stage. A pedunculated skin flap is grafted from the thigh to the hand. After union to its new bed the blood supply from the thigh is gradually diminished by partial constriction of the pedicle.

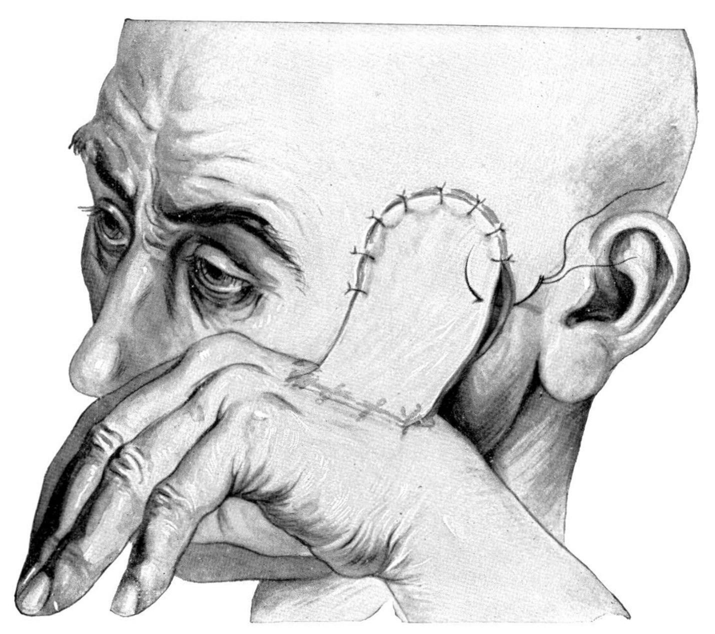

FIG. 416. Migratory flap, second stage. After separation of the flap from the thigh, the flap now with the pedicle attached to the hand is transplanted to the face.

cles, and how much reactive hyperemia results when the pedicle is released again.

A flap that is to be transferred to a distant site can be first transplanted to an intermediate location and then to its final site. Thus it is possible to transfer a pedunculated flap from the abdomen or thigh to the forearm, and after it has been vascularized in this site, to transfer it to the face (migratory

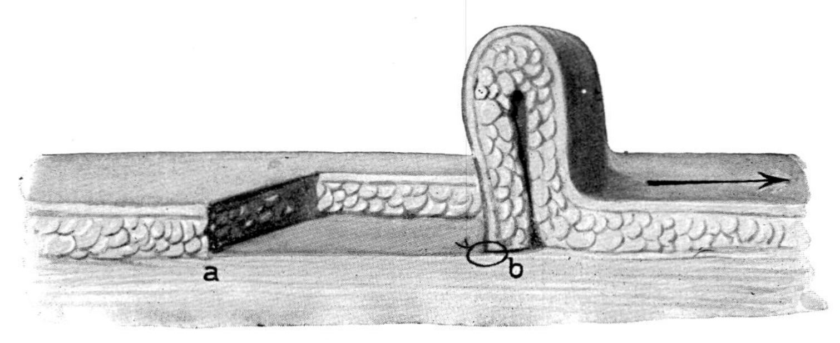

Fig. 417. Creeping flap. The margin of the skin flap separated at "a" is sutured at "b." After healing, the front part of the flap is detached from this base "b" and displaced in the direction of the arrow.

flap, Figs. 415 and 416). A special form of migratory flap is the creeping flap (Fig. 417), in which the free margin of an oblong pedunculated flap is implanted in the immediate proximity of its base. After the flap has united at its new site, the old base is detached, so that the flap is receiving its blood supply at the site of primary implantation and the detached portion can be shifted. Tissues for covering a defect can be carried over still greater dis-

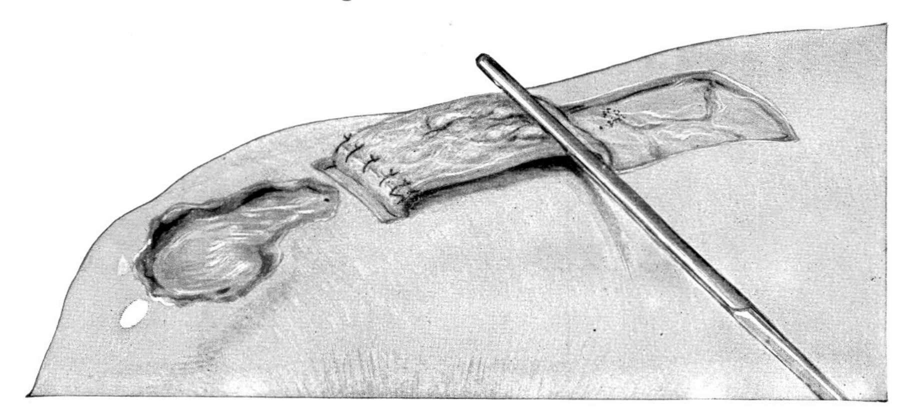

Fig. 418. Rolling flap. The border of the flap is released and turned over at its base. It is then planted with the loose end in a freshly made wound. After healing, the flap is separated from its original base, turned over and used to cover the defect.

tances by means of a rolling flap (Fig. 418), which is made in the following manner: a rectangular skin flap is elevated on both its long sides and on one short side. It is then turned over in the direction of the defect that is to be closed in such a way that its deep surface faces upwards, and the short free edge is sutured to a small flap which is elevated for this purpose. After the flap has healed in this position, the old base is divided, the flap is turned over on its new base so that its deep surface faces downward, and it is then sutured into the defect. Since this maneuver can be frequently repeated it is possible to move such a flap over long distances. It is more practical, however, to

Fig. 419 Fig. 420 Fig. 421

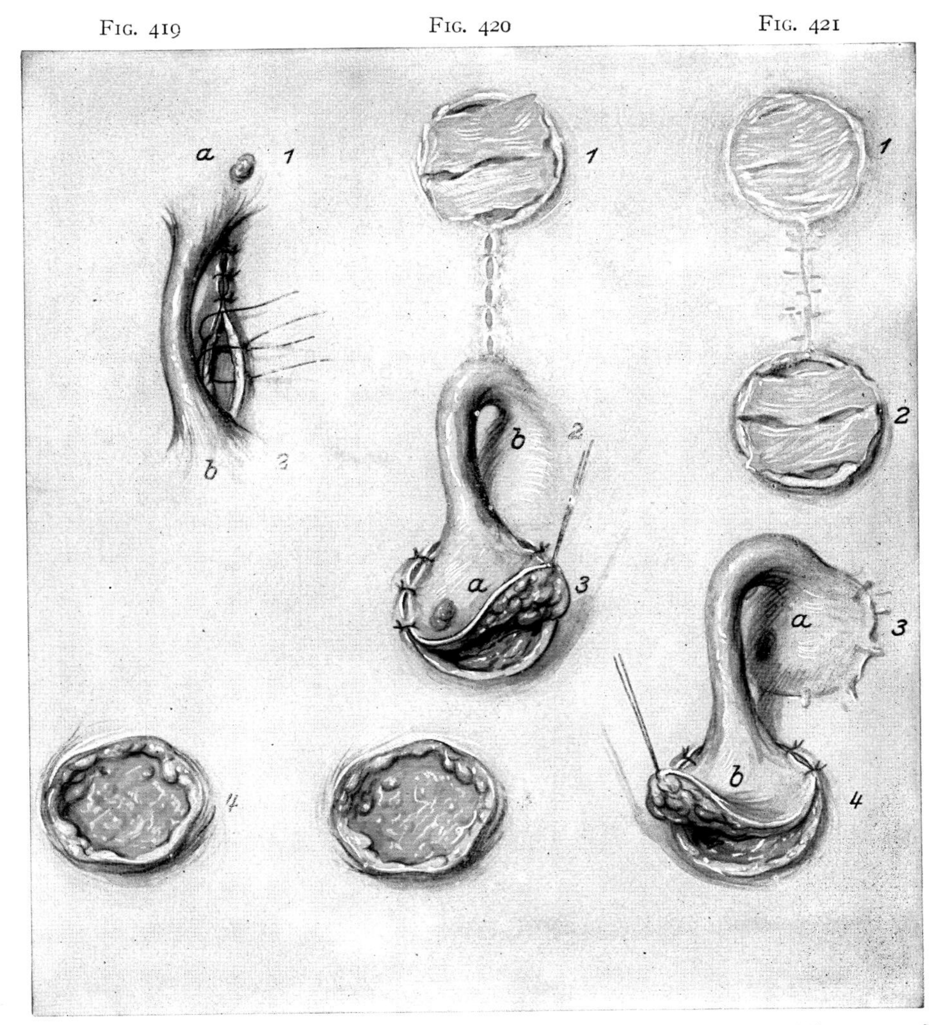

Fig. 419. Migratory flap with tubular pedicle. Stage 1. The future pedicle of the migratory flap is sutured to form a tube. The defect caused by its elevation is sutured.

Fig. 420. Migratory flap with tubular pedicle. Stage 2. The tubular pedicle is mobilized with an attached flap and is reimplanted in the direction of the defect to be covered.

Fig. 421. Migratory flap with tubular pedicle. Stage 3. Another flap is mobilized at the base of the pedicle and is used to cover the primary defect. If the length of the pedicle is insufficient, the procedure may be repeated.

suture the pedicle of the creeping flap into a tube, at the start (Filatow) (Figs. 419, 420 and 421). By freeing and implanting the ends of this tubular flap alternately, the flap may be carried over a considerable distance, as caliper compasses are moved. When the flap is to be sutured in place the pedicle may be opened, if necessary, and used to help cover the defect.

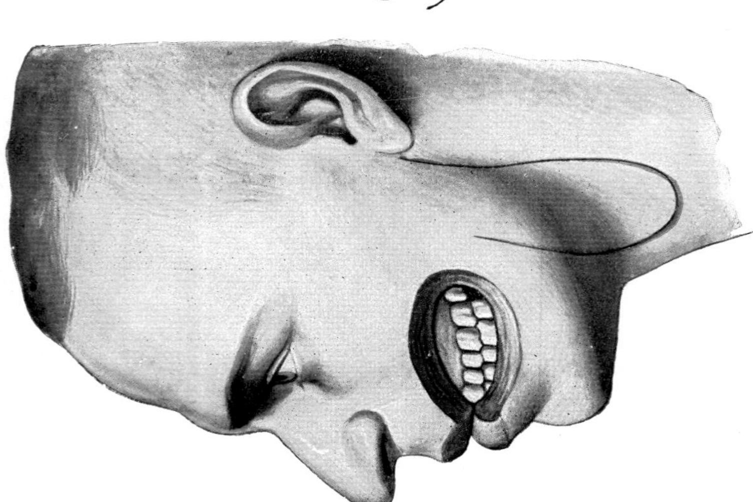

Fig. 422. Epithelization of both sides of a flap. Stage 1. A long, pedunculated flap is formed over the area of the sternocleidomastoid muscle.

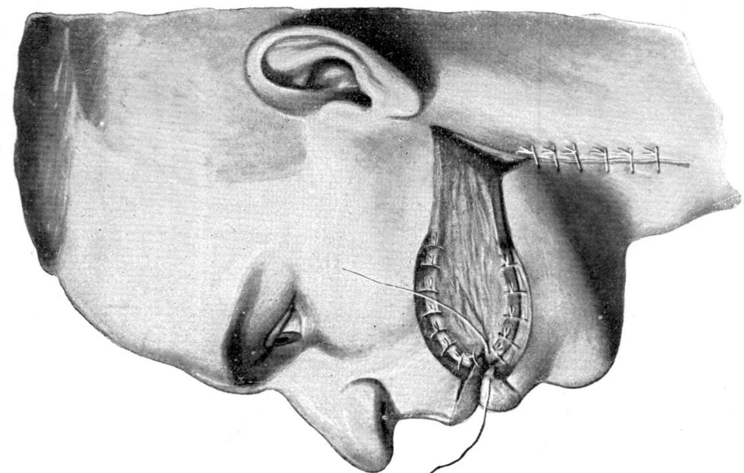

Fig. 423. Epithelization of both sides of a flap. Stage 2. The flap is inserted in the defect with the epithelium inward, so that its epithelium replaces the mucous membrane. The defect resulting from the removal of the flap is closed by suture.

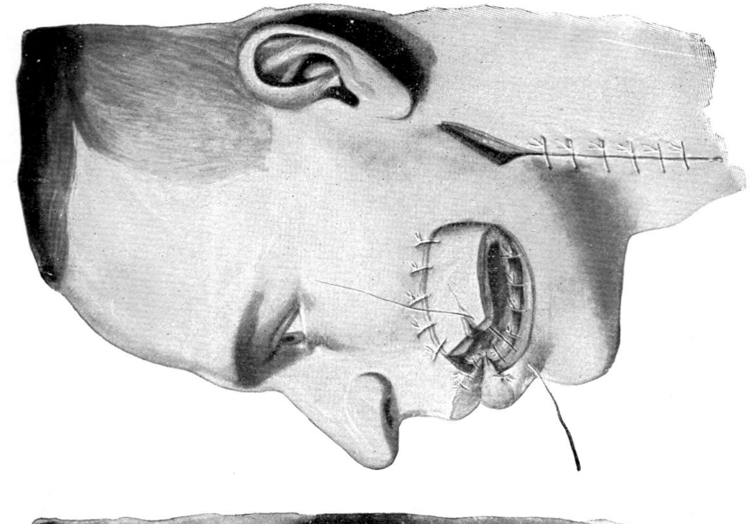

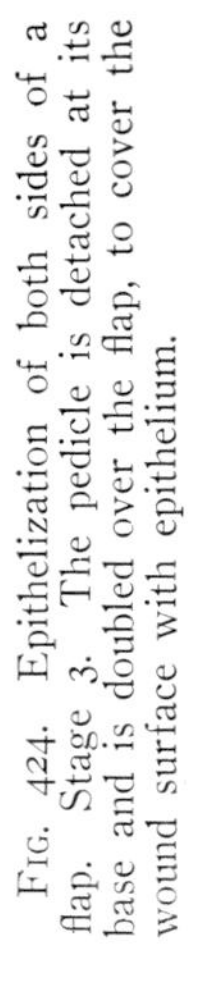

Fig. 424. Epithelization of both sides of a flap. Stage 3. The pedicle is detached at its base and is doubled over the flap, to cover the wound surface with epithelium.

Epithelization of Flaps. When skin flaps are to be used to replace a defect which requires epithelium on both sides (nose, cheek, ear), provision must be made for this. It can be accomplished in various ways. A pedunculated flap may be used and its pedicle, after separation, folded over the flap (Figs. 422, 423, 424 and 425). This does not usually give satisfactory results, for the double flap forms a thick pad that is difficult to shape properly. Two flaps may be cut from neighboring areas, their wound surfaces placed against each other, and after union the pedicle of one flap is divided. The double flap, supplied by only one pedicle, is then transplanted in the usual manner. The best and simplest epithelization of both sides of a flap results

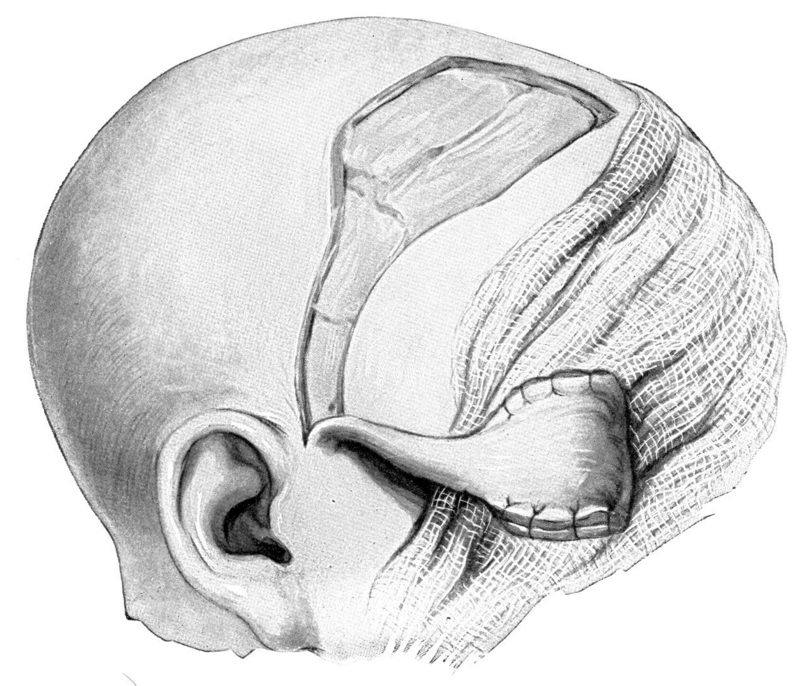

FIG. 425. Epithelization of both sides of a flap by primary doubling. A temporal flap with tubular pedicle is made and the flap is doubled on itself. The secondary defect is covered by Thiersch grafts.

from the use of Thiersch skin grafts (Figs. 426 and 427). The desired flap is raised, both the flap and the wound are covered with Thiersch grafts, a few layers of paraffin gauze, a rubber plate, or a plate of sterile composition, is placed between the flap and its wound bed; the flap is turned back in its old bed, and held in place with a few sutures, to prevent shrinking. As a rule after eight days the Thiersch grafts have become firmly attached, and the flap may then be used.

Transplantation of bone or cartilage may be combined with the transplantation of pedunculated skin flaps. Occasionally, it is possible to remove the skin and bone as one flap, for example, skin from the ulnar edge of the forearm with a bone splinter from the ulna; skin from the forehead with a splinter of the external table of the skull (Fig. 428); or, skin of the chest wall with a superficial portion of the sternum. Otherwise, the bone or cartilage

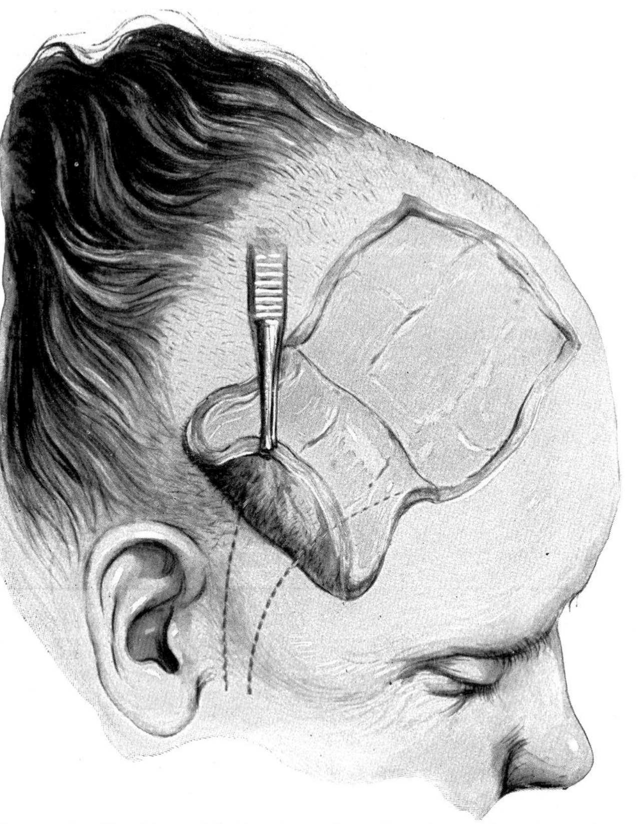

Fig. 426. Double epithelization of a flap by Thiersch grafts. The flap is first loosened only so far as it will be doubly epithelized. Thiersch grafts are placed on the wound side of the flap and on the defect resulting from its removal. The flap is sewed in again over a layer of paraffin gauze for 10 days. The illustration shows the double epithelized flap after it is elevated the second time. The temporal pedicle is indicated by the dotted line.

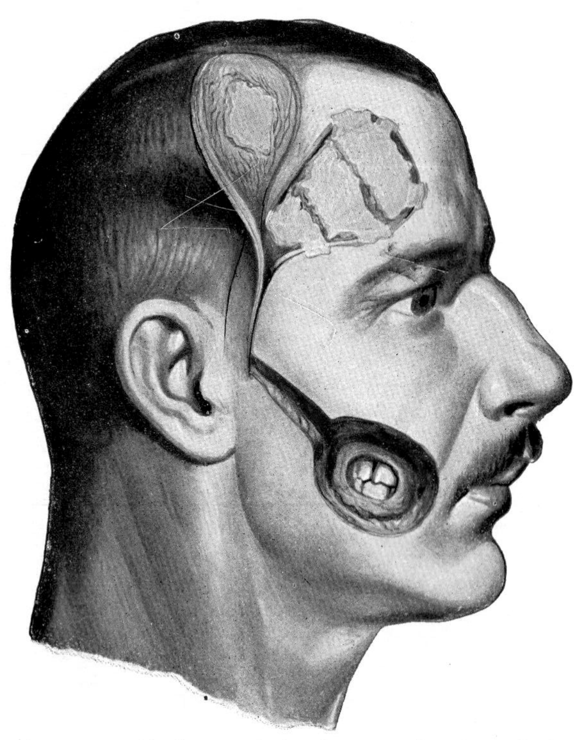

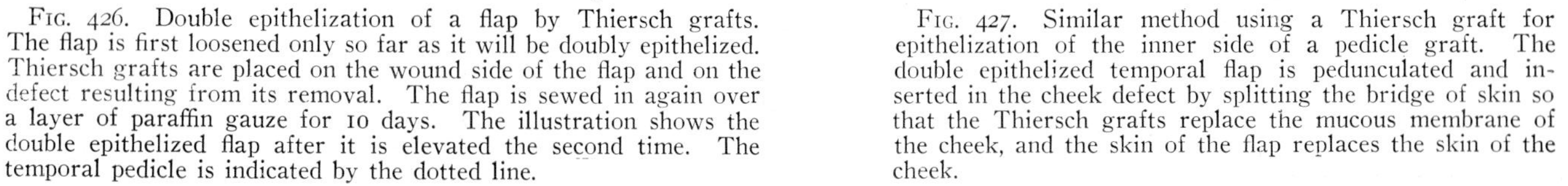

Fig. 427. Similar method using a Thiersch graft for epithelization of the inner side of a pedicle graft. The double epithelized temporal flap is pedunculated and inserted in the cheek defect by splitting the bridge of skin so that the Thiersch grafts replace the mucous membrane of the cheek, and the skin of the flap replaces the skin of the cheek.

must be placed as a free transplant under the skin to be used for a flap (Fig. 429). When it has become accustomed to its new site it is transplanted as part of the skin flap.

5. Repair of Skin Defects by Free Grafts

For free skin transplants either the superficial layer of the skin, the epidermis, or its entire thickness may be used. Small islands of various thicknesses may be transplanted, or epithelial pulp may be used. Autoplasty alone has a chance for success (Fig. 430).

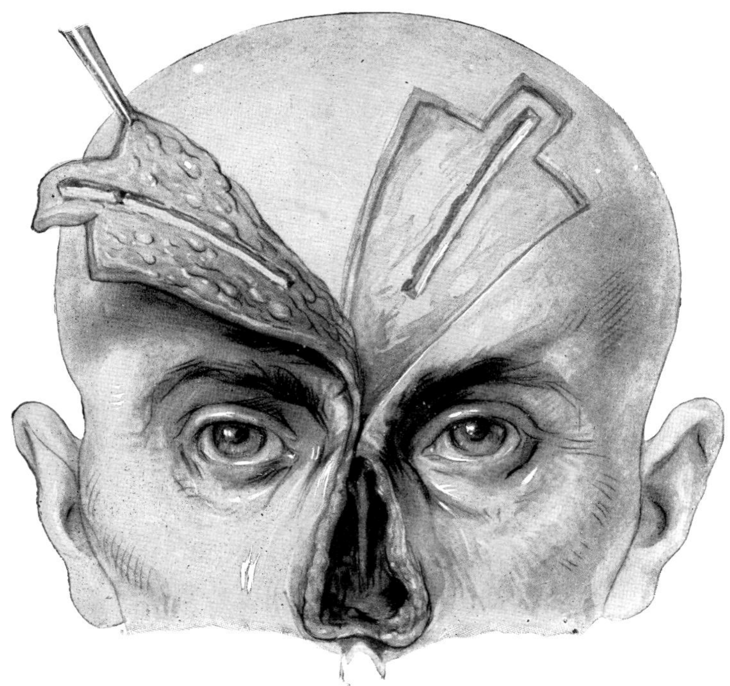

Fig. 428. Formation of a pedunculated skin flap containing a narrow piece of bone. A skin flap supplied by the frontal artery is taken from the forehead, and a small piece of bone from the outer table of the skull is included in it. It is used for reconstruction of the nose.

Whole Thickness Grafts (Wolfe-Krause)

These grafts are very sensitive; their healing remains doubtful even under the most favorable conditions and after scrupulous observance of all principles. When transplanted on granulating surfaces they are seldom successful for they require a bacteria free, recently made wound surface for a bed. The skin may be taken from the abdomen, the chest wall, the back, or the thigh. Elliptical grafts are removed which are of such size that the resulting defect can be united by suture, or a graft is cut out according to a rubber model without considering the closure of the new defect (Fig. 431). The new wound may then be covered with Thiersch grafts. The skin graft must be cut relatively large, since it shrinks about one-third its size after it is removed. The graft is detached from the underlying tissue by cutting vertically against its under surface, care being taken to separate it from all subcutaneous fat (Fig. 432).

If any fat remains adherent, it should be removed later with a razor. It is very important to press the graft firmly into the new bed, continuing the pressure for some moments. It then adheres firmly and as a rule needs no sutures to hold it in place. Even if the graft takes, its surface will become purplish within the next few days and blebs will often form.

A more extensive form of whole skin transplantation is the grafting of part of the pinna of the ear which is covered with skin on both sides and which has cartilage within it. As a rule, a wedge-shaped graft is removed

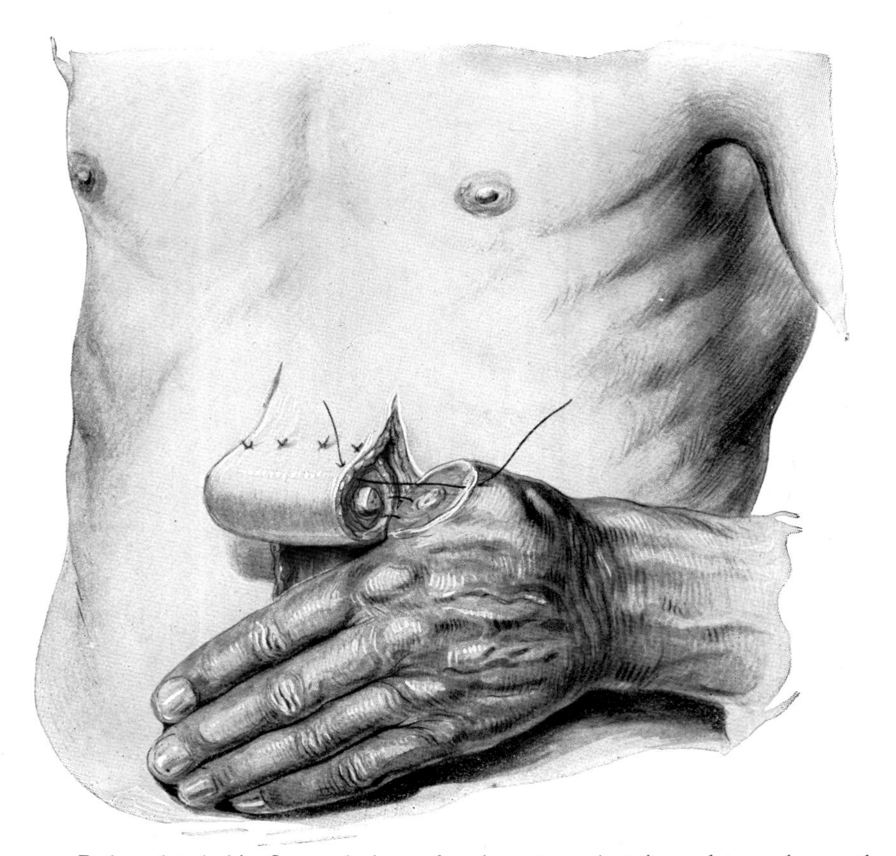

FIG. 429. Pedunculated skin flap enclosing a free bone transplant is used to replace a thumb.

from the pinna to replace a defect in the ala nasi. The pinna is drawn together immediately by sutures (Fig. 433).

Mucous membrane can also be transplanted, as, for example, to cover defects of the conjunctiva or of the oral mucous membrane. There is a choice here, between this procedure and the use of Thiersch grafts.

EPIDERMAL GRAFTS

Transplantation of the epidermis by the method of Thiersch is by far the most important method of skin transference. The grafts require little preparation, and they are almost sure to heal if the general rules for transference of tissue are not grossly disregarded. The grafts grow best on fresh, aseptic wound surfaces, but also do well on healthy granulation tissue. If it is not possible to promote healthy, deep red, fresh appearing granulations, it is best to remove them with a sharp curette or knife. Because the resulting hemorrhage

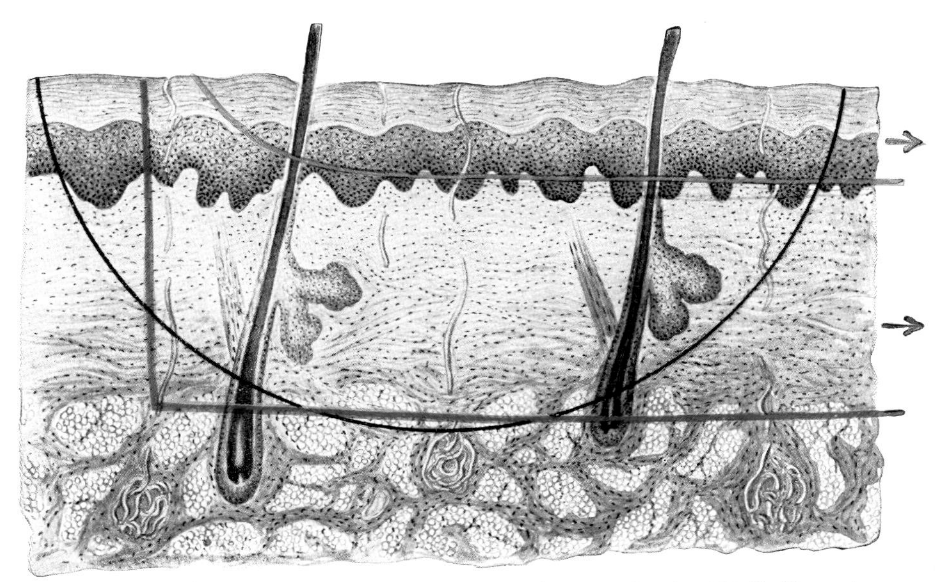

FIG. 430. Skin-grafting. Red: transplant of entire thickness of skin (Wolfe-Krause). Blue: epidermis transplant (Thiersch). Black: cuticle transplant (Reverdin).

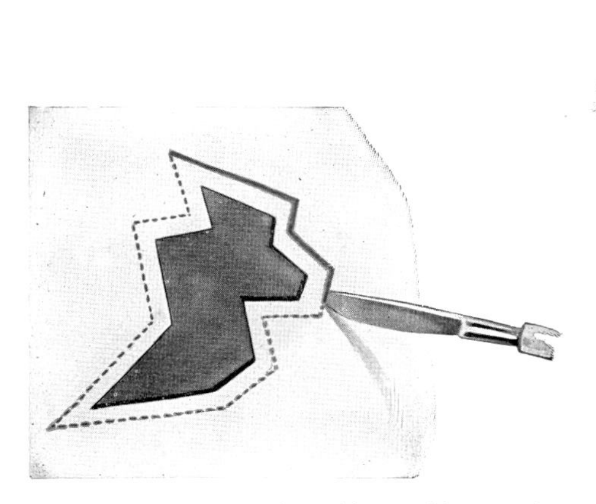

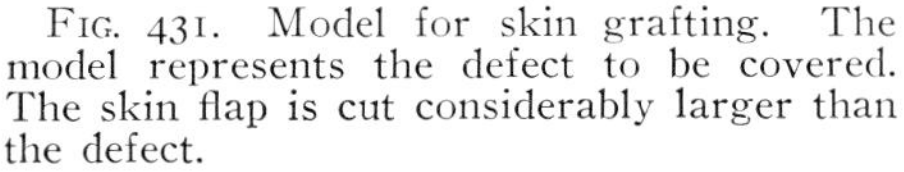

FIG. 431. Model for skin grafting. The model represents the defect to be covered. The skin flap is cut considerably larger than the defect.

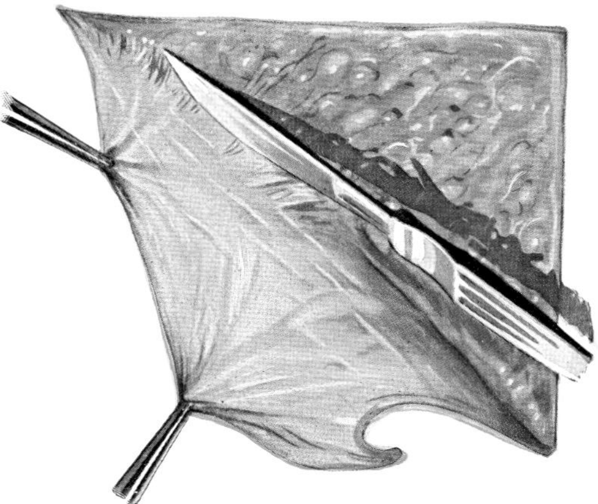

FIG. 432. Removing skin flap for free transplant. The edge of the knife is directed against the skin, which removes every particle of fatty tissue.

can not be controlled at once, I apply the Thiersch grafts the following day in such cases, after the oozing has been checked by a pressure dressing.

Thiersch grafts are usually taken from the lateral and anterior aspects of the thigh, though small grafts can be taken from the immediate vicinity of the field of operation. I do not disinfect the place from which they are to be taken, but wash it carefully with salt solution. When the main operation is not done under general or lumbar anæsthesia, the place from which they are to be taken is injected with 0.5 percent novocain-adrenalin solution, in parallel lines, about 2 cm. apart (Fig. 434), after outlining the area in the form of a rectangle with a colored solution. Blocking the lateral cutaneous nerve of the thigh, as a rule, is not enough, if large grafts are to be removed.

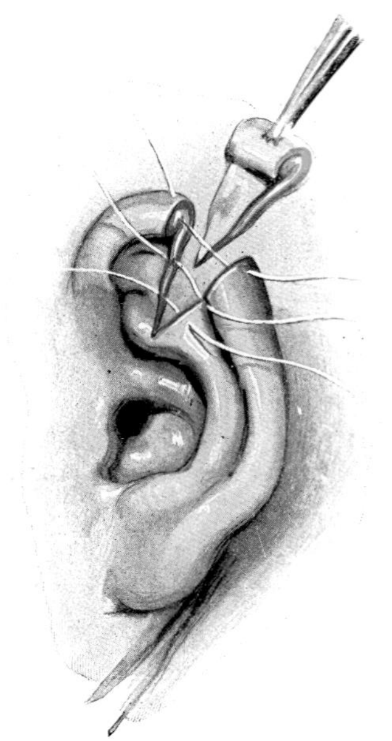

FIG. 433. Removing a piece from the pinna which is to be used as a free transplant. The resulting defect is sutured.

No great skill is required to cut Thiersch grafts if the knife is very sharp and the skin is tightly stretched. The shape of the knife is of no great importance, whether hollow ground or plain, wide or narrow. It is impossible to immobolize the skin of the thigh by the methods generally recommended, such as stretching it lengthwise with two hands or with two brushes. It moves laterally then, like a violin string. It is only possible to hold it firm by stretching it transversely. To do this, an assistant grasps the skin firmly with both hands opposite the place where it is to be excised, holding a fold of it at right angles to the long axis of the thigh, as if he were attempting to remove this fold from the bone with his fingers (Fig. 435). To prevent his hands from slipping off the skin, the assistant should wear cotton gloves and the skin of this portion of the thigh should be painted with mastic. Olive oil may be wiped over the skin to make the knife slide easily and to prevent the strips of skin adhering to the knife as they are cut. In this

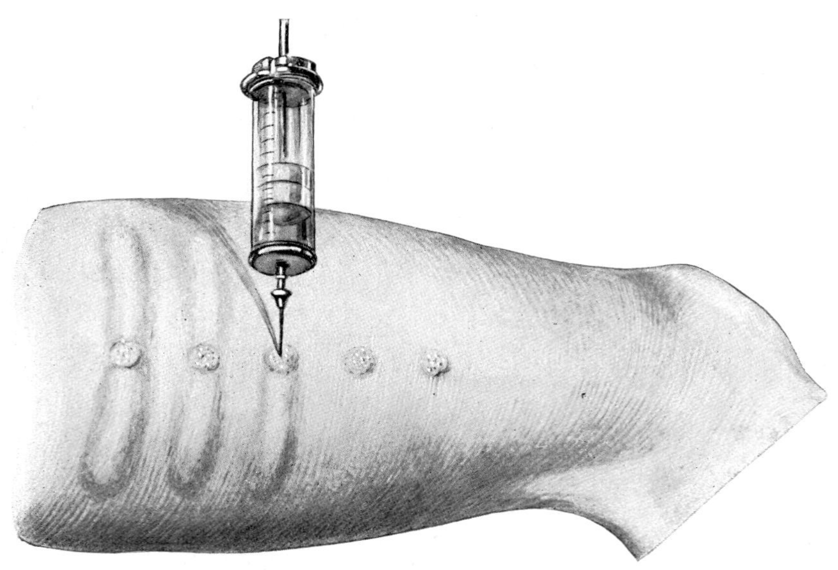

FIG. 434. Parallel areas injected with local anæsthesia on the lateral side of the thigh, before removing Thiersch grafts.

manner, flaps of epidermis can be cut easily in any length desired. I do not attempt to cut the thinnest possible grafts, but purposely try to get somewhat thicker ones, so that the vascular loops of the skin may be included (Fig. 430). In some cases where thicker skin seems to be important, as

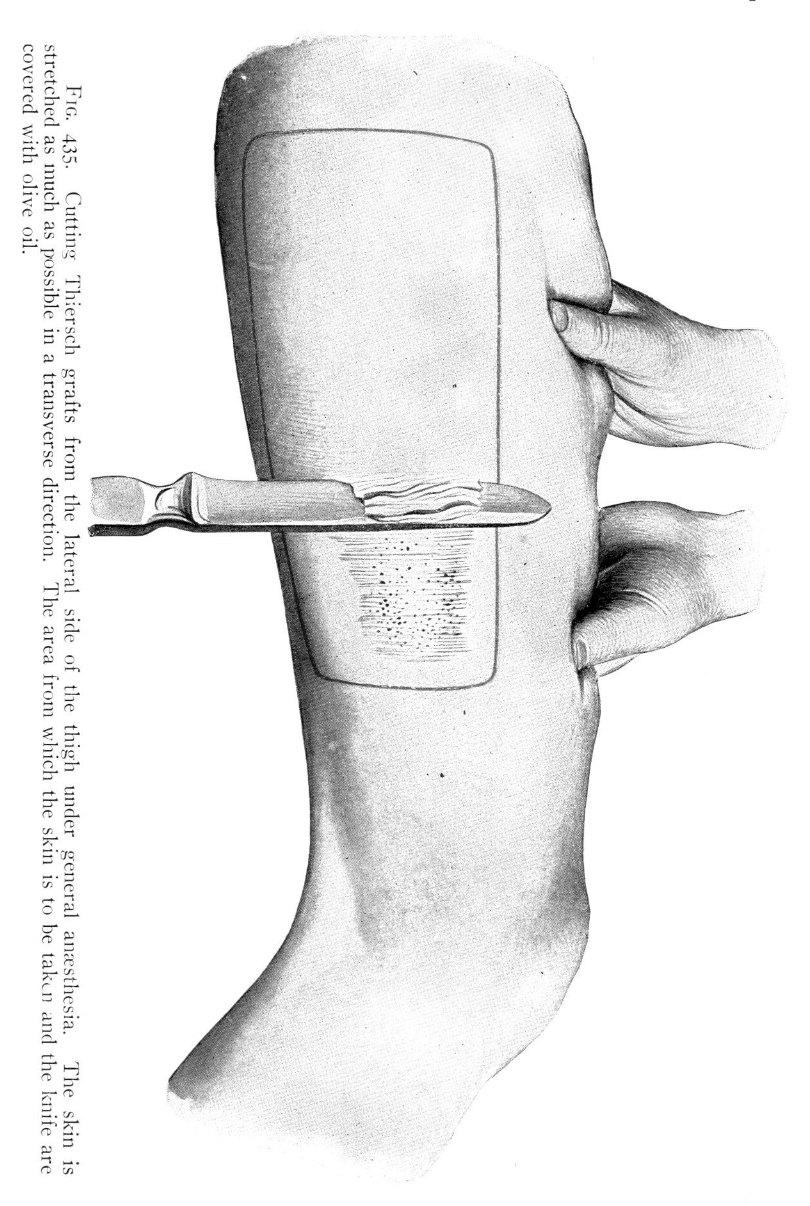

Fig. 435. Cutting Thiersch grafts from the lateral side of the thigh under general anæsthesia. The skin is stretched as much as possible in a transverse direction. The area from which the skin is to be taken and the knife are covered with olive oil.

for example in plastics about the face or for covering finger stumps, Thiersch grafts may be so thick that they are intermediate between the true Thiersch and the Wolfe-Krause grafts.

The cut epidermis is transferred from the knife directly to the wound surface (Fig. 436) without the aid of forceps or spatula. It is important to emphasize the harmfulness of using saline solution to float the grafts between cutting and transplantation. After the graft is transferred directly to the wound surface, it is correctly placed and spread with the aid of olive tipped directors. The graft is held firmly with one director, while the edges are smoothed out with the other, until the graft is completely unfolded.

The complete smoothing out of the graft is important, because if the flap is not perfectly flat it will not unite to the granulation tissue. Thiersch grafts are placed at a distance of about 1 to 3 mm. from the wound margin, and about the same distance from each other, so that secretions from the

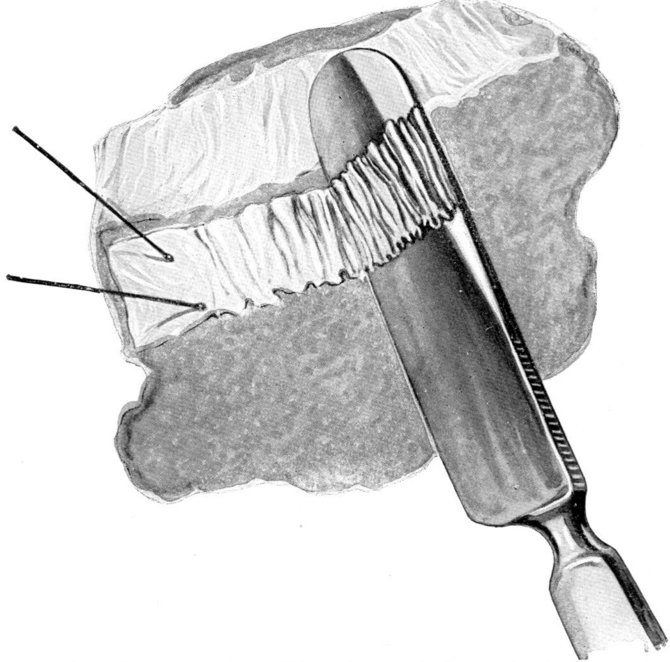

FIG. 436. Transferring the epidermis (Thiersch) graft from the knife to the surface to be covered.

granulations may have an exit without raising the graft. After the grafts are placed they are pressed firmly against the wound.

The Dressing. The simplest method is to apply no dressing over the grafts. If this is done, care must be taken that the grafts do not become mechanically displaced and are protected from flies. It is frequently sufficient, in grafts on the extremities, to place the limb at rest by applying traction and then placing it under a protective cradle. Or the grafts may be protected by cotton rings, netting (Fig. 385), cardboard or wooden hoops fastened to the part with adhesive plaster or skin sutures. When no direct dressing is used it is advisable to retard the drying of the grafts by placing moistened layers of gauze over the protecting frame. If these measures appear too uncertain, the area surrounding the site of transplantation is painted with mastic and a double layer of gauze is applied. Thiersch covered the grafts with perforated silk. Some surgeons use small plates of cork or silver over the grafts. The first dressing should not be removed for five days, and it is preferable to permit it to remain for eight days. Dressing materials that have become adherent to the grafts should be softened with olive oil for several hours before attempting their removal. I have found Lassar's zinc paste useful in subsequent dressings.

Thiersch grafts are so successful in cavities when they are subjected to constant pressure and temperature, that they have a definite place in the epithelization of artificially produced cavities (Esser). This principle is

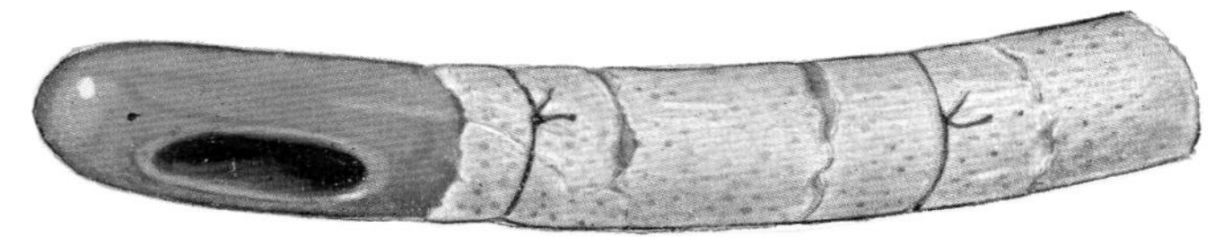

FIG. 437. Prosthesis prepared with epidermis for the restoration of an epithelial lined tube. The flaps of epidermis are fastened around a tube with fine catgut so that the deep surface of the graft is exposed.

used in making subcutaneous epithelial tubes, as for example, an artificial esophagus, or epithelial pockets, as an artificial bladder. The skin under which the tube or pocket is to be made is released from the subcutaneous tissue to the necessary extent, by undermining, rather than by broad splitting incisions. The wound cavity is packed with dry gauze until hemorrhage has entirely ceased. A prosthesis is made to fit the skin pocket, which can be easily introduced under the detached skin. To line a tube with epithelium,

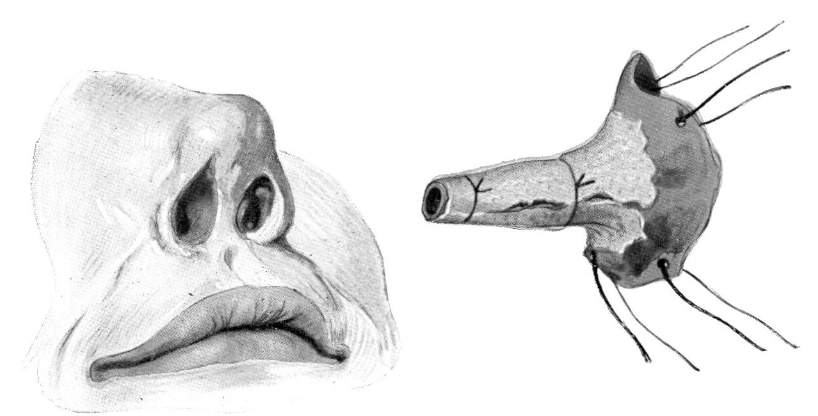

FIG. 438. Prosthesis prepared with Thiersch grafts for the restoration of a nasal passage. The prosthesis covered in this manner is placed in the freshly prepared nasal canal and fastened by sutures.

a soft rubber tube of a corresponding size serves as a prosthesis (Fig. 437); to make a pocket, the prosthesis is made of Stent's dental compound, which becomes soft in warm water and hardens again at body temperature. The prosthesis is completely covered with Thiersch grafts whose deep side is placed outward. The flaps are firmly tied or sewed on with fine catgut. The prosthesis so prepared is inserted into the prepared pocket, and is fastened in place with a few sutures. The necessary holes in the modeling compound are made with a hot needle. The skin incision is sutured over the prosthesis, leaving small openings for the escape of wound secretions, and the part involved is placed at rest. The prosthesis is removed after 8 days. The cavity is then epithelized if the grafts have taken.

The procedure may also be used to enlarge and epithelize certain orifices (Fig. 438), for example, the nasal cavities. The narrowed orifice is enlarged by direct incision. A Stent prosthesis is fitted, covered with epithelial grafts, and inserted into the cavity, where it is fastened with sutures. The nasal prosthesis is open at the ends, so that nasal breathing is not obstructed.

The areas from which Thiersch grafts have been taken, and which at most ooze only slightly, should be covered with a zinc ointment dressing, which can be removed after about 8 days. Nothing remains then except a slight discoloration of the skin. If there is any delay in healing, the ointment dressings are reapplied.

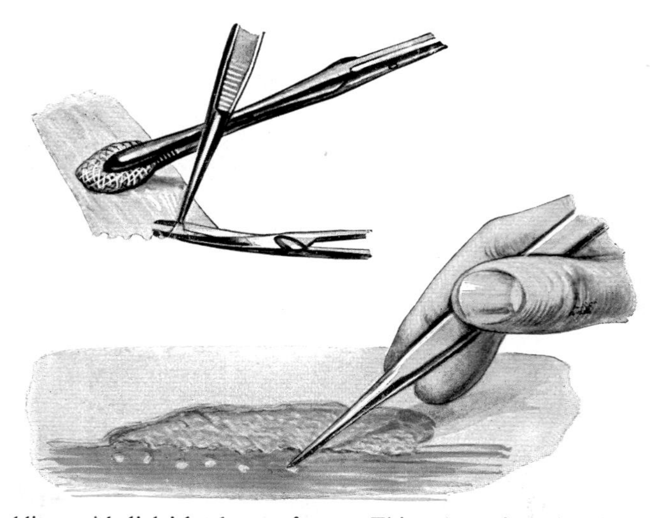

FIG. 439. Imbedding epithelial islands, cut from a Thiersch graft under the granulations of a wound (Braun).

Transplantation of Epithelial Islands. Because Thiersch grafts are occasionally raised from the wound bed as the result of unfavorable conditions of the grafted surface and therefore do not heal, the epidermis has been transplanted in small islands, instead of large grafts, and anchored firmly in the wound. According to the method of Braun, small pieces, about one mm. in diameter, are cut from Thiersch grafts and are imbedded obliquely under the granulations with a tissue forceps (Fig. 439). These islands are placed over the entire surface to be epithelized about ½ cm. apart. It is alleged that these germinating islands also heal well in infected granulations, but of this there is some doubt. My assistant, Kurtzahn, reported on this procedure before the German Surgical Congress in 1925.

Injections of Epithelial Pulp. According to the method of Pels-Leusden, tightly stretched skin is scraped with a sharp knife, as is done in Mangold's transplantation of epithelium, and the epithelium, blood, and lymph pulp obtained, are placed in a syringe and injected forcibly by means of a thread on the piston (Fig. 109), under the granulations. The needle should not be too fine. If the epithelial pulp, placed in this manner, grows there will appear after a time small epithelial foci, in the form of white dots, over

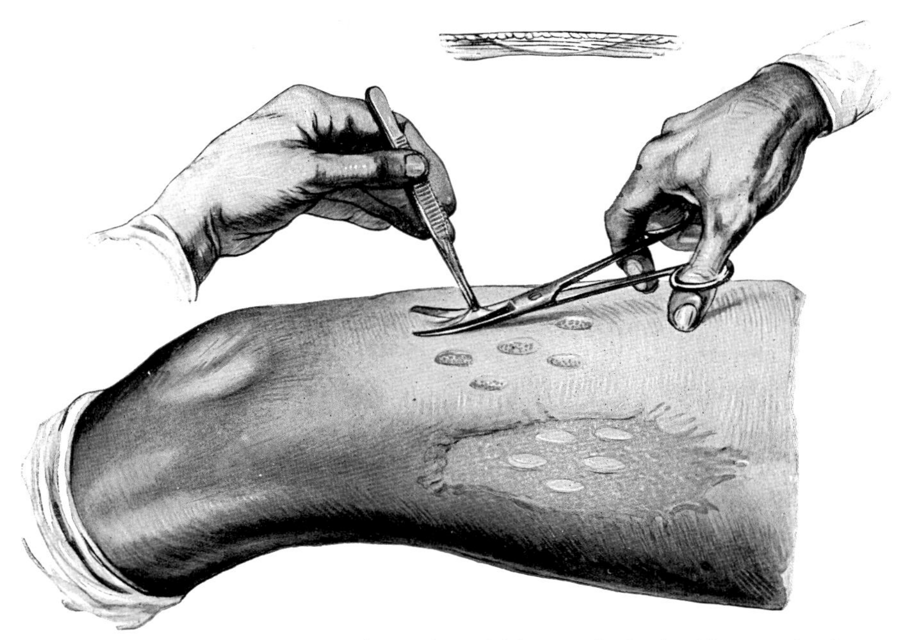

Fig. 440. Skin-grafting with Reverdin grafts, which are obtained with curved scissors and tissue forceps.

the granulating surface. These points grow rapidly, fuse and epithelize the entire wound surface. I do not believe that this procedure can compare with the Thiersch method for transplantation of skin, because the transplanted cells are certainly damaged.

Kurtzahn, in my clinic, has developed the transplantation of tissue pulp by utilizing other kinds of tissue, such as the pulp of parenchymatous organs, the thyroid, ovary, testis (Kurtzahn, German Surgical Congress, 1923). This procedure is advantageous in that the material is easily transferred and the patients are ambulatory. It may be repeated frequently. It has the disadvantage, however, of damaging the injected cells through crushing, preparatory to injection.

Reverdin Grafts. In certain cases Reverdin grafts are preferable for covering granulating surfaces. This method has the advantage of

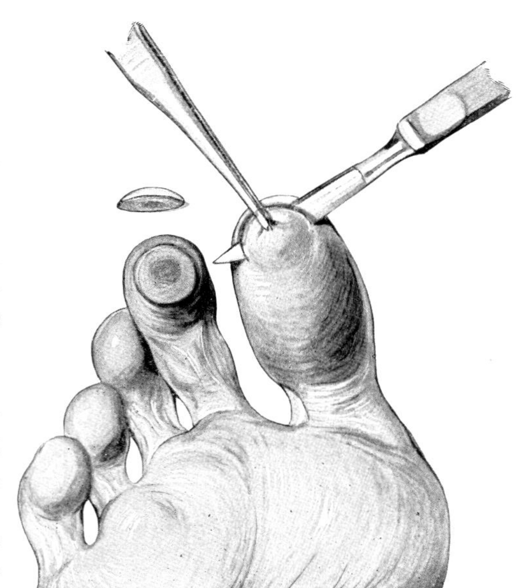

Fig. 441. Removal of a toe pad which may be used as a substitute for the tip of the nose.

permitting the application of further grafts at each dressing without additional preparation. After the skin over the area from which the grafts are to be taken is anæsthetized, a small area of skin is lifted with a forceps or with a needle and is then excised with a sharp curved scissors, or a knife (Fig. 440). The small oval piece of skin, about 1.5 cm. long and 1/4 to 1/2 cm. wide, is placed on the surface of the granulations and firmly pressed in place. These bits of skin are placed at a regular distance from each other, so that the wound surface looks like gingerbread covered with almonds. The grafts, which are the thickness of the whole skin in the center but become thinner as they reach the edges (Fig. 430), usually heal well even on poor granulations. Complete healing takes place rapidly, as a rule. A special form of Reverdin graft is the transplantation of a toe pad to replace the tip of the nose (Fig. 441). The pad is cut off a suitable toe with a sharp knife and is placed under firm pressure on the wound surface of the tip of the nose.

B. SURGERY OF THE SKIN AND OF THE SUBCUTANEOUS TISSUE

1. Management of Contractures of the Skin and Keloids

Contractures of the skin occur after injuries, especially after burns, after sluggish healing of an ulcer, or as a constitutional disease (Dupuytren's contracture). The firmness of the cicatricial band is freqquently so great that an attempt to stretch it by mechanical means, such as traction, is fruitless, in spite of great force and a great deal of patience.

The overgrowth of cicatricial tissue, in the form of keloids, results likewise in contractures. On the other hand, keloids may be annoying for cosmetic reasons, or because of their size, or because their surfaces are so easily injured. Keloids are as a rule treated with little success. They are not local conditions, but manifestations of a constitutional disorder.

Attempts to soften cicatricial bands or keloids by chemicals are usually unsuccessful. Fibrolysin (Merck), the sodium salt of thiosinamin, is the remedy most frequently used, both locally and generally. For local use, an ampoule of a 15 percent alcoholic or a 10 percent glycerinated solution is injected under the cicatrix, in quantities of about 1 cc. at each point of injection. The injections are rather painful, so that previous local anæsthetization is often necessary. For general use, the contents of one ampoule are injected subcutaneously, or intramuscularly. The treatment must be continued for months, at intervals of several days.

Cholin chloride (Fränkel), in a 2 to 10 percent solution, is injected into and under the cicatrix in quantities up to 30 cc. Following this, local hyperemia of the diseased part is induced by means of heat cabinets, heating pads, hot baths, etc. The treatment is continued for a long time, at intervals of a few days.

Stoeltzner recommends the injection of 6 to 10 cc. of a 50 percent solution of urea under the scar tissue. The treatment must be repeated over a long period of time.

Von Payr recommends a mixture of hydrochloric acid, pepsin and Pregl's solution for softening the cicatrix. Two percent pepsin is added to Pregl's solution (a solution of hydriotic acid, iodic acid and metallic iodine .04 percent) 24 hours before its use. Shortly before injecting, a mixture is made of 3 parts of this solution and 1 part of a 2 percent novocain solution. The cicatrix is saturated with this solution. The treatment must be repeated frequently.

If these remedies fail, which usually is the case, the cicatricial contractures can still be treated surgically. Simple excision of the cicatrix with

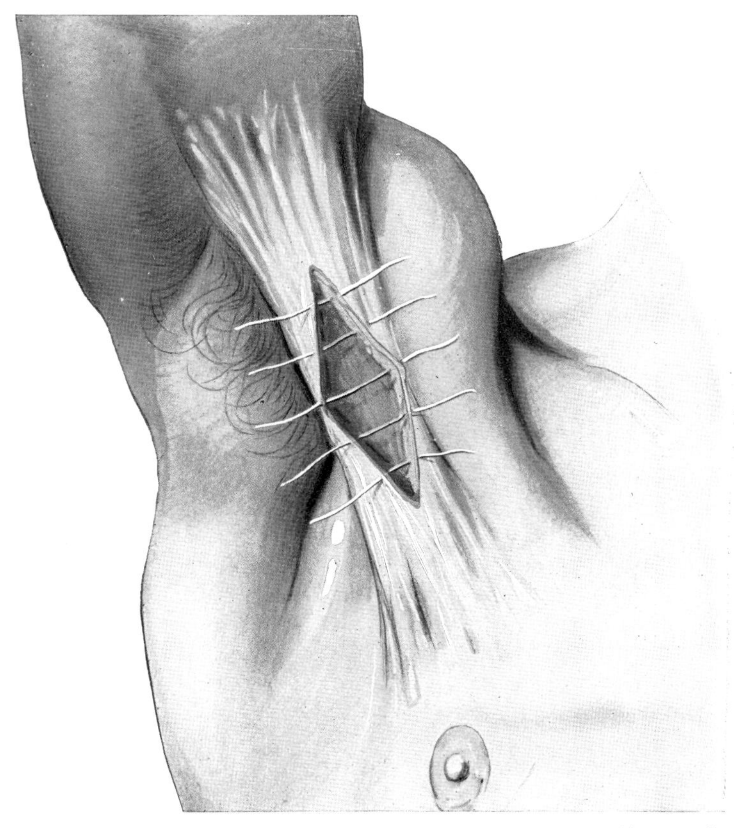

FIG. 442. Splitting a cicatrix which restricts motion. After making an incision across the contracting band and stretching the wound by forced motion, the wound is sutured in a longitudinal direction. This is only to be used when there exists a contraindication to complete excision of the contracting band.

subsequent suture frequently accomplishes nothing, but plastic operations may lead to good results.

The old rule, to split in a transverse direction and suture lengthwise (Fig. 442) but seldom brings success, for there is not always enough material for longitudinal suture, and the rigidity of the tissue may prevent its uniting. When the contracture has been released by a transverse incision, it is better to cover the resulting defect by a plastic operation. It is still better to excise the cicatrix, particularly when it consists of tissue of poor quality with a tendency to ulcer formation or to further contracture. This is encountered in the surgical treatment of Dupuytren's contracture of the hand.

The only procedure that is of value in such cases is complete excision of all the affected skin, as well as the subcutaneous and fascial tissue. Free skin transplants should not be used to cover the ensuing defect, for they do not heal well on the base of the scar tissue, nor do they offer sufficient resistance to further contractions of scar tissue. Only a flap from adjacent skin with either a permanent or temporary pedicle should be considered. For the correction of Dupuytren's contracture in men I usually use the skin of the scrotum (Figs. 406 and 407).

In dealing with contractions which are due to cicatricial webs between the fingers, there may be difficulty in covering the whole surface on both sides. The least that should be done is to epithelize completely the sulcus between the fingers by a skin flap. It is best to use a pointed flap that is

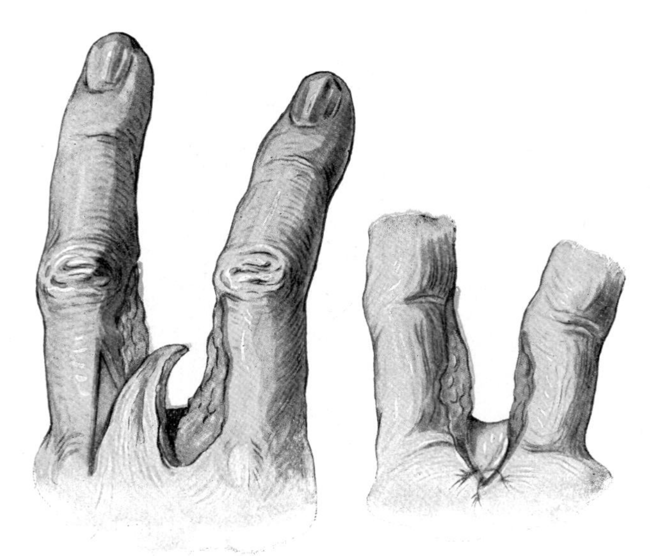

FIG. 443. Roser's flaps for epithelization of a wound angle. Very useful in operations for webbed fingers.

cut from the edge of the defect for this (Roser's flap, Fig. 443), and draw it straight through the angle so as to cover it completely.

Good results are often obtained in a simple way by plastic prolongation of a cicatricial band. One may use either a Z-shaped incision, or the incision devised by Morestin for finger contractures, which divides the cicatrix like a harmonica, and which has also been used successfully for elongating cicatricial bands over the larger joints. The operation in either case is begun by splitting the cicatrix for its entire length by an incision which extends into the healthy tissue beneath the scar, so that the band is divided into a right and left half.

For the Z-shaped elongation, one of the two transverse incisions is made at the upper end, the other, in the opposite direction, at the lower end of the lengthwise incision (Fig. 444). The distance between the two transverse incisions should be a little more than the final elongation desired. The triangular skin flaps formed in this manner are excised down to the healthy tissue, and any subcutaneous cicatricial bands are divided, after forcible stretching. The wound is closed by suturing together the margins which form right angles with one another and then closing the central portion of the incision.

In elongation of a scar by Morestin's method, the two marginal flaps formed by the longitudinal incision are indented by numerous transverse incisions, from one to several centimeters long. This is done in such a way that an incision on one side is opposite a point midway between two incisions on the other side (Fig. 445). When the contracture is now stretched, the

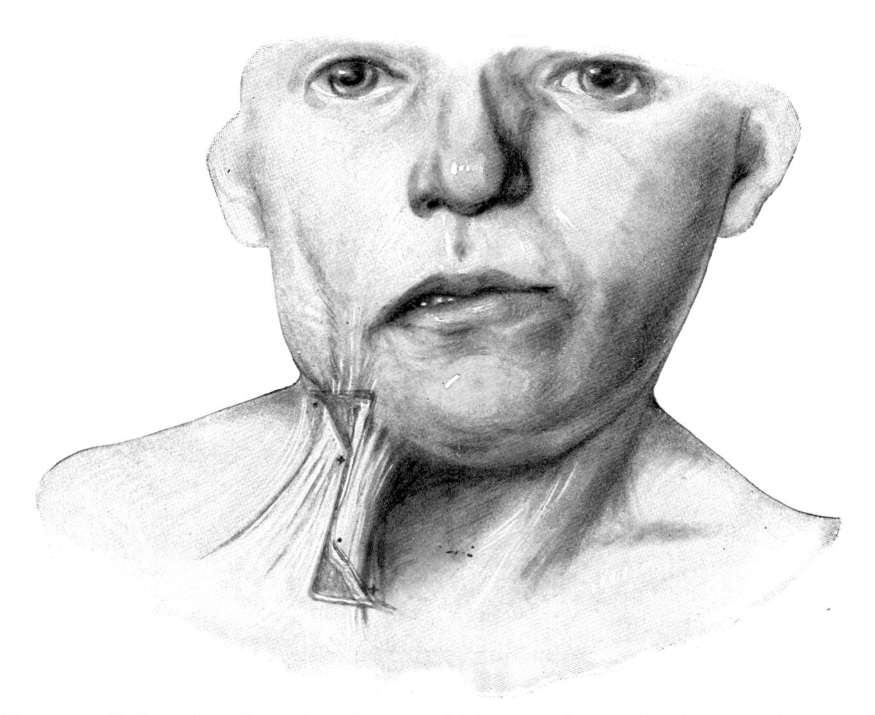

FIG. 444. Z-plasty for elongation of a cicatricial band. An incision is made along the tense band and from each end of this, incisions are carried across the band in opposite directions. The points indicated are approximated after elevating the flaps.

transverse incisions extend triangularly, like a harmonica, and the rectangles of skin bounded by two incisions likewise become triangular in shape. The dentations should fit into the opposite notches, so that the skin wound can be completely closed by suture. The results with this procedure have been good.

In the surgery of keloids satisfactory results are not obtained from simple excision of the keloid, since the new cicatrix degenerates in the same way within a short time. Temporary results are obtained by treating the cicatricial contractures with local injections, as described previously. One may also excise the keloid and after repeated irradiation with radium or x-ray allow the wound to heal by granulation.

2. Removal of Nevi, Angiomata and Papillomata from the Skin

These affections of the skin should be removed not alone for cosmetic and functional reasons, but also because of the possibility of later degeneration, as for example, to melanosarcoma.

Permanent **depilation** of an area of skin has been accomplished by Rethi by elevating the whole thickness of the skin, carefully dissecting the

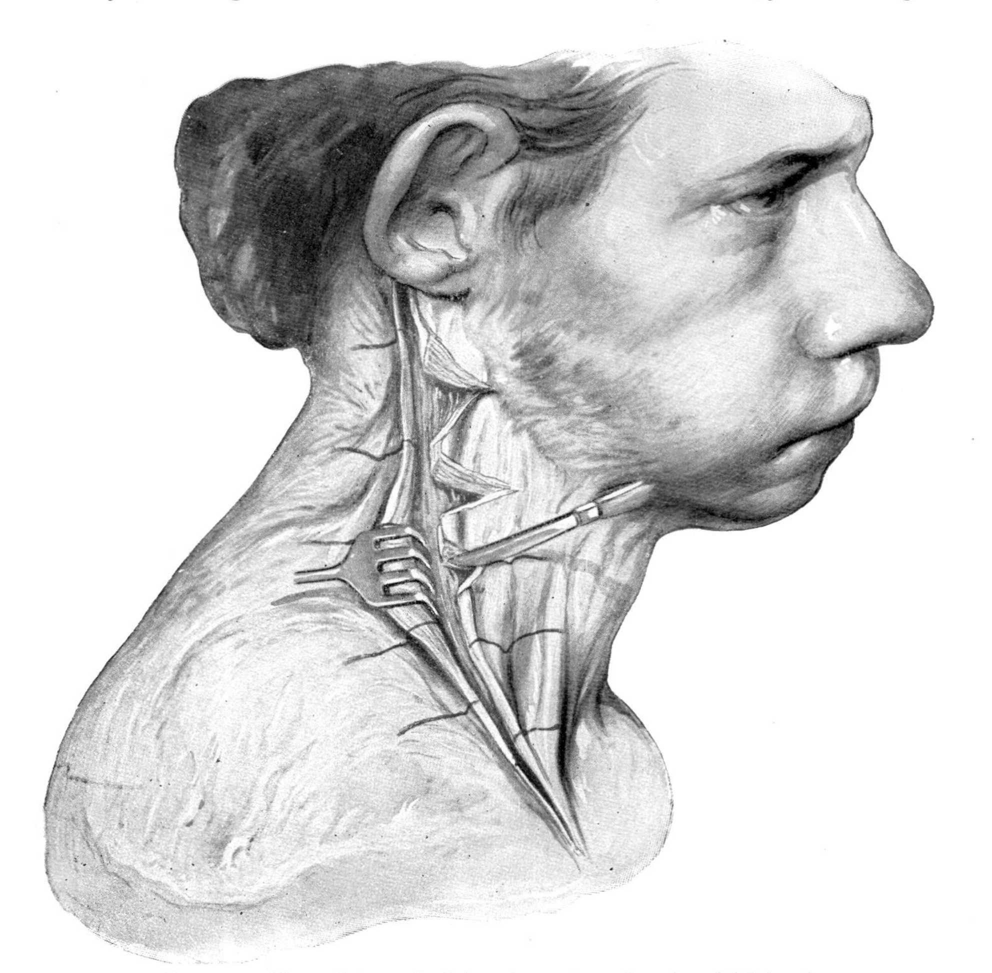

Fig. 445. Morestin's method for elongation of a cicatricial band.

layer containing the hair papillæ from its under surface (Fig. 446), and replacing the skin flap. A cicatrix results from the skin incision, of course. For this reason, it is preferable to excise the hairy area, when the defect can be covered in a simpler way. Electrolysis and x-ray irradiation have only a temporary effect, unless the irradiation is so extensive that it may cause permanent injury to the skin. It is useless to pull the hair out.

Nevi should be excised. If possible the resulting defect should be of such a shape that it may be closed by suture. If direct union by suture is not possible, the defect should be covered immediately by a pedunculated flap or free graft. Large birth marks about the face in children may some-

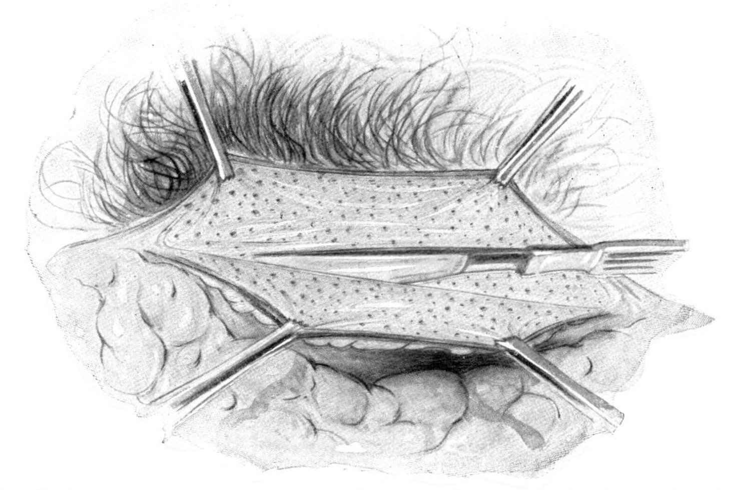

FIG. 446. Depilation (Rethi). The whole thickness of the skin is elevated and by careful dissection the layer bearing the hair papillæ is excised from the under surface of the flap.

times be replaced with Krause grafts. Thick Thiersch grafts also give satisfactory cosmetic results. Tattoo-marks may be removed in the same manner.

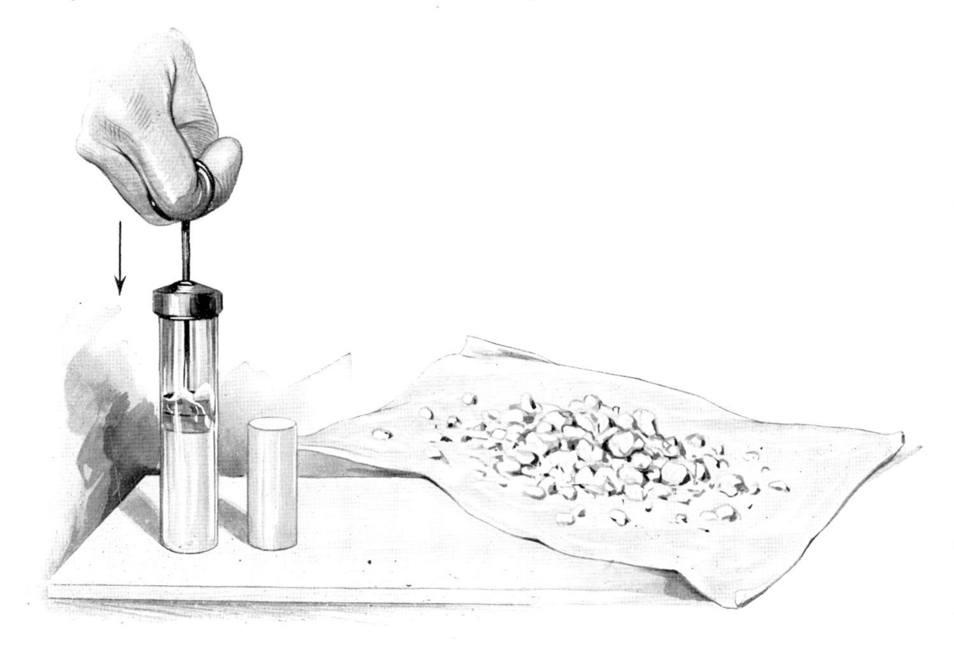

FIG. 447. Making a cylinder of carbon dioxide snow with a glass syringe.

For **skin angiomata** also, excision is the simplest and surest procedure. The cavernous sinuses are best removed from the tissue with a sharp curette.

Lexer advises the use of alcoholic injections a few days before operation to coagulate the blood in the sinuses. Because excision always leaves a scar, it is better to try conservative measures first in an attempt to remove an angioma from the face. The most promising procedure is the use of carbon dioxide snow, which is often successful, and furthermore leaves a minimum scar. The angioma is frozen three times for 1 to 2 minutes at a time, with an interval for thawing between. These treatments are given every 1 to 3 weeks, until the angioma has disappeared. Caution in the duration of the freezing period is necessary at first, but later, when the skin has

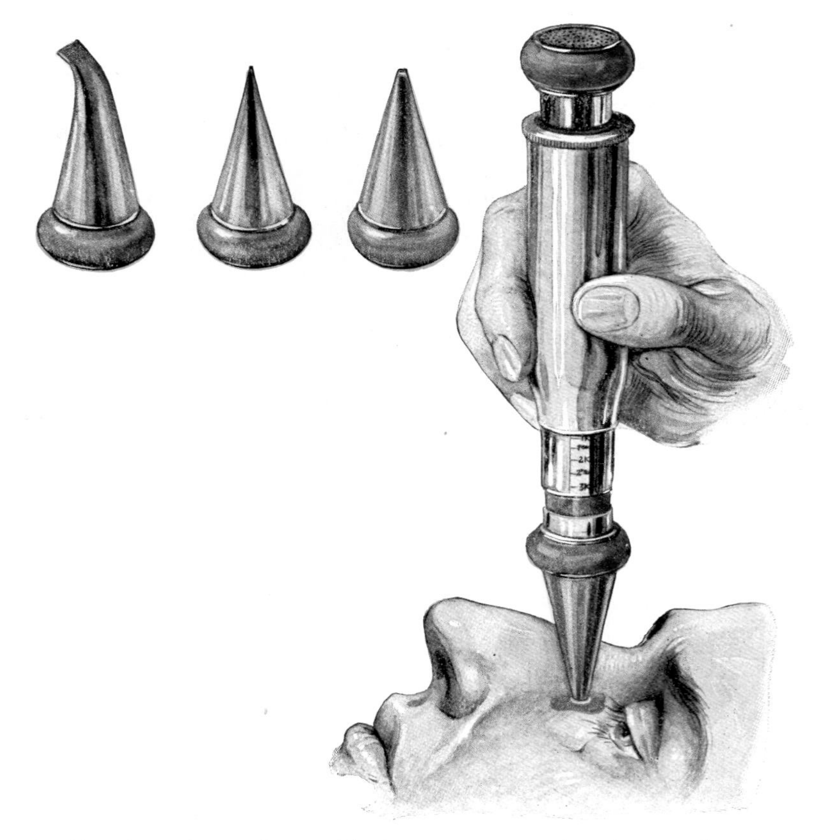

Fig. 448. Freezing a hemangioma with the cryocautery. Attachments of various shapes.

become accustomed to the influence of cold, the period of freezing may be extended. The carbon dioxide snow, which will form on a sterile towel held in front of the outlet of a carbon dioxide cylinder, can be shaped to a form corresponding to the skin area that is to be frozen. A carbon dioxide pencil can also be made by packing the snow into a glass cylinder (Fig. 447). A cryocautery (Vignat) gives remarkably good results (Fig. 448). The apparatus consists of a hollow inner tube, a surrounding fiber handle controlled by a spring, and various attachments of thin sheet copper that screw on to act as tips. The inner tube is filled with carbon dioxide snow and a little acetone, the appropriate attachment screwed on, and the apparatus pressed over the place to be frozen, the pressure used being indicated by a scale on the inner tube.

Injections of hot water are also used in the treatment of hemangiomata (Reder). The operator, his hands protected from the heat by heavy rubber gloves, draws boiling water into a porcelain or metal syringe, inserts a fine needle at the edge or outer side of the angioma, and injects the hot water first under and later into the angioma. The operator attempts to limit the injection to the angioma by pressure, as for example, by pressure around it with a beaker (Fig. 449). Several injections may be made at one sitting. Up to 100 cc. of water may be used, depending upon the size of the tumor. Care must be exercised not to damage the skin too severely, otherwise it

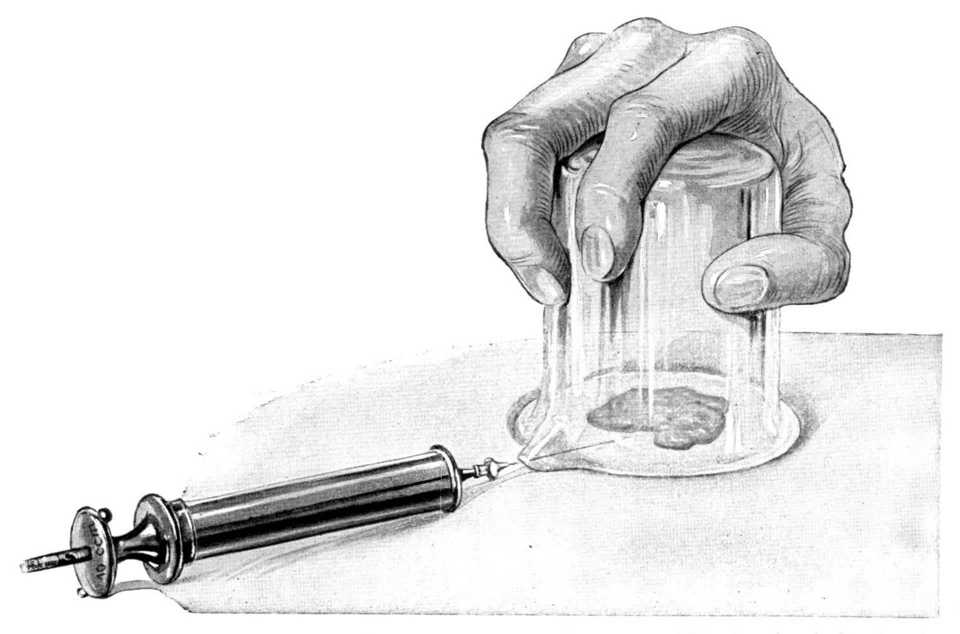

FIG. 449. Injecting hot water or alcohol into a hemangioma, to which the circulation has been restricted by pressure with a glass beaker.

becomes necrotic. The injections may be repeated at intervals of days and weeks. Instead of hot water, several cubic centimeters of 70 percent alcohol or of 30 percent liquor ferri sesquichlorate may be used.

Other methods for the treatment of angioma make use of the Paquelin cautery, the electric needle, Forest's needle, x-ray, and radium. If a cautery is used the skin should be constantly protected and the punctures should not be too close together, in order to prevent extensive tissue necrosis.

Verrucæ and other skin appendages, such as fibroma molluscum, are removed more quickly and completely by excision, the skin at their bases being closed by suture. When the appendages have a pedicle of considerable diameter, the flap used to cover the resulting defect is cut from the skin over the tumor in the same way that flaps are made in the amputation of a limb. If there is any suspicion of malignancy in the growth, it should be widely excised and all possible regional lymph nodes should be removed. When it is impractical to excise the verrucæ because of their large number, the individual lesions may be frozen with carbon dioxide snow or ethyl chloride (Blendermann) and shelled out while frozen with a sharp curette. The wound bed should be cauterized with a crystal of trichloracetic acid. The small wound heals by granulation. Shaving off the anæsthetized wart and subsequent cauterization of the wound bed is hardly to be recommended.

3. Removal of Lipomata, Atheromata, Cysts of the Subcutaneous Tissue and Ganglia

Before injecting a local anæsthetic, I always mark the site of the lesion and the line of incision with a dye, since after the anæsthetic is injected even a tumor of moderate size can not be clearly seen or felt. If it is acceptable on cosmetic grounds the skin incision should be made along the natural folds of the skin directly over the tumor. In excising lipomata, the incision should best be made into the tumor substance, so that the border between tumor and healthy tissue can be visualized (Fig. 94).

By placing a sharp hook beneath the skin on one side and another in the tumor on the same side, the tumor may be removed by sharp or by blunt dissection. All bleeding vessels should be ligated. The other side of the tumor is shelled out in the same manner. After the tumor is removed, the wound bed is examined for tumor tissue, any vessels that are still bleeding are tied and the wound is closed in layers, being careful to obliterate any dead spaces.

In excising cysts the surface is first exposed. The best evidence of its complete removal is obtained when the posterior side of the cyst is shelled out without opening the cyst cavity. However, the removal of the posterior wall is apparently easier when the cyst is emptied previously by puncture or incision, so that the deeper surfaces can be more easily approached (Fig. 93).

Although etiologically ganglia do not belong with subcutaneous tissue tumors, since they originate from joint capsules, tendon sheaths and tendons, they may be discussed here because of their superficial position. The rupture of a ganglion by force, such as a blow from a wooden mallet, or a large book, or the use of a pressure bandage seldom gives permanent results. Complete excision is a surer means of cure. The ganglion, whose position has been previously marked on the skin, is freely exposed under local anæsthesia in the manner described for the removal of lipomata and cysts. A transverse skin incision should be used on the dorsum of the hand. When difficulties arise the cyst is opened, its contents evacuated and the sac followed into the deeper tissues. The tendons between which the ganglion has forced its way to the surface are exposed and are retracted with blunt hooks. Diverticula between the tendons must be followed up carefully. The greatest care should be taken to avoid injuring any nerves in the field of operation, as for example, the peroneal nerve during the excision of a ganglion in the popliteal space. Even trauma from retraction should be limited in order to prevent paralysis.

Joint ganglia almost always have a pedicle which is attached to the joint capsule. In many cases a communication exists between the joint and the cyst. The strictest asepsis must be maintained in every ganglionectomy. The pedicle must be divided close to the joint capsule, and if the point is opened the capsule should be sutured. If a portion of the cyst wall can not be removed, it should be everted, so that the secretions can flow into the surrounding tissues. The subcutaneous tissue should be closed with a continuous catgut suture, the skin with silk. The involved limb should be placed at rest in a splint for eight days.

4. The Surgical Treatment of Elephantiasis

The surgical treatment of elephantiasis consists in the removal of as much excess tissue as possible, and the provision of new channels for the removal of tissue fluids.

Every operation is to be preceded by prolonged elevation of the affected part (thigh vertical, leg at 135°, Fig. 287), and careful treatment of any existing eruption or ulcers. Elevation of the part is also important after the operation, during the period of healing.

1. The reduction of the limb's circumference is accomplished by excising elliptical sections of the tissues down to the muscle fascia. They should not be too small. In addition to this, large sections of the fascia covering the muscles are excised in order to provide a connection between the deep and superficial lymphatics (Fig. 450). The superficial wound, including the skin, is carefully sutured.

2. New channels for drainage may be established in various ways. The fenestration of muscular fascia (Lanz, Condoleon, Payr) is not limited to the leg alone, but can also be used advantageously in the thigh and arm.

In an attempt to establish new channels for drainage through the bone marrow, the lateral side of the femur has been opened for several centimeters. Pedunculated flaps of fascia lata have been placed in the bone marrow, where they are held by catgut sutures, in order to keep the channel open.

According to Handley it is possible to obtain drainage (Fig. 451) by inserting subcutaneously heavy silk threads from the site of elephantiasis to non-affected parts of the body. A small incision is made at the distal end of the lesion and a long, slender dressing forceps, a director with an eye, or a wire, when the tissue is not too firm, is carried as far as possible in the subcutaneous tissue, in a proximal direction. Another incision is made at the end of the dressing forceps or wire, and a heavy, doubled silk thread is drawn with the instrument through the tunnel, the thread's end being anchored in the subcutaneous tissue at the site of the first incision. The procedure is repeated through the second incision proximally, and the thread is drawn upwards, until it extends above the diseased area. In the lower extremity it should extend above Poupart's ligament. The ends of the thread are anchored here also. The skin incisions are sutured. Similar threads are placed over various parts of the limb. The success of the operative treatment of elephantiasis is very doubtful.

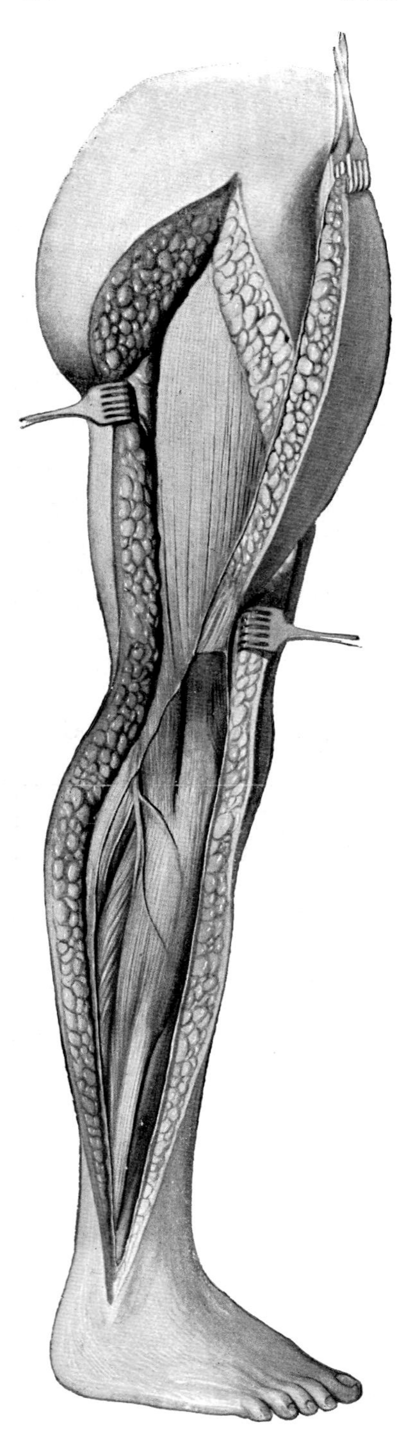

FIG. 450. Treatment of elephantiasis by excising segments of skin and subcutaneous tissue and establishing fenestrations in the fascia. The peroneal nerve must be protected.

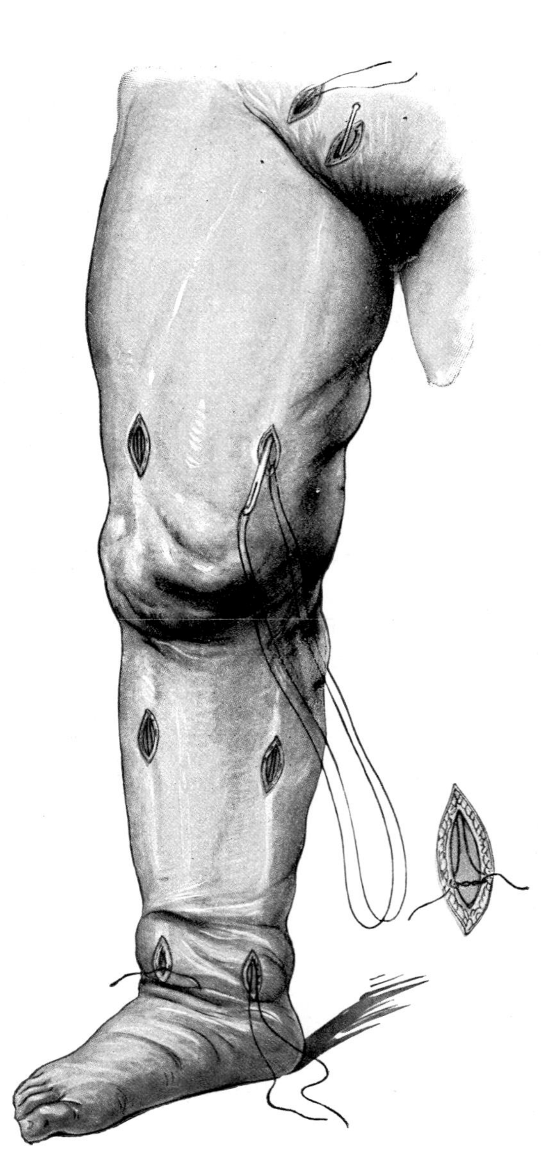

FIG. 451. Lymphangioplasty. Treatment of elephantiasis with subcutaneous threads. Long strands of silk are inserted in the subcutaneous tissue from the foot to the groin to act as capillary drains. This has not been very successful.

The treatment of scrotal elephantiasis is described under operations on the scrotum.

5. Surgical Management of Furuncle and Carbuncle

When furuncles require surgical treatment, they should be excised with a circular incision. A solution of 2 percent novocain-adrenalin is injected around and beneath the infected area. I have not observed an extension of the infection as a result of its use. Only when considerable oozing occurs is the cavity packed with iodoform gauze, otherwise the wound is merely covered with plain dry gauze, after the surrounding skin has been covered with a thick layer of zinc oxide ointment. When the inflammation extends into sur-

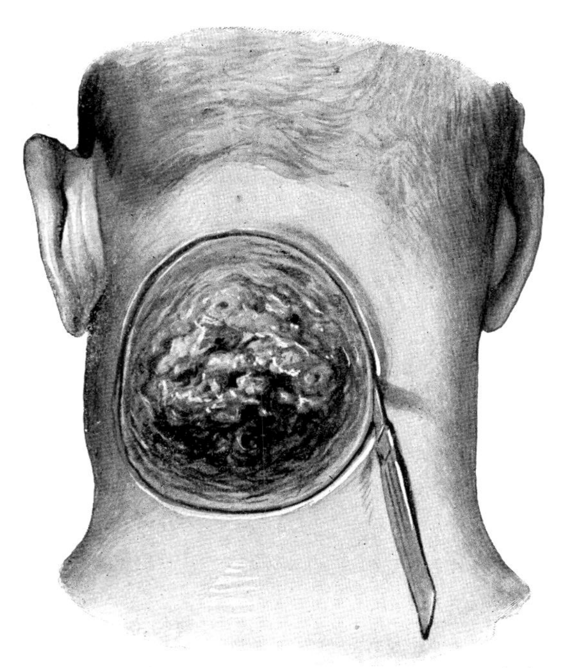

Fig. 452. Circular excision of a carbuncle of the neck. First step, incision.

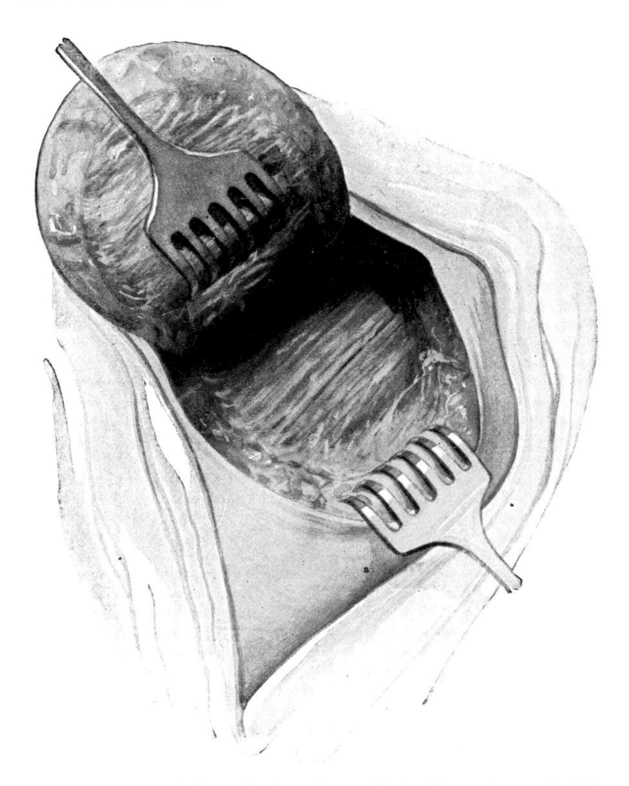

Fig. 453. Second step. Excision of the tissue, including the underlying deep fascia.

rounding tissues radial incisions are made from the edge of the circular excision. Thrombosed veins are incised. It is not advisable to cauterize the furuncle, because the necrotic crust prevents the discharge of inflammatory products.

Radical surgical treatment of a carbuncle requires a general anæsthetic. The best treatment is radical excision. The infected and necrotic area should be quickly excised by a circular incision, the base being freed from the non-necrotic tissues (Fig. 452). It is desirable that the excision include the fascia over the muscle. Although the excision is followed by profuse bleeding, not much time need be lost in ligating the vessels, because the hemorrhage can

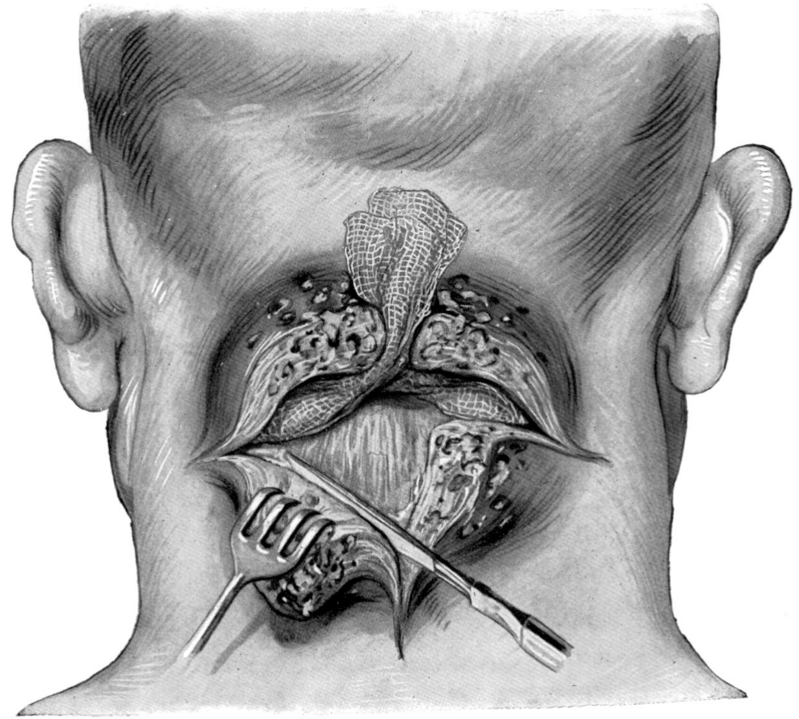

Fig. 454. Carbuncle treated by crucial incisions and the packing of iodoform gauze under the elevated margins.

soon be stopped by packing the cavity with iodoform gauze. When tissue infiltration around the lesion is so extensive that it can not be included in the excision, the margin should be split perpendicularly in several places, the edges raised and iodoform gauze packed beneath them. The cavity produced in this manner closes surprisingly quickly in spite of its size, and no other operation is as a rule necessary to cover the skin defect.

Another method for treating a carbuncle consists in crucial incisions (Fig. 454), made perpendicular to one another, which extend from the healthy tissue on one side to healthy tissue on the other, and which penetrate the entire thickness of the inflamed tissue. The four points thus formed are elevated with sharp hook retractors, released from the underlying healthy tissue, including the muscle fascia, by extensive undercutting, and the pockets packed with iodoform gauze. The points of the flaps usually become necrotic, and these may be cut away with scissors at the time of the original incision. The resulting defect heals rapidly after the wound has become clean.

In the after-treatment of furuncle and carbuncle, the use of force to squeeze out pus or core is absolutely to be condemned. Local aggravation and metastatic spreading of the infection may result from it. The accumulated pus may be safely removed by very gentle pressure over the surround-

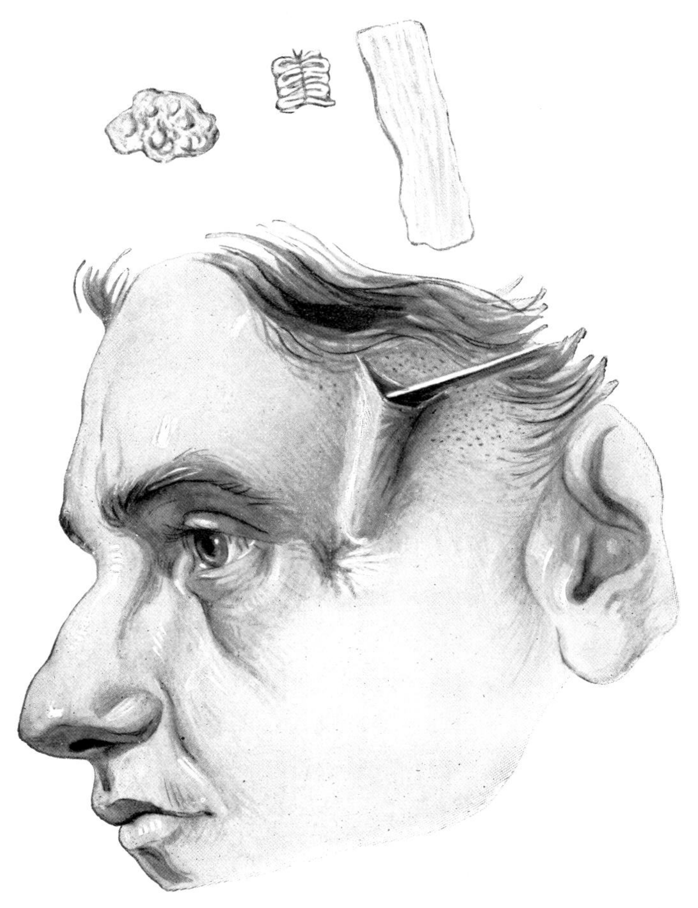

FIG. 455. Elevating a retracted scar, by introducing tissue through an incision made at a distance. The depression is padded with a cushion of tissue (fat, fascia tampon, laced fascia cushion, a piece of cartilage, or a piece of bone).

ing skin or through cautious suction with Klapp's cups (Fig. 296). These measures should be used with such great care that no pain is caused. Necrotic material is usually discharged without artificial help. The surrounding skin may be protected by a thick layer of zinc ointment.

C. RESTORATION OF CONTOUR BY TISSUE TRANSPLANTATION AND PARAFFIN INJECTION

Disfiguring depressions of the surface from scars, tissue losses, etc., can be elevated by padding with free transplants of fat (E. Rehn). In the same way, fat transplants may be used primarily as supports for subcutaneous defects surgically produced, or as protection from surrounding cicatricial tissue formation during the repair of certain tissues after operation (treatment of brain and dural defects, nerve suture, and cartilage defects). The fat is usually taken from the lateral side of the thigh, the abdominal wall, or in women from the breasts. It is often difficult to get the required quantity of fat from very thin individuals. After the bed is prepared, the fat is inserted and sometimes fastened in place with catgut sutures. The general rules relating to free transplantation of tissue must be scrupulously observed (Chapter I, page 119). The fat is inserted through the smallest possible incision, which is made in the skin as far from the area to be elevated as is practical, and is pushed into its bed (Fig. 455). The skin wound should be closed without drainage.

Strips of fascia lata may be advantageously used to fill in some tissue defects (Kirschner); these are used either in the form of small bundles tied with catgut or strips are packed in (Fig. 455).

Other deformities of contour, such as saddle nose, are preferably elevated by free grafts of bone or cartilage, the technic of which is discussed elsewhere.

Small depressions, as for instance sunken cicatrices (pock marks), can be raised by injections of paraffin. Gersuny recommends for this purpose white vaseline, which may be diluted with olive oil in the proportion of 1 to 4, or 1 to 8. Eckstein used paraffin with a melting point of 58°C. The paraffin is liquefied by careful heating, and is injected from one side with a warm syringe and needle. Pressure is made on the needle hole for a few moments after the cannula is withdrawn, until the mass hardens.

Paraffin may be injected if there will be but slight pressure on it, particularly for elevating small cosmetic defects, but it should not be used to fill in larger defects, such as hernial openings. The introduction of large amounts of paraffin into the pleural cavity to compress the lung is for many reasons interdicted. If lung compression is desired it can be obtained by safer means. The fate of injected paraffin varies. It may be absorbed; it may be infiltrated with fibrous tissue; it may be the nidus for tumor formation; or it may be extruded as the result of suppuration.

CHAPTER VI

OPERATIONS ON MUSCLES, TENDONS AND FASCIA

A. DIVISION AND SUTURE OF MUSCLES AND TENDONS

Muscles and tendons are exposed by incisions parallel to their course. It is advisable to make the skin incision slightly to one side of the tendon but, if necessary, to extend it over the tendon, at one or both ends (Fig. 456), so that the motility of the tendon will not be interfered with by adhesions to the whole of the skin cicatrix. The sheath of a tendon is usually opened laterally. I can not recommend complete extirpation of tendon sheaths, as suggested by Salomon, to further the healing of sutured tendons.

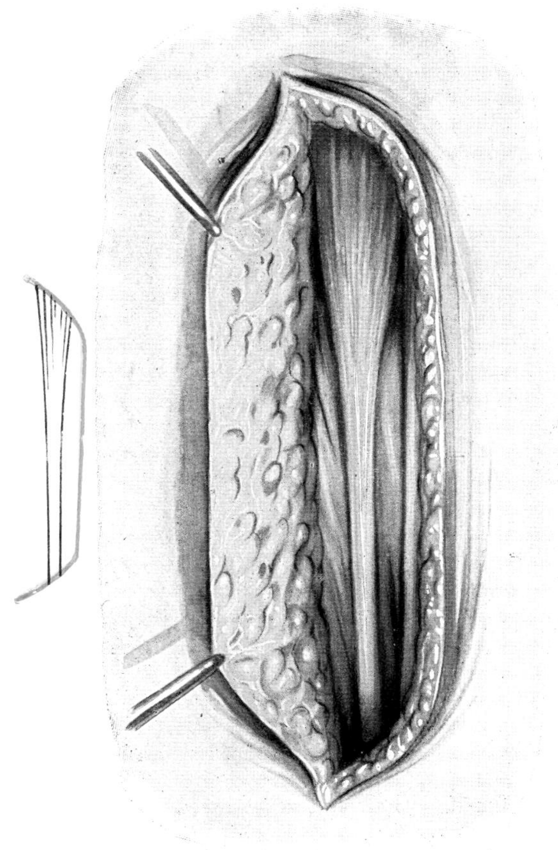

FIG. 456. Exposing a tendon by an incision to one side of the tendon.

When tendons or muscles prevent easy access to deeper structures, they should be exposed and retracted to the side. If the tendons are relaxed by placing the joints in suitable positions the retraction is facilitated. Only when absolutely necessary should tendons and muscles be divided. The most favorable method of incising a muscle is in the direction of its fibers (Fig. 457), penetrating partly by blunt, partly by sharp dissection between the muscle fibers. The muscle is closed subsequently with a few catgut sutures. When it is impossible to avoid cutting across the muscle, or when it has been injured, the muscle should be relaxed by posture and the divided fibers closed with strong catgut sutures. The catgut sutures must include the fascia, otherwise they will cut through the soft muscle tissue. Some surgeons prefer mattress sutures (Perthes' suture for the rectus abdominis muscle). In any event, it is of prime importance to use a musculo-fascial suture, since the fascia insures most of the support.

If the area of operation is beneath a broad muscle, it may be exposed more adequately by turning back the muscle temporarily (Fig. 458). For this purpose it should either be divided and turned back at its insertion or at its origin, leaving sufficient tissue attached to the bone for subsequent suture, or a portion of bone may be removed with the origin or insertion of the

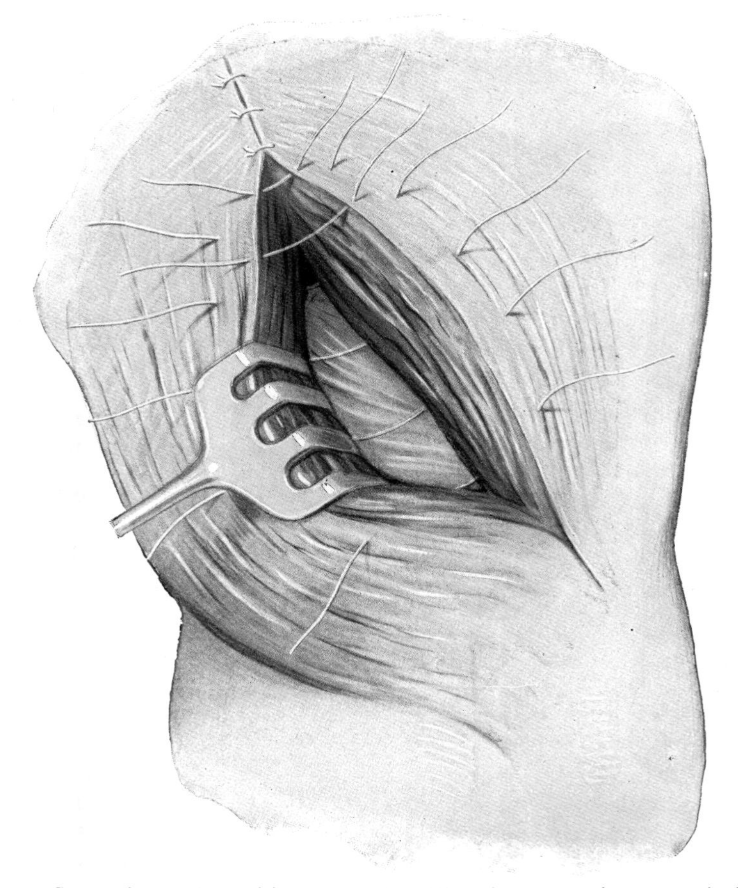

FIG. 457. Separating and reuniting a muscle. The gluteus maximus muscle is separated in the direction of its fibers. It is sutured with deep and superficial interrupted stitches which include the fascia.

muscle. In turning back the muscle, one must protect the nerves which supply it, and if possible also the blood vessels. In this way the sterno-cleidomastoid, the pectoralis major and minor, and the gluteus maximus may be turned back to expose the underlying structures. After the completion of the major operative procedure the continuity of the muscle is restored by careful suturing of the muscle.

When attempting to suture a muscle which has been divided for some time it will be found that the ends have retracted considerably and the gap between the ends replaced by cicatricial tissue. Therefore, the ends must first be located and amply exposed. It may be difficult to bring the ends together, even though the extremity is fixed in a position which relaxes the muscle. It is frequently advisable to protect the suture line, which is under

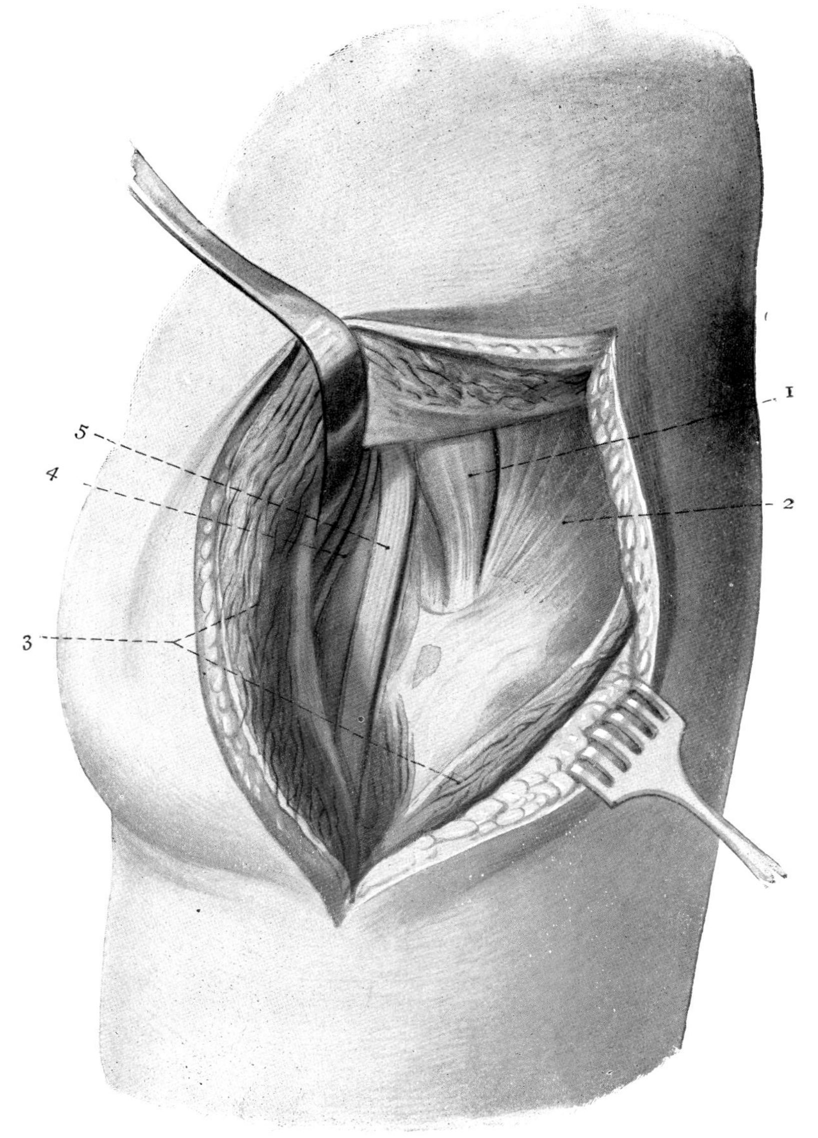

FIG. 458. Retraction of part of a muscle to expose underlying structures. The gluteus maximus muscle is cut through near the greater trochanter and is retracted together with its nerves and vessels. 1. Piriformis muscle. 2. Gluteus medius muscle. 3. Incised surface of the gluteus maximus muscle. 4. Pudendal nerve. 5. Sciatic nerve.

tension, by suturing a free fascia lata transplant around it, like a cuff (Kirschner) (Fig. 463). If it is impossible to bring the muscle stumps together, a fascial tube attached to both stumps may be used as a means of indirect union. In those instances where the direct union of tendon stumps

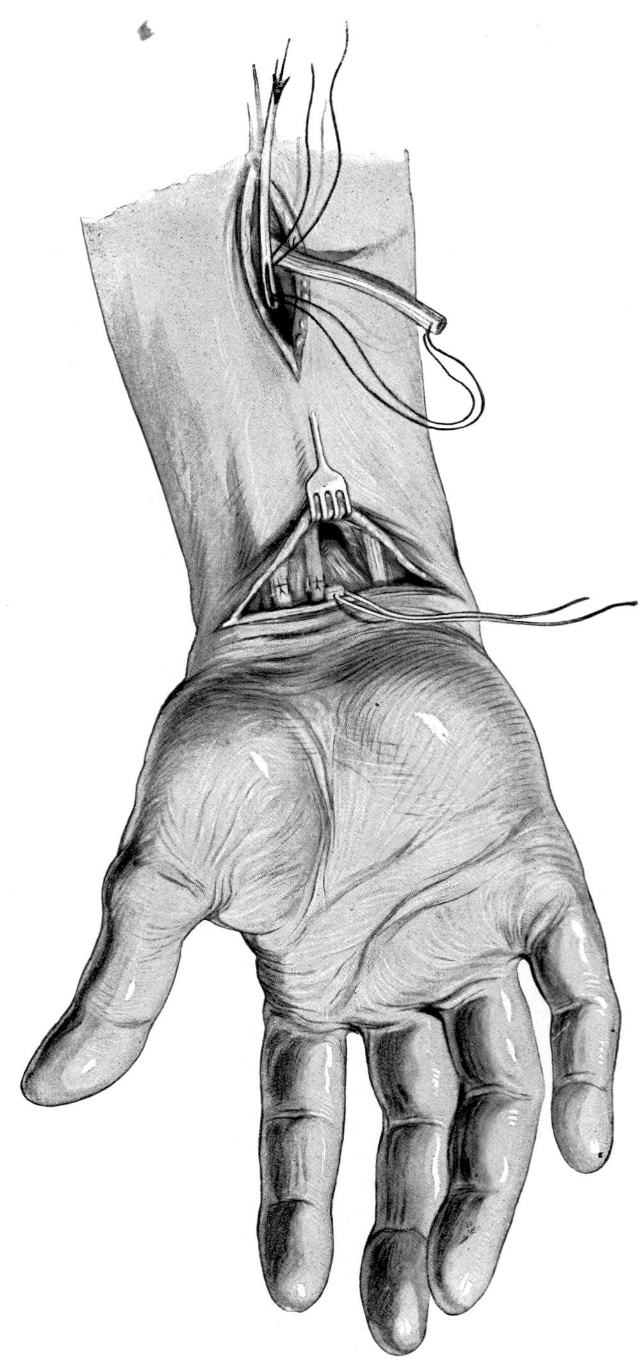

FIG. 459. A tendon which has retracted after being cut may be found through a proximal incision. It can then be attached to a director and carried to the point of injury where the ends are sutured.

appears impossible, the question must arise whether ascending or descending tendon transplantation will not restore function.

When tendons must be divided in order to expose deeper structures, for example, the tendon of Achillis for a posterior exposure of the ankle-joint; the patellar ligament for anterior exposure of the knee-joint; or the peroneal tendons in a resection of the ankle-joint (Kocher), the method of subsequent suture must be considered at the time the tendons are divided, if good function is to be obtained. The line of division should be oblique or in the shape of a Z.

Considerable difficulty may arise in reuniting tendons, even a short time after injury, which have been divided transversely, because of the retrac-

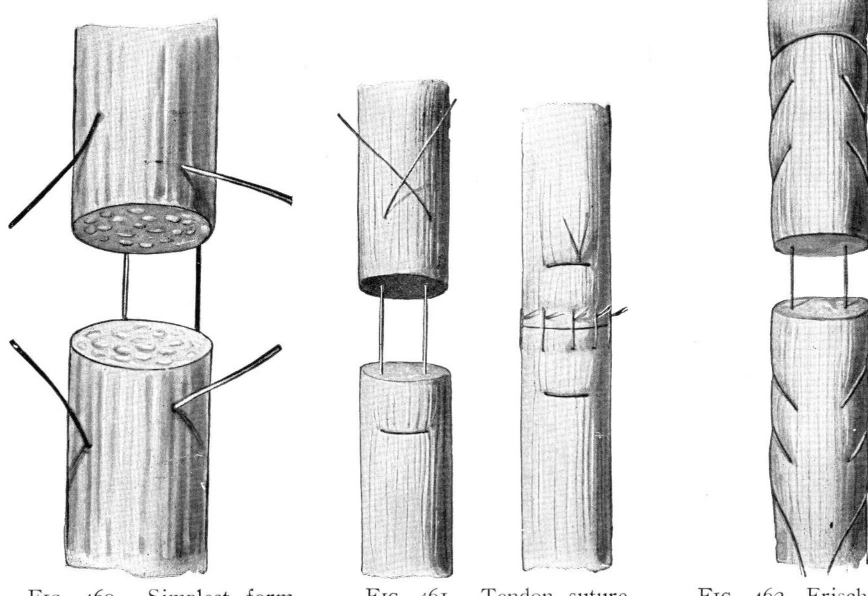

FIG. 460. Simplest form of tendon suture, by two vertical, interrupted sutures.

FIG. 461. Tendon suture with mattress sutures, and subsequent circular interrupted sutures.

FIG. 462. Frisch's tendon suture. After the sutures illustrated are placed, circular interrupted sutures are inserted to reinforce the union.

tion of the ends and because of the disproportion between the tension and the small cross-section of the cut tendon. These difficulties may increase greatly when the tendon is surrounded by a sheath. The distal end of the tendon can usually be easily found by flexing or extending the distal joint. On the contrary, it is rather difficult to locate the proximal end. If it can not be located by extreme flexion or extension of a joint, by freeing the wound margins, and by stroking towards the wound or by the pressure of elastic bandages, the wound must either be enlarged, or the tendon exposed through a new incision proximal to the wound (Fig. 459). The tendon is then drawn out of the new wound, its end, fastened to a silk thread is drawn by means of the thread through the tendon sheath into the original wound, where it is sutured to the distal end.

Fine silk is usually used for tendon suture. A number of methods of tendon suture have been devised in order to prevent the sutures from tearing out. They attempt to serve a double purpose, on the one hand, to anchor the thread in the tendon so firmly that it will neither tear out nor cut through, and on the other hand, will not interfere with the vitality of the issue through crushing. It is impossible to fulfil both conditions, so that in every tendon suture some sacrifice of each ideal is necessary. From among the many

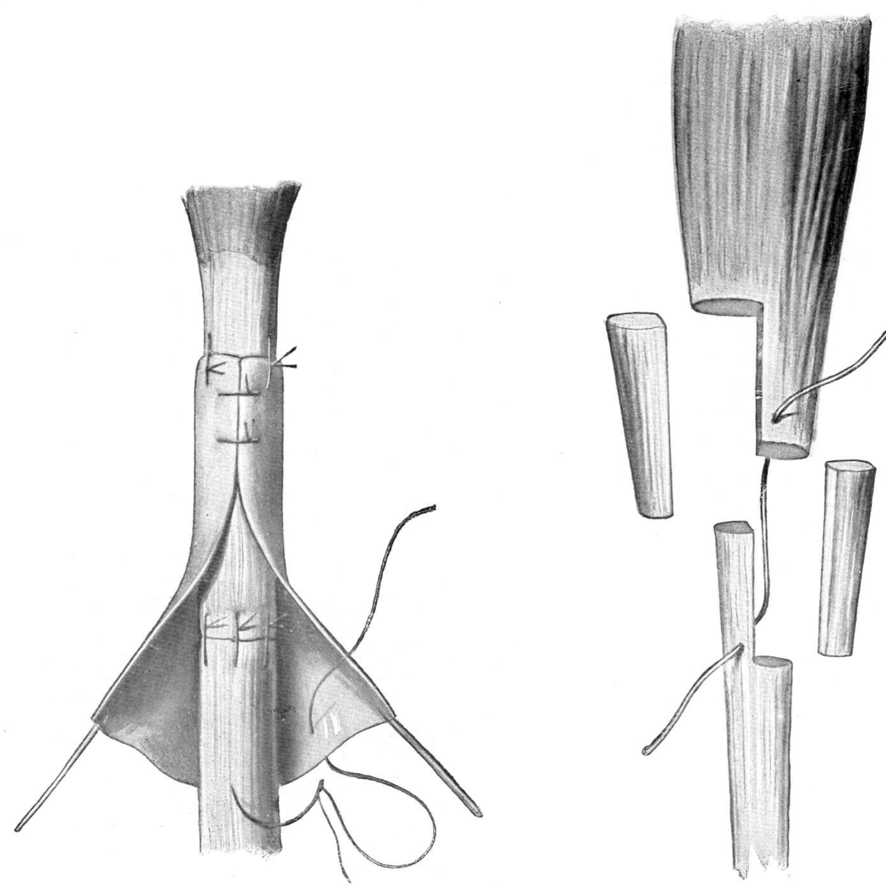

FIG. 463. Fascial graft for reinforcing a tendon suture.

FIG. 464. Uniting two tendon stumps by overlapping.

methods of tendon suture I recommend that of Frisch. I use it when simple interrupted sutures in two perpendicular planes are not sufficient (Figs. 460 and 461). Both ends of a silk thread are attached to fine needles; beginning a few centimeters from one of the tendon ends, a continuous suture is run along the margin of the tendon to its end, where it emerges on the cut surface. The other end of the thread is carried along the parallel margin of the tendon (Fig. 462). Then each of the two threads is carried through the cut surface of the distal portion of the tendon and a continuous suture is inserted in an inverse direction. The ends are tied together under sufficient tension to approximate accurately the two cut surfaces. The line of union is reinforced with fine interrupted sutures.

In some cases even this type of suture does not hold, the threads cut through, and in spite of the efforts to bring them together, the tendon stumps again retract. Under such conditions, and when one wishes to be sure of the tendon suture it is best to reinforce the line of union by a fascial transplant (Fig. 463). A piece of fascia of suitable size is drawn under the sutured tendon by threads in the four corners. It is placed so that half will cover one end and half the other end of the tendon. It is sutured around the united tendon like a cylinder, and fastened to both the proximal and distal portions by fine silk sutures. After this cuff is completed, a continuous suture through the tendon and fascia may be inserted.

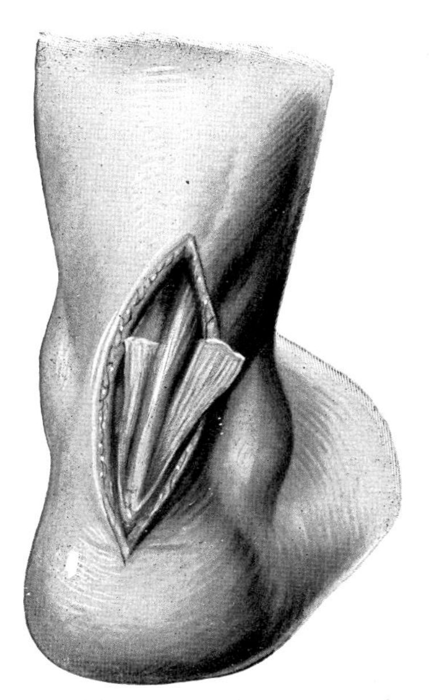

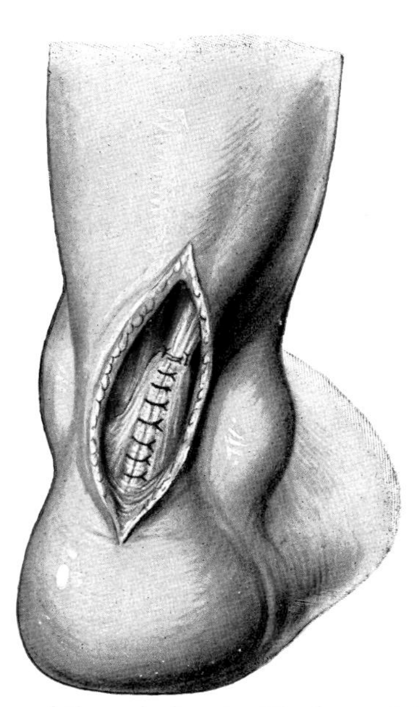

Fig. 465. Uniting two tendon stumps where an excess of tissue is found. The lower tendon is split and after suture of the tendons the split end is sutured around the upper tendon.

Where there is an excess of tendon tissue, as often occurs when a tendon that is too long is to be shortened, or in the transplantation of a tendon, the two ends of the tendon can be united far more securely if they are joined not only by their small transverse surfaces but also lengthwise. Three methods may be used: first, the tendon ends may be recut in the form of steps, and these fitted together, so that a wider surface for union is afforded (Fig. 464). Second, the thicker end of the tendon may be split for a short distance vertically, the smaller end laid within it, and the split tendon sutured around it (Fig. 465). Third, two or three longitudinal button-holes can be made in the thicker tendon stump, and the thinner end laced through these slits and sutured in place (Fig. 466).

After the tendon is sutured, the limb should be immobilized in such a position that there will be no tension on the sutured tendon. After 8 to 14 days the splint is removed for short periods and active and passive movements cautiously begun, to avoid the formation of adhesions.

The success of a tendon suture always remains doubtful. The prognosis is more unfavorable for flexor tendons than for extensor tendons; the prospects are less favorable for tendons with sheaths than for those which have no sheaths. Long, narrow tendons offer more technical difficulties. The prognosis is more favorable if the tendon is sutured soon after the injury; secondary suture of the long flexor tendons of the finger within the sheath, furnishes a particularly unfavorable prognosis.

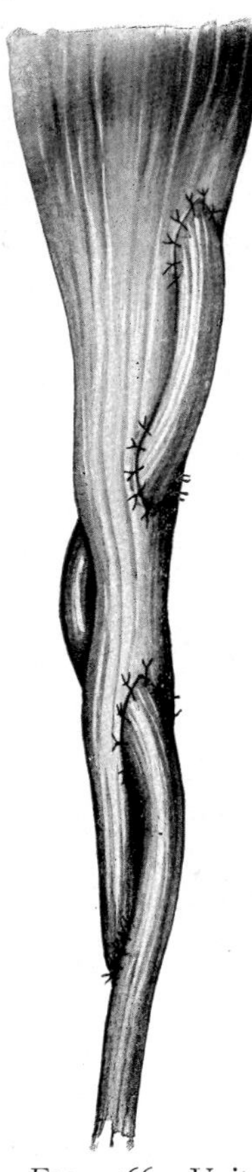

Fig. 466. Uniting two tendon stumps by braiding the end of one stump through button-holes in the other tendon. This can only be done when there is an excess of tissue present.

B. LENGTHENING AND SHORTENING OF MUSCLES AND TENDONS

An abnormal shortening of a muscle can be relieved by tenotomy, with or without subsequent suture. Subcutaneous tenotomy is generally done only for large tendons, which possess no tendon sheaths, as for example, the adductors of the thigh, the tendon Achillis, the fascia plantaris pedis. Such tendons unite without suture, after division. Open tenotomy is, however, a preferable method and the only method to be used for smaller tendons or for those surrounded by sheaths.

In subcutaneous tenotomy the surgeon grasps a tenotome with the four fingers of his right hand, introduces it through the skin under the strongly stretched tendon, but parallel to it, and turns it at an angle of 90°, so that the blade is perpendicular to the tendon. The right thumb is placed on the skin over the tendon, and the tendon cut through, with a sawing motion, the skin being carefully protected. The tense tendon snaps apart. If the tendon has not been entirely divided, any remaining strands are torn apart by force or are divided subsequently.

In open tenotomy, the tendon is exposed by an incision to one side of the tendon. Its sheath is slit and the tendon is divided by a Z-shaped incision. The tendon is split in the center by a longitudinal incision, several centimeters longer than the proposed lengthening. The two tendon halves thus formed are divided transversely in one direction at one end, and in the opposite direction at the other end, so that the tendon ends are cut in steps. The ends of the tendons are shifted to provide the necessary length and then sutured (Fig. 470).

Another method of lengthening a tendon is by forming a flap on each tendon stump, turning it down and suturing it to the opposite flap (Fig. 471).

The method of making a number of alternating incisions from the right and the left margins to the midline of the tendon and opening them lengthwise by force is less efficient (Fig. 472). The muscle can frequently be lengthened

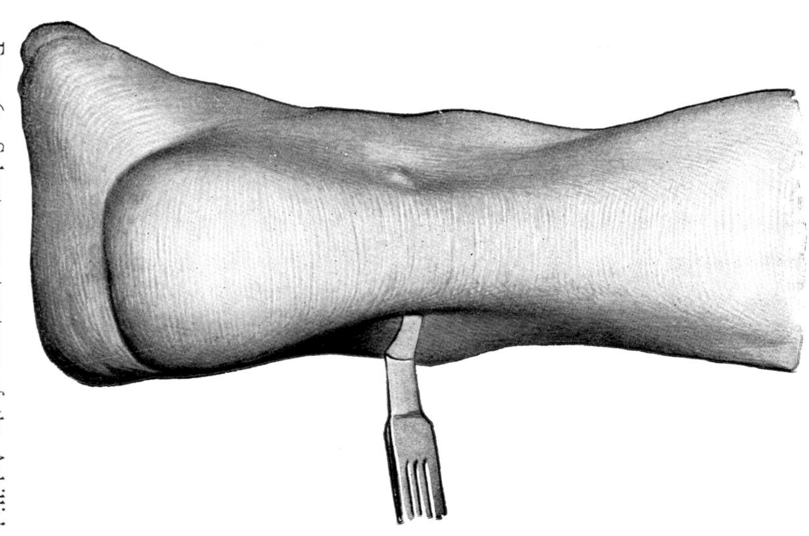

Fig. 467. Subcutaneous tenotomy of the Achillis' tendon. 1st stage: the tenotome is inserted under the tendon, parallel to the direction of the tendon.

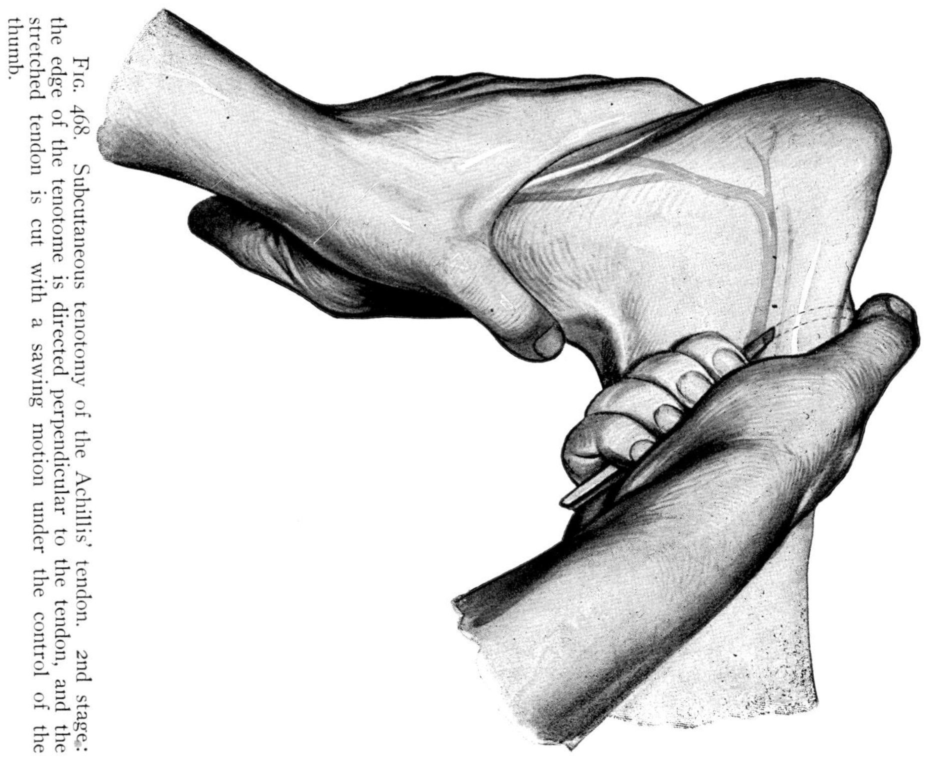

Fig. 468. Subcutaneous tenotomy of the Achillis' tendon. 2nd stage: the edge of the tenotome is directed perpendicular to the tendon, and the stretched tendon is cut with a sawing motion under the control of the thumb.

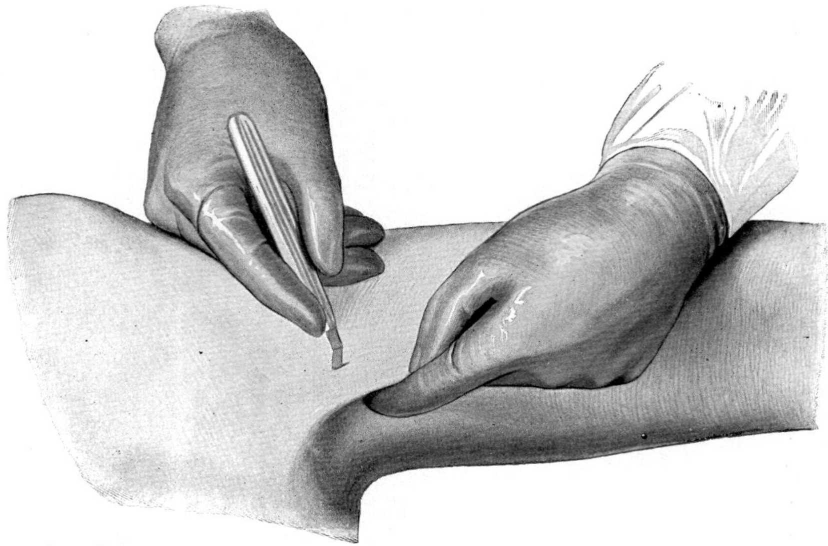

Fig. 469. Subcutaneous tenotomy of the adductor tendon. The tenotome is introduced under the tendon parallel to the direction of the tendon. The tenotomy is done under the control of the left index finger after the blade of the tenotome is turned perpendicular to the sheath.

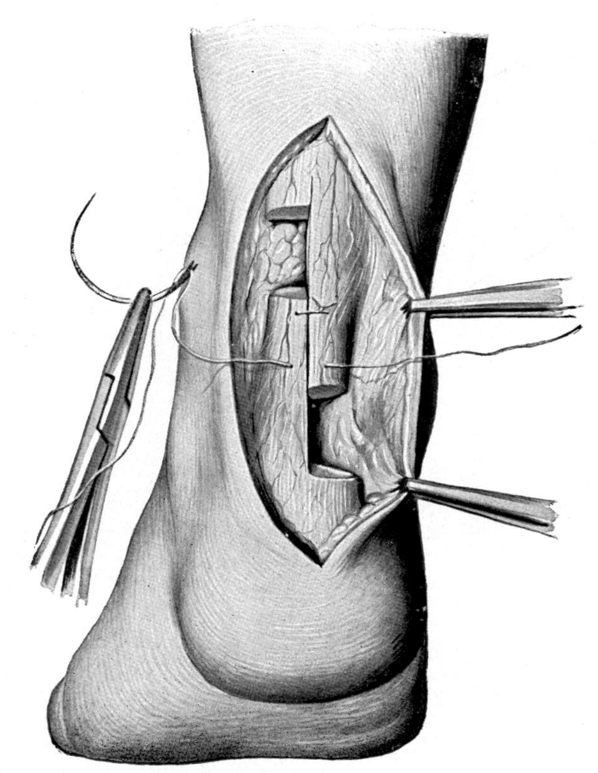

Fig. 470. Open elongation of a tendon by a Z-shaped incision.

without an interruption of its continuity by a notch at the junction of tendon and muscle and forcible extension (Vulpius) (Fig. 473).

When a pronounced shortening of a muscle is combined with muscular degeneration, as in ischemic contraction, the Z-shaped incision can be extended into the muscle tissue. It is remarkable how function may be restored to such a muscle after its length is properly adjusted (Kirschner).

When sufficient elongation of a contracture can not be accomplished by these procedures, there is one last resort, the shortening of the whole extremity by removing a section of bone. Thus, in a badly contracted finger there may be partial restoration of function by the resection of a phalanx.

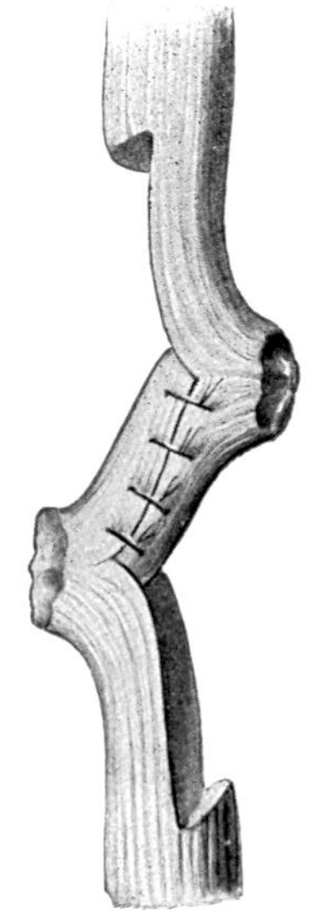

FIG. 471. Open elongation of a tendon by bilateral flap formation.

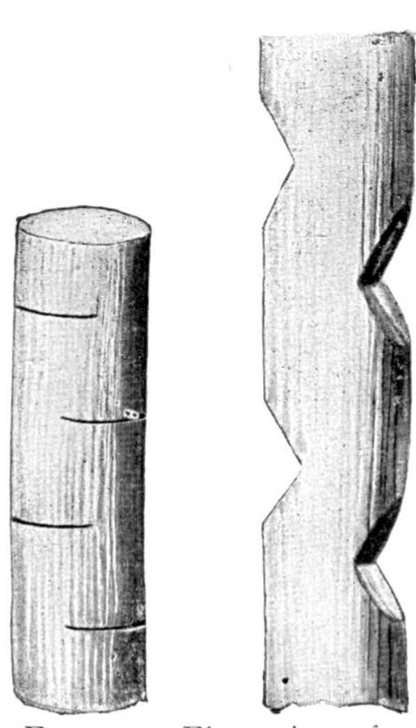

FIG. 472. Elongation of a tendon by incisions made on alternate sides and forcible extension.

A tendon that is too long may be shortened in several ways. The tendon can be pleated by braiding it longitudinally with two ends of a thread and then drawing up the thread, as a result of which the tendon draws together in pleats or folds, or a loop can be sutured in the tendon (Fig. 474). In either case the thickening of the tendon is not to the advantage of tendon motion. To avoid such thickening, the tendon must be divided, shortened, and sutured together. The ends are reunited by overlapping, by interlacing, or by enveloping one end in the other (Figs. 464, 465, 466).

C. TRANSPLANTATION OF TENDONS (NIKOLADONI)

Tendon transplantation does not imply free transplantation, but simply a displacement of tendons. The term no longer corresponds to present-day usage, but it has been used for so many years that it can not be lightly discarded.

It is but seldom that disease or injury of a muscle itself requires a tendon plastic. Usually this operation is required for paralysis following disease of the nervous system. Apart from irreparable peripheral nerve injuries, anterior poliomyelitis is the most frequent cause of such conditions.

Several preliminary conditions must be fulfilled before a tendon plastic is undertaken. If these are disregarded the results will be doubtful.

The paralysis of the muscle that is to be restored must be conclusively established. It takes a long time for the function of a nerve to be restored after trauma, or after disease (infantile paralysis, peripheral neuritis). When

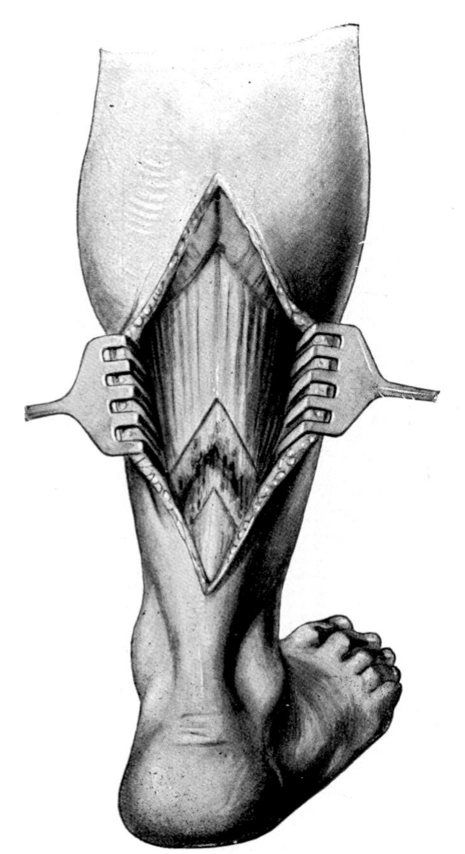

FIG. 473. Lengthening of the tendon of Achillis (Vulpius) by incision at the junction of the muscle and its tendon, and forcible extension.

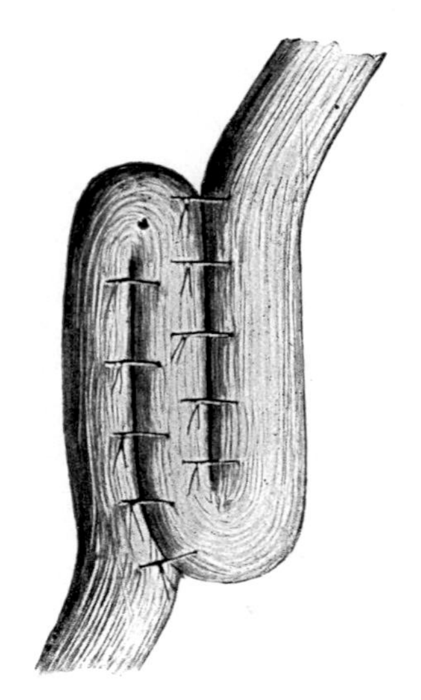

FIG. 474. Shortening a tendon by forming a loop.

the affection of the nerve is of such a type that the final outcome can not be predicted with certainty, it is necessary to wait a year or two before any surgical interference is undertaken. During this period the patient should have exercise, massage, and electrical stimulation to prevent contractures and build up his general condition. A tendon plastic should then be done only if the extremity can be placed, with no resistance, in the position to which the new muscular attachment will draw it. If this is not possible, the limb should be brought to the correct position and gradually immobilized by plaster bandages, before the plastic operation is attempted. It is generally not advisable to operate on children under four years of age, because of the great difficulty in determining in small children the functional capacity of the muscle to be replaced, as well as the muscle to be used, and also, because of the lack of coöperation of such children, after the transplantation.

The best way to determine which muscles are strong enough to be used to replace the paralyzed muscle, is to test their capacity for work by active

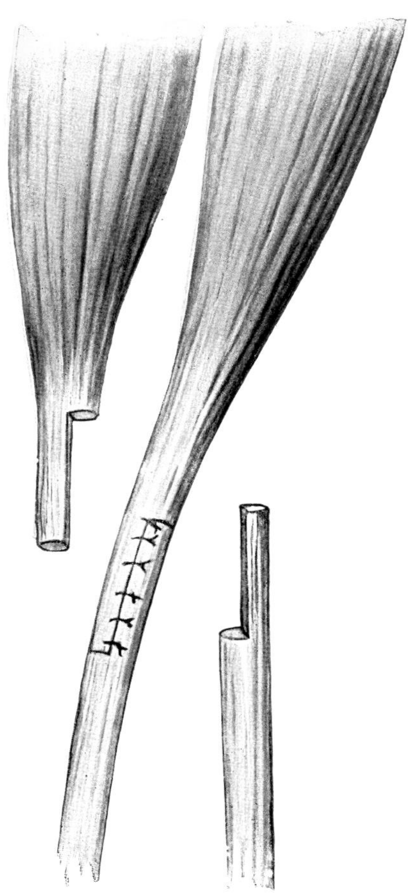

FIG. 475. Tendon transplantation. A healthy muscle (red) is attached by its tendon to the distal segment of the divided tendon of a paralyzed muscle (yellow). This method is to be preferred.

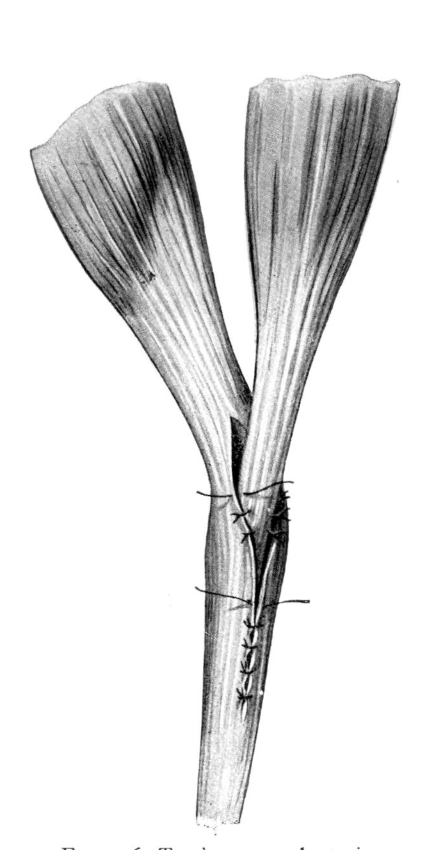

FIG. 476. Tendon transplantation. The proximal end of the divided tendon of the healthy muscle is inserted into the tendon of the paralyzed muscle. If the recipient is not completely degenerated this method is useful.

motion and thus establish the power of the available muscles. Electrical reactions are inferior to this. The appearance of an exposed muscle is of great value in estimating the functional capacity; a pale, yellow color is a sign of degeneration. For successful transplantation only a muscle which has a healthy deep red color should be used.

The simpler the plan of operation, the more promising the result. The muscle used for transplantation should not be less than half of its new antagonist in diameter, otherwise it will be inadequate within a short time. Its length should not be less than that of the paralyzed muscle. The donor should not be detached, during its exposure, further than the middle of its belly, because the blood vessels enter above this. Tendon transplantation succeeds not only when muscles with a similar action are transferred, which is of course preferable, but also when muscles with an antagonistic action

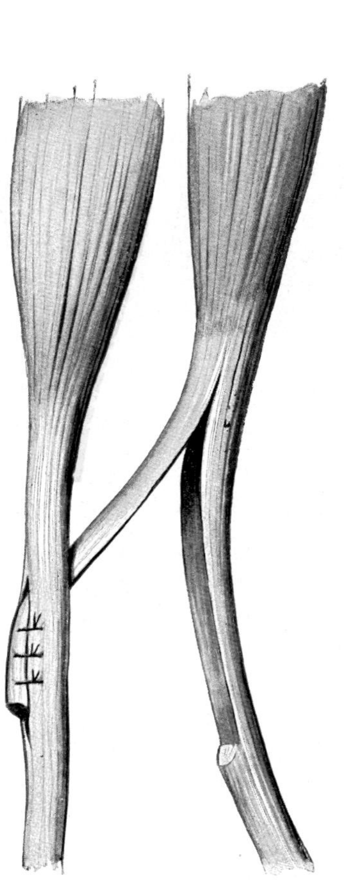

FIG. 477. Partial tendon transplantation. A part of the tendon of the healthy muscle is attached to the tendon of the paralyzed muscle. This is not a very good method.

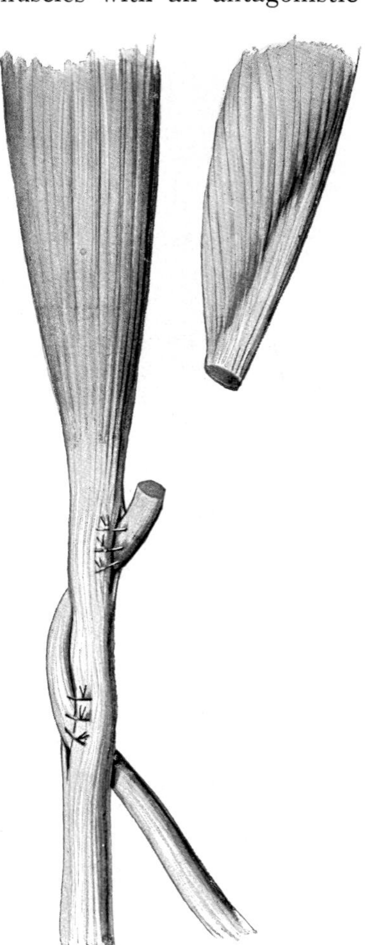

FIG. 478. Tendon transplantation. The tendon of the paralyzed muscle is passed through two slits made in the tendon of the healthy muscle. This procedure is not very successful.

are used. This last procedure has the advantage that though the predominant group of antagonists is weakened, the strength of the group of muscles with a similar function to the paralyzed muscle is not affected.

Of all the various methods of tendon transplantation, the most effective is the one in which the transplanted muscle is drawn upon for the new task in its entirety, and the paralyzed muscle is eliminated completely; and in which there is end to end union between the new muscle and the paralyzed one, total tendon displacement (Fig. 475). When there is reason to believe that the receiver possesses some activity, it should not be entirely eliminated, but the entire donor tendon should be grafted laterally on the receiver, which is left intact, total descending tendon transplantation (Fig. 476). Lateral transplantation of a longitudinal section of the donor tendon on the receiver, partial descending tendon transplantation (Fig. 477), does not give as good results, nor does ascending tendon transplantation (Fig. 478), in which the distal end of the divided tendon of the receiver is attached laterally to the intact donor tendon. The results are also just as poor in lateral union between undivided donor and receiver tendons (Fig. 479).

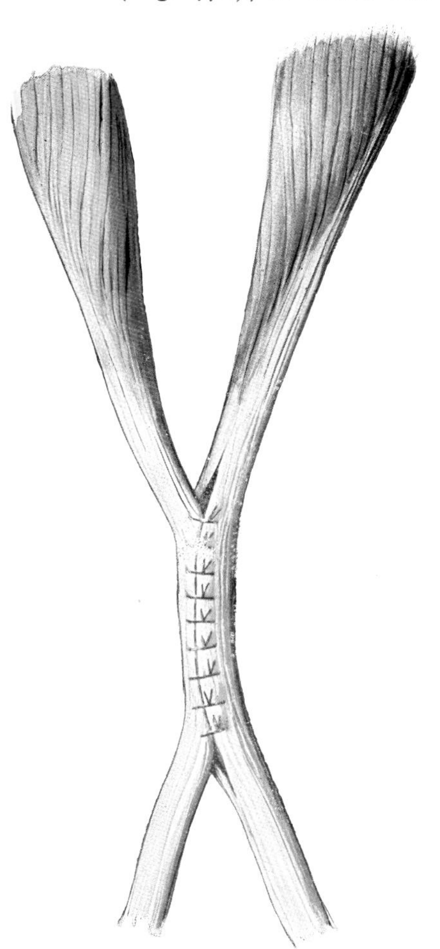

Fig. 479. Lateral suture of tendons.

The donor tendon should be displaced so that the new muscle may run as directly as possible to its insertion, since any angulation has a definite effect upon its action. For this reason, the tendon that is to be transplanted should, as a rule, be freed close to its insertion, divided, and traced proximally, where it is drawn out through either an extension of the original incision or through a second, proximal incision. From here it is carried as directly as possible to the new point of insertion. A straight tunnel can be made by boring through the subcutaneous tissue with a strong dressing forceps. The tendon is then drawn through this tunnel, subcutaneous tendon displacement (Fig. 480), or, if the tendon of a muscle that is to be replaced passes through a sheath, the new tendon can be drawn through this sheath, after resection of a portion of the tendon of the paralyzed muscle (physiologic transplantation of tendons, Biesalski).

It is of great advantage in tendon transplantation to fasten the tendon itself to the new point of insertion. If it is too short, it must then be either united to the distal end of the tendon of the paralyzed muscle, or prolonged by transplanted fascia or silk threads.

A tendon can be inserted on a bone by incising the periosteum, elevating it on either side, and chiseling a groove in the bone (Lange), in which the tendon is placed. The periosteum is closed by sutures which include the tendon, and in addition, several silk sutures are placed through the periosteum and tendon, penetrating even the bone if possible (Fig. 481). The insertion will be more secure if a piece of bone is left on the donor tendon when it is removed, which can be united with the freshened surface of the bone at the site of implantation. The tendon may also be carried through a canal drilled in the bone and simply sutured in a loop (Fig. 482), or fastened by interlacing as previously described. Codivilla fastens the tendon to the bone with a nail, after drawing the end under a periosteal bridge and

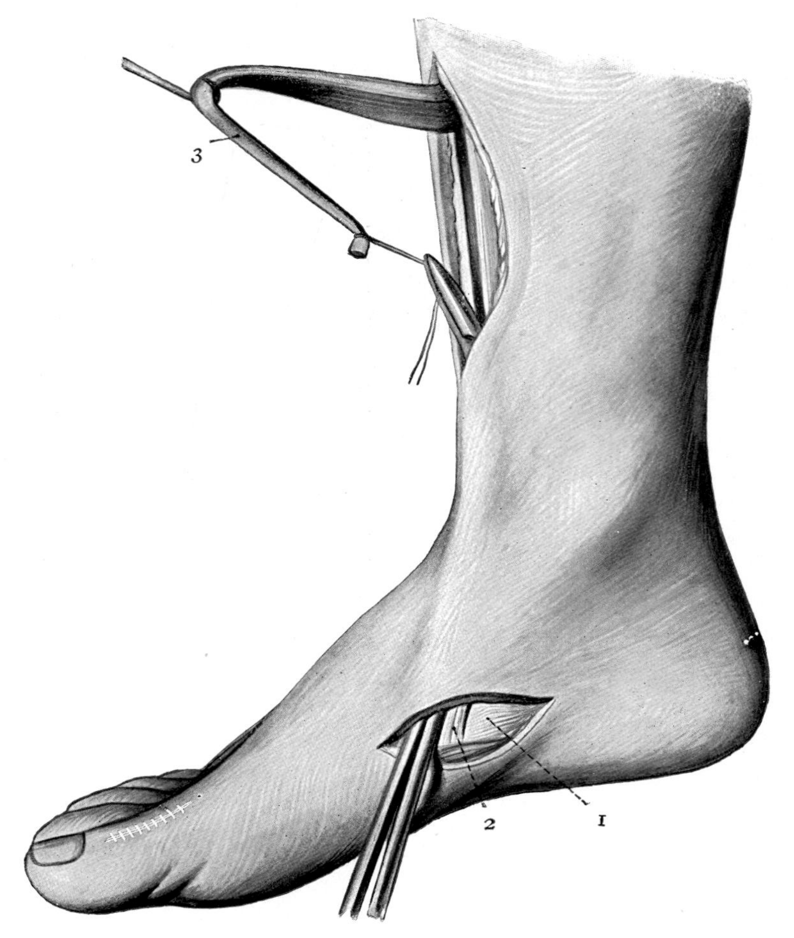

Fig. 480. Subcutaneous tendon transplantation. The donor extensor hallucis longus muscle (3) is separated from its original insertion. It is then exposed somewhat distal to its origin, pulled out and provided with a silk thread. The new site of insertion, os naviculare (1), is exposed. A straight tunnel is made with a dressing forceps under the skin between the new place of insertion and the muscle. The tendon is pulled with the dressing forceps to the new site of insertion. (2) Tendon of the paralyzed tibialis ant. muscle.

wrapping it with wire or silk. We have had frequent success with this procedure (Fig. 483). For a permanent union of donor and receiver tendons, when there is sufficient length, any of the methods described for joining tendons when an excess of tendon is available may be used, such as the steplike union, interlacing, or insertion of one end in the other which has been slit open.

When the tendon is not long enough for direct union of tendons it may be necessary to build an "artificial tendon." Silk or free fascia or tendon

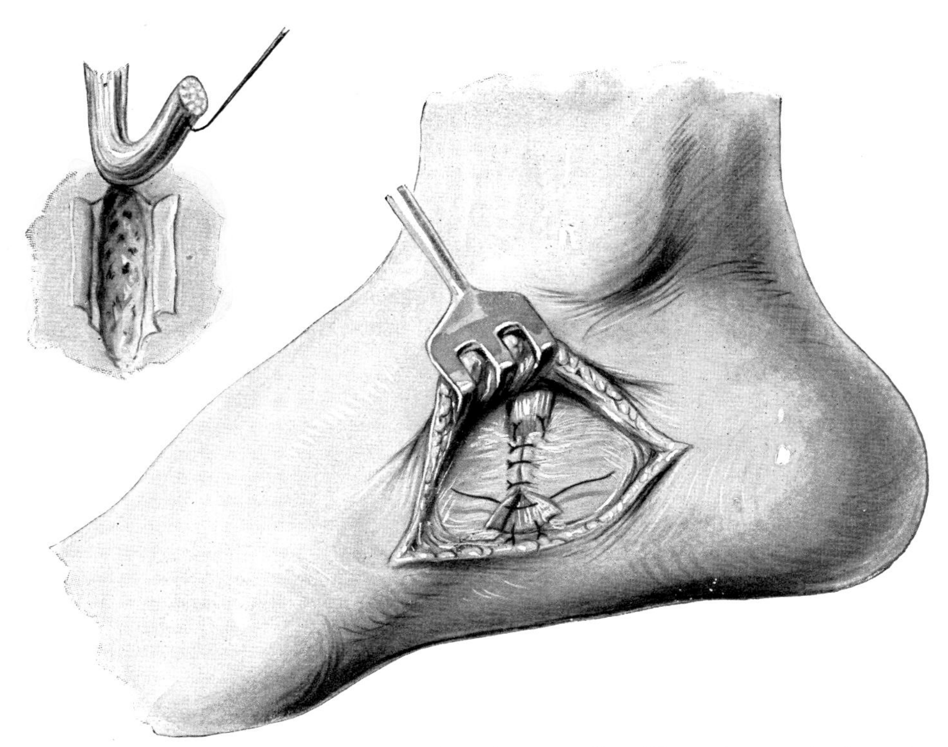

FIG. 481. Method for attaching a tendon subperiosteally. The periosteum is elevated and the tendon is placed in a groove in the bone and after reposition of the periosteum is fixed by suture.

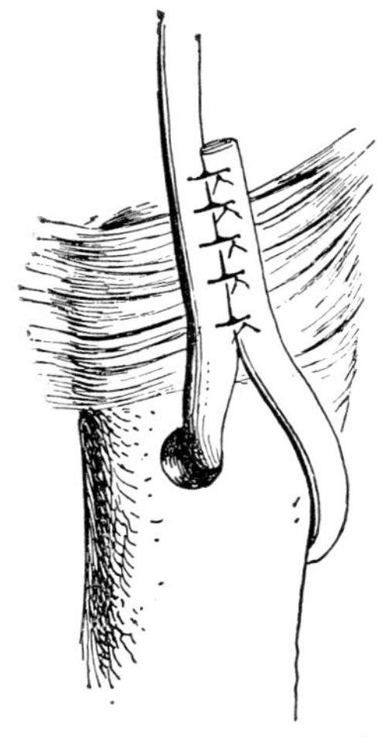

FIG. 482. Method of retaining a tendon by carrying it through a canal in the bone and then suturing it so as to form a loop.

transplants may be used to establish union. Fascia is distinctly superior to the other substitutes.

The proper length of the muscle is a deciding factor in its later capacity for work. At the end of the operation it must be somewhat stretched when in the position of greatest relaxation, so that there will be no excess length to overcome during contraction. This is accomplished by placing the limb in a position to completely relax the muscle when the new union is established, and the length of the muscle is adjusted so that it is just slightly stretched. The overcorrected position must be maintained throughout the operation and for several weeks thereafter. The limb should then be placed in a relaxed position for a period of three weeks longer. The plaster cast or splint is the

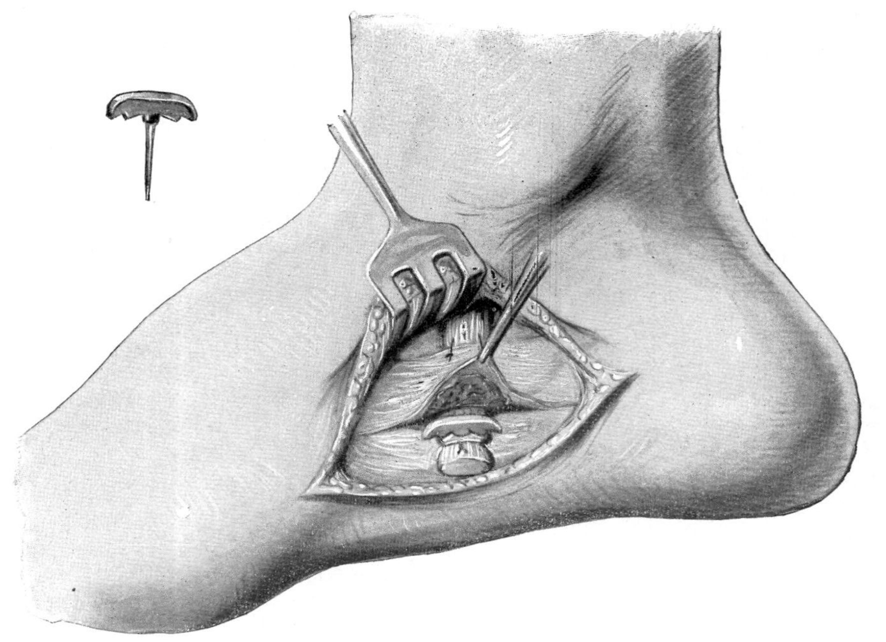

FIG. 483. Tendon retention with Codivilla's nail. The end of the tendon which has a piece of wire around it is pulled through a periosteal tunnel and nailed to the bone.

most satisfactory means of maintaining the position desired. After a period of from 5 to 8 weeks passive and active motion is cautiously begun.

D. CONSTRUCTION OF ARTIFICIAL TENDONS. FREE TRANSPLANTATION OF FASCIA AND TENDONS

When artificial tendons are to be substituted it is even less advisable than in tendon transplantation to open the entire course of the tract in which they are to lie. A tunnel should be made through the tissues and the artificial tendon drawn through it with the aid of a director or heavy silk thread. For this only two transverse incisions are necessary, one for the attachment and one for the insertion of the tendon.

Artificial tendons can be formed from inert or from living material. When forming an artificial tendon from silk (Gluck, Lange), a number of silk threads of suitable strength and length are fastened, as previously described, at the junction of muscle and tendon, and at the end of the tendon they are braided together for the desired length (Fig. 484). The ends of this braid are fastened to the other end of the tendon or to the bone. This artificial tendon must be immobilized for from 6 to 8 weeks.

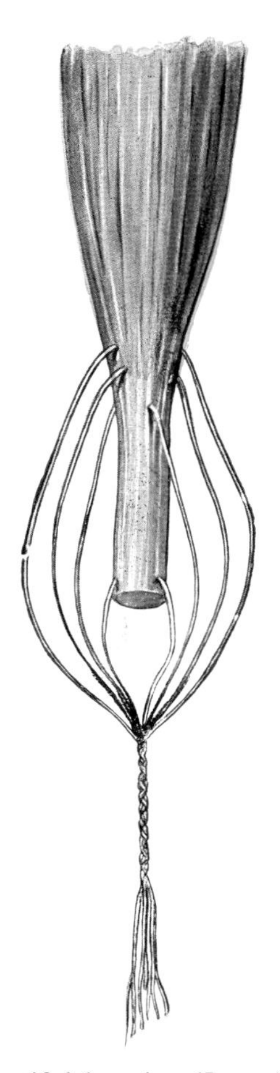

FIG. 484. Construction of an artificial tendon (Lange), with the use of silk thread.

It is difficult to obtain tendons for autoplastic grafts. The tendon of the palmaris longus is the most available one. Because of this difficulty and because of the superiority of fascia for this purpose, the free transplantation of tendon tissue (Kirschner, E. Rehn) is of no great importance. E. Rehn recommends the use of homoioplastic tendons or of autoplastic strips of skin as tendon substitutes.

Autoplastic transplants of fascia (Kirschner), on the other hand, have a wide use at present, in practical surgery. The fascia lata, which is very strong in its distal and dorsal sections, gives an accessible and inexhaustible supply of material. The fascia of the thigh is exposed by an arched, longitudinal incision on the posterolateral aspect of the thigh. The fascia is removed in the form of bands or strips. Two longitudinal incisions are first made in the fascia and their ends then are joined by two transverse incisions (Fig. 485). The fascia can then be removed by blunt dissection from the

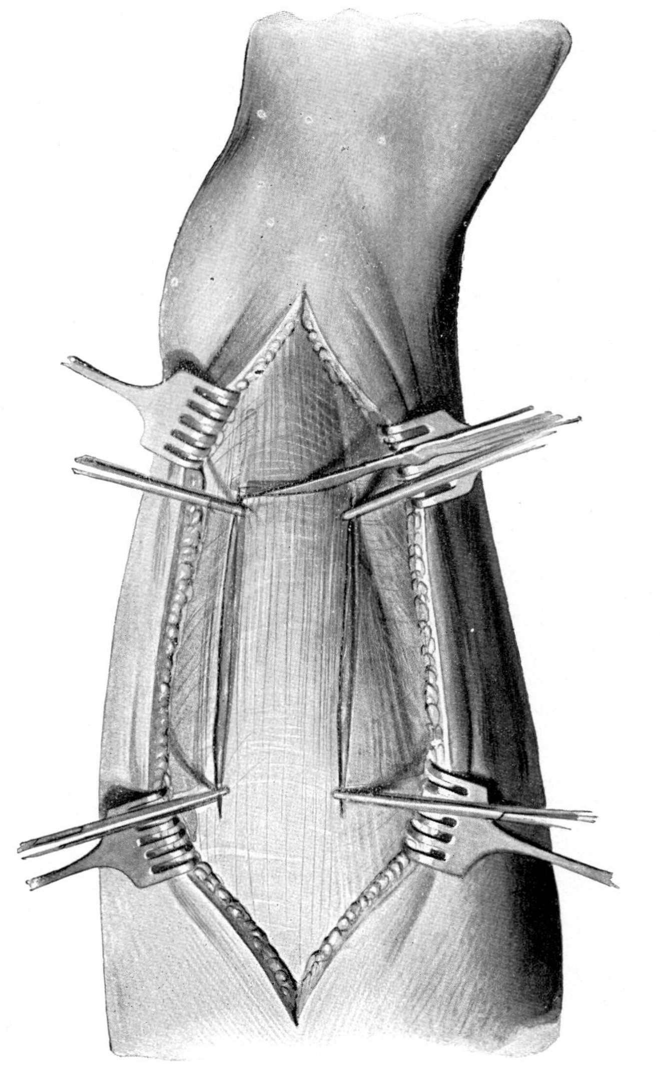

Fig. 485. Removing a free transplant from the fascia lata (Kirschner).

underlying muscles. It can be transferred by threads or Kocher clamps placed in its four corners. The subcutaneous fatty tissue may be left with the fascia if necessary. The gap resulting from the removal of the fascia requires no suturing or covering to prevent herniation of the muscles.

An artificial tendon from fascia (Kirschner) is made in the following manner; after a narrow rectangle of a suitable length is excised from the fascia lata it is provided with four threads in the corners, by which it can be held. It is sutured in the form of a cylinder around the tendon ends, which lie a few centimeters apart. The tube is then fastened to the ends of the tendon (Fig. 486).

The indications for the use of free fascial transplants are extraordinarily numerous. Many of these possibilities, where it was demonstrated that fascia could be utilized, were quite obvious, but were offered as distinct discoveries

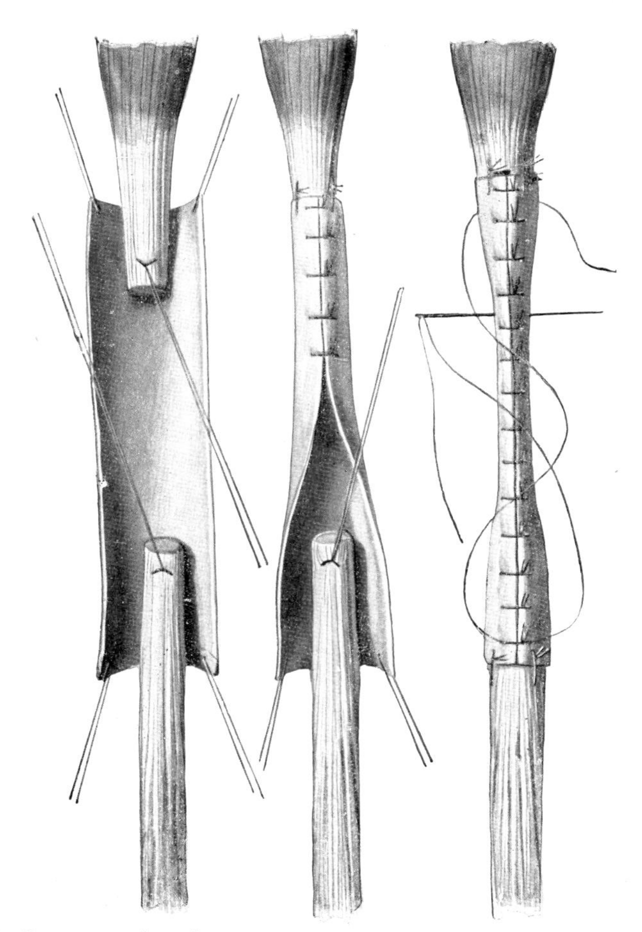

FIG. 486. Reconstruction of a tendon by the use of a fascial graft (Kirschner).

by zealous authors. Free transplants of fascia have proven their usefulness as substitutes for tendons, as reinforcement for tendon and other suture lines, as living sutures in the repair of hernia, in the treatment of ptosis, in facial palsy, as substitutes for articular ligaments, as sutures for parenchymatous organs, in the treatment of rectal prolapse, in the repair of defects of the abdominal and chest walls, as a dural substitute, as inlays in joint mobilization, etc.

CHAPTER VII

THE SURGERY OF BLOOD VESSELS

Every operation in which a scalpel is used involves "The Surgery of Blood Vessels," since many vessels are incised, and demand the surgeon's attention. Procedures referring to this are covered in Chapter IV: "The Control of Hemorrhage and the Loss of Blood." In that chapter are discussed the measures to be taken in massive hemorrhage, as well as the methods for blood transfusion.

A. MANAGEMENT OF CONGENITAL VASCULAR TUMORS (ANGIOMATA)

The management of capillary vascular tumors of the skin, which are, in reality, dermatological, rather than surgical lesions, is described in Chapter V: "Removal of Nevi, Cutaneous Angiomata, etc." This chapter is concerned only with the control and management of arterial and venous tumors, such as cirsoid aneurysms and cavernous angiomata.

In arterial tumors, complete extirpation undoubtedly gives the best results. To prevent hemorrhage Esmarch's constriction is used if possible. When this is not possible, as in operations about the head, excessive bleeding may be prevented by ligation or by temporary constriction of the principal arteries supplying the region, and of all the major vessels connected with the tumor. The tumor should be extirpated in the direction of the blood stream. The tumor is, if possible, released first from the underlying tissue, and then shelled off the skin. When the tumor is attached so intimately to the skin that it can not be separated from it, the skin should be removed with it and the defect immediately repaired by a plastic operation or skin graft (Fig. 487).

When **arterial tumors** can not be removed in their entirety, alleviating measures should be attempted. Ligation of the main arteries and all other vessels entering the tumor seldom gives lasting results. These are tied with heavy, mass ligatures carried through the tumor and, if necessary, including the skin. They may also be treated with injections of alcohol, Linser's bichloride of mercury solution (3 cc. of a 1 percent solution), 30 percent sodium chloride solution, or boiling water, as described for the treatment of nevi.

Venous tumors should also be excised, if possible, and by the same method. Cavernous tumors that have invaded surrounding tissues, so that all parts can not be cut out, can often be removed by radical curettement with a sharp curette. When it is not possible to remove the tumor entirely, mass ligation, and the injection of alcohol, of a solution of bichloride of mercury, of sodium chloride, or boiling water may be tried. These measures may also be used a day prior to the operation for prophylactic hemostasis.

Considerable importance has been attached to Payr's treatment of cavernous angiomata by the insertion of magnesium needles (Fig. 488). Needles, 1.5 centimeters long and 2 millimeters wide at their bases are cut from plates of pure metallic magnesium, boiled immediately before being used, and rinsed in dilute acetic acid. A needle is grasped with a fine hemostat and pushed into the tumor through a small slit in the healthy skin. A number of these needles are distributed throughout the tumor. If the tissue of the tumor is

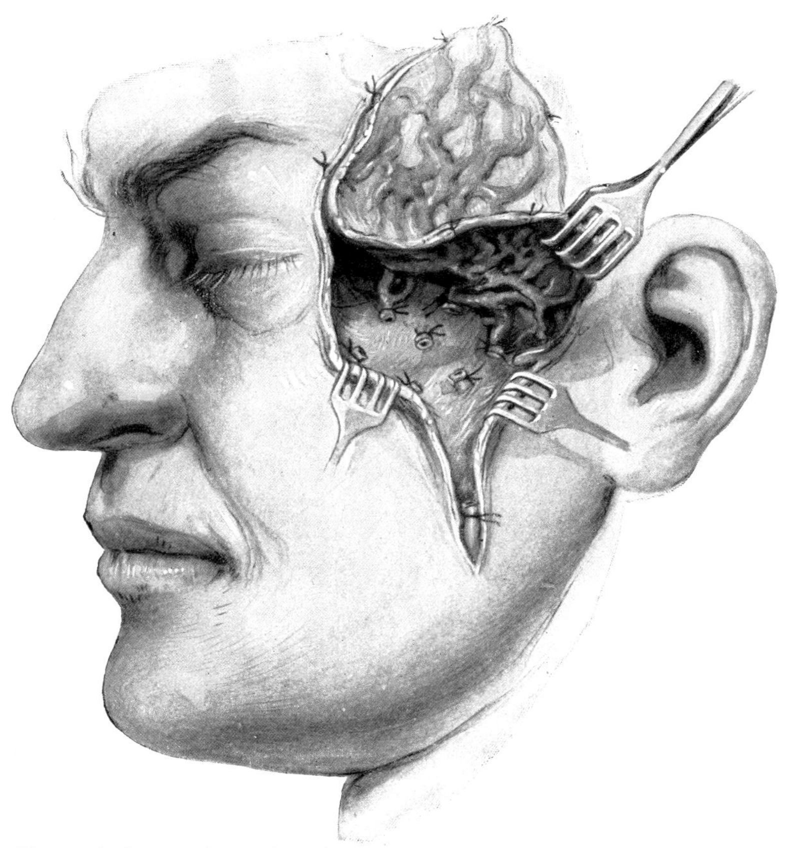

FIG. 487. Removal of an angioma of the head. The temporal artery is first exposed, ligated and divided. The other vessels are then exposed by dissection and ligated.

dense, small stab wounds are made in it with a fine knife or a tenotome and the needles inserted in these. In large tumors, 20 to 30 arrows may be inserted at one time, through several openings. The small skin incisions are sutured and a pressure dressing applied. The magnesium gradually forms a salt during which hydrogen is given off. More needles may be inserted at intervals of several weeks.

B. VESSEL SUTURE

In the surgical treatment of injury or disease of a large vessel, there are two possible courses open. Either the vessel can be ligated at either side of the injury, or, continuity of the blood stream can be restored, usually by vessel suture. Ligation of large vessels is very apt to be followed by the immediate or gradual development of serious consequences.

Occasionally, after a large artery is ligated, gangrene may develop in the tissues supplied by the artery. Even if gangrene does not develop, it does not mean that ligation does no harm. The blood supply may be sufficient to keep the tissue alive, and yet not enough to always maintain the part's full capacity for work. Babinski and Heitz have clearly demonstrated the clinical results of ligating the brachial artery. Gangrene of the fingers and hand was rare, but such symptoms as chronic cyanosis, edema, reduction of temperature, intermittent claudication, atrophy and induration of the muscles developed frequently in the forearm and hand. In addition to these, there may be sensory, motor or vasomotor disturbances, pain, decrease in strength, easy fatigue, paralysis and contractures.

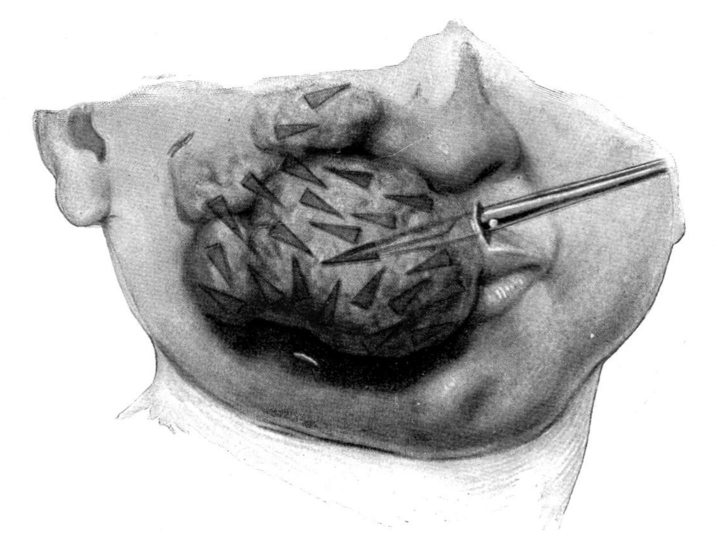

FIG. 488. Placing magnesium needles in a cavernous angioma (Payr). The needles are introduced into the tumor through puncture holes made through healthy tissue.

These last symptoms remind one of ischemic muscular contractures. Such devitalized tissues are less resistant to external conditions that may be injurious, as for example cold. Similar conditions arise when the femoral artery is ligated. The more highly differentiated specialized cells of various tissues are more quickly and seriously damaged from the nutritional disturbances following arterial ligation. Ganglia cells, particularly those of the brain, are specially sensitive. It is, therefore, easy to understand why ligation of the common carotid, or internal carotid artery may bring about irreparable damage to the brain.

All the unfavorable sequelæ of injury or disease of a large arterial trunk are avoided, if, instead of ligating the vessel, it is repaired by arterial suture and its continuity restored.

Every ligation of a large artery must, therefore, be considered unphysiological. It should be done only in exceptional cases, as when technical difficulties preclude other measures, in severe infection, or when it is necessary to terminate an operation rapidly.

After an artery is ligated, the local disturbance is relatively more severe the larger the cross-section of the vessel, the fewer the branches, and the nearer the ligature is proximally to a large branch. It would be of great value to be able to determine in advance the precise effect of a ligation on the function, or at least, on the nutrition, of the tissues supplied by the artery. Several methods have been developed for this.

Hotz, after blocking the artery in question, makes small incisions in a finger, or a toe. If there is definite bleeding from the wound, he concludes that the collateral circulation is sufficient, otherwise there is danger of tissue necrosis. Frisch's sign is positive when there is evidence that venous blood from the part supplied by the artery to be ligated flows towards the body. Korrotkoff measures the arterial blood pressure below the temporarily closed artery; when the arterial blood pressure falls below 30 mm. Hg., he believes that the collateral circulation is insufficient. For Coenen's sign, one observes during the operation, whether a strong stream of blood comes from the peripheral end of the incised vessel. If this occurs, the circulation of blood should be sufficient for nutrition. Dreyer's method involves a collateral branch, which is certainly hazardous, since he sacrifices a valuable pathway for blood from another source. Moskowicz's sign is based on the assumption that a part has a sufficient blood supply when, after Esmarch's anemia, there develops a reactive hyperemia. To demonstrate Moskowicz's sign, Esmarch's anemia is produced by bandaging the extremity, if necessary after elevation, and the anemia is maintained for at least 2 minutes. The artery is compressed at the site chosen for ligation while the bandage is removed. If the reactive hyperemia extends to the distal end of the extremity, the collateral circulation should suffice. Unfortunately, all these signs demonstrate neither the vitality nor the later functional capacity of the tissues. However, even if these tests indicate a good collateral circulation, every attempt should be made to avoid ligation and to repair the vessel.

The fundamental considerations in every vessel suture are that a permanent blood channel through the artery is reestablished and that it accomplishes not merely an external union without an inner channel. Because of the technical difficulties of end to end vessel suture and because small thrombi continually form on the sutures, the needle holes, and the line of union, only vessels of a caliber over a certain minimum size should be sutured, if the operation is to be of any advantage to the patient. Accessory branches, for example, the profunda femoris artery, or the arteries of the forearm and leg, need not be sutured after their main branches are given off. Suture of such small vessels may be a technical triumph for the surgeon, but it does the patient no good.

We know from experience the effect that ligation of certain arteries will have on the tissues. The external carotid, the hypogastric or the profunda femoris may be ligated without subsequent tissue damage. In the majority of cases, ligation of the axillary, the external iliac, or the femoral artery below the exit of the profunda, is not followed by gangrene, but a more or less severe functional derangement will occur. On the other hand, it is dangerous to ligate the subclavian, the common iliac, the femoral above the origin of the profunda, in the lower end of the adductor canal, or in the popliteal space, or, above all, the common and internal carotid. These latter are to be especially avoided in elderly people.

When a main artery is ligated, it has been suggested that the accompanying vein also should be ligated in order to prevent emptying of the vessel and impoverishment of the tissues which it drains. I do not believe that this theoretical procedure is true in practice, and, therefore, I advise against the simultaneous ligation of the artery and vein.

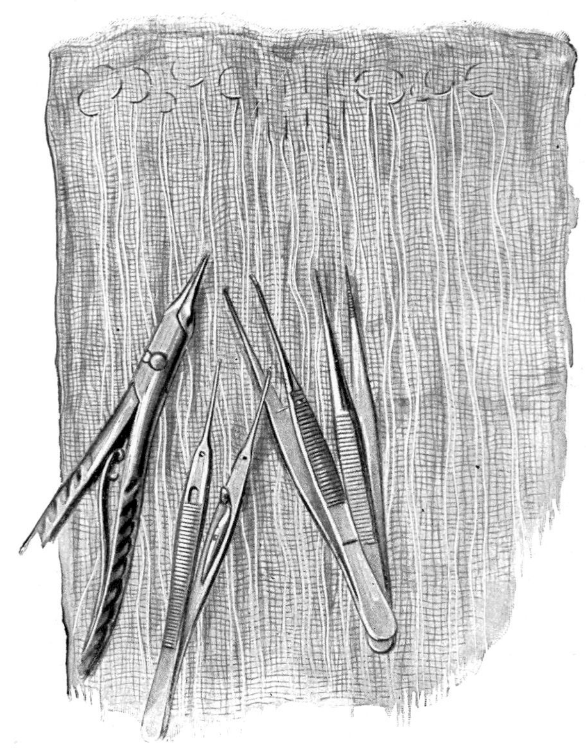

FIG. 489. Delicate instruments for suturing vessels; straight and curved needles, needle holder, anatomical and surgical forceps, the latter provided with a retention lock.

Particularly fine instruments are necessary for vessel suture because of the delicacy of these tissues. The instruments used for blood vessel surgery should be kept separate and used for nothing else. The only indispensable special instruments are the needles, which are very fine, with taper points. They are either curved, when they are handled with a needle holder, or better, they are straight, and handled with a tissue forceps (Fig. 489). For temporarily clamping vessels which are to be sutured, light spring clamps (Höpfner's, Fig. 490) or Carrel's clamps are used. The blades are covered with rubber to protect the vessel walls. They should be pressed together until the circulation is occluded, but the vessel wall should not be crushed. Haberland occludes the vessel with a rubber tube and an ordinary hemostat (Fig.

491). If necessary, a gauze may be placed around the vessel and a heavy catgut ligature tied around it, firmly enough to close the vessel (Fig. 492). The vessel can also be occluded with a strip of gauze fastened by a hemostat (Fig. 493), or the vessel may be compressed by an assistant between his index finger and thumb.

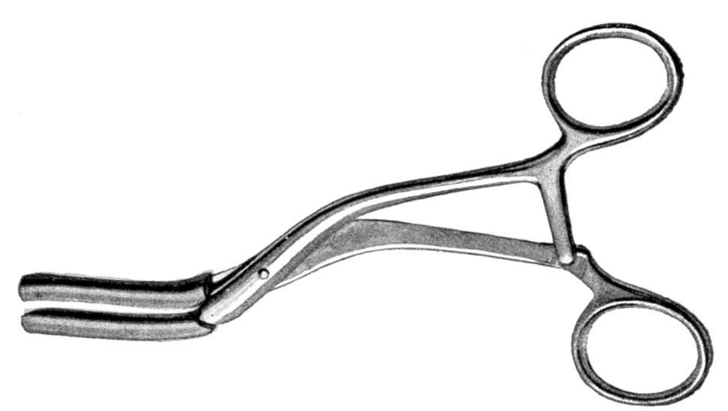

FIG. 490. Vessel clamp with rubber covered blades (Höpfner).

The sutures are of the finest silk thread. They are soaked in sterile vaseline or sterile citrate ointment. Because the needles are so fine, it takes some time to thread them. They should be threaded before operation, inserted in a piece of gauze and sterilized (Fig. 489). All the instruments used for vessel suture should be kept in a 2 percent sodium citrate solution after they are sterilized, and lubricated with citrate ointment if they are to come in

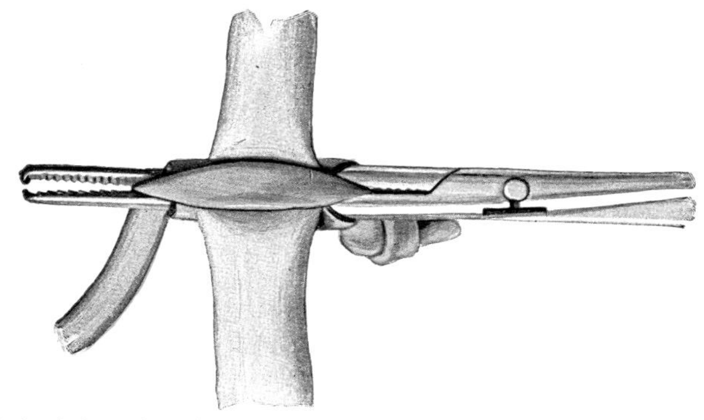

FIG. 491. Method for clamping vessels (Haberland). The blades of the hemostat are covered with rubber tubing and pressure on the vessel is made against these by a rubber tube drawn through them and over the vessel.

contact with the intima. The sponges should also be moistened with the 2 percent citrate solution. The citrate ointment is made up of lanolin, sodium citrate, distilled water, āā 50.0, liquid petrolatum 350.0, and sterilized.

The success of vessel suture, whether arterial or venous, depends upon the union of itima with itima. Vessel suture resembles intestinal suture, in that there must be accurate end to end approximation, but while in intestinal suture the serosa is inverted, in vessel suture the intima is everted (Fig. 495). Every stitch should pierce the entire thickness of the vessel wall. Eversion of the walls and approximation of both intimae is accomplished by U or mattress sutures (Fig. 494). The suture is carried through the first vessel wall from without inward, from within outward on the second vessel, again from without inward on this wall, and then to the first vessel, to pass from within

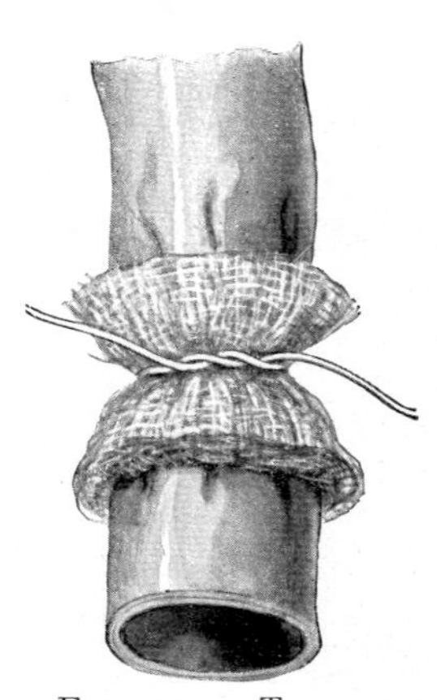

Fig. 492. Temporary constriction of a vessel by tying over a piece of gauze.

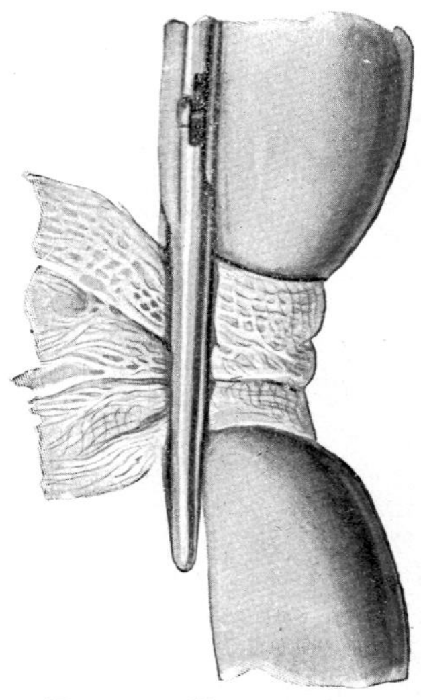

Fig. 493. Temporary constriction of a vessel with a strip of gauze fastened by a hemostat.

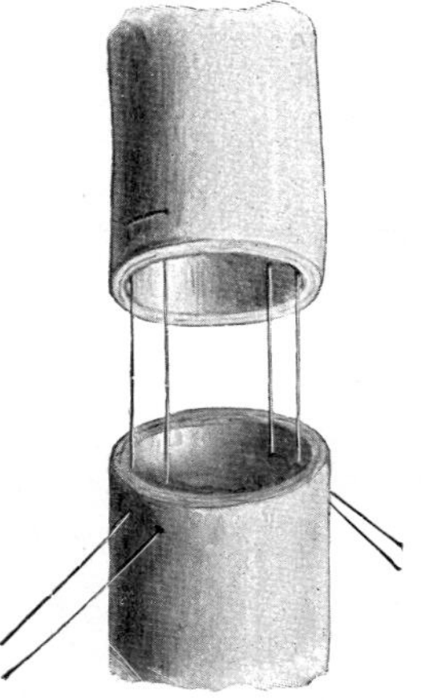

Fig. 494. End to end suture of a vessel. Placing two mattress retention sutures.

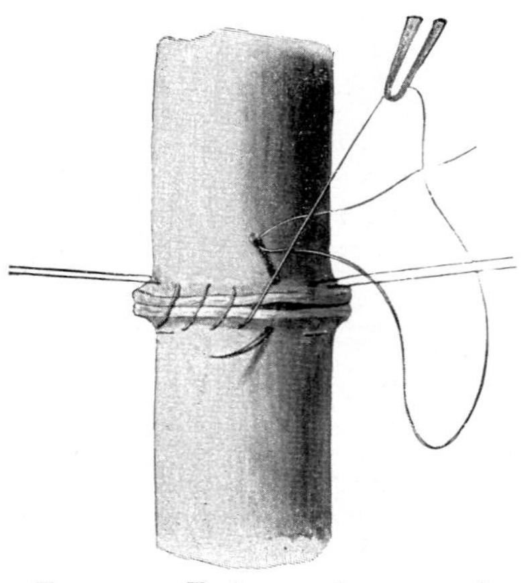

Fig. 495. End to end suture of a vessel with continuous suture between the two mattress sutures. Intima is sutured to intima.

outward. It is then tied. In restoring the continuity of a vessel by circular suture (Fig. 495) two or three mattress sutures are inserted after the ends of the vessel have been freshened so as to provide easily approximated surfaces. If two mattress sutures are used these are placed at opposite points, while if three are necessary these should be placed at equidistant points.

When vessels are very delicate, it is better to use three mattress sutures for drawing the vessels together and everting the margins. The approximated, everted margins are then sutured continuously with the ends of each mattress

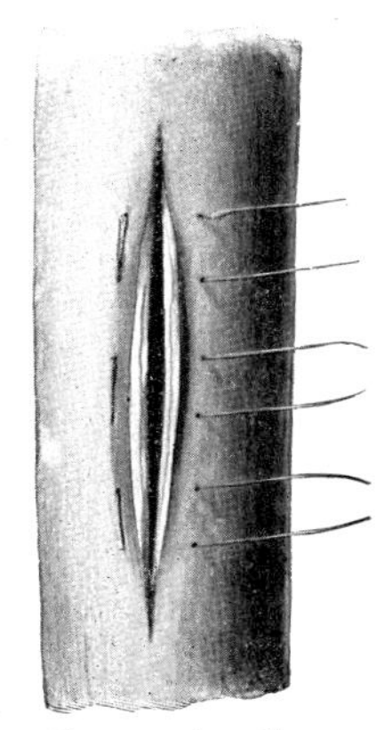

FIG. 496. Closure of an incision in a vessel with mattress sutures, which approximate intima to intima.

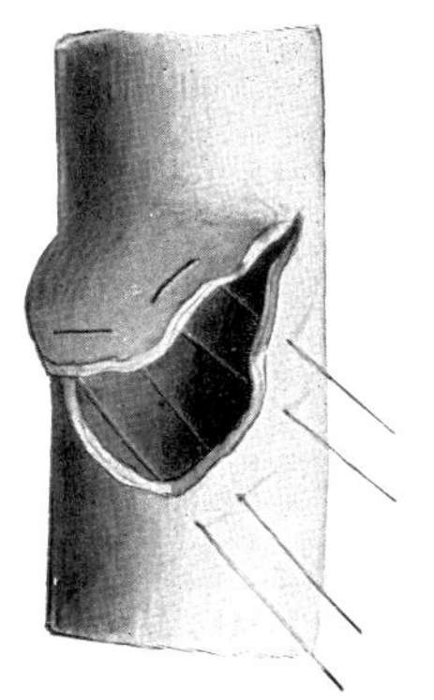

FIG. 497. Closure of a flap-shaped injury to a vessel with mattress sutures which approximate intima to intima.

suture, the stitches lying 1 mm. apart and 1 mm. from the margin. When this is finished, the ends are tied with one another. The additional suture of the periarterial tissues increases the security of the vessel suture, but it is not absolutely necessary. When the suturing is terminated the peripheral clamp is taken off the artery first, and then the central clamp is slowly released. After venous suture the clamps are removed in reverse order. There is frequently some hemorrhage from the individual needle punctures. This bleeding can be checked by pressure within a short time, if the suture line is compressed between sponges for a few moments to diminish the force of the blood stream. This direct method of vessel suture is simpler and more dependable than a method involving the use of a prosthesis (Payr).

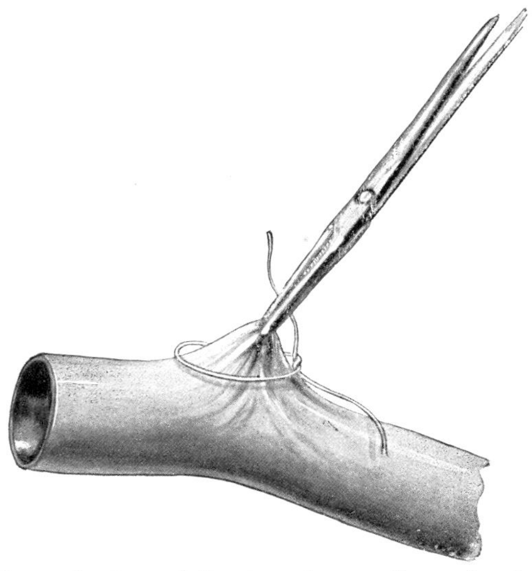

FIG. 498. Lateral ligation of a small opening in a vein.

Injuries to the lateral wall of an artery are sutured on the same principles (Figs. 496 and 497). Fairly large openings in the walls of veins can be closed by drawing the site of injury to a point and ligating it (Fig 498). Generally, veins that have been cut across need not be sutured, but can be ligated. Occlusion of even the principal veins does not, as a rule, give rise to any lasting disturbance.

When the ends of a divided vessel lie some distance apart, they can often be brought together by placing the extremity in a suitable position. This position of relaxation must be maintained by splints for at least ten days after the vessel has been sutured, and should be discontinued gradually and with the aid of supportive bandages. Wide exposure of both ends of the vessel is also helpful in their approximation, since the elastic arteries can be considerably stretched.

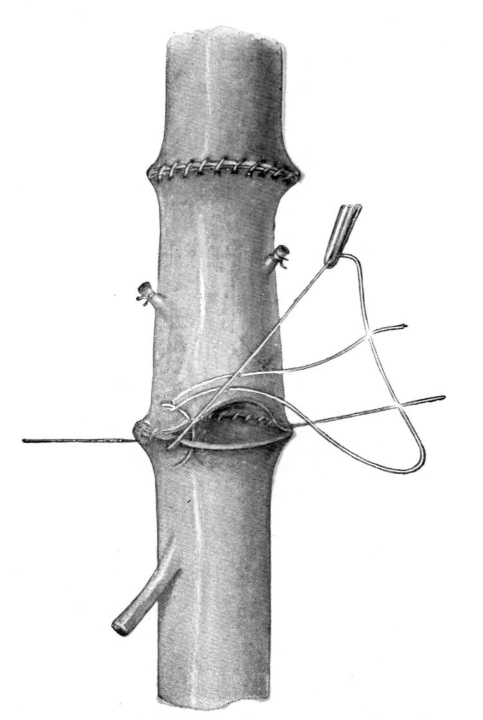

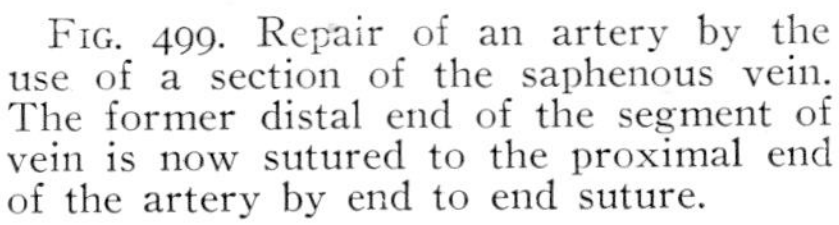

Fig. 499. Repair of an artery by the use of a section of the saphenous vein. The former distal end of the segment of vein is now sutured to the proximal end of the artery by end to end suture.

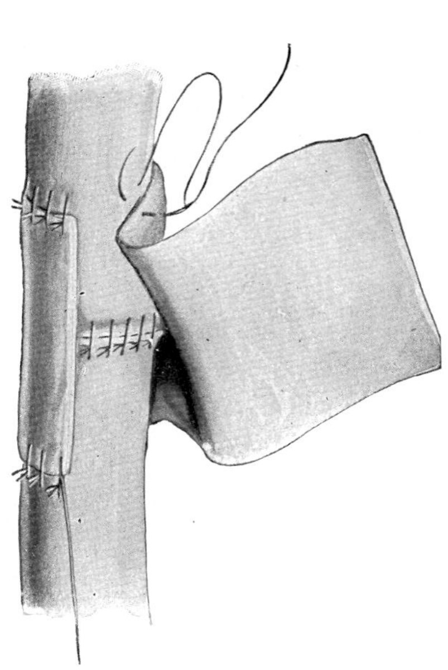

Fig. 500. Reinforcing a circular suture of a vessel by a fascial transplant (Kirschner).

If the ends of an important artery can not be brought together by any method, for example, the ends of a torn popliteal artery, they may be united by inserting a free transplant from another vessel. As a rule, a section of the saphenous vein is used. After exposing and freshening the two ends of the divided artery, a section of the saphenous vein in the thigh is removed and the arterial continuity is reestablished with a circular suture at either end. If any valves are present in the section they must be placed in the reverse direction (Fig. 499). Because of the arterial pressure the vein will at first become spindle-shaped, but in time the shape adjusts itself, due to thickening of the wall. Bridging the vessel gap by a free venous transplant is so much simpler and safer than direct arterial suture under great tension, and is much more physiologic than ligation, that this method should be used oftener than it has been.

It is worth noting that vessel suture is so successful due apparently to the excellent blood supply of the tissues involved. The suture line withstands considerable tension, and as a rule it remains intact in an infected area where it is necessary to drain or pack the wound. In such a case, an attempt should be made to cover at least the line of suture with some of the surrounding tissues. A suture line that is under tension can be reinforced considerably and safeguarded by surrounding it with a free transplant of fascia lata (Kirschner, Fig. 500). Patients who have undergone such an operation must be constantly watched, so that in case the suture line gives way serious hemorrhage may be forestalled by immediate constriction and ligation. A loose Esmarch tourniquet, or a pneumatic cuff may be left in place around the extremity so that in case of secondary hemorrhage it can be used immediately. It is well to have on hand a compression apparatus for the aorta, in case it should be needed.

C. SURGICAL TREATMENT OF ANEURYSMS

Every aneurysm finally forms an obstruction to the circulation. The conditions essential to the life of the tissues of the region are interfered with. In many cases the entire limb may show evidences of disturbance as a result of the obstruction. In addition, the vascular tumor often presses upon the adjoining nerve trunks and muscles. Sometimes emboli lodge in the peripheral arteries and nutritional derangements follow. It is but seldom that an aneurysm remains quiescent. In most instances they enlarge slowly or give rise to repeated hemorrhages in the tissues, which results in inflammatory and pressure symptoms. There is always the threatening danger of rupture. Besides the local symptoms, larger aneurysms, especially arterio-venous aneurysms, will in time damage the heart. In arterio-venous aneurysm, the blood thrown into the arteries does not reach the capillaries, but passes through the fistula directly into the vein, and returns at once to the heart. More work is thrown on the heart in handling this increased quantity of blood, and it enlarges and hypertrophies under the constant strain of overwork.

The conservative treatment of aneurysms, which consists in continuous or temporary compression of the aneurysm or of the artery proximal to it, is of little value in most cases. It should be limited to inoperable aneurysms. Every aneurysm should, if possible, be treated surgically.

Theoretically, the following procedures might be useful:

1. Proximal ligation of the artery.
2. Distal ligation of the artery (Brasdor-Wradrop).
3. Ligation of all vessels communicating with the sac.
4. Ligation of all vessels communicating with the sac, opening and cleaning out the sac.
5. Ligation of all vessels communicating with the sac and resection of the sac, or endo-aneurysmorrhaphy.
6. Division of the proximal and distal arteries, removal of the sac, and restoration of the continuity of the vessel by suture.

The vein involved in an arterio-venous aneurysm must be taken care of separately.

Practically, nearly all of these procedures have but a historical value. The restoration of continuity by vessel suture is the procedure of choice (Fig. 501). The other procedures are to be considered only as possible alternatives if there is difficulty with this one.

In many cases there is great difficulty in restoring the normal continuity of the artery; in some cases the difficulties are insurmountable. Experience has taught that when an aneurysm is present the circulation is always obstructed to a certain extent, and as a result there has been a gradual increase in the collateral circulation. It is often possible, because of this, to ligate arteries with impunity, though their sudden ligation would, otherwise, certainly cause severe disturbances. This does not mean that operation for an aneurysm should be deferred, because the technical difficulties of operation increase daily. Among these difficulties are the increasing calcification and enlargement of the sac, injury to adjacent muscles and nerves by pressure, and the invasion of the surrounding area by fibrous tissue which later hinders rapid dissection. An aneurysm may enlarge noticeably in three weeks from the onset. Difficulties arising from waiting far outweigh the advantages gained in the formation of collateral circulation.

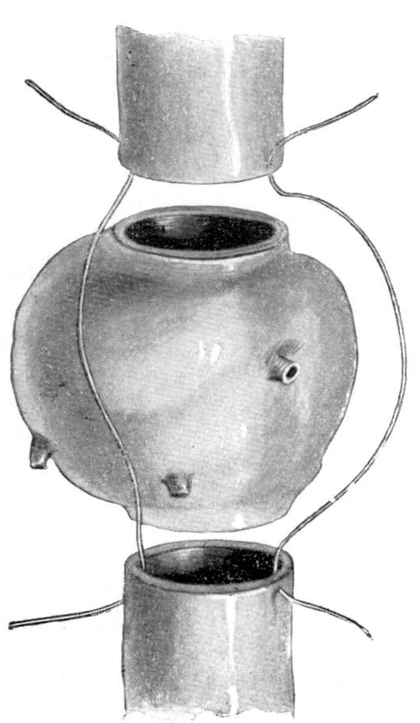

FIG. 501. Ideal operation for aneurysm. The sac is excised and the continuity of the lumen is restored by end to end anastomosis.

Esmarch's anemia is of great aid in operations for aneurysm and should be used whenever possible. With its protection the aneurysm may be directly incised, and the blood-clot removed, which will expose from within the existing anatomical conditions. The connection between the sac and the large blood vessels can then be located without difficulty. The vessels can be dissected out, and the operation concluded by the most suitable method.

An operation that must be done without Esmarch's method of hemostasis is much more difficult. The aneurysm should be exposed by a large incision parallel to the course of the vessel and directly over the tumor, or by a modified flap incision. It is important that the incision be of sufficient size. The healthy portions of the artery are freed first proximal to the aneurysm, then distal to it, and narrow tapes, such as are used to hold a tracheotomy cannula, are passed under them. The section of the vessel which lies between the tapes and which contains the sac of the aneurysm is carefully exposed, beginning as a rule at the central end and working toward the peripheral end. Any arterial branches which are found near the sac must be carefully preserved, since they may play an important rôle in the collateral circulation after the main artery is ligated. Tapes or heavy silk ligatures should be passed around these branches. If, however, the branches can be

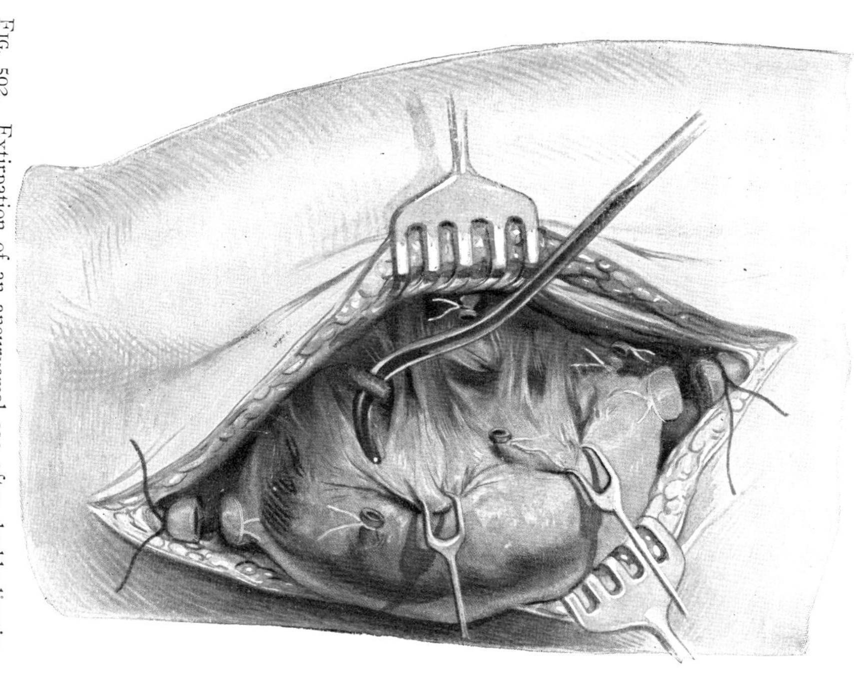

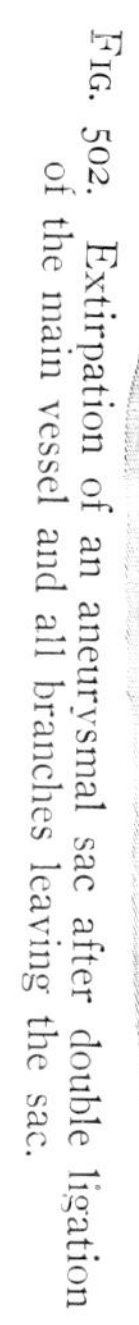

Fig. 502. Extirpation of an aneurysmal sac after double ligation of the main vessel and all branches leaving the sac.

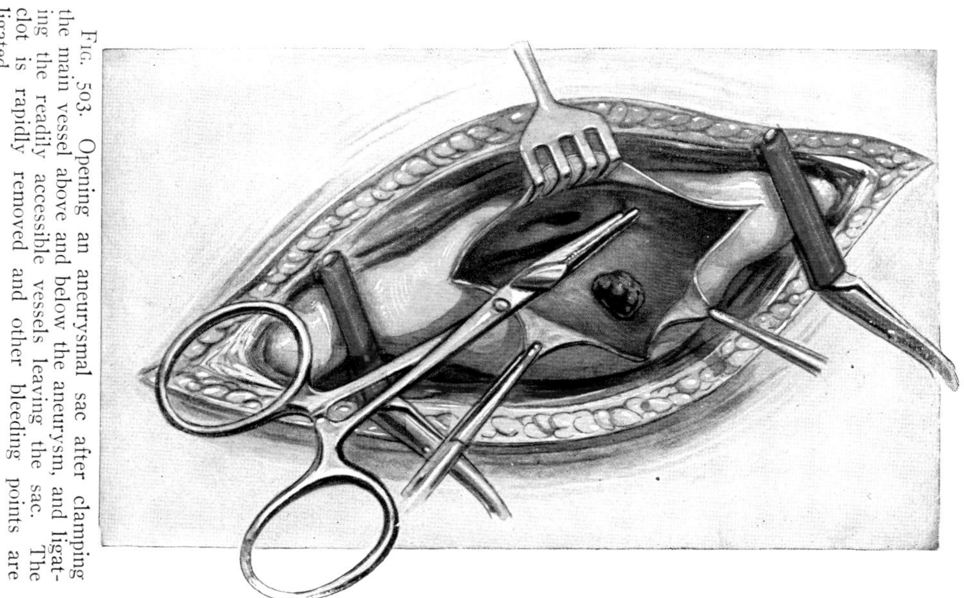

Fig. 503. Opening an aneurysmal sac after clamping the main vessel above and below the aneurysm, and ligating the readily accessible vessels leaving the sac. The clot is rapidly removed and other bleeding points are ligated.

seen to emerge from the aneurysmal sac, they should be doubly ligated and divided (Fig. 502). When the vein forms an integral part of the aneurysm, or if such a connection is suspected, it should be exposed both proximally and distally, its branches ligated, and tapes passed around it, in the same manner.

If an unexpected hemorrhage occurs during the exposure of the aneurysm, all the tapes lying under the individual vessels are drawn tight by the assistant, until the blood stream is interrupted. It is not always possible to check the bleeding because there may be several unnoticed vessels running into the aneurysmal sac. In such instances the bleeding point should be grasped temporarily. If this fails, too much time may be wasted, as a rule, in trying to locate and clamp the remainder of the vessels emptying into the sac. It is better to split the aneurysm summarily, quickly remove the blood-clot, grasp the mouths of the bleeding vessels, and, if necessary, check the hemorrhage temporarily by packing or with the finger (Fig. 503). As soon as the aneurysm is completely exposed as far as the normal vessel at either end, clamps are placed on the vessel, both distal and proximal to the aneurysm, as well as on any branches that have not been ligated. The vein is also clamped on both sides in an arterio-venous aneurysm. The sac can now be opened lengthwise. If any bleeding should come from an overlooked posterior vessel, the vessel should be seized quickly from the inside (Fig. 503). The lining of the sac can be easily examined after the clot is removed. If it is a true aneurysm, the proximal and distal portions of the artery are divided through healthy tissue, or, after the suggestion of Hohlbaum, one end may be divided nearer the aneurysm, and that portion of the artery used to form a cuff over the suture line of the vessel for reinforcement. The same method is used for a false aneurysm which has such a wide attachment that lateral arterial suture is impossible. When the false aneurysm has only a narrow attachment to the artery, the small hole in the arterial wall left by its excision may be closed by lateral suture (Fig. 504). In arterio-venous aneurysm the connection between the artery and vein must by all means be separated (Fig. 505). When the connection is narrow a piece of the wall of the vein can be left attached to the artery to be used for lateral closure of the artery. Otherwise, the artery must be divided transversely at two levels.

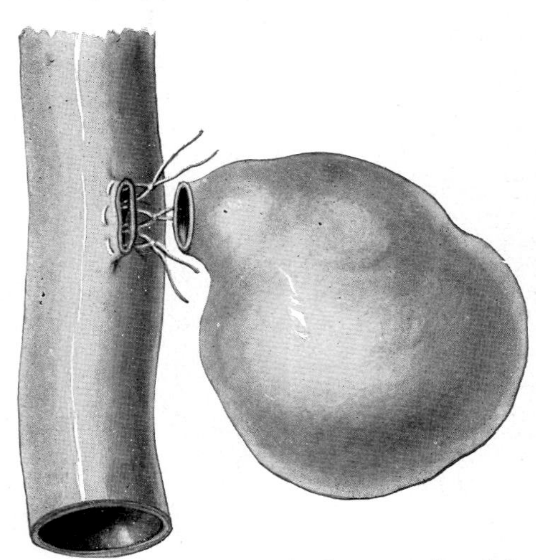

FIG. 504. Removal of a saccular, false aneurysm with a small opening into the vessel lumen. The opening into the vessel is closed with sutures which approximate the intima.

The methods by which a divided artery, or an artery with a lateral opening, is repaired are discussed in section B of this chapter. A vein which is involved in an arterio-venous aneurysm may be divided between two ligatures.

When the aneurysmal sac can not be exposed on all sides, the artery is divided close to the sac at either end and the sac is incised in its entire length. If it has not been possible to use a tourniquet, profuse hemorrhage may result, which should be controlled by the measures previously described. An aneurysmal sac which is intimately connected with the surrounding tissues may be left in situ, after the clot has been removed and all collateral branches have been ligated. It should be obliterated, as far as possible, by suturing together the intima and by drawing into it adjacent tissues (Fig. 506).

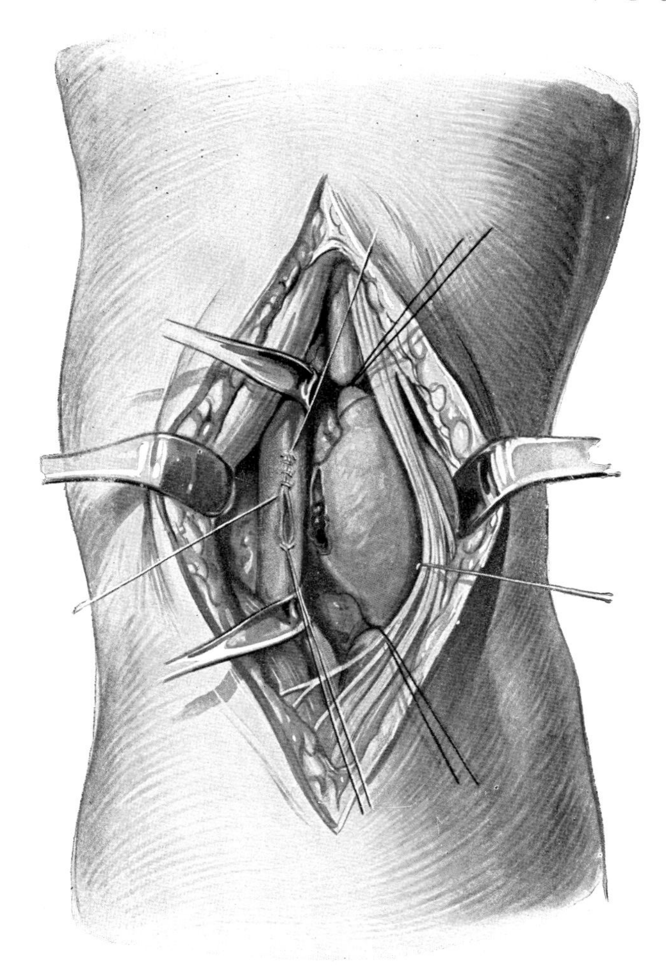

FIG. 505. Arterio-venous aneurysm. The vein is permanently ligated above and below the opening connecting the two vessels. The artery is clamped until the opening has been closed.

When, because of the location of the aneurysm, the proximal vessel (as in aneurysm of the first portion of the subclavian) or the distal vessel (as in aneurysm of the internal carotid at the base of the skull) is inaccessible, an attempt may be made to ameliorate the condition by ligation of the distal or proximal afferent vessel. The results are not very good. Another palliative measure is to try to reinforce the wall of the aneurysm by several layers of fascia lata which is extended as far as possible at both ends (Kirschner) (Fig.

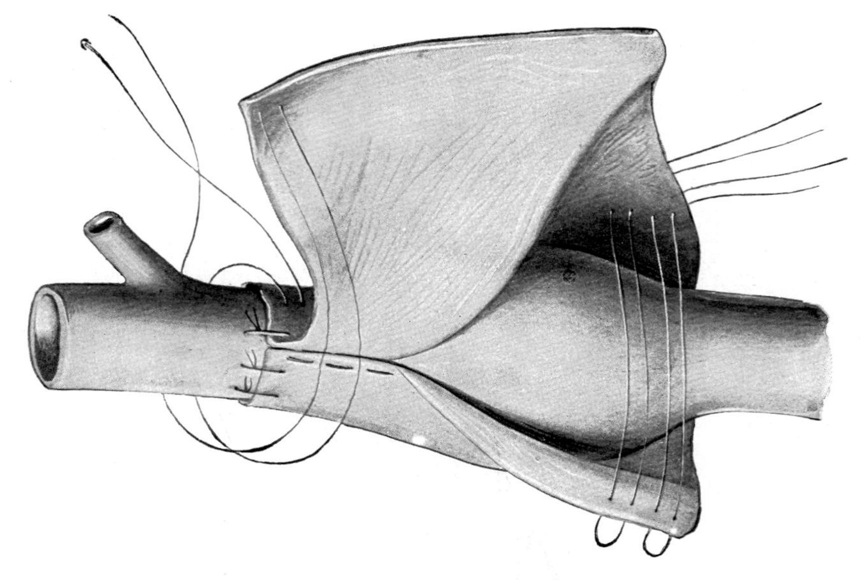

Fig. 507. The use of a fascial transplant to reinforce the walls of an aneurysm which cannot be removed (Kirschner).

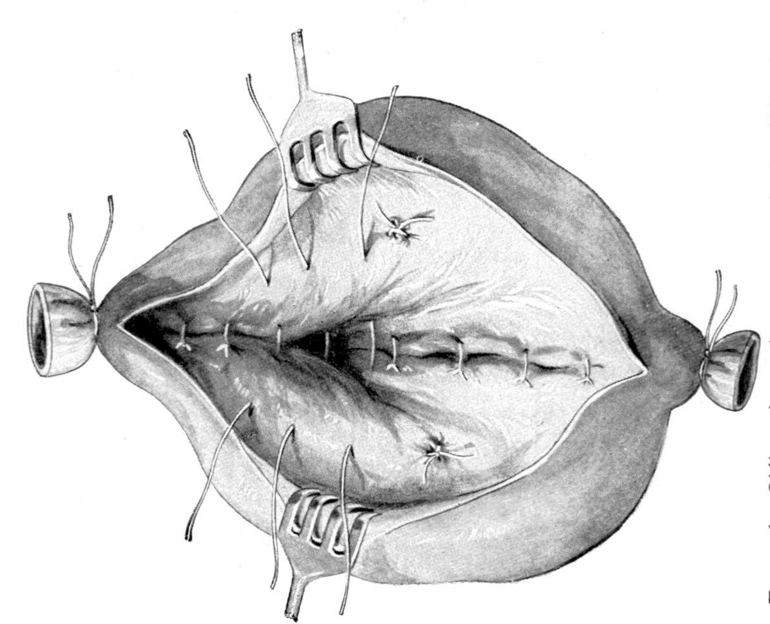

Fig. 506. Obliterative endo-aneurysmorrhaphy (Matas).

507). When an aneurysm has been exposed and is found to be quite inaccessible, it may be impossible to check the hemorrhage by any of the usual methods. As a last resort, the sac may be packed with pieces of muscle tissue (Fig. 508), the wound sutured in layers, and a pressure dressing applied (Küttner).

In all aneurysm operations, in which a tourniquet has been used, the constriction should be released before closing the wound and the field of operation examined for hemorrhage.

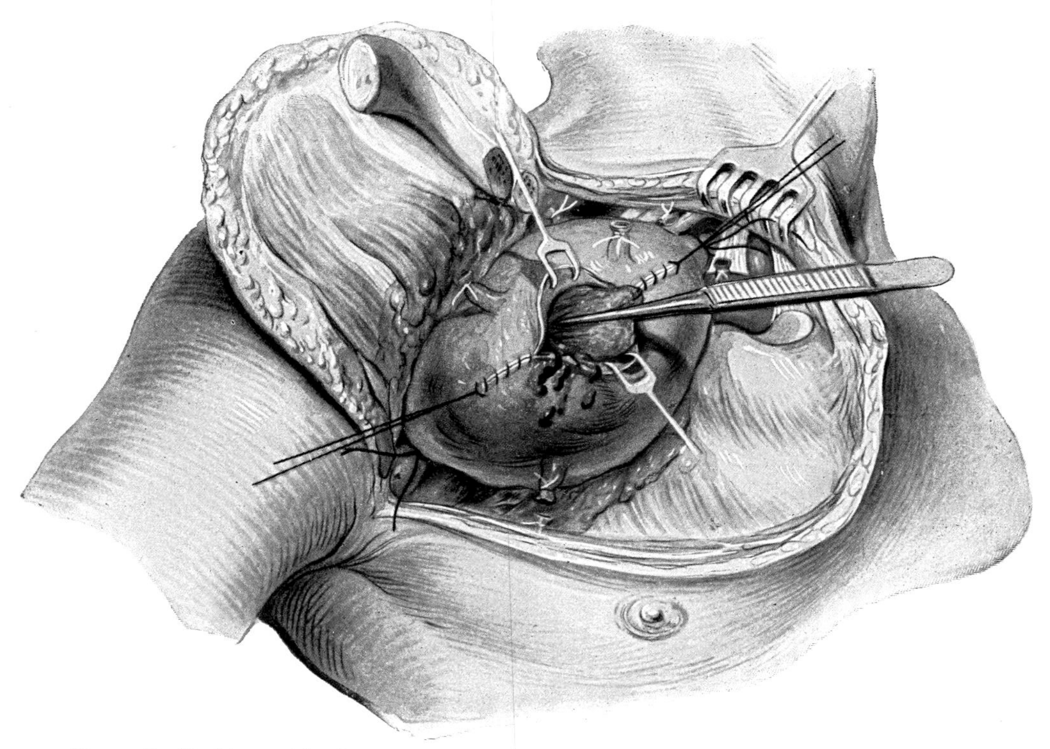

FIG. 508. Packing a bleeding aneurysm, which cannot be removed, with pieces of muscle.

After an aneurysm operation, as in every other operation, on a blood vessel, the limb should be immobilized in such a position that there will be no tension on the sutured vessel.

D. ARTERIOTOMY

An artery is opened and closed only for the removal of an embolus.

Although obstruction of an artery by an embolus can not be compared to obstruction from a tourniquet, since there is no interference with the veins or lymphatics, and no tissue changes from pressure on nerves, it causes, nevertheless, severe nutritional disturbances in many instances. The degree of tissue damage will depend on the size of the embolus which is a major factor in determining where it will lodge. The effect on the tissues can be seen within a few hours. As a rule, secondary thrombosis develops in the vessel, distal to the embolus, making the outlook less favorable for an embolectomy. The chances for saving the endangered tissues and restoring the continuity of the vessel vary with the time of operation; the earlier it is done, the more favorable is the prognosis. Within the first five hours the outlook is good, but it rapidly becomes less so. In the absence of any very definite contraindication, the operation should always take place within the first 24

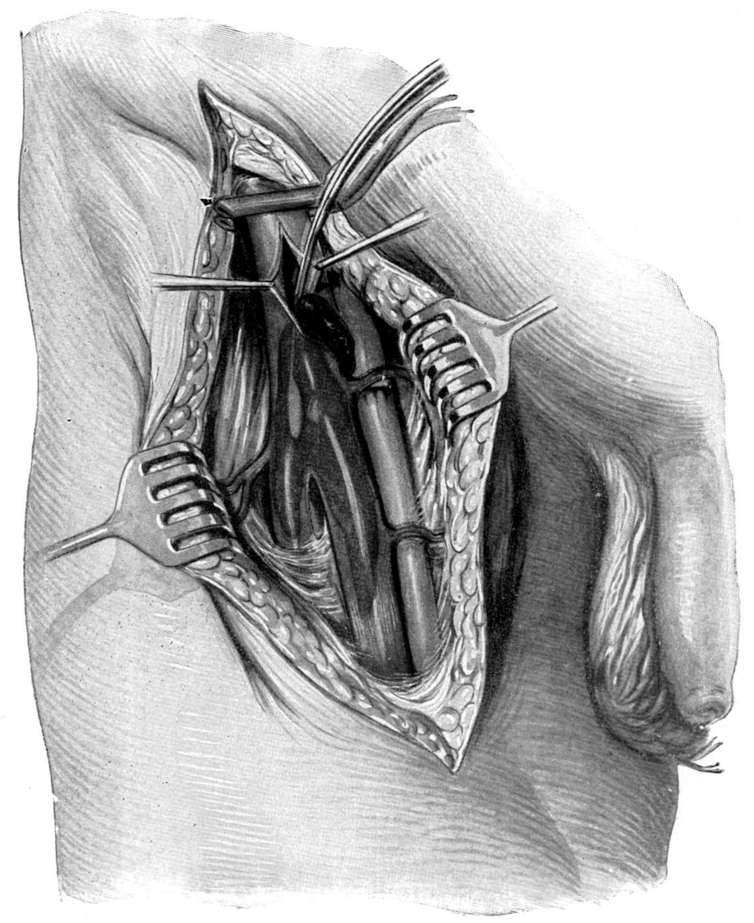

Fig. 509. Embolectomy. The artery is clamped above the clot and is opened by a longitudinal incision. The clot is removed with a slender dressing forceps.

hours, for within this period of time the tissue necrosis can be limited, and the extension of the arterial obstruction prevented by removal of the embolus. The development of secondary thrombosis in the vessel is a complication which makes the operation more difficult and the prognosis much less favorable. According to Key, the operation was successful in 24 percent of all the cases he collected, and in 60 percent of Key's own cases.

It is frequently difficult to locate the exact position of the embolus. The point at which the pulse is perceptible, and the one at which it disappears, the exact location of pain and resistance along the course of the vessel, the extent of possible skin temperature changes, disturbances of color, nutrition, sensation and motion, which start usually distal to the seat of the embolus, all give valuable information. When necessary, the artery should be exposed in several places and exploratory punctures made to determine its patency. When there are several emboli in the same vessel it may only be possible to locate the proximal embolus at first.

Arteriotomy should be performed under local anæsthesia, whenever possible. An attempt should be made to expose the point of lodgment of the embolus. If this is not accessible, the nearest artery peripheral to it should be exposed. If the abdominal aorta is the site of the embolus, for example, it should not be exposed directly, but an attempt may be made to remove the embolus through an incision in the common or external iliac artery.

After the artery is exposed in the region of the obstruction, the exact location of the embolus and its extent must be determined. When the embolus lies at a bifurcation, the three branches forming the bifurcation must be exposed as far as necessary to reach healthy tissue. After the proximal vessel is caught with a protected elastic clamp, the artery is opened with a longitudinal incision, preferably just proximal to the site of the embolus, or just distal to it. Only if absolutely necessary is the incision made at the exact site of the embolus (Fig. 509). If the embolus is not extruded spontaneously, it should be carefully removed with a blunt sound, a blunt forceps, or a dull curette. The intima must be protected against any trauma. It is not advisable to open the artery at the site of the embolus, because the damaged wall favors the formation of thrombi and repair in this area is not so good. A hair-pin, a bent wire, or a small gall-stone curette may be used as the curette. All instruments coming in contact with the intima should be lubricated with citrate ointment. It is difficult and sometimes impossible to remove entirely all the blood clot when a secondary thrombus has formed. Sometimes the artery must be opened in several places and an attempt made to remove the thrombus with a curette, to break it up and, by opening the proximal or distal clamp, to allow the blood to wash the fragments out of the vessel. The same procedure is used to remove an embolus from a vessel that is not directly accessible. Before breaking up an embolus that lies at the bifurcation of a vessel, through an incision in one branch, the other branch should be exposed distal to the bifurcation and be clamped, to prevent loose clots entering this branch. If an embolus lying in the aorta is to be removed, the common iliacs, or the opposite external iliac should be exposed and clamped.

In any case, before closing the opened vessel, the proximal clamp should be released to make sure that the blood stream is unobstructed. After the vessel is closed with the usual arterial suture, the extremity should be examined. If there is evidence of interference in the blood supply, a further search for clots should be made.

The removal of emboli obstructing the pulmonary arteries before their entrance into the lungs has already been discussed (Chapter I).

E. TREATMENT OF VARICOSE VEINS

Varicose veins are a constitutional disease, if they are not caused by a local obstruction to venous return. They are found in the extremities, usually the legs, seldom in the arms or trunk, in the region of the hemorrhoidal plexus, and in the pampiniform plexus. The treatment of varicosities in the last two regions will be discussed separately.

The method of treatment varies with the extent of the process. The first step in the surgical treatment of varicosities of the lower extremity is always ligation of the saphenous vein. Only rarely, and then only when dealing with small varicose veins, clearly showing Trendelenburg's sign, is this treatment effective in itself. Surgical extirpation is the surest procedure for all extensive varicosities, and particularly in the presence of thrombosed veins. Babcock's subcutaneous stripping of the vein is the proper treatment for elongated, dilated saphenous vein or other skin veins. Isolated varices are obliterated by injection. Multiple subcutaneous ligation, though sometimes followed by brilliant results, is so apt to fail completely that it should be used only when other surer methods can not be employed. I have had no experience with circular or spiral incisions through the skin and subcutaneous tissue. The extent of these procedures and the prolonged convalescence should restrict their use to severe cases, to which other methods of treatment are not applicable. Transplantation of the point of junction of the saphenous vein with the femoral, in order to obtain the benefit of competent femoral valves, is in my opinion, aside from the question of correctness of the theory, not a suitable operation, nor is the transplantation of the varicose veins under the deep fascia (Cecca).

If an ulcer is present in the region to be operated on, an extensive operation should, if possible, be deferred until the ulcer is healed. If the ulcer has not healed previously, especially if it is extensive, any operation should be done with care because of the danger of infection. The ulcer should be thoroughly disinfected, the operation should be as simple as possible, and the incision should be made as far from the ulcer as it is practical to make it. The ulcer should finally be excised as one piece from the subcutaneous tissues and all the instruments used in this part of the operation should be discarded. The best treatment for leg ulcer is continuous high elevation of the limb, the thigh vertical, the leg obliquely upward (Fig. 287). Because varicose veins are often invisible after emptying and are concealed by the color of the solution used for skin disinfection, I always mark with a dye the line of the vein and the intended line of incision before the operation. To do this, the patient is seated erect on a chair and the surgeon on a low foot stool.

It is not necessary to keep the extremity at rest and the patient in bed for a longer time after an operation for varicose veins than after any other aseptic operation. A pressure dressing is applied and the limb elevated with the knee slightly bent for a few days. The patient is usually kept in bed for eight days, though for any special reason I do not hesitate to allow him to leave the bed even the first day. The injection treatment requires no rest. The danger of embolus is no greater than after any other operation.

1. Injection Treatment

The actual purpose of the injection treatment is to destroy the endothelium of the vein by introducing an irritating fluid and thus obliterate the varicose veins. It is not the primary purpose of the injection to cause thrombosis in the vein. The formation of a thrombus should be regarded as a coincidental phenomenon. The patient is seated on a high chair or across a high operating table, so that the limbs hang down. The operator, sitting on a footstool, places the foot of the limb to be treated on his knee (Fig. 510). The needle of a 2 cc. syringe containing 1 cc. of the solution to be injected

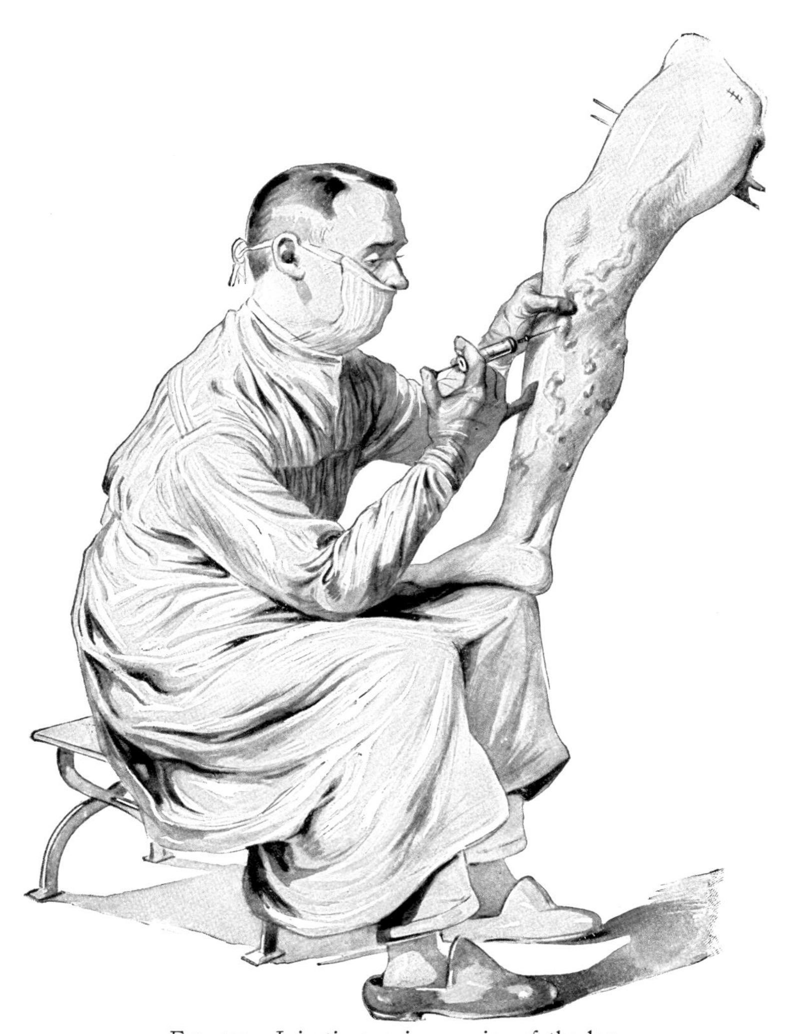

FIG. 510. Injecting varicose veins of the leg.

is inserted into the region of the previously marked varices. Blood is first aspirated from a distended varix, to make sure that the needle point lies in the vein. When the blood flows freely into the syringe, the varix is pressed with the left hand until it becomes exsanguinated, and refilling is prevented by pressure below it. The solution is injected slowly into the vein. It is allowed to remain in the vein for a few seconds before the pressure is released and the blood admitted. If a wheal forms during the injection it indicates that the point of the needle is outside the vein, and the injection should be immediately stopped, otherwise necrosis of the skin may ensue. (Instead of using the fingers, a tourniquet may be applied above and below the varix to be injected. I. S. R.) A 20 to 30 percent saline solution in quantities of 1 to 2 cc. is preferable to the more toxic remedies (for example: a 1 percent solution of bichloride of mercury). This solution is combined with an anæsthetic and is marketed under the name of Varicophtin. Fifty percent glucose solutions are also very useful, being used in amounts of from 5 to 15 cc. (Saline or glucose solutions separately or mixed are so satisfactory that there seems to be no actual necessity for the use of quinine and urea, etc. I. S. R.)

The injection treatment does not confine the patient to bed. It can be administered to ambulatory patients. Embolus occasionally occurs, but the incidence is extremely low. I ligate the saphenous vein before beginning the injection treatment. (This procedure of ligation has not been generally adopted. I. S. R.)

2. Multiple Subcutaneous Ligation (Kurzmik, Scheede, Kocher)

The saphenous vein is ligated just below its junction with the femoral before ligation is begun. The patient lies on a table with the limbs lowered, to allow the veins, which have previously been marked with a dye, to stand out. A fine, curved needle is passed through the skin, beneath each visible vein and varix. The ligature is immediately tied over the skin. All branches of each individual varix should be tied, if possible. From 100 to 200 ligatures are often placed in one limb. Fine silk is used for ligation (Kocher), since it is more durable than catgut. The ligatures are removed on the fifth day. Kocher allows his patients to get up on the second day. I have observed occasional instances of marked temporary improvement when this method was used, only to be followed by exaggerated recurrences.

3. Ligation of the Saphenous Vein (Trendelenburg)

The position of the saphenous vein can be seen frequently as a prominent cord or as a brown line. Otherwise its location must be determined. Its course is on a line drawn from the point where the femoral vein passes under Poupart's ligament to the medial condyle of the femur. The position of the vessel is often located too far laterally. The course of the vein and the line of the skin incision are marked in advance. I place the ligature close to the junction with the femoral vein, and exactly a hand's breadth below Poupart's ligament, through a transverse incision from 10 to 15 cm. long. I make a transverse incision in order to be sure to find any accessory veins (lateral and median saphenous veins), which are frequently present. This is done under local anæsthesia using a 0.5 percent solution of novocain-adrenalin. Hemostasis by constriction is unnecessary, as well as difficult to obtain because of the high location. The extremities, however, should be elevated above the level of the body. The thigh is rotated laterally and the skin and subcutanous tissue is divided until the saphenous vein lying directly on the fascia is exposed. If it is not located by the time that the deep fascia is exposed, it must lie further medially. When the vein is exposed, a search is

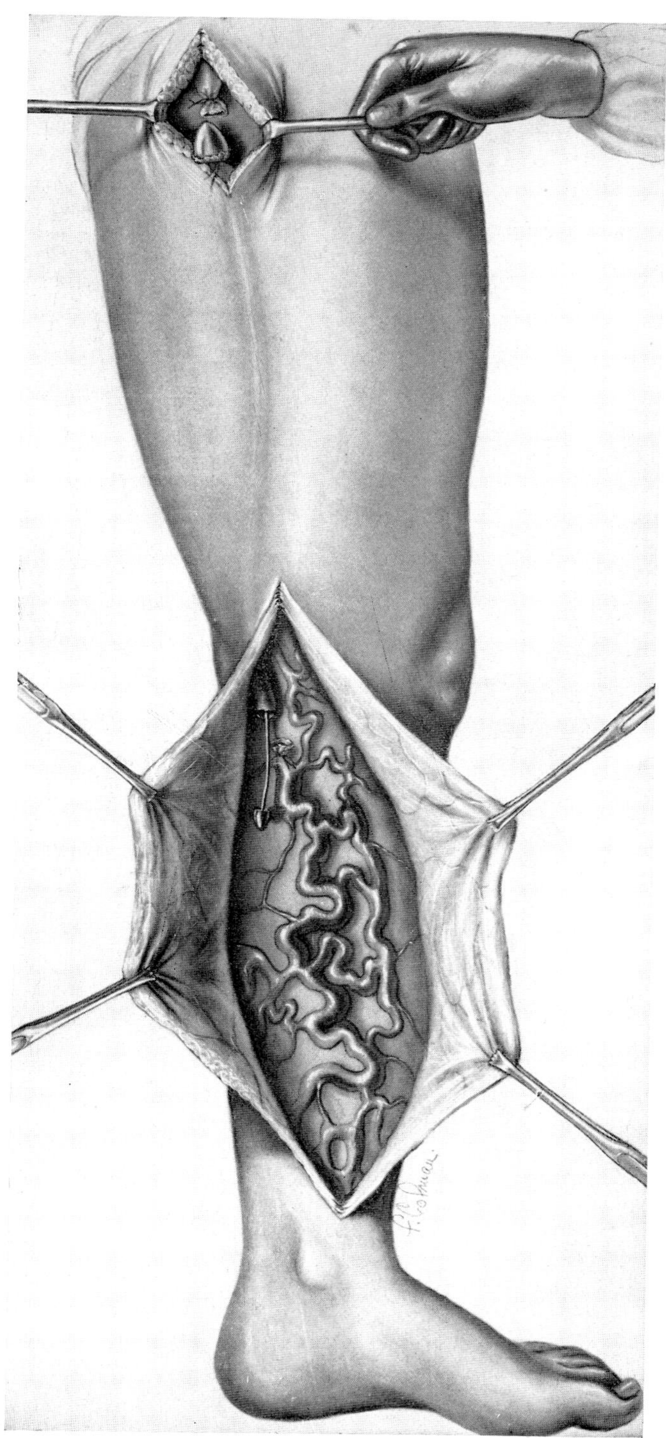

FIG. 511. Stripping of the saphenous vein (Babcock) and dissection of the veins below the knee.

made for accessory vessels, which are likewise ligated. A grooved director is passed under the vein, which is then ligated peripherally, while proximally it is grasped with a hemostat and the vein is divided between these two points. While the proximal wound margin is retracted with a sharp hook the upper limits of the vein are exposed by making traction on the central end of the vein. Accessory branches are ligated and divided as they are exposed (Fig. 512). Some authors stress the danger of thrombus formation in the saphenous stump which may extend into the femoral vein. They therefore advise

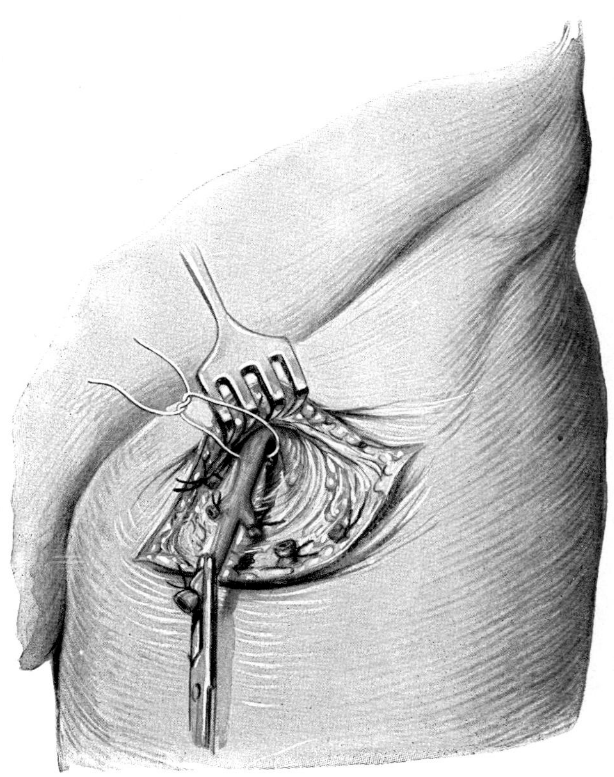

FIG. 512. Ligating the saphenous vein just before it empties into the femoral vein. The tributary veins entering it at this level are also doubly ligated and divided.

ligation at the point of junction of the femoral and saphenous veins. I consider it harmless to leave a small stump.

4. Subcutaneous Removal (Babcock)

A slightly tortuous varicosed saphenous vein can be removed in its entire length by two or three small skin incisions. The operation requires a flexible probe, about 65 cm. long, made of annealed copper-wire, as described by Babcock (Figs. 511 and 513). The probe is provided with an acorn tip 1 cm. in diameter at one end, and with a smaller one at the other end. General or spinal anæsthesia is usually used, although the pain is tolerable under local anæsthesia. A tourniquet is applied at the upper end of the thigh. The saphenous vein is exposed at its upper end, and ligated centrally. It is not

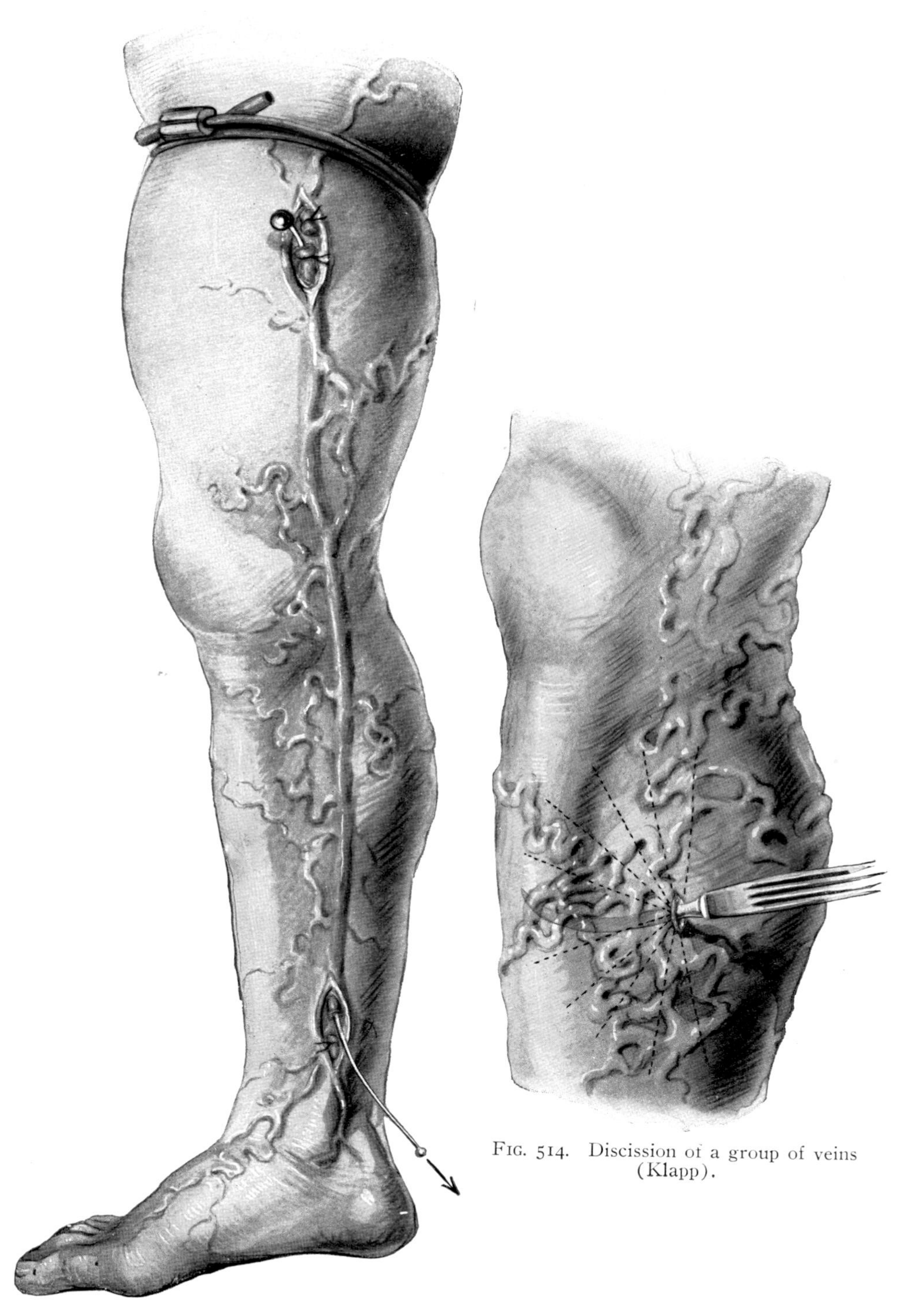

FIG. 513. Subcutaneous removal of the saphenous vein (Babcock).

FIG. 514. Discission of a group of veins (Klapp).

divided but simply opened peripheral to the ligature. The small tip of the Babcock vein extractor is inserted into the opening and pushed peripherally as far as it will go, even as far as the medial malleolus. As a matter of fact the probe can be pushed into the vein but a moderate distance, so that the procedure must be repeated. The site at which the small acorn tip has become lodged is palpated and a small incision is made over this point. The vein is ligated peripheral to the small acorn tip, and is divided between the ligature and the tip of the probe. The end of the probe is carried into the open wound. Through the upper incision the peripheral end of the vein is tied tightly to the probe just below the large acorn and divided (Fig. 513). By traction combined with short jerks the vein is withdrawn, all side branches being torn as it is removed. The procedure may then be repeated if necessary. The skin wounds are closed and a pressure bandage is applied to the entire limb. The limb is elevated and the tourniquet is taken off. Secondary hemorrhage from the torn branches is slight, if it occurs at all.

5. Discission (Klapp)

After ligating the saphenous vein the limb is suspended vertically. A particularly strong tenotome (saphenotome) (Fig. 514) is inserted at about 3 cm. distance from the veins to be treated and these are divided by several radiating incisions close under the skin (Fig. 514). Finally, through the same incision the vessels are divided parallel to the skin so that their deep connections are destroyed. Similar divisions are made progressively through several puncture points from the foot to the thigh.

After applying a compression bandage, the limb can be placed in the horizontal position. Motion should be begun on the first day; on the third day the extremity should be allowed to hang over the edge of the bed at intervals, and the patient should be out of bed in from 8 to 10 days. I have had no experience with this procedure. Bange reports two deaths from emboli following the operation.

6. Excision (Madelung)

The excision of varicose veins should be done with Esmarch's tourniquet, after the veins have been emptied as previously described. A longitudinal incision is made after marking the vein which is to be removed. The incision must be carefully made to avoid cutting directly into the veins, because the skin is frequently paper thin. The extirpation should begin centrally and extend peripherally. While the skin is retracted with hook retractors, the main trunk is exposed, tied centrally, caught peripherally with a hemostat, and divided between them. While strong traction is made on the peripheral end, the mass of veins is dissected free with scissors or scalpel from the surrounding tissue, which may be very dense because of fibrous tissue formation (Fig. 515). The excision should be thorough and sweeping rather than neat. The deep connections are ligated and divided, and every accessory superficial vein which can be exposed should be removed. So as not to make the skin incision too long, in places where the varicosities are trifling, several incisions may at times be used and between these a bridge of skin may be left. The varicose veins can often be drawn under the skin bridge. When the varicosities extend laterally beyond the limits of the wound, a second incision may be made and the dissection continued. It does little harm if a single varicose vein is left between the various fields of operation, since these small sections atrophy. From this standpoint, the plan of operation is to remove first sec-

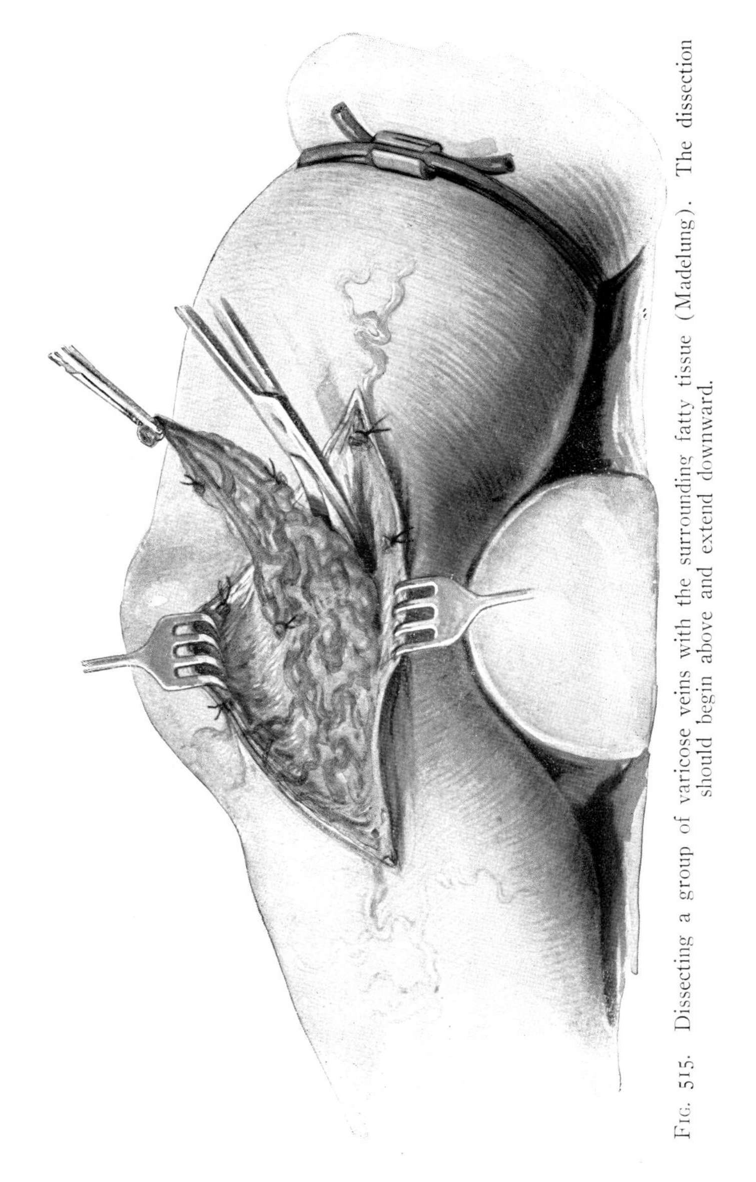

Fig. 515. Dissecting a group of varicose veins with the surrounding fatty tissue (Madelung). The dissection should begin above and extend downward.

tions of veins which are markedly affected, while less affected portions may be left behind. The skin wounds, which are as a rule of considerable length, are closed by continuous suture. Hemorrhage does not occur if a compression bandage is applied and the limb elevated, even though every vein has not been ligated.

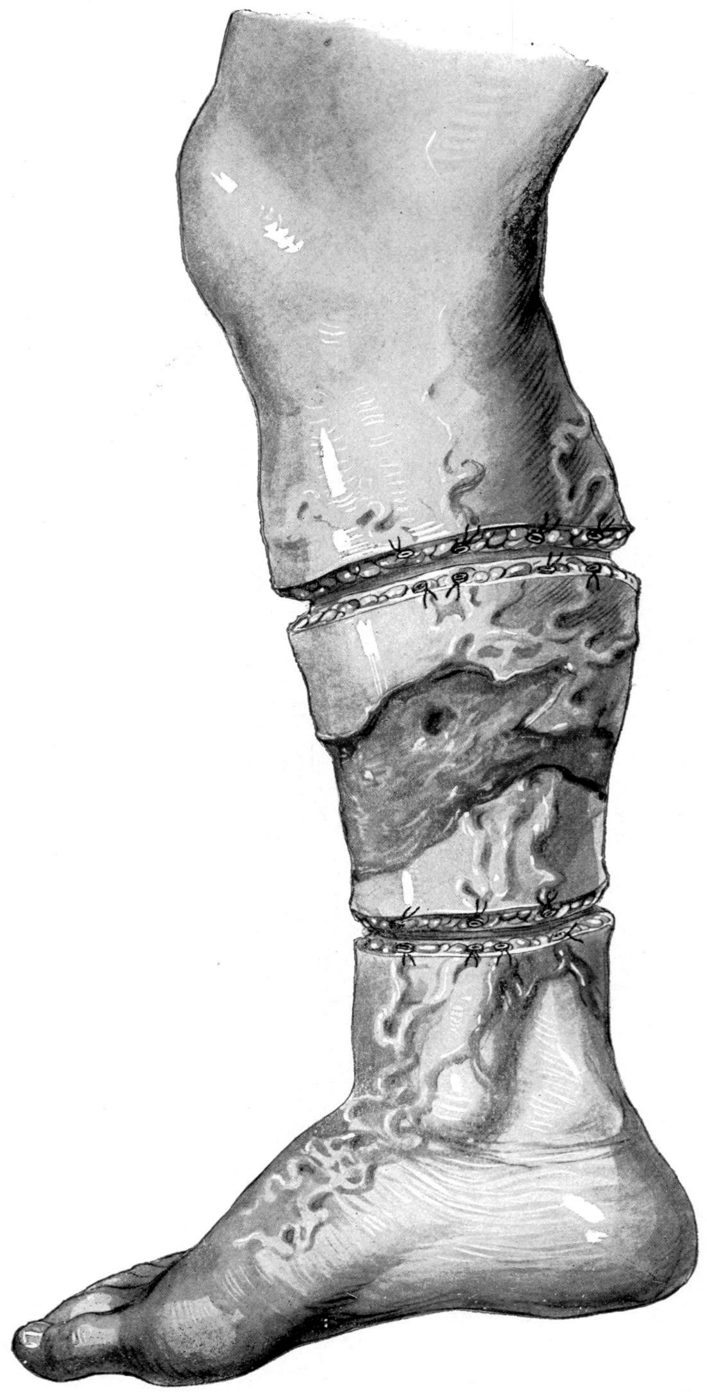

FIG. 516. Circular incision dividing the skin, the subcutaneous tissue and the muscle fascia. All divided vessels are ligated and the skin sutured.

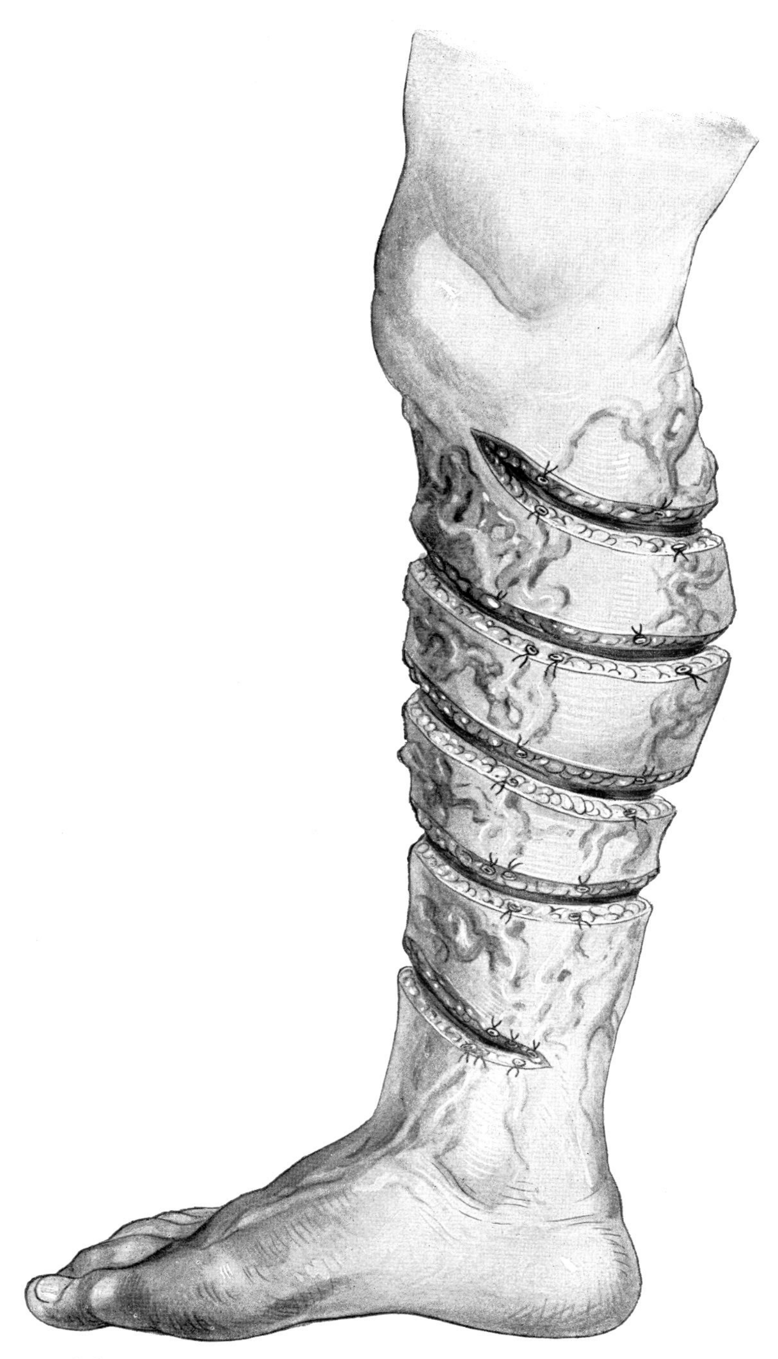

FIG. 517. Spiral incision, dividing the skin, the subcutaneous tissue and the muscle fascia. The divided vessels are ligated and the skin left open to heal by granulation. This operation is rarely done.

7. Circular and Spiral Incisions of the Skin and Subcutaneous Tissue (Moreschi, Rindfleisch)

Circular and spiral incisions are made without regard to the position of the varicose veins. Their purpose is to obliterate the veins of the subcutaneous tissues, to prevent their reconstruction by circular or spiral cicatricial bands, and to shunt the flow of lymph from the superficial tissues to deeper

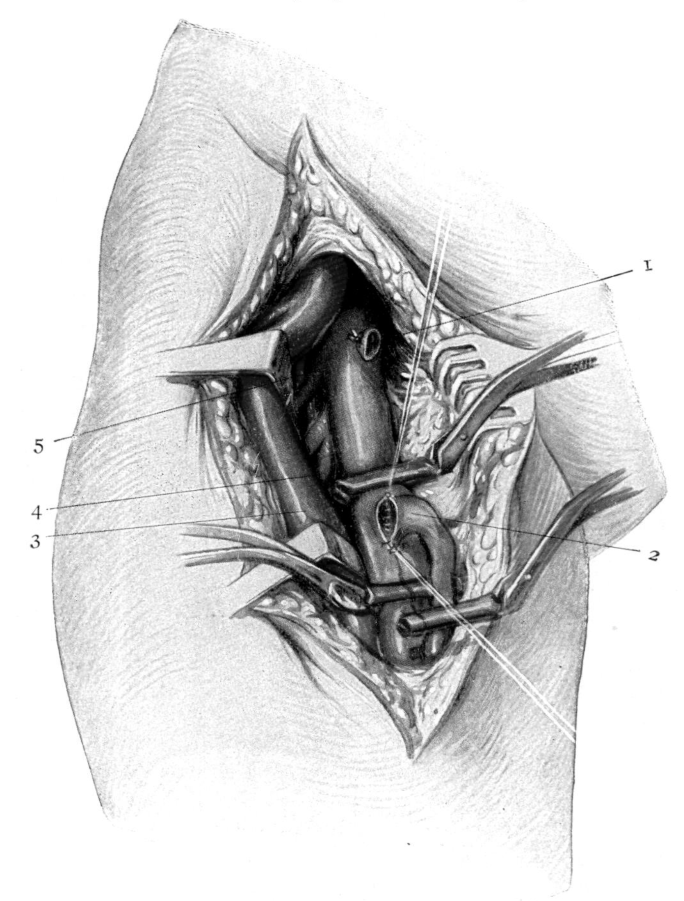

Fig. 518. Transplantation of the saphenous vein into the femoral vein, distal to a valve of the femoral vein (Delbet). 1. Tied, primary anastomosis of the saphenous vein in the femoral vein. 2. Saphenous vein. 3. Femoral artery. 4. Vena femoris profunda. 5. Vena circumflex femoris lateralis.

tissues through incisions in the muscle fascia. The incisions divide the skin, subcutaneous tissue and muscle fascia (Figs. 516 and 517). All vessels met are divided, pulled out as far as possible, grasped and ligated. The wound is not sutured, nor are the incisions in the muscle fascia. They are packed and healing takes place by granulation. Moreschi's circular incisions (Fig. 516) are used close above and below a leg ulcer. Rindfleisch's spiral incision (Fig. 517) begins at the knee and runs spirally to the malleoli, the incisions being about 10 cm. apart, so that, as a rule, four or five incisions are made on each side of the leg. The patient must remain in bed for a month following the operation. Favorable results have been reported in desperate cases, but I have had no personal experience with either of these procedures. (The operation which combines Babcock's method with that of excision of the veins in the leg (Fig. 511) has given very excellent results. I. S. R.)

8. TRANSPLANTATION OF THE ORIFICE OF THE SAPHENOUS VEIN (DELBET)

This operation is based on the theory that varicose veins primarily result from incompetency of the valve guarding the orifice of the saphenous vein. The femoral vein has a valve a few centimeters peripheral to the junction of the saphenous with it. The saphenous vein may have the benefit of this valve, if it is detached from its usual site of junction with the femoral and is transplanted below the valve. If the theory is correct the major cause of the varicosities should be eliminated.

The operative technic is as follows: without the aid of a tourniquet a longitudinal incision of about 15 cm. is made, beginning at Poupart's ligament and extending downward along the femoral vein. The point where the saphenous vein empties into the femoral vein is exposed. After ligating the lateral branches, both veins are exposed sufficiently to be clamped about 8 cm. peripheral to the site of junction (Fig. 518). It may be difficult to expose the veins in the presence of many lateral branches. The saphenous vein is ligated close to its orifice and is divided peripheral to the ligature in an oblique direction, approximately parallel to the femoral vein. The peripheral end of the saphenous vein is transplanted into a lateral opening in the femoral vein, which is now clamped centrally, 5 to 7 cm. peripheral to the point of its usual junction. The clamps are removed, any bleeding is checked, and the wound closed.

CHAPTER VIII

OPERATIONS ON THE NERVES

A. GENERAL CONSIDERATIONS

Peripheral nerve surgery, in particular nerve suture, is distinct from other types of surgery in that wound healing may be uncomplicated, the anatomic conditions may be fully restored, and yet there is no certainty that functional activity will result. There is no adequate explanation of the fact that perfect function occurs in one case, and fails to do so in another, where the conditions of suture have been the same. It is impossible to prognosticate the end-results of any peripheral nerve operation with certainty. The most that can be done is to restore carefully the anatomical structure and attempt to find an explanation for the unknown factors governing end-results.

In spite of this uncertainty, there are however numerous known factors of prognostic importance. That technic plays an important role is evident from a comparison of the results in civil and military surgery. In the former good results are obtained in about 80 percent of the cases, while in the latter in about 40 percent. The length of time between injury and suture is of considerable importance. Nerve suture done within 1 to 2 months after injury is the most successful, some authors reporting approximately 100 percent good results; after 6 months the operative prognosis is much less favorable; after 12 months the successful results of suture may be placed at 25 percent; while later they approach 0 percent. The prognosis is more favorable if the injury occurs in the middle third of the nerve than in its proximal or distal third. The individual nerves differ also in their power of regeneration; suture of the brachial plexus and of the radial nerve should give an average of 70 percent good results, of the median 50 percent, of the ulnar 30 percent, of the sciatic and tibial nerves 40 percent, and of the peroneal 20 percent.

The return of function after nerve suture may be observed at the earliest after a few weeks, as a rule after about three months; no further improvement should be expected after one year, and if function has not returned within two years, none should be expected. In the reestablishment of function volitional impulses seem to exert a substantial influence. The patient must make continuous efforts to execute the motions dependent on the affected nerve, and he should be assisted in this as far as possible by the use of mechanical appliances. Also passive exercises, massage, alternating hot and cold baths, heat, and electricity with a mild galvanic current should be used frequently in the after care.

Most of the operations on nerves can be performed under local anæsthesia. Nevertheless, general anæsthesia is as a rule preferable, because electrical excitability can not be elicited if nerve conduction has been interrupted by a local anæsthetic, and because involuntary motions of the unanæsthetized patient may tear the delicate nerve sutures which are frequently under considerable tension.

I never use a tourniquet when operating on nerves. There is no great need for a tourniquet because the exposure of the nerve is nearly always a problem of anatomical dissection through muscle interspaces, without the division of very vascular structures. Moreover, the success of a peripheral nerve operation is at best so doubtful, that every complication should be avoided, such as secondary hemorrhage and hematoma, which may occur if the operation is done after the application of a tourniquet. There is also the danger of damaging the nerve by pressure. It is most distressing to operate upon a patient for partial nerve injury and have complete paralysis develop after the operation.

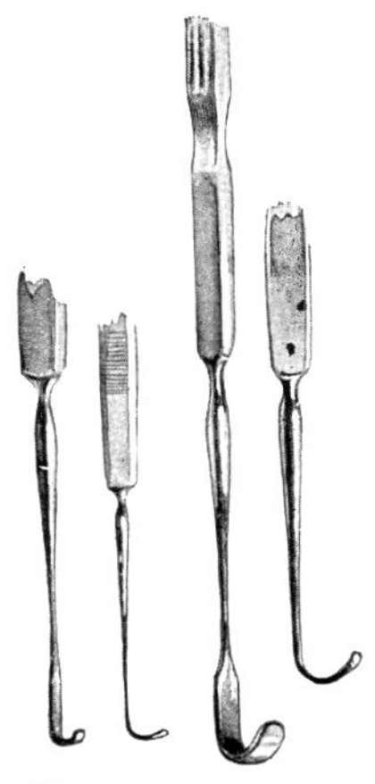

FIG. 519. Nerve hooks.

The incision for exposure of a nerve follows in general the direction of the course of the nerve but should lie over the line of the muscle interspaces through which the nerve is exposed. The incision is made somewhat laterally when

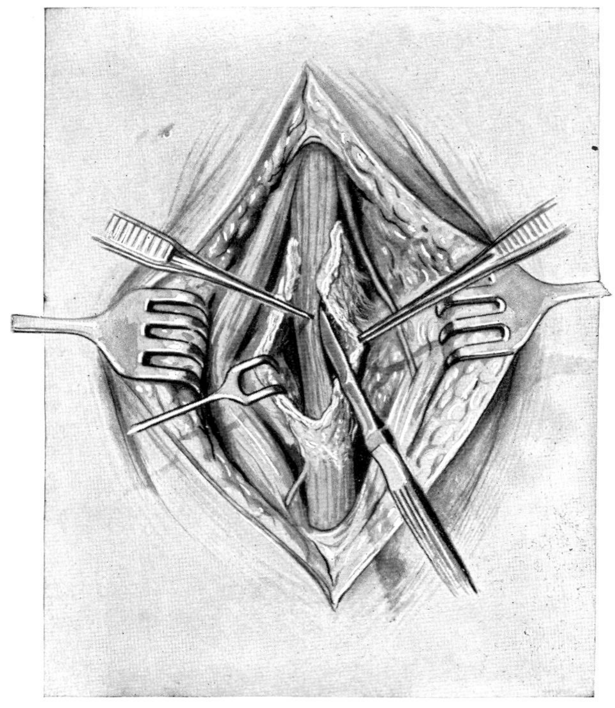

FIG. 520. Perineurolysis. The nerve is dissected from the surrounding cicatricial tissue which is removed.

the nerve lies directly under the skin (ulnar, tibial), similar to the exposure of tendons, to prevent the skin cicatrix from adhering to the nerve.

When exposing nerves that are covered by large muscles, musculo-plastic incisions are made to form large flaps which can be turned to one side, as is done with the pectoralis major muscle or the gluteus maximus muscle. The

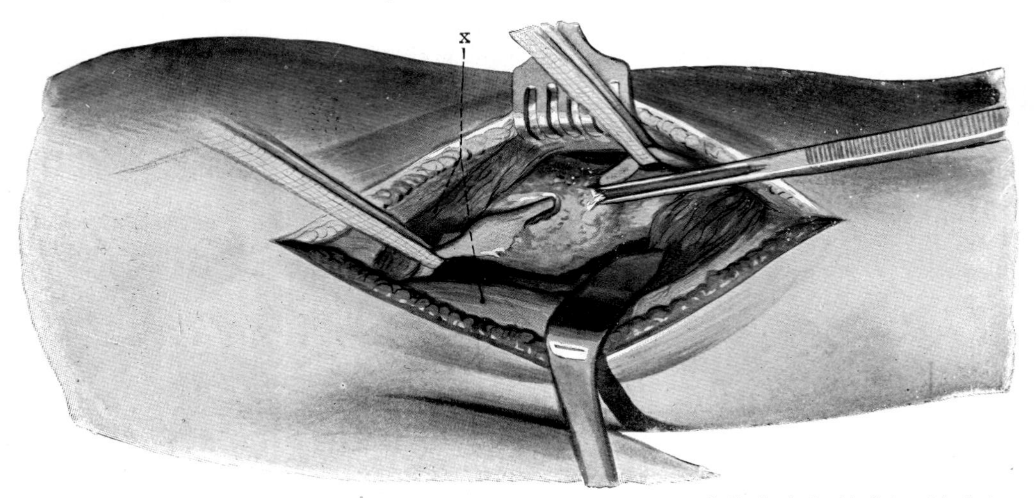

FIG. 521. Neurolysis. The bone callus in which the nerve (radial) is imbedded is chiseled away. x. The divided triceps muscle.

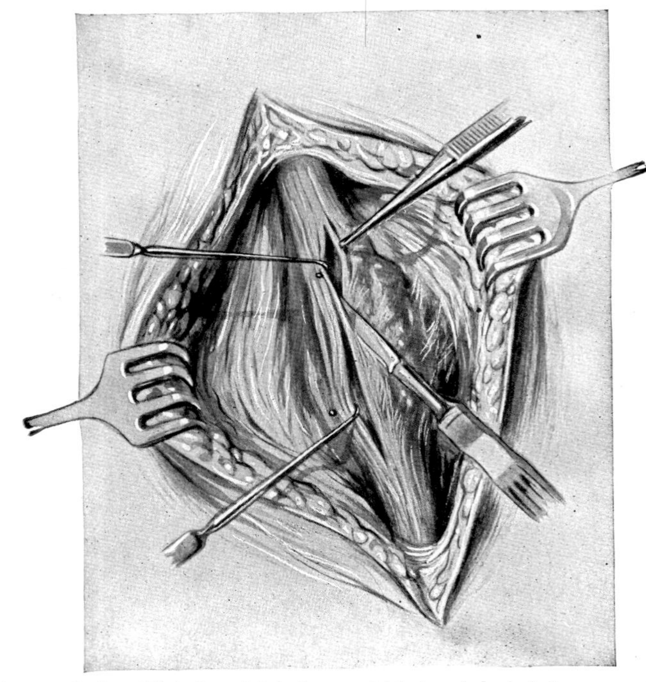

FIG. 522. Endoneurolysis. The cicatricial tissue which has invaded the nerve trunk is dissected out and removed.

nerve itself must be handled with the greatest gentleness. To free it from its bed, its sheath is carefully grasped with fine forceps and the nerve is gently dissected free with a sharp knife (Fig. 520). A nerve is never released by blunt dissection, nor should force be used to free it. As soon as the nerve is free at one place it is laid over a nerve hook (Fig. 519), which should be fairly wide to avoid bruising the nerve. Vein retractors may be used for larger nerves. The nerve can also be elevated or retracted by placing a broad tape under it (Fig. 521). Only the most gentle traction should be made on a nerve. If the nerve is imbedded in scar tissue, it should first be freed above and below the cicatrix, then beginning at either end, it is cautiously dissected free (exoneurolysis) (Fig. 520). Any branches should be carefully guarded from injury. If the nerve is included in callus, it should be freed by gently chiseling off the overlying callus, exercising extreme caution so as not to injure the nerve (Fig. 521).

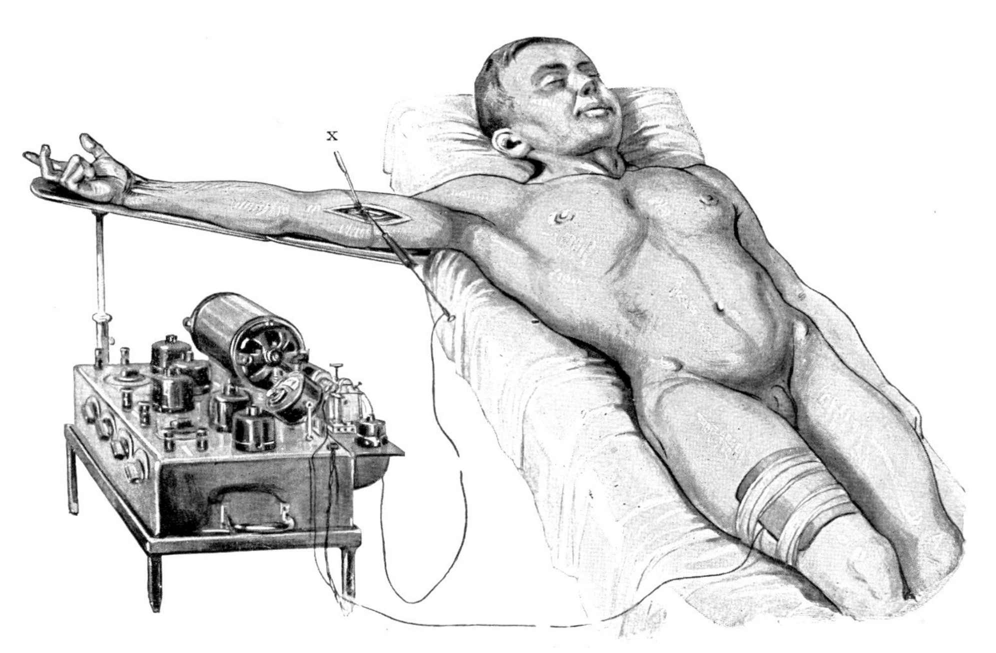

FIG. 523. Electrical stimulation of an exposed nerve. One moist electrode is fastened to the leg, the sterile electrode is applied to the nerve. The nerve lies on a rubber covered hook (x).

If, when the nerve is freed from its bed, it is still surrounded by scar tissue, longitudinal incisions should be made in the fibrous tissue, splitting it and releasing the nerve from the constriction (perineurotomy). The constricting tissue should then be dissected off the nerve (perineurolysis). When the scar tissue penetrates the nerve trunk and extends between the nerve tracts, as is the case in neuromata or adhesions, the individual nerve tracts should be freed separately from the scar tissue (endoneurolysis) (Fig. 522). This is done by separating the nerve fibers from one another just above and below the affected section, elevating fibers with a fine nerve retractor, and freeing them as they pass around the lesion into the normal section. The use of salt solution, described later, will facilitate this procedure. The longitudinal splitting of a neuroma for diagnosis, as described subsequently, may become the first step in endoneurolysis in many cases. If this procedure for freeing most of the nerve fibers proves unsuccessful, excision of this section of the nerve can not, as a rule, be avoided.

The most difficult question to decide in nerve surgery is whether a diseased section still possesses tracts which function or can be restored to function, and whether therefore they can be retained or must be excised. Regardless of clinical tests made previously, the following tests should always be made:

1. Palpation. The firmer the affected area feels to the touch, the more plentiful and dense the cicatricial tissue present, the less can one count upon the conductibility of the nerve fibers or on later regeneration.

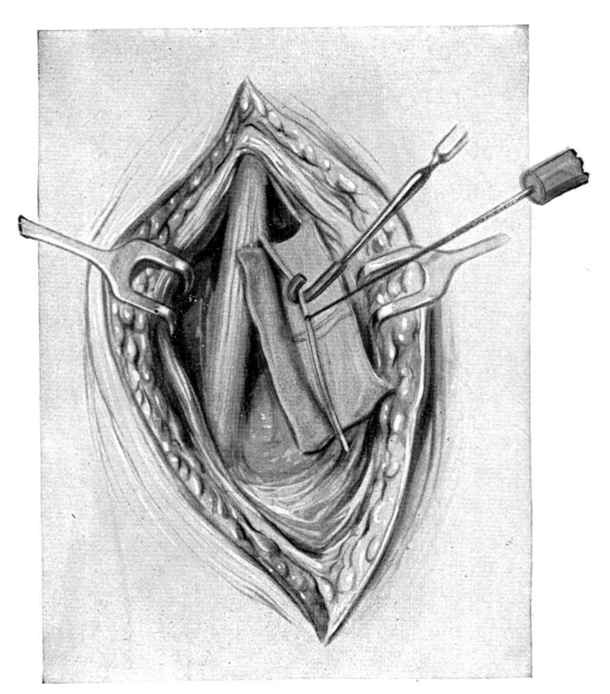

FIG. 524. Application of the electrode to a nerve.

2. Electrical Reaction (Fig. 524). Electrical excitability may be determined with either the unipolar or bipolar method, with a weak faradic current. In the unipolar method a moist electrode is applied to the skin, which has been moistened with salt solution, at some distance from the site of operation and held in place by a rubber bandage. The other electrode, which is sterile and which consists of a platinum wire inserted in an insulating fiber holder, is placed in contact with the exposed nerve. The nerve should be protected against side currents by rubber tissue placed beneath it, or it should be elevated by a rubber covered retractor. For bipolar stimulation, the nerve is in contact with two platinum electrodes, about 1 cm. apart. Very weak currents are used at first, and their effects are tested on the muscles lying within the field of operation. The strength of the current may be increased gradually. The exposed nerve responds frequently to direct stimulation, when indirect stimulation through the skin causes no reaction. When the muscles respond

to stimulation of the nerve central to the affected section, nerve conduction is certainly present. When the muscles do not respond to stimulation of the nerve central to the lesion, electric conduction is absent at that time and the reestablishment of nerve function becomes problematical at best. Recovery without surgical interference is less apt to occur the longer the duration of the lesion. If muscular contraction results from stimulation peripheral to the lesion, it is improbable that there is complete interruption of conductivity, because the excitability of a peripheral nerve section is rapidly lost, usually within 14 days. When stimulation peripheral to the lesion produces no reaction, nerve conduction is interrupted, but its reestablishment is possible.

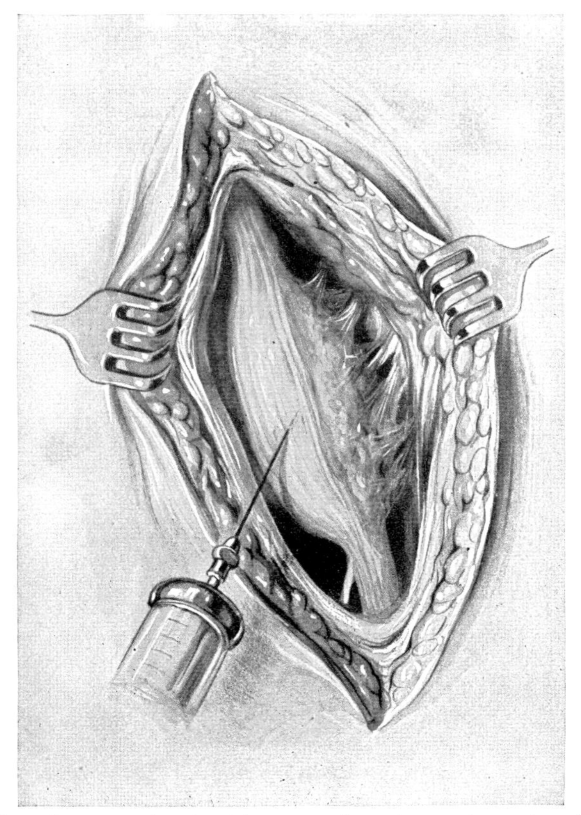

FIG. 525. Infiltration of a nerve involved in a scar in order to determine the condition of the individual components.

Electrical stimulation during operation is of value in determining individual nerves and nerve sections, and for distinguishing sensory and motor branches, which is often of great aid in view of the frequent difficulty and uncertainty of identifying them anatomically. However, the results are disappointing when attempts are made to identify individual nerve tracts in an intact nerve by means of electrical reactions. This would be an invaluable aid in Stoffel's operation. Only individual nerve fibers which are separated from the main trunk can be recognized by this means.

3. Infiltration with normal saline (Hofmeister). About 10 cc. of physi-

ologic salt solution are injected at the site of the lesion directly into the nerve with a fine needle. If the solution extends through the affected region to reach the healthy section beyond it, it is evidence of a relative lack of density of the cicatricial tissue (Fig. 525), which probably can be traversed by the new outgrowth of nerve fibers.

4. After incising the affected section of nerve longitudinally, the incised surface should be examined closely with a magnifying glass if necessary. It may be possible in many cases to differentiate the cicatricial tissue from the nerve fibers and to determine the extent and density of the cicatrix, as well as the connection, the distance apart, and the progress of the nerve fibers. By extending the longitudinal incision the individual nerve fibers may be followed through the scar (endoneurolysis).

B. RESECTION AND SUTURE OF NERVES

When it seems improbable that conduction will be reestablished, either spontaneously or by neurolysis, the section of nerve involved should be re-

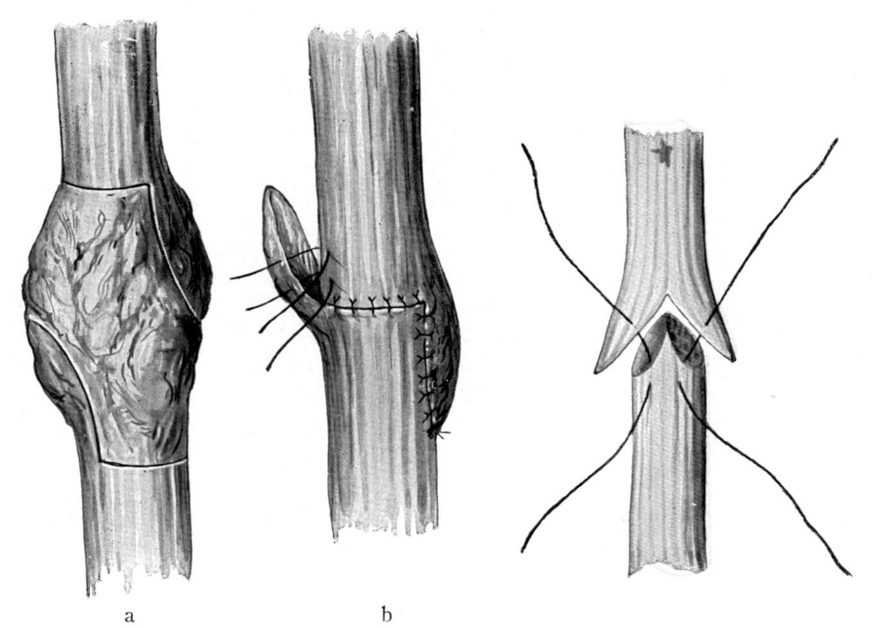

Fig. 526 a and b. Excision of a neuroma and restoration of the nerve by end to end suture using portions of the capsule of the neuroma for reinforcement of the line of suture.

Fig. 527. Another method for end to end suture of a nerve.

sected. The nerve is laid over a wooden spatula and is cut directly across with a very sharp knife. An occasional spurting vessel may be encountered which will usually stop bleeding of itself. If not, it is grasped with a delicate hemostat, avoiding the nerve tissue, ligated with fine catgut, which is tied but once, and the ends cut short. Though it would be desirable to remove all the affected tissue, the resection must be done sparingly, since direct nerve suture should be done if the best results are to be obtained. Before dividing the nerve two corresponding points are marked with methylene blue on the nerve so that there will be no rotation when the ends are approximated. To reinforce the subsequent suture after closing large gaps, a flap can be taken from each side of the neuroma, one attached to the central, the other to the peripheral end of the nerve (Fig. 526). These flaps can be used in drawing the ends of

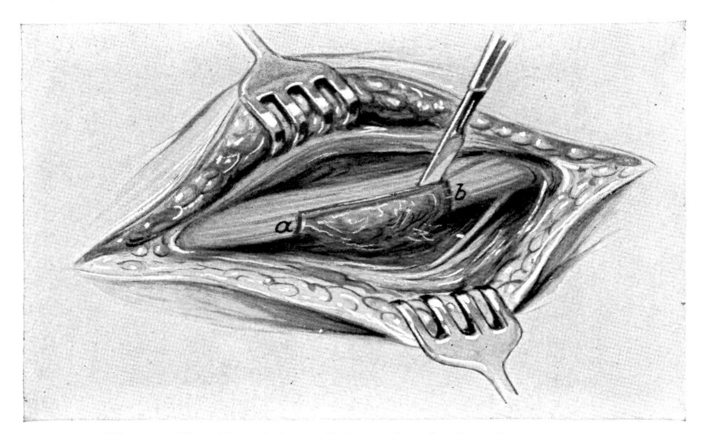

FIG. 528. Partial excision of a lesion in a nerve.

the nerve together and then sutured laterally on opposite sides of the nerve, to reinforce the suture. Or the central end of the nerve may be notched, the other end beveled, and the two surfaces fitted together (Fig. 527). When only part of the nerve is involved and the rest is normal and capable of con-

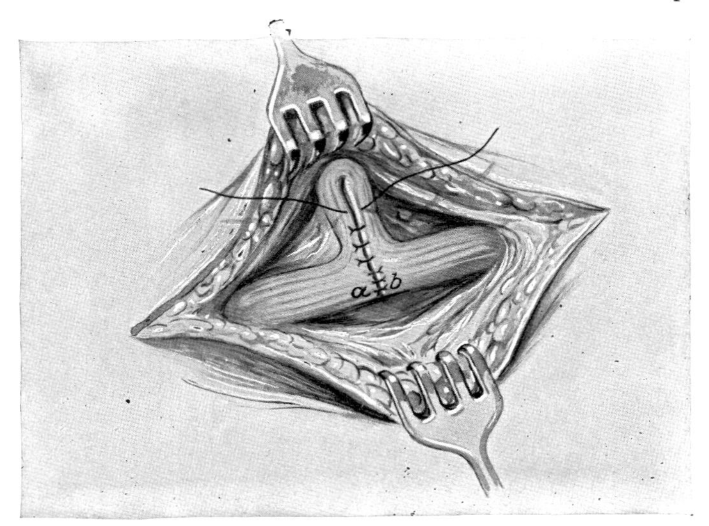

FIG. 529. Closure of the defect caused by the excision.

duction, only the affected portion should be excised. The incised surfaces are then sutured together so that the divided tracts are in continuity (Figs. 528 and 529).

Suture of a nerve divided by operation or injury is for the purpose of permanent restoration of the continuity of the healthy nerve fibers. The perineurium of the nerve stumps is sutured with fine catgut or fine silk. Small needles are used in order to avoid injury to the nerve itself (Fig. 530). Sutures are placed first at opposite points on the circumference, drawing together the divided perineurium. The intervening spaces are then sutured closely so that no nerve tissue protrudes between the sutures.

To protect the suture line, or the section of nerve released from cicatricial tissue or callous, from renewed inclusion in fibrous tissue or callous, the area should be surrounded by healthy tissue. Autoplastic material alone should be used for this purpose. It is best to use pedunculated muscle flaps from the vicinity, and these are always available. If necessary, free fat transplants may be used, or even grafts taken from the great omentum, which latter is impractical. There have been many warnings against the use of free fascial

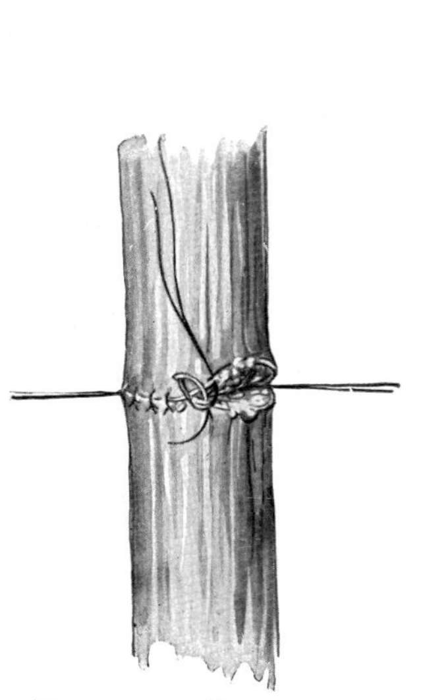

Fig. 530. Circular nerve suture. Two tension sutures are introduced on opposite sides of nerve. The perineural sheath is then sutured.

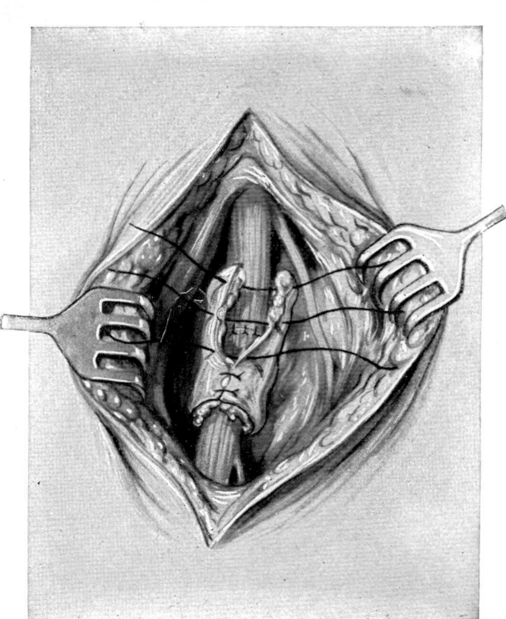

Fig. 531. Surrounding the site of suture with a fat-lined fascial graft (Kirschner).

transplants, because of the possibility of constriction from shrinking of the graft. I have, however, obtained good results from their use, though care was taken to leave a layer of fat on the side of the fascia turned toward the nerve, and the graft was large (Fig. 531).

C. MANAGEMENT OF NERVE DEFECTS

An attempt should be made to draw together the ends of a nerve which has been divided transversely, by steady, gentle traction on both ends. It has been observed that a nerve stretched repeatedly or by a sudden jerk loses much of its elasticity, so that it can not even be stretched again to its original length. The extremity should be placed in the position most favorable to relaxation of the nerve, for by posture gaps as long as 7 cm. may be overcome. Such a position of the extremity must be maintained for 14 days after operation by splint or cast, and should be only gradually discontinued. When the ends of the nerve can not be brought together in this manner, both parts of the nerve should be freed for a distance, leaving attached to them, however, the connective tissue which is important for their nutrition. Extension of this dissection leads to interference with nutrition and therefore to a less favorable prognosis. Occasionally, a nerve which does not have a direct course can be

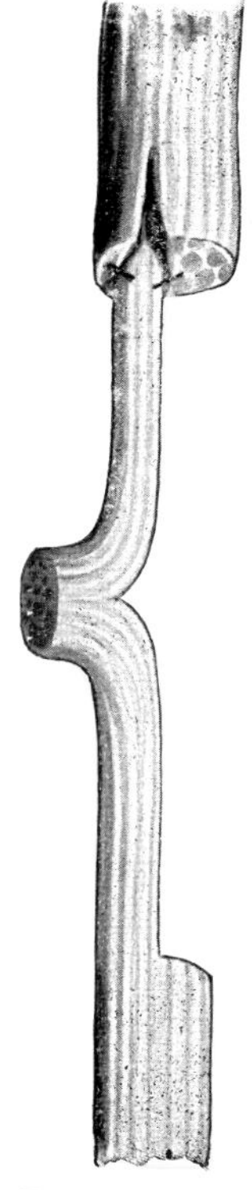

FIG. 532. Nerve implantation. Bridging a nerve defect with a slip turned up from the peripheral end.

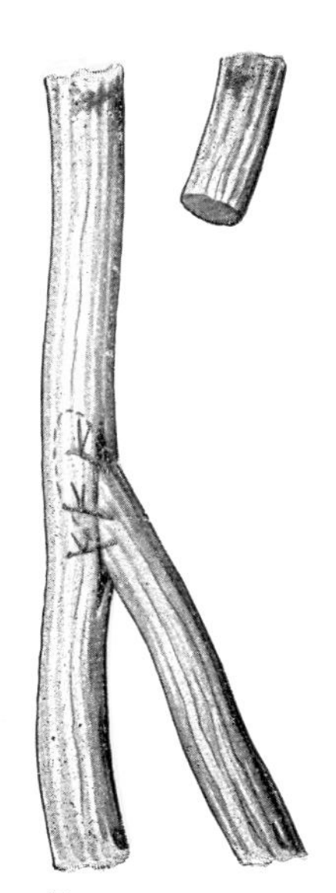

FIG. 533. Nerve implantation. The peripheral part of the paralyzed nerve is implanted laterally in the healthy nerve. The ends marked red are the central ends.

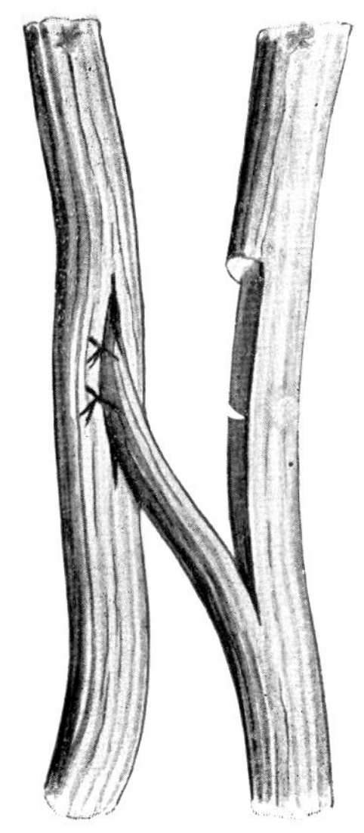

FIG. 534. Nerve implantation. A peripheral flap of the paralyzed nerve is implanted laterally in the healthy nerve.

displaced so that its course will be more direct and thus shorter. The ulnar nerve can be displaced from behind the medial condyle to the flexor surface of the forearm, thus shortening its course by as much as 3 cm. An extreme measure to permit direct union of a nerve, especially in the arm, is to shorten the entire arm by removing a section of bone. The suggestion has also been made that in these desperate cases (Kirschner, Loeb) the bone may be divided to allow direct nerve suture and subsequent healing, but after 2 or 3 weeks to put extension on the still ununited bone and gradually restore it to its original length.

Any procedure which does not involve direct approximation of the nerve ends has a decidedly less favorable outlook. The attempts to bridge nerve defects and secure conduction by free nerve transplants have thus far not led to encouraging results. Since a single suture in the course of a nerve has a very uncertain outcome, the results are just twice as doubtful when two lines of suture are necessary in an implantation of a nerve transplant, even should the free transplant be as viable as the nerve itself. Theoretically, autoplastic nerve tissue offers the best prospects, but it is almost impossible to procure and is limited to the use of unimportant, small superficial nerves which are unsuitable. For a homoioplastic graft a nerve from a recently amputated

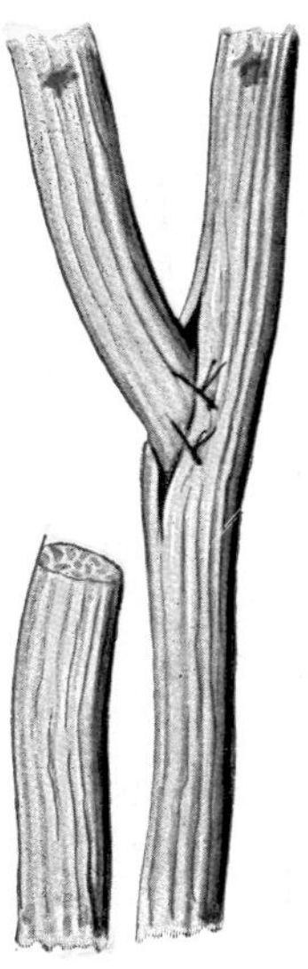

FIG. 535. Nerve implantation. The central part of the divided healthy nerve is implanted laterally in the paralyzed nerve.

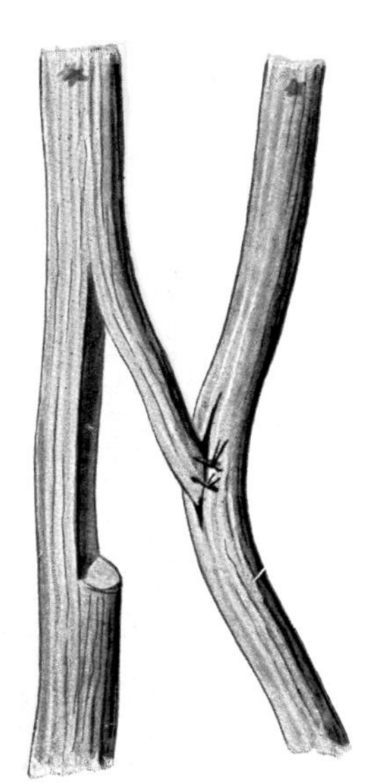

FIG. 536. Nerve implantation. A central slip of the healthy nerve is implanted laterally in the paralyzed nerve.

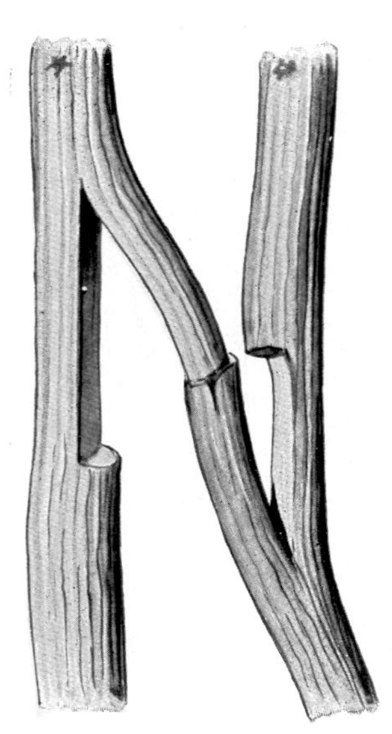

FIG. 537. Nerve implantation. A central slip of the healthy nerve is united end to end with a peripheral flap of the paralyzed nerve.

limb or one from a person that has just succumbed has been suggested. The use of tubes, either hollow or filled with agar, to bridge a nerve gap (tubulization) was much heralded for a time but the results were so disappointing that it is no longer used.

It is better, though even this has not too encouraging results, to bridge the gap with a pedunculated nerve flap, which is taken from either one or both ends of the divided nerve. Because the return of nerve function depends principally upon the regeneration of the central end, it is better to take the flap from the peripheral end only, so as not to damage the central end (Fig. 532).

When a nerve defect can not be bridged by any available method, or when the affected section is inaccessible, a last resource is nerve grafting or anastomosis (Figs. 533-539). Because of the uncertainty of success, an important healthy motor nerve should never be injured or divided for the sake of a damaged nerve. An unessential, superficial sensory nerve should be used for anastomosis. The only exception to this rule is the anastomosis of the hypoglossal or the spinal accessory to the peripheral end of the facial nerve, though their use is also hardly justifiable. When such operations are successful, disturbing simultaneous movements are very apt to result. It is advisable in anastomosing not to divide the paralyzed nerve entirely, if there is any possibility of any remaining function. The possibility of restoration of func-

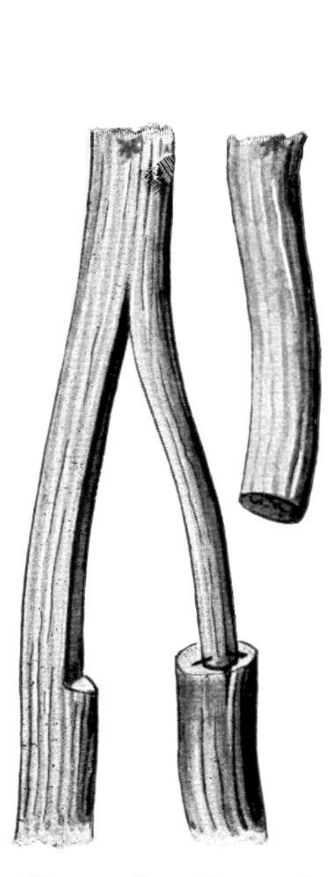

FIG. 538. Nerve implantation. A central slip of the healthy nerve is implanted in the peripheral end of the divided paralyzed nerve.

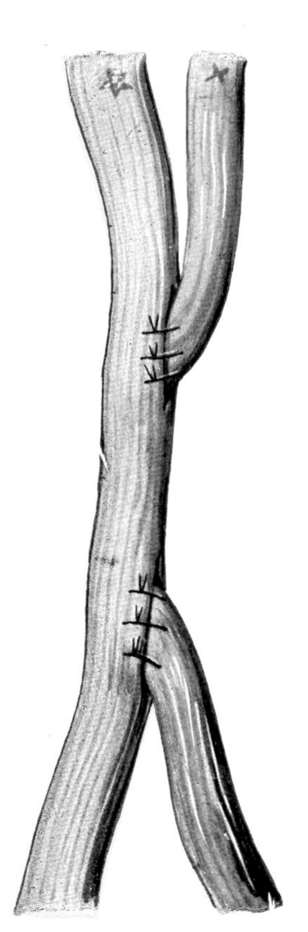

FIG. 539. Double nerve implantation. The central and the peripheral ends of the divided paralyzed nerve are planted laterally in the healthy nerve.

tion should not be removed. On the basis of these two principles, if there is not available an unimportant sensory nerve for an end to end graft lateral anastomosis of the damaged nerve to a healthy nerve is the preferable procedure (Fig. 534). Either a lateral flap, about 1/3 the thickness of the nerve is split off as a bridge from the peripheral end of the diseased nerve (Fig. 534), or its entire peripheral end (Fig. 533), or its entire peripheral and entire central ends (Fig. 539) (double grafting, Hofmeister), are implanted laterally in the healthy nerve.

The lateral implantation of one nerve into another is done by making a small transverse cut and a T-shaped longitudinal incision in the receiving nerve, the nerve to be implanted is placed in this incision so that its transverse incision lies against the transverse incision of the healthy nerve. The T slit is closed with fine sutures (Fig. 540).

For paralysis, which can not be relieved by the procedures described, healthy nerves have been planted directly in the muscles, for the purpose of neurotisation of the paralyzed muscles (Heineke); or, pedunculated flaps have been taken from healthy neighboring muscles, split and planted in the paralysed muscles, in order to lead nerve fibers to them (Erlacher). It is extremely doubtful whether either of these procedures ever yield satisfactory results.

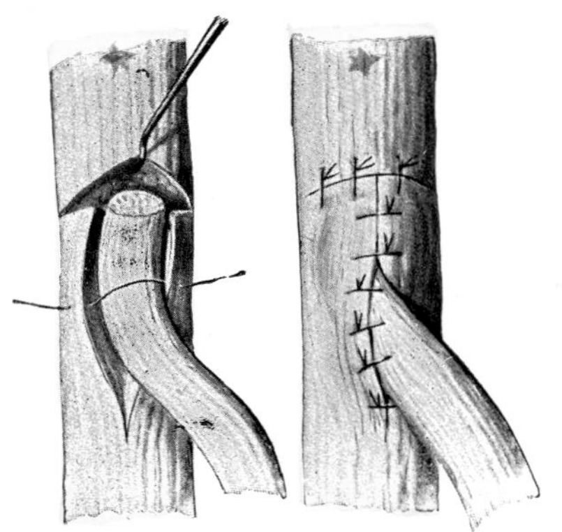

FIG. 540. Lateral implantation of a nerve after a T-shaped incision of the receptor nerve, so that the cut section of both nerves come into direct contact.

D. TREATMENT OF PATHOLOGIC IRRITABILITY OF NERVES

The irritation of a peripheral nerve may involve its motor, sensory or trophic portions or a combination of these.

Mechanical pressure on sensory nerves from constriction or pressure of malignant tumors, callus, by perineural or endoneural cicatricial tissue (neuroma, amputation neuroma), or actual diseases of the nerves (neuralgias) may lead to unbearable pain, which demands surgical treatment, if all other forms of treatment have failed to relieve it. Surgical treatment is first directed toward the removal of possible mechanical causes responsible for irritation. In many cases the irritability can be relieved by the various types of neurolysis and subsequent measures to prevent recurrence of cicatricial overgrowth. When these procedures are not applicable, are ineffectual, or are followed by relapses, the diseased section of nerve should be excised, as for example, a neuroma of the ends or in the course of a nerve, and the nerve, if divided, should be sutured immediately. When this measure also fails or is not feasible, the nerve should be interrupted temporarily, or even permanently, central to the diseased area. In a mixed nerve, the disadvantage of motor paralysis should always be weighed against the advantage of the relief of pain.

Nerve conduction can be blocked for months, or sometimes permanently by injecting the nerve with 1 to 3 cc. of 70 to 95 percent alcohol. Alcoholic injection has an advantage in that the nerve need not always be exposed, but can be often reached with a needle. Alcoholic injection is indicated when the area affected is inaccessible or can be reached only with difficulty, as for example, the ganglion of the trigeminal nerve or its branches. The stronger the alcohol is, the more severely does it damage the activity of the nerve, so that many surgeons prefer using absolute alcohol. In mixed nerves, sensory conduction is abolished more easily than is motor conduction. Sixty percent alcohol eliminates usually only the sensory pathways, and affects to only a slight degree the motor pathways. This is important in the control of pain in mixed nerves. Seventy percent alcohol is used as a rule for injection of the sensory trigeminal nerve. (Frazier uses absolute alcohol. I. S. R.)

Freezing a section of nerve (Trendelenburg) enjoys greater popularity for temporary interruption of conduction. Perthes has devised a special apparatus for this, in which the nerve is enclosed in a cooling device (Fig.

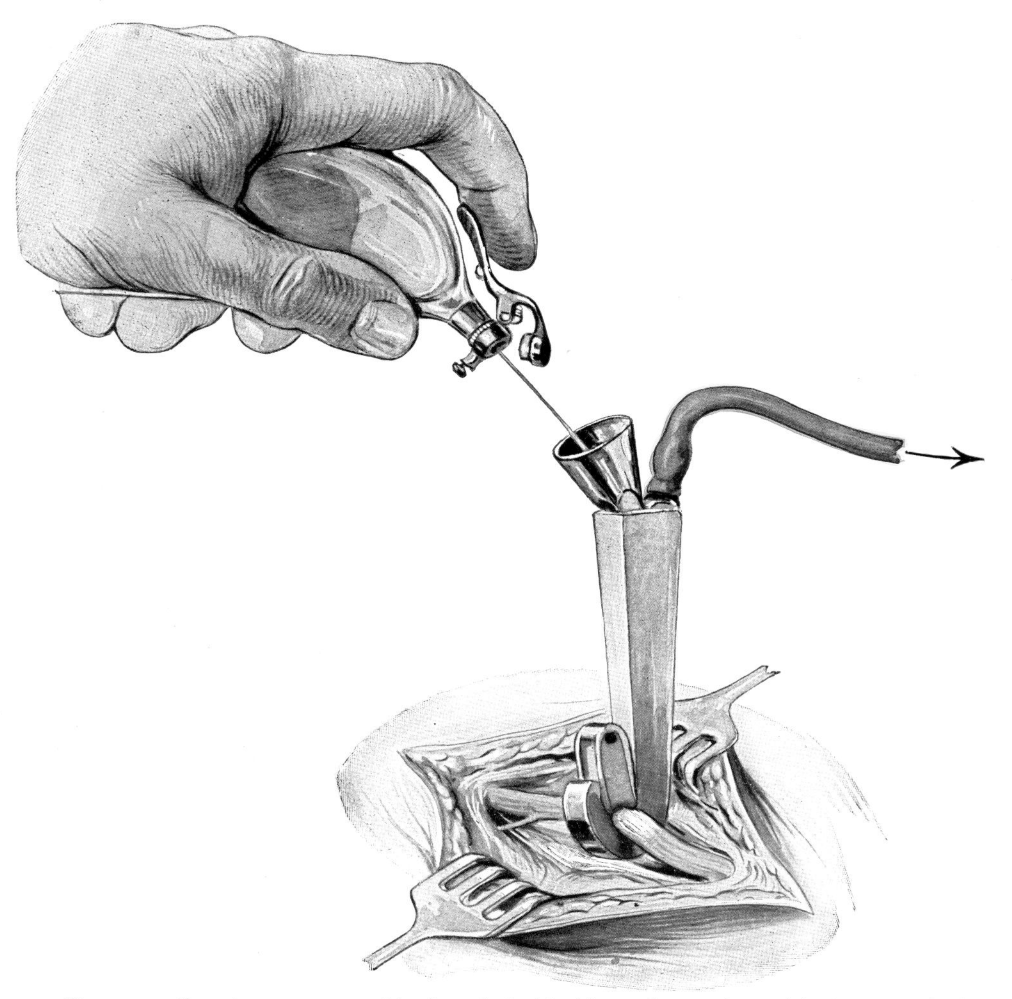

FIG. 541. Freezing a nerve with the ethyl chloride aspirator (Trendelenburg-Perthes). The nerve is passed over the hook on the apparatus and then kept in place with a wedge. Ethyl chloride is sprayed in above. Aspiration of this causes rapid evaporation and cooling of the container.

541), through which ethyl chloride (— 15°) mixed with air is passed with the aid of a suction pump. I freeze the nerve in a simpler and more rapid way by surrounding it on all sides with carbonic acid snow (— 80°) (Fig. 542). The carbonic acid snow is collected on a sterile towel, and is sterile. I also use the cryocautery (Fig. 448), which was described in Chapter V. The motor paralysis resulting after freezing should disappear in the course of months, while the pain frequently does not recur, although such results are by no means constant. I have experienced failure in several cases. Other authors as well, seem to have had similar experiences. The time for freezing has had to be extended from 2 or 3 minutes to as much as 20 minutes.

Transverse division of a nerve central to the lesion eliminates the pain immediately and with certainty. Motor nerve conduction is, of course, interrupted by this method and immediate nerve suture offers no certainty of its return. When motor conduction is reestablished, the pain may also, of course, recur. The same is true when the nerve is crushed with an angiotribe above the level of the lesion (Fig. 543). To eliminate the pain, and, of course, the motor function as well, with certainty and permanently it is not enough simply to divide the nerve, but a section several centimeters long should be excised or twisted out central to the lesion (trigeminal, phrenic).

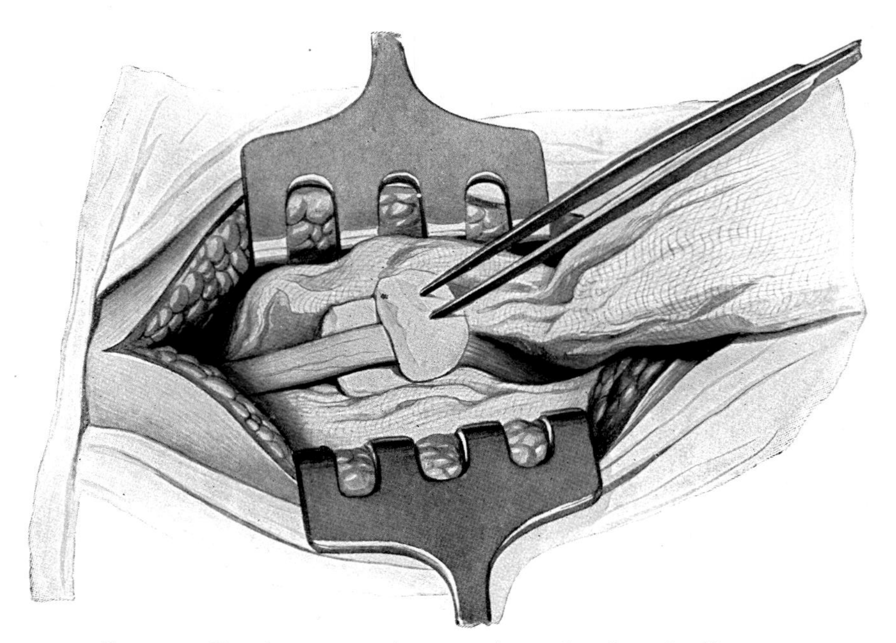

FIG. 542. Freezing a nerve between pieces of carbon dioxide snow.

When the nerve trunk above the site of the lesion is not accessible, or when the lesion involves an extensive section of the nerve, other surgical measures are possible. Occasionally the nerve, exposed peripherally, can be pulled carefully from its bed for a considerable distance (trigeminal and phrenic nerve). The nerve is seized transversely with a longitudinally grooved Thiersch forceps; the forceps is turned slowly (one turn in from 1 to 3 minutes) around its longitudinal axis (Fig. 544), so that the nerve is wound gradually around the forceps and is torn from its attachments (exoresis).

In Förster's operation the sensory nerve conduction is interrupted directly at the spinal cord. By this method, after laminectomy the posterior roots of the spinal nerves are resected. Chordotomy, the division of the antero-lateral column in the spinal cord, gives even better results in the more severe types of pain. It is followed by immediate cessation of all pain sensation, while the sensations of touch and temperature and motor conduction are preserved. (This latter operation has been popularized in this country by Frazier, and the Spiller-Frazier operation for chordotomy has been extensively employed. I. S. R.)

The etiology of trophoneurotic ulcers is considered at present to be due not to a deficiency, but to irritation of a sensory nerve, which acts reflexly on the vascular supply. To promote healing of such ulcers, therefore, the irritating condition should be surgically removed, or the diseased nerve should be interrupted central to the site of the lesion.

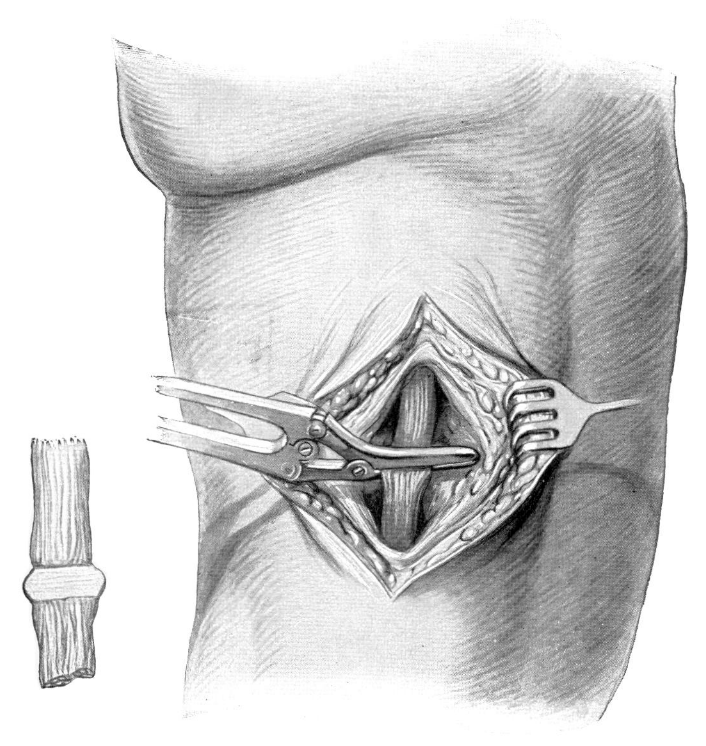

FIG. 543. Crushing a nerve.

In every nerve injury, whether the result of accident or operation, whether it has damaged the nerve laterally or has completely divided it, there arises the danger of the development of a neuroma. In operations which involve the nerves, for example, in excision, an attempt should be made to prevent the formation of such amputation neuromata by special measures. The peripheral end of the nerve may be implanted laterally in its trunk, forming in this way a loop (Fig. 545) (Bardenheuer); the end of the nerve may be notched and the tips sutured together (Fig. 546); the nerve may be crushed with an angiotribe somewhat centrally or in the region of the division (Krüger) (Fig. 543), or infiltrated with 90 percent alcohol, formalin, or phenol, or frozen. The nerve may also be divided with the Paquelin cautery instead of with the knife, to counteract the development of neuromata (Payr, Hedri). None of these procedures are, however, certain.

In spasticity of central origin which interferes with the free movement of the limbs, the spasticity may be relieved by resecting the nerves supplying the muscles, with resulting paralysis. The paralysis of the muscles caused by this results in most cases in a more or less severe impairment of motion,

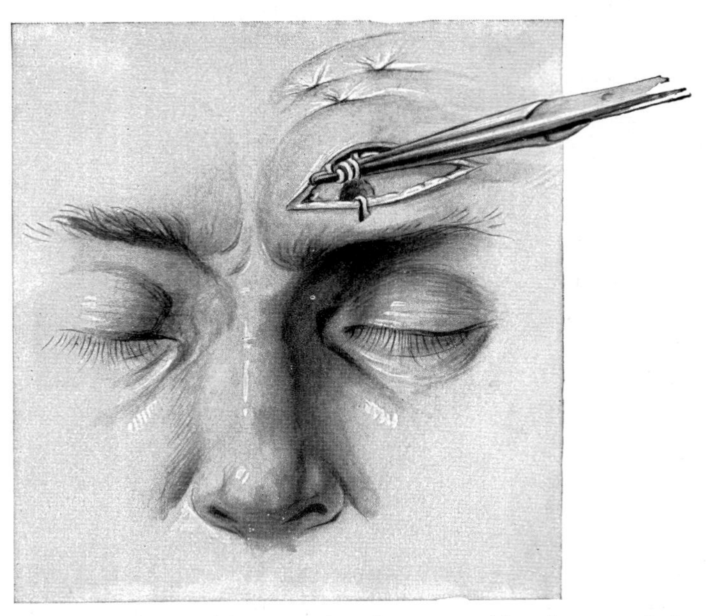

FIG. 544. Exoresis of a nerve. After grasping the nerve with a hemostat it is twisted from its attachments.

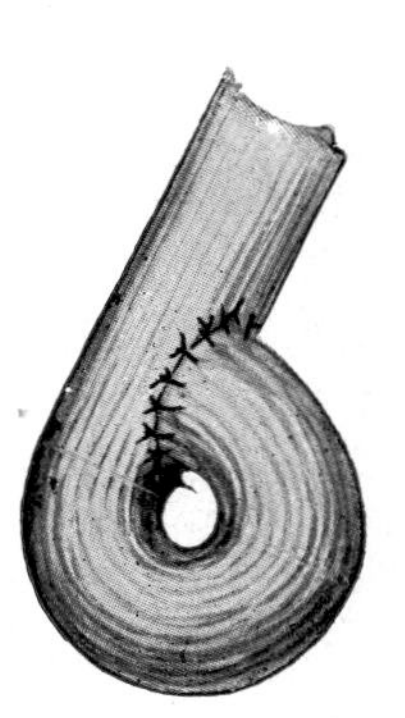

FIG. 545. Sling formation to prevent amputation neuromata.

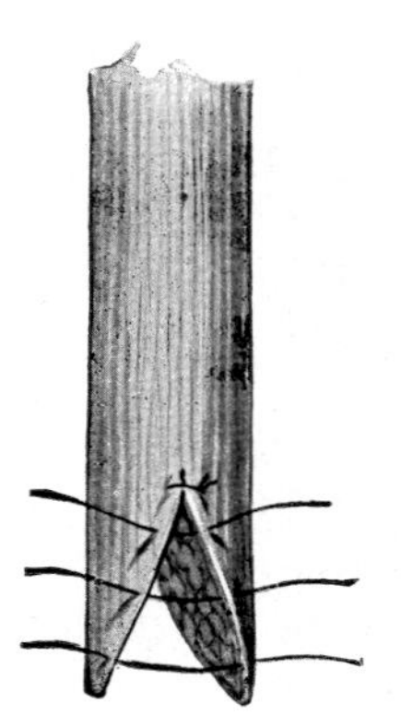

FIG. 546. V-shaped resection and suture of a nerve to prevent amputation neuromata.

so that the indications are for a lessening rather than complete interruption of motor conduction. This can be accomplished by dividing only a part of the motor nerve tracts supplying the muscle group (Stoffel's operation), or by interrupting the single reflex arc causing the spasticity in the posterior sensory nerve roots of the spinal cord (Förster's operation).

In Stoffel's operation (Fig. 547), the peripheral nerve trunk is exposed and the separate bundles are identified by their anatomical location and connection with the individual muscles and by electrical stimulation. One-third to one-half of the nerve bundle supplying the spastic group of muscles is divided or a section several centimeters long may be excised. The operation, according to Stoffel, is indicated for the relief of spasticity in hemiplegia and diplegia, when it is limited to individual muscles and groups of muscles. The contra-indications to the operation are extensive spasticity, considerable athetosis, youth, and severe mental disturbances. Subsequent regulated exercise and education are of decided value.

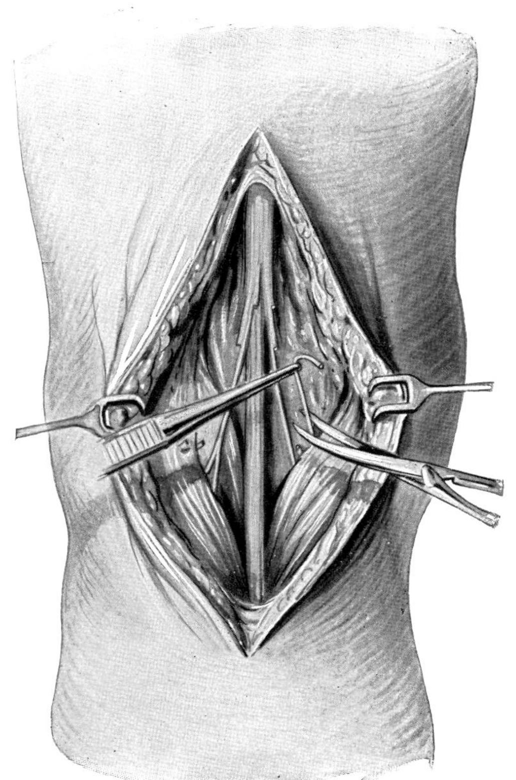

FIG. 547. Stoffel's Operation. Individual nerve tracts are divided so as to lessen the innervation of a muscle and thus relieve spasticity.

E. PERIARTERIAL SYMPATHECTOMY

On the theory that the centrifugal sympathetic fibers run longitudinally in the adventitia of the large arteries, Lëriche, Brüning and others, recommended, in cases of vasomotor disturbances of the distal portion of the extremities, the removal of a ring of adventitia about 10 cm. long to remove the vasoconstrictor control and thus produce hyperemia. If this can be accomplished it will have a favorable influence on trophic disturbances. While this theory is no longer tenable in its entirety, since the vessels are known to be supplied by nerve fibers entering various segments and not by longitudinally running fibers, there occurs, nevertheless, hyperemia and increased temperature of the extremity distal to the site of periarterial sympathectomy which lasts for a period of weeks. There is little to be said for the temporary or prolonged effects of such hyperemia upon the particular lesion. Opinions concerning this are greatly at variance, enthusiastic support being counterbalanced by flat opposition. The procedure has been recommended in all lesions in which nutritional (trophoneurotic) disturbances or painful conditions (causalgia) of distal sections of the extremity can be traced back to a primary or to a nervous diminution of the arterial blood supply. The advocates of the operation claim that the reflex arc involving the diseased or irritated nerve section is broken by interrupting the sympathetic tracts running with the blood vessels, and as a result pain and nutritional disturbances caused by vessel spasm no longer occur. They are relieved by paralysis of the vessel musculature with the resulting beneficial hyperemia. Such primary vasomotor trophic neuroses are or may be Raynaud's disease, erythromelalgia, scleroderma, angioneurotic edema, acroparæsthesia, migraine, trigeminal neuralgia,

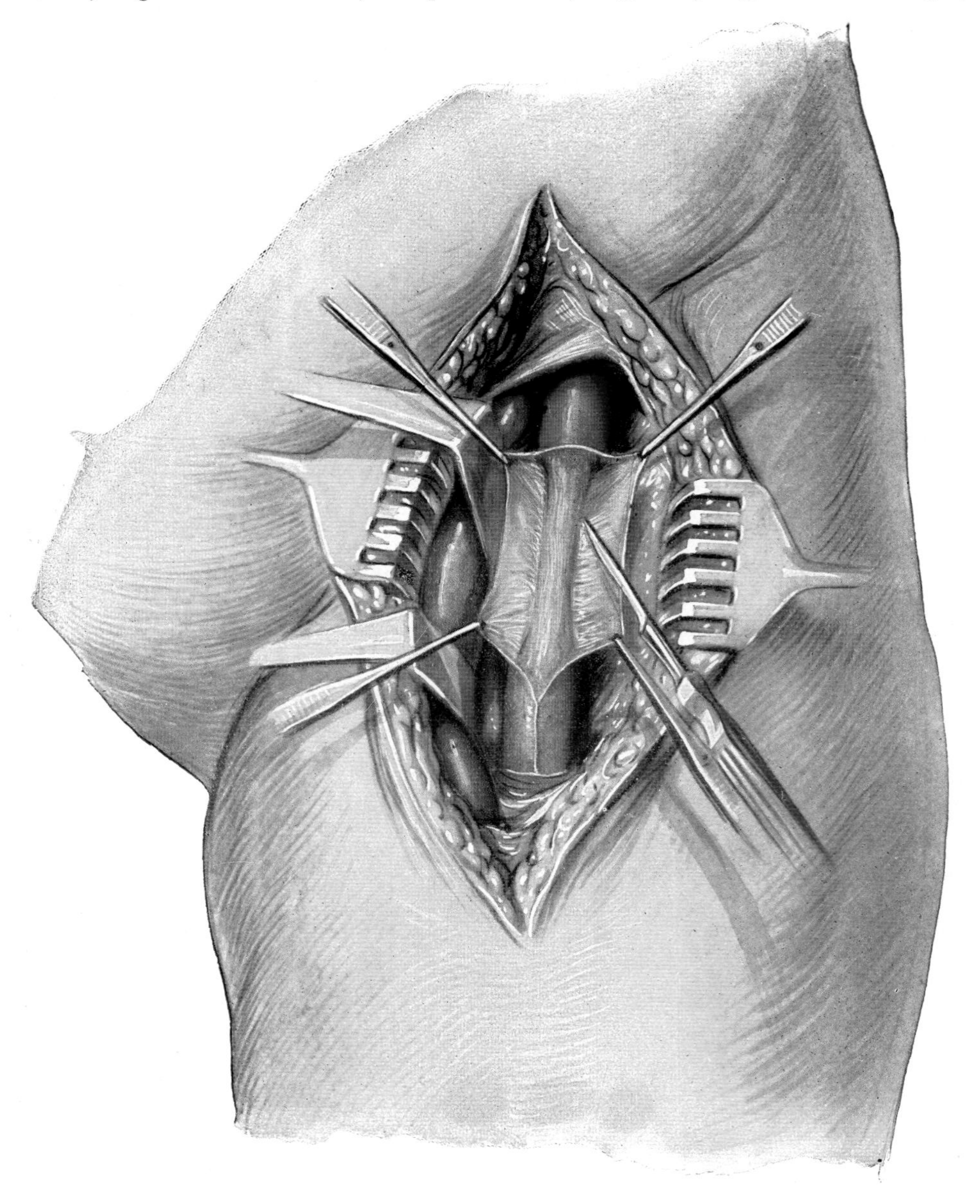

FIG. 548. Periarterial Sympathectomy. The adventitia of the femoral artery, exposed over a length of 10 cm., is split longitudinally, carefully dissected from the vessel for a distance of at least 7 cm., and removed. The vessel contracts considerably while this is being done.

etc. (The limitations of periarterial sympathectomy are being more and more realized and it is being replaced by various types of sympathetic ganglionectomy and ramisection. I. S. R.)

Other lesions resulting in nerve irritation which are supposedly relieved by periarterial sympathectomy are amputation neuromata, constriction of individual nerve trunks by cicatricial masses, pressure on nerves by the callus surrounding chronic ulcers (ulcera cruris, x-ray ulcers, perforating ulcer of the foot), through tissue induration and edema following freezing, burns, amputation of a limb, cicatrices, etc. Successful results were expected even in arteriosclerotic nutritional disturbances (intermittent claudication), and when the lumen of the vessel was organically narrowed, and the walls had lost their elasticity. The procedure was also recommended for the cure of pseudo-arthrosis.

Part of the direct results in ulcerative diseases and other nutritional disturbances is to be credited, in my opinion, to rest following the intervention, to elevation, good care, etc., of the affected part, to the effect of the incipient hyperemia, which, in my experience, is as transitory as the results dependent upon it. The result is more comprehensible when the pain depends on vascular spasm, though it has been observed that after one side was operated upon improvement has occurred on both sides. I believe, therefore, that periarterial sympathectomy is indicated only when all palliative measures have been exhausted, to which may be added, besides rest and elevation of the diseased limb, the removal of possible neuromata, neurolysis, and the division of the involved nerves. It should never be used in arteriosclerotic disturbances, in severe infection of the distal section of the extremity, or in tuberculosis of the bones and joints. (When it seems imperative to prevent sympathetic stimuli from reaching a part, sympathetic ganglionectomy is a more rational procedure. I. S. R.)

To perform the operation (Fig. 548) the main artery of the limb involved is first exposed under local anæsthesia for a distance of 8 to 10 cm., and in order to include the particularly numerous nerve tracts entering near the proximal section, the exposure is made as far proximally as possible. The brachial artery is exposed just distal to the axilla, the femoral artery directly below Poupart's ligament. Small lateral branches, as well as vessels running over the artery are divided between ligatures. The adventitia of the exposed artery is cautiously split longitudinally with a sharp knife, lifted with delicate toothed forceps, and carefully dissected free with a sharp knife on both sides. If possible, it should be removed in one piece. To accomplish this an effort should be made to follow the line of cleavage between adventitia and media. If any of the vessel sheath remains it should be removed, so that the artery is freed entirely of the adventitia, for a distance of from 7 to 10 cm. While the adventitia is being dissected free, the vessel contracts, sometimes to one-half of its original size. Removal of the sheath may be more difficult because of this. The wound is closed in the usual manner, by suturing the muscle, fascia, and skin. The limb is placed at rest, slightly elevated. The pulse may be absent for several hours distal to the site of operation as the result of the vessel spasm produced by the trauma. Hyperemia and rise in temperature do not occur until the return of the pulse. These may last for several weeks.

There are two postoperative dangers that may occur. The vessel may rupture subsequently because of calcification of the lumen or injury to the media, with a resulting sudden, severe arterial hemorrhage with its serious sequelæ. Second, infection of the field of operation may occur and Pels-Leusden thinks this is especially frequent. This may be the result of opening, during the operation, the lymph vessels accompanying the large blood vessels, which often contain bacteria from distal infected areas. All infected areas should if possible be allowed to heal or should be thoroughly cleaned up before the operation.

CHAPTER IX

BONE SURGERY

A. GENERAL PRINCIPLES

Surgery of the bones is distinct from other types of surgery because of the hardness of the material. A disadvantage of this increased hardness is that the usual instruments intended for the soft parts can not be used. Very strong, special instruments are required, and considerable strength is necessary in their application. The instruments and the way in which they are used resemble closely those used by mechanics for working on wood, iron and stone. An advantage of the increased solidity is that bony tissue has an exact form and allows a good reciprocal fitting of fragments; also that bone sutures and other means of fastening find an excellent hold.

The bones form the rigid, elastic support of the body; they are constantly subjected to pressure, bending and traction. A more or less pronounced displacement of the fragments occurs, as a rule, when a bone is fractured as the result of an injury or operation. In surgical procedures on bones, the bones should be kept as intact as possible. A bone that is markedly weakened or broken should be protected by the application of a plaster cast, a splint, or traction bandages, and by careful handling of the limb, especially during the dressings, until its structure has been restored, in order to avoid spontaneous fracture, or displacement of the fractured ends. The injured limb, however, must also be treated as soon as possible with active and passive motion, massage, electricity, baths, etc., to prevent ankylosis of the joints and atrophy of the muscles, the occurrence of which would nullify the results of an otherwise successful bone operation.

In all operations on bones in which there is no purulent infection, especially in correction of position and bone transplantation, meticulous asepsis is necessary. Bone abscesses, fistulæ, sequestra, granulating wound surfaces must therefore be taken care of in a previous operation. Even though there is no evidence of infection, the sterility of such areas is not certain. Latent infection, including tetanus, has a particular predilection for bony tissue. There are numerous cases in which pyogenic organisms have lived for decades in bone, without giving evidence of their presence. A period of six months should, as a rule, elapse between the last manifestation of infection and an operation for the correction of position. Before extensive operations, a period of twelve months at least should elapse. If there has been a previous infection, a careful examination should be made before any operative procedure, to determine if there is any sign of latency. The temperature should be watched for several days and the area subjected to massage, percussion, heat, and strain. If the operative site is covered with thin, cicatricial skin which may cause nutritional disturbance after operation, this skin should be replaced by a healthy skin flap or graft before any operation on the bone is attempted.

Bone is insensitive. If the soft parts covering the bone and in the field of operation are anæsthetized, a bone operation may be performed under local anæsthesia. The skull, for example, can be operated upon without pain after the scalp has been anæsthetized and incised. This is of particular value in operations on the brain, since the meninges, at least over the convexity of the brain, and the brain itself are insensitive to pain. Local anæsthesia in bone operations has one drawback, in that the patient receives the disagreeable

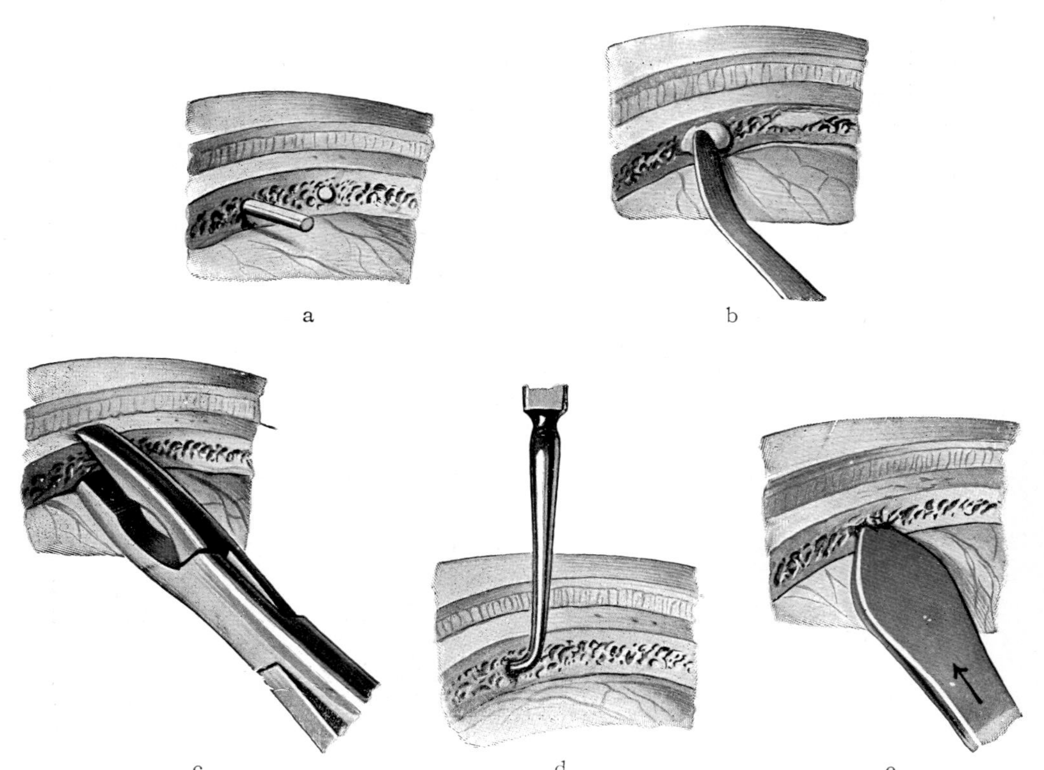

FIG. 549 a–e. Methods used for checking hemorrhage from diploic vessels, (a) by introducing a small ivory peg, (b) by pressing in little pieces of wax or muscle, (c) by bone compression, (d) by twisting in Krause's hooks, (e) by pressure with an elevator.

impulses of the instrument on the bone, especially on the skull, and is aware of the chiseling, drilling, rongeuring, or breaking of the bone.

Though a tourniquet is used to control hemorrhage in the soft tissues, it may have no effect on bleeding from the bone marrow. External constriction of the soft parts can not always arrest the blood supply of the medullary space. To avoid secondary hemorrhage in plastic operations on bone, it is better not to use a tourniquet. Bleeding vessels running in the bone itself can not be caught and ligated in the usual way. Hemorrhage from a large vessel in a bone may therefore be fairly extensive, and even dangerous when from an emissary vein. It rarely stops spontaneously because the vessels can not contract in the rigid channels. A good method for checking the hemorrhage is by driving in a tapered ivory peg (Fig. 549 a) or small pegs of hardwood (oak), whose projecting portion can be cut off. One may also use bone wax, small pieces of muscle or gauze, which are pressed into the opening (Fig. 549 b). Twisting a blunt bone hook into the canal, pressing into it with an elevator (Figs. 549 d and e), or crushing the layers of bone surrounding it are less dependable methods (Fig. 549 c). The jarring which occurs during bone surgery, particularly during chiseling, can, to some extent, be mitigated by carefully supporting the bone. Sandbags are not suitable for this purpose for, aside from the danger of sepsis from blood and pus retained from previous operations, they are apt to give off dust during hammering, even though wrapped in moist cloths. Thick sponge-rubber cushions make the best padding. They possess such great elasticity that they form the best means for avoiding the well-known "hammering phenomena" when chiseling the skull, which are, in reality, a manifestation of a more or less severe concussion of the brain.

Fat embolism is another possible complication in bone surgery. It may occur at any time from a few hours to eight days after the operation. It results when fat enters an open vein at the site of operation or injury and is carried to the lungs, brain or other organs. In pulmonary embolism there are symptoms of unrest, distress, shortness of breath, cyanosis, cough, and bloody expectoration. In cerebral embolism brain symptoms are most marked, and it is necessary to differentiate between the effects of narcosis and coma. Occasionally there are symptoms of irritation of the cerebral cortex. When the renal vessels are blocked by an embolus, uremic symptoms may arise and the urine may contain considerable quantities of fat. The treatment consists in venesection and replacement of the lost blood by salt solution or blood. Stimulants may also be indicated.

A bone is exposed, as a rule, by a longitudinal lateral incision, when it lies close to the surface and is not covered by important structures. It is frequently advisable to expose the bone by two opposite longitudinal incisions, and the bridge of tissue thus formed is held back with wide retractors so that the bone may be reached from all sides. If the bone is covered with muscles, it should, if possible, be exposed through an interspace which does not contain the principal vessels and nerves. If these structures lie near the site of operation, they should be exposed and retracted in order to avoid injuring them. The bone may also be exposed by turning aside a muscular flap from above it. In order to determine the extent and exact location of diseased bone before operation, a roentgenogram is taken with markers placed on the skin. The exact location of the disease can then be determined from its relation to the skin markers, and the most suitable site for the skin incision chosen.

The periosteum is of greater importance than the marrow for the vitality and reconstruction of bone. The periosteum is very sensitive to nutritional disturbances. According to Lexer, its osteogenetic function is most perfectly retained when it remains attached to its nourishing muscles. For the sake of bone formation, extensive detachment of the periosteum on one side of the bone should be avoided. When the bone must be divided transversely, it should, as a rule, be exposed on all sides. This can be done either extra-periosteally or subperiosteally. In subperiosteal exposure (Figs. 551 and 552), the periosteum is split by a longitudinal incision, with transverse incisions

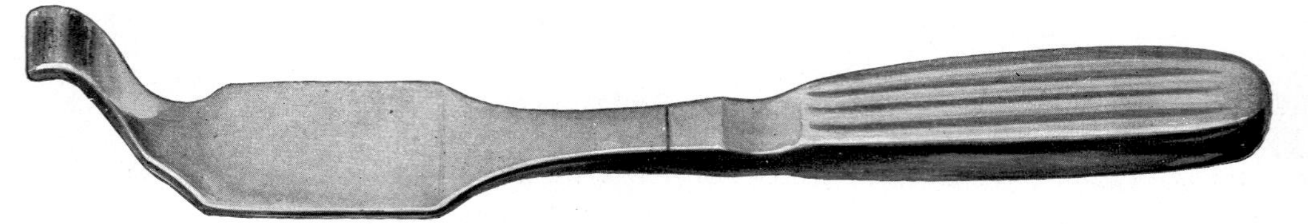

FIG. 550. Combined muscle hook and elevator.

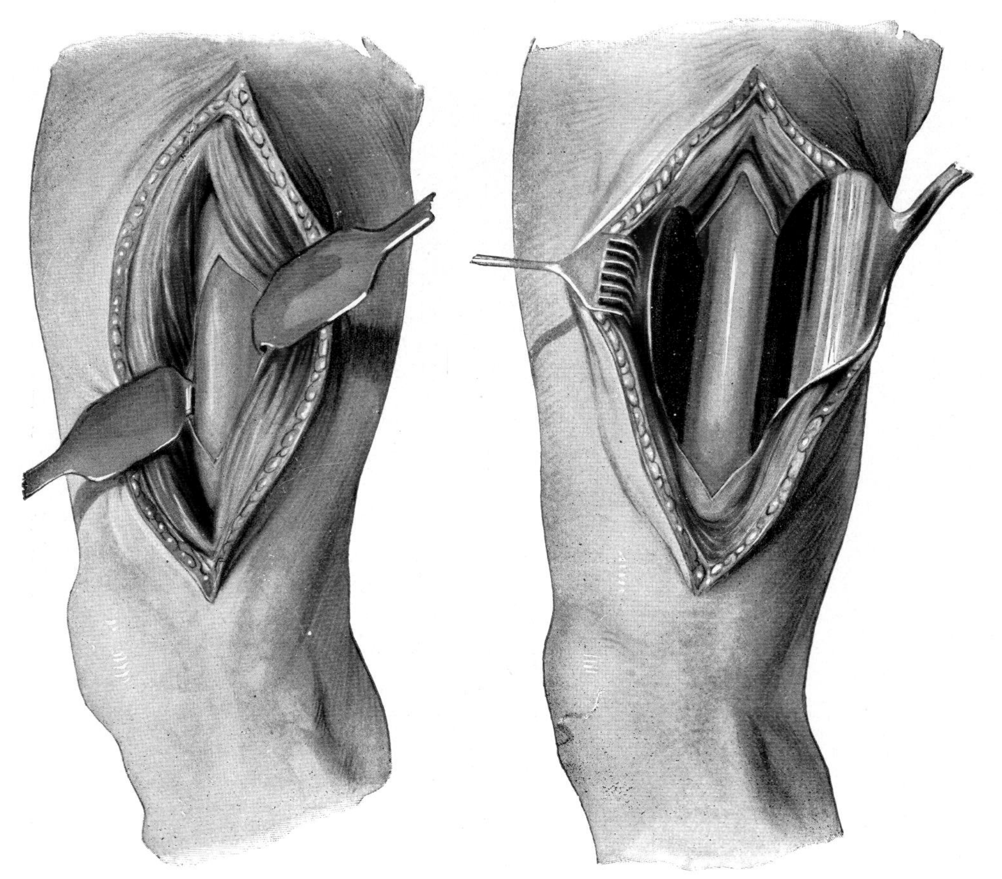

FIG. 551. Subperiosteal exposure of the femur with the aid of two combined muscle hooks and elevators.

FIG. 552. Subperiosteal exposure of the femur with the aid of a bent scoop.

at either end, if necessary, and carefully separated from the bone by the use of rugines or suitably curved elevators. The scoop or elevator is passed under the periosteum in the region of the muscle insertions, and carried in the direction the muscle fibers take in leaving the bone, as for example, in the direction of the intercostal muscles on the ribs. When the periosteum has been raised at one place, so that the instrument can be carried safely between it and the bone, further separation is, as a rule, rapid and uniform. In subperiosteal exposure, the periosteum is raised without disturbing its uninterrupted connection with the overlying muscles. In extraperiosteal exposure, the periosteum remains on the bone and the surrounding soft parts are detached from the periosteum. At points of insertion of muscles, this becomes difficult and there is a rich blood supply to be dealt with. Because of its simplicity, the subperiosteal exposure is generally preferred. Extra-periosteal exposure is used mainly in malignant disease.

During the further course of the operation the detached soft parts are protected and retracted with curved retractors. The soft parts lying under the bone must also be protected when the bone is to be divided, and this may be done by inserting under the bone at each side a curved elevator. A combined muscle retractor and elevator (Figs. 550 and 551) is useful for this. The soft parts must be particularly well protected when saws are used, especially the circular saw. For this purpose broad lead scoops (Fig. 552), which can be bent in any way desired, are particularly adapted. They were made originally for transferring Thiersch grafts.

When the operation on the bone is completed and the bleeding has been carefully checked, the soft parts are carefully sutured in layers in aseptic cases. If the wound is infected, drains are inserted, or the wound is left wide open. Movement can and should be begun before healing is complete.

B. BONE SURGERY

In all work on bones, the bone must be kept free from the soft parts and held securely. Since this can not be done by grasping the extremity

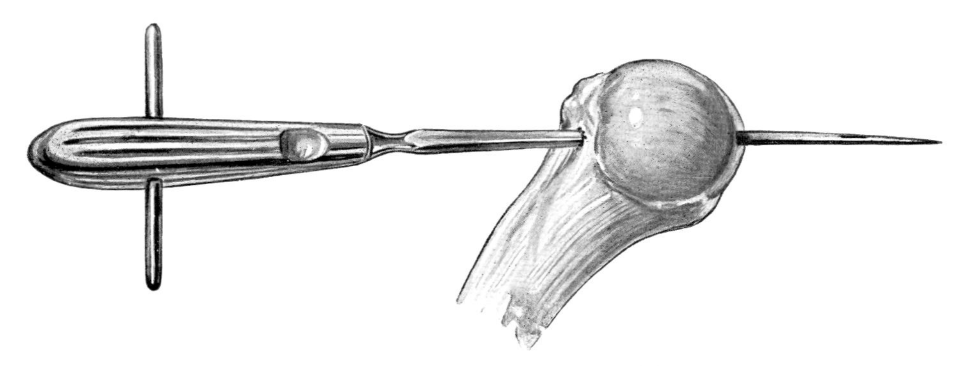

FIG. 553. Bone perforator and needle.

outside the region of operation, the bones may be drawn forward and hooked firmly with pointed or dull bone hooks (Fig. 606), or held with bone-holding forceps, made with sharp prongs (v. Langenbeck, Fig. 554) or with tubular mouths (Lambotte, Fig. 555). Special sequestrum forceps serve to seize the sequestrum (Fig. 556).

For making holes, drills or tapered flat borers of various diameters are used. When soft parts which must be avoided lie beneath the bone, such as the meninges, a spherical or oval (Fig. 557) drill is best. These push the

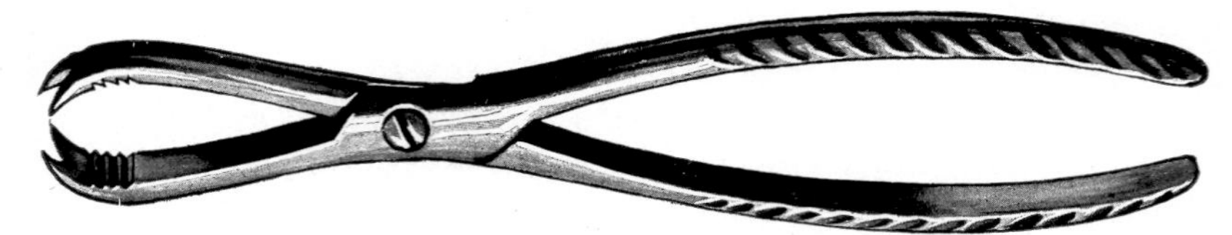

FIG. 554. Bone-grasping forceps (Langenbeck).

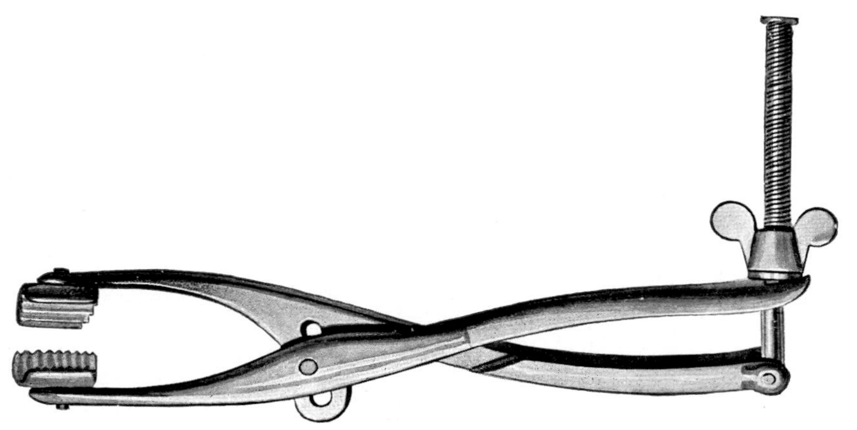

FIG. 555. Bone-grasping forceps with tubular mouth (Lambotte).

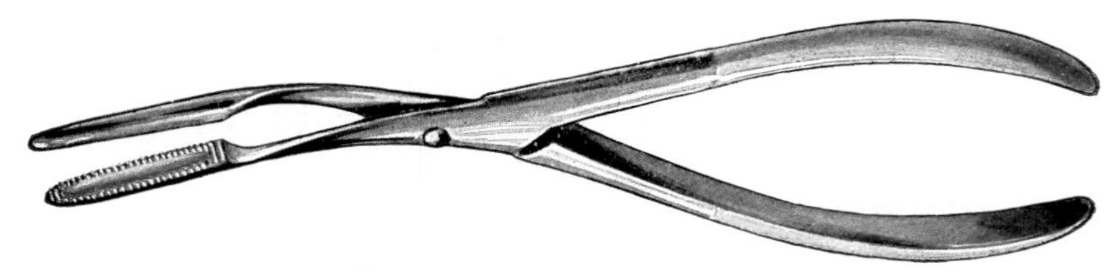

FIG. 556. Sequestrum forceps.

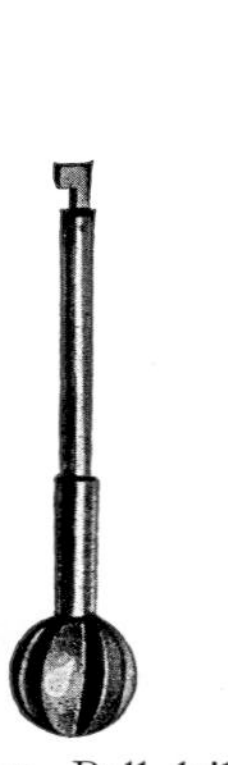

FIG. 557. Ball drill.

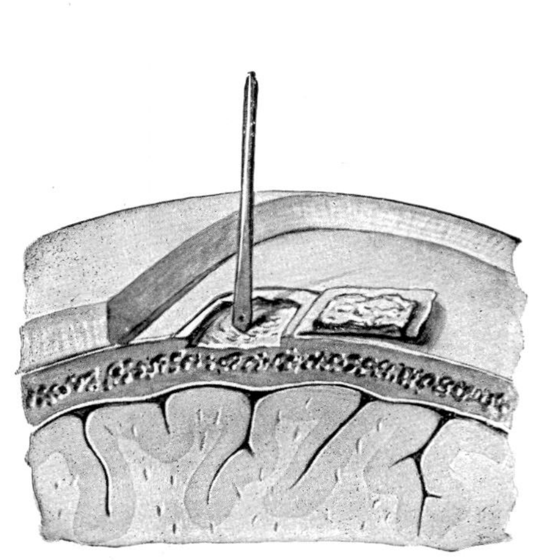

FIG. 558. Osteoplastic perforation of a bone. Before the drill bores through the skull an osteoperiosteal flap is raised, which closes the hole later.

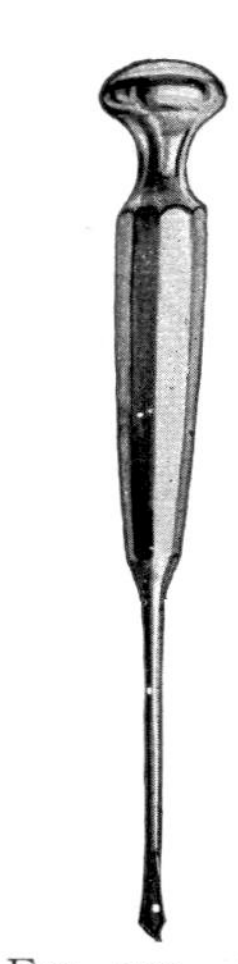

FIG. 559. Hand awl with eye for drawing through a wire.

soft parts before them, especially the tough meninges. The best instrument of this kind is Martel's trephine, which automatically blocks itself after penetrating the skull. Drills may also be used for enlarging existing holes, for example, the medullary cavity of the long bones. If it is desired to drill

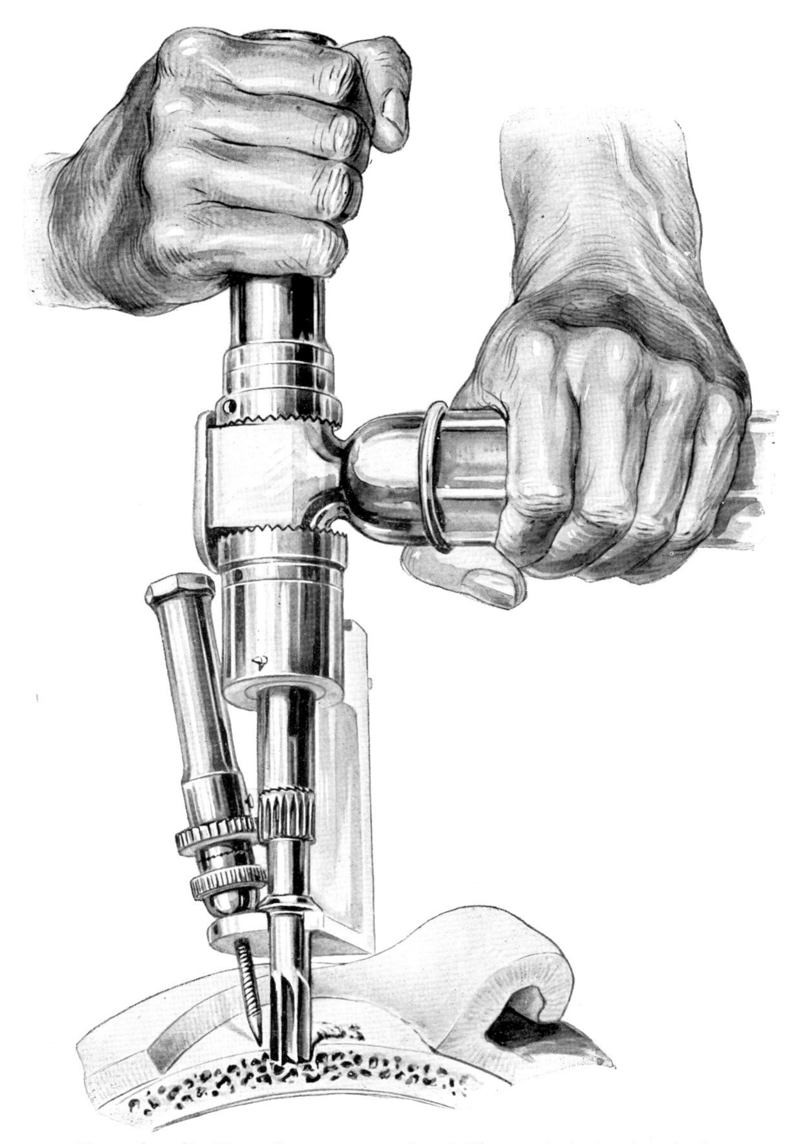

Fig. 560. DeMartel's apparatus for drilling a hole in the skull.

through a bone, as for instance the skull, but leave no defect, a chip of bone with attached periosteum is chiseled out as a flap before applying the drill. The small bone flap is subsequently laid back over the holes (Fig. 558). This is not necessary as a rule, for even large holes rapidly close.

Because the bone, with the exception of its spongy tissue, offers considerable resistance to drilling, the drills are usually driven by motors. Hand awls are also used, however (Figs. 559 and 560). A drill with a flat borer (Fig. 561) which is constantly being turned backward and forward is suitable for its own attachments only. It is superfluous and should be replaced by a drilling machine which turns in one direction. The most commonly used

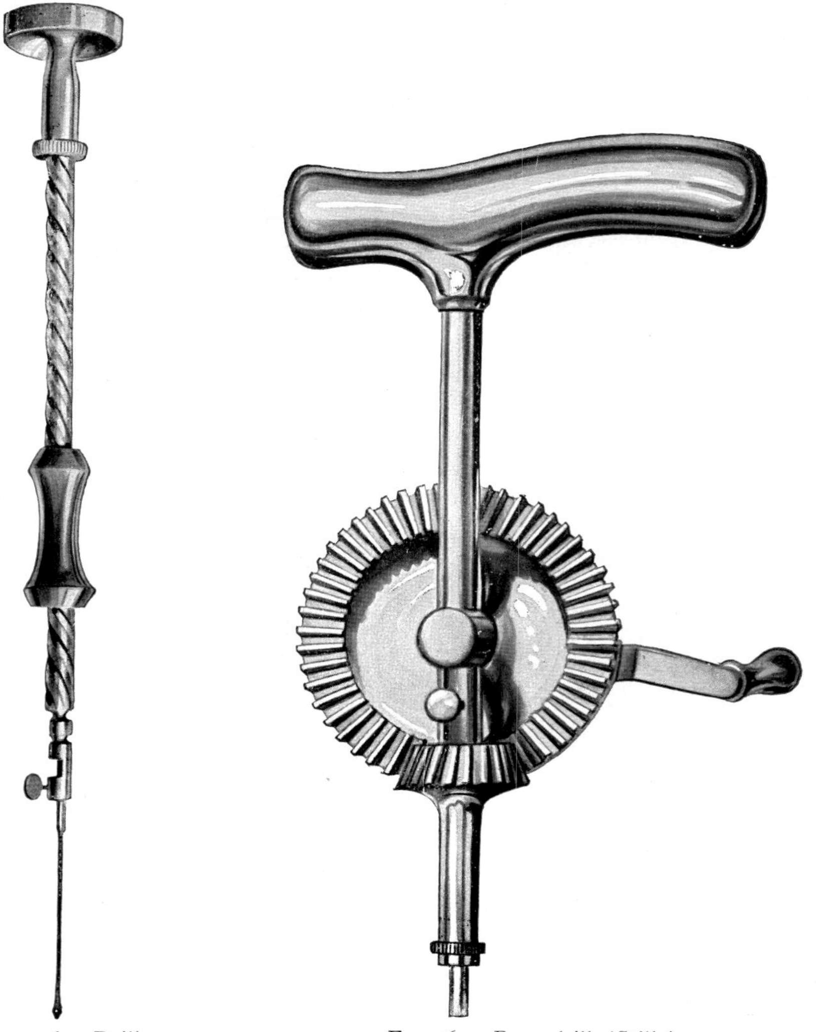

Fig. 561. Drilling machine with flat borer.

Fig. 562. Bone drill (Stille).

hand drill is Stille's bone drill (Fig. 562). It should not be considered as the ideal machine, for the ball-bearing hand drills used by metal workers (Fig. 563) are better and may be used in surgery as well. An electrical drill (Fig. 564) saves time and effort. Its handle is shaped like the butt of a revolver (Fig. 565), and the trigger serves as the switch for starting and stopping the drill. An electrical drill must be cooled by a continuous stream of water, to prevent overheating the adjacent bone which may result in necrosis and sequestration (Fig. 581).

In many cases a wire is to be drawn through the hole drilled in the bone. Many drills are provided with an eye at the point for threading the wire, so that the wire may be drawn through the bone, as the drill is withdrawn. It is often difficult to pass the wire through holes drilled in long bones, because the soft marrow affords no guidance and the hole on the far side of it can not be easily found as the wire is pushed through. An awl with an eye may be passed through the hole to draw the wire through (Fig. 559). A loop of fine wire may be inserted and attached to the wire to be used, thus acting as a guide through the hole (Fig. 606).

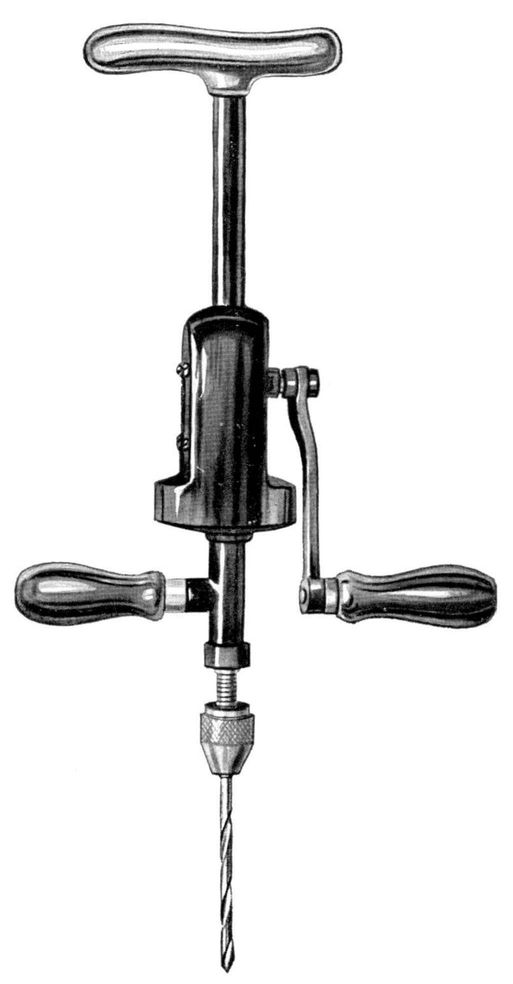

Fig. 563. Bone drill equipped with ball bearings and wimble.

Other procedures in dealing with bone, such as shaping the ends of the bone, making or removing angles and edges, the forming or flattening of grooves, are accomplished with the aid of gouge forceps (Figs. 566 to 570), chisels (Figs. 571 to 574) and saws (Figs. 583 to 585). The mouth of Luer's forceps, which is made so as to use the principle of leverage, may be either circular or oval (Figs. 566 and 567). One lip may be flat (Fig. 568), by means of which the instrument may be slipped into a small space, as between the meninges and the skull. When using gouge forceps, the bone should be sharply cut through as the forceps are closed. Since thick layers of bone can not always be cut through in this manner, even with great effort, the surgeon may have to combine a leverage action with cutting, thus breaking through the bone.

Great force can be exerted with Harvey's forceps (Fig. 569), the jaws of which are short and the arms lengthened by an interpolated joint.

The punches (Fig. 570) are a modification of Luer's forceps. A small oval plate is pushed against a cutting frame and in this way punches or cuts interposed tissue. The jaws are connected with the handle by a long, narrow shank which conveys the force. Being long and narrow, the punches are particularly adapted for work in narrow passages, such as the nose, mouth, larynx and ear.

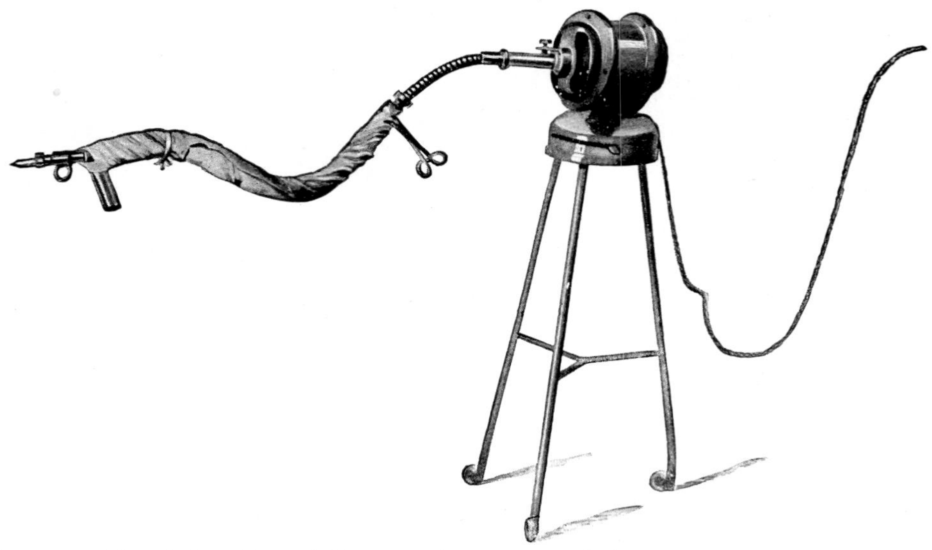

FIG. 564. Electrically driven drilling machine. The shaft is protected by a boilable metal tube and by a sterile cloth.

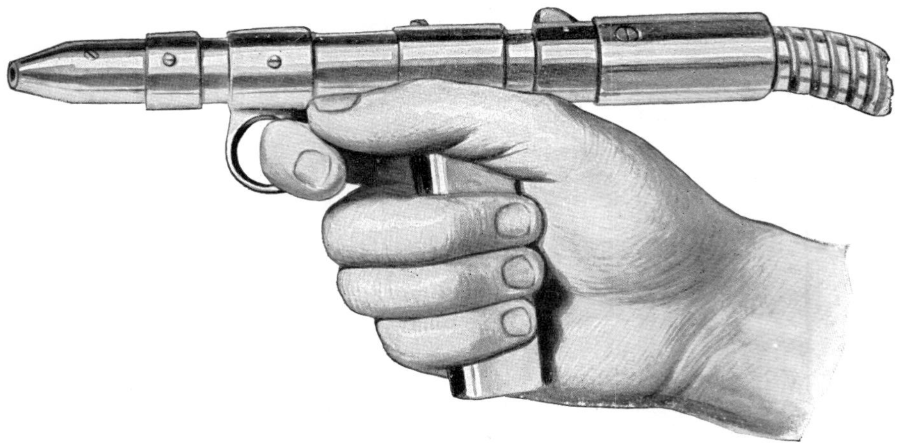

FIG. 565. Hand-piece of the electrically driven drilling machine with trigger for starting and stopping.

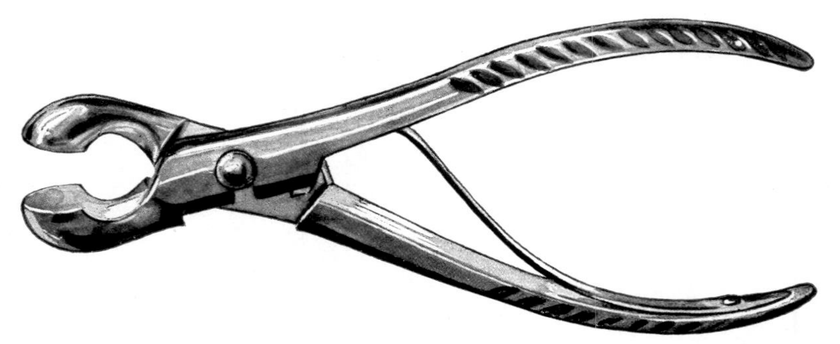

FIG. 566. Luer's gouge forceps with circular tip.

The handle of a chisel must be grasped firmly in the hand, if it is not held in the finger tips, as an ear chisel is held. The handle should be fairly

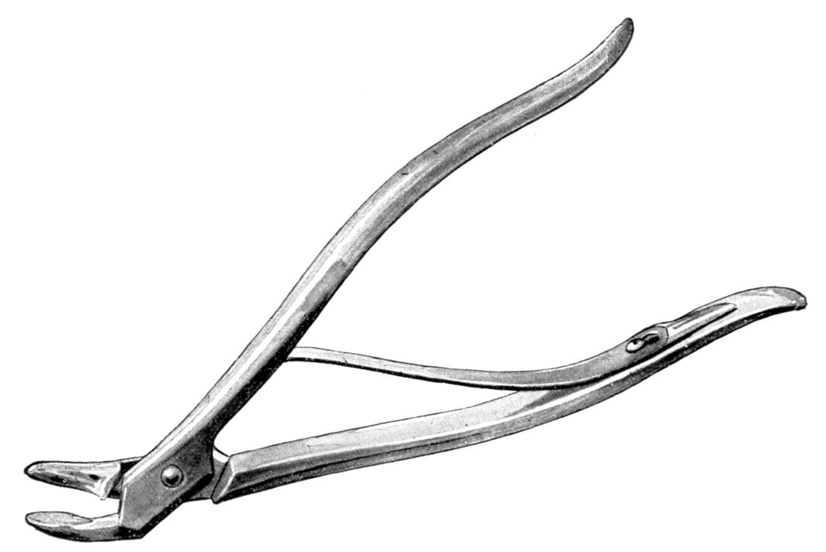

Fig. 567. Gouge forceps with pointed tip.

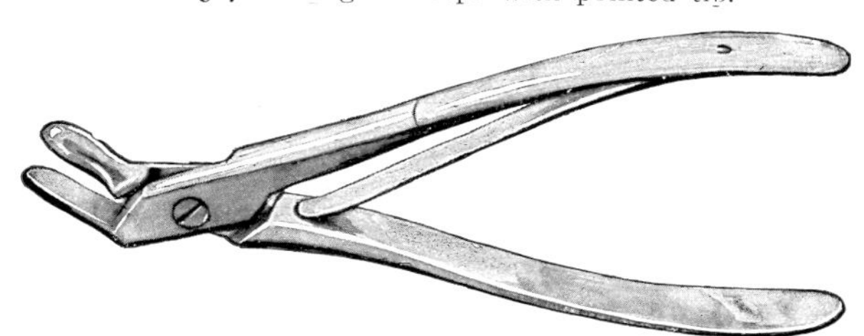

Fig. 568. Gouge forceps, whose lower lip is flat.

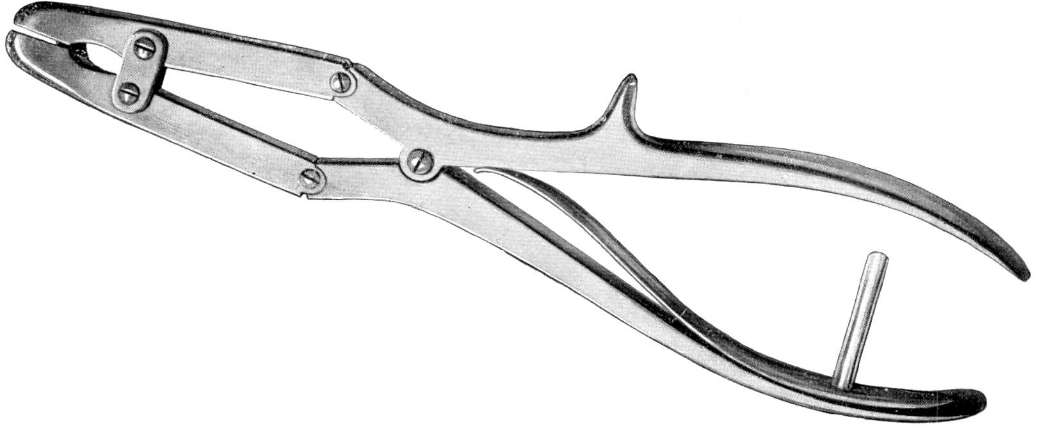

Fig. 569. Harvey's gouge forceps.

thick if it is to be held easily in the hand without tiring the surgeon. The thin handles usually found on chisels can be enlarged by covering them with rubber tubing or wrapping them with rubber bandages (Fig. 571). Chisels, which may be either straight or grooved (gouge), are made in various lengths, widths and thicknesses. In most work requiring a straight chisel, the osteotome edge (Fig. 572) is preferable to the chisel beveled on one side (Fig. 573).

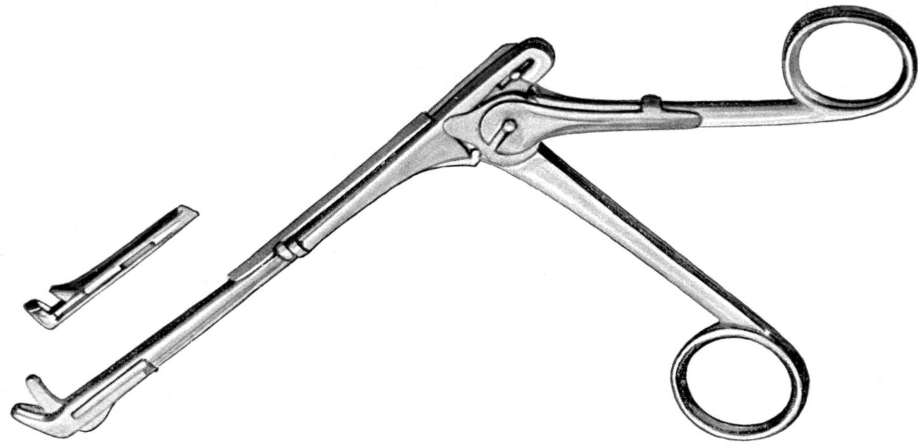

Fig. 570. Bone punch with various punches.

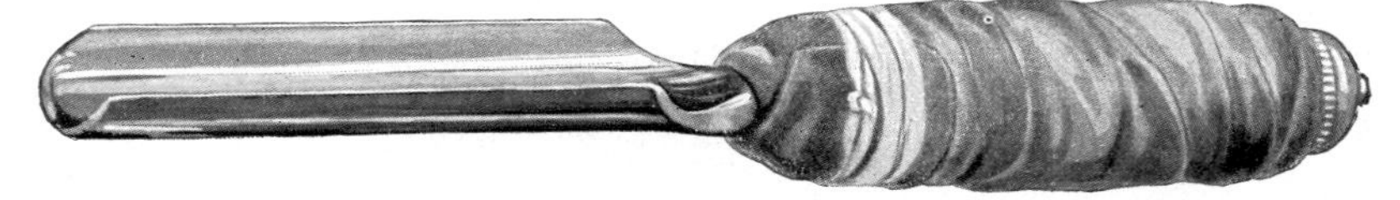

Fig. 571. Gouge, whose handle is wrapped with rubber to render its hold more secure.

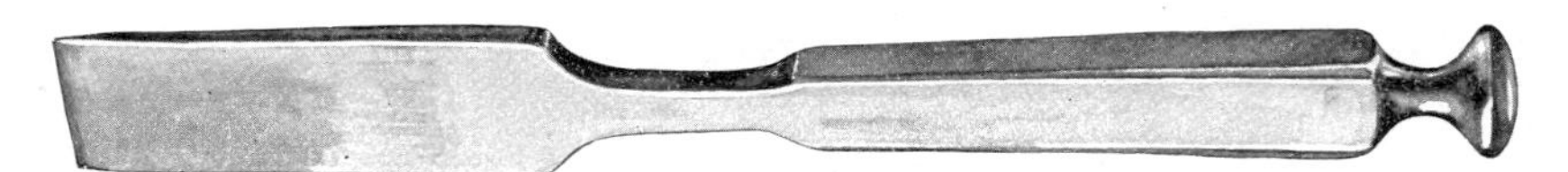

Fig. 572. Straight chisel, osteotome edge.

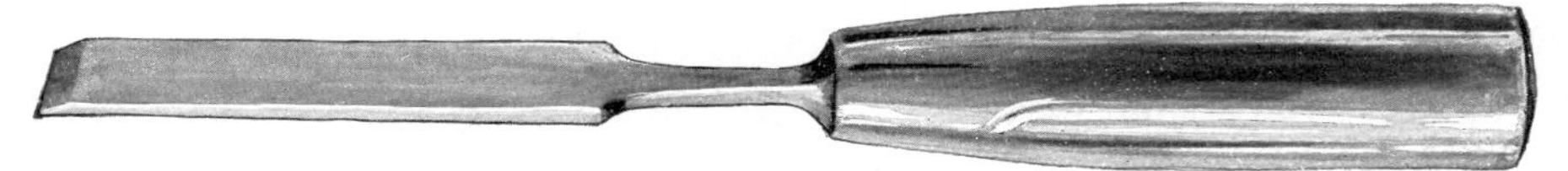

Fig. 573. Straight chisel, beveled on one side.

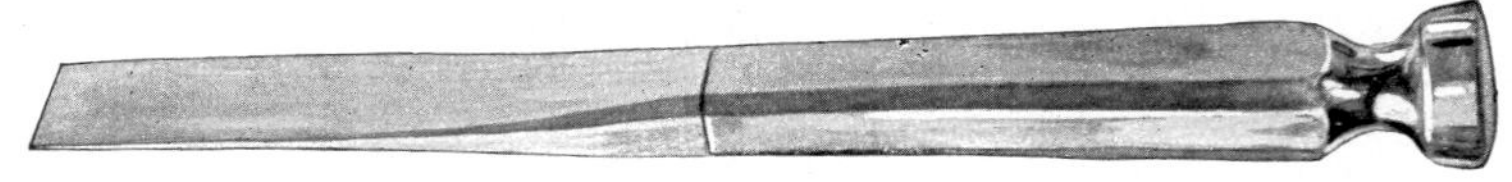

Fig. 574. Knife chisel.

The thinner the cutting edge of the chisel, the more easily is the bone cut, the smoother the groove, the less the danger of splintering, and also the more sensitive is the instrument. I reserve the fine knife chisels (Fig. 574) for particularly delicate work. The edge of the chisel is placed against the bone, and the chisel is held nearly parallel to the surface of the bone (Fig. 577; incorrect example Fig. 578). One thin splinter after another is carefully chiseled away, thus avoiding great jarring, and sudden unintentional penetration of the chisel into deeper tissue. Wooden mallets (Figs. 575 and 576) do not produce as much jarring as the metal ones. They can be boiled and therefore do not endanger the asepsis. If metal hammers are used they should be provided with rubber caps. As previously stated, suitable cushions should be used to support the part of the body involved.

Because of the great resistance of bone, if it is to be divided by chiseling, it must be done gradually. The edge of the chisel is held obliquely and a groove is chiseled in the bone, which is gradually deepened (Fig. 579). There are special chisels for each purpose. A bone is seldom divided by driving a chisel directly into it. For making furrows that must not exceed a certain depth, for instance, on the skull, there are chisels provided with a nose-piece on one corner. If the surgeon is skillful he does not need such special instruments of this type.

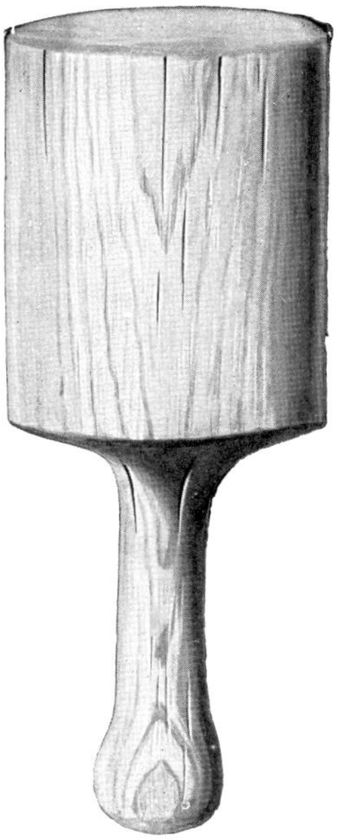

To divide a bone along a particular line with the aid of the chisel requires skill, effort and time. This may be done much more easily if holes are drilled at short intervals (Fig. 580) and the bone then cut through with the chisel between the holes. This procedure, which has usually been used on the flat bones of the skull, has been recommended by Perthes for the division of other bones, as for example, for the angular division of the inferior maxilla.

Gouges (Fig. 571) of various sizes and widths are used mainly for making grooves and eliminating cavities, and for laying open the bone after sequestrectomy.

FIG. 575. Wooden mallet for chiseling.

Several types of saws are used: the handsaw (Figs. 583 and 584), the wire saw (Fig. 587), and the circular saw (Fig. 588). The chain saw, formerly so popular, is rarely used at present. In sawing, as in drilling, considerable heat is developed, which may lead to necrosis and sequestration of the adjacent bone. A continuous stream of salt solution should be

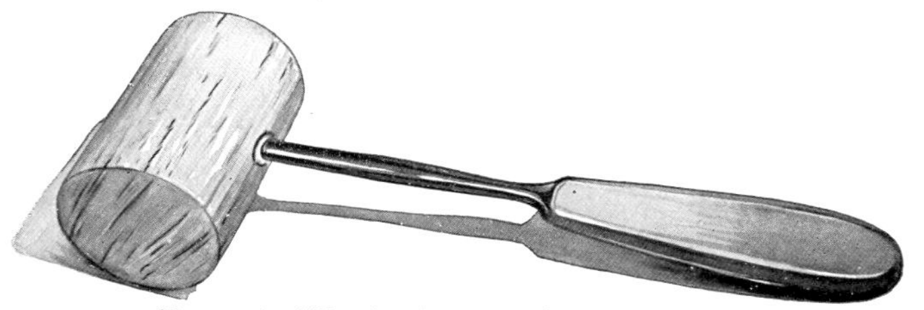

FIG. 576. Wooden hammer for chiseling.

allowed to run over the saw and bone to cool them (Fig. 581). Even in spite of this, sufficient heat may develop to produce marginal sequestra (Fig. 582) and interfere with callus formation, especially if there is further damage by resulting infection. Because of this, I avoid the use of the electrical circular saw as much as possible, but use it always when it is desirable to discourage regeneration of bone.

There are two types of hand saw commonly used: the fret saw (Fig. 584) and the bow saw (Fig. 583). The teeth should be bent as in a cross-

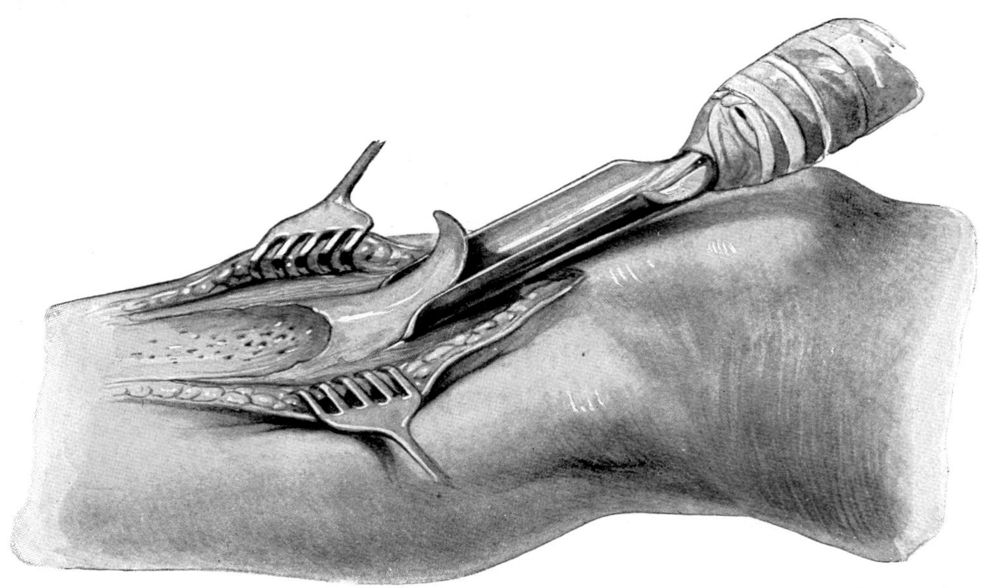

FIG. 577. Correct method of chiseling a bone. Thin chips are chiseled out one after another with the chisel lying nearly parallel to the bone.

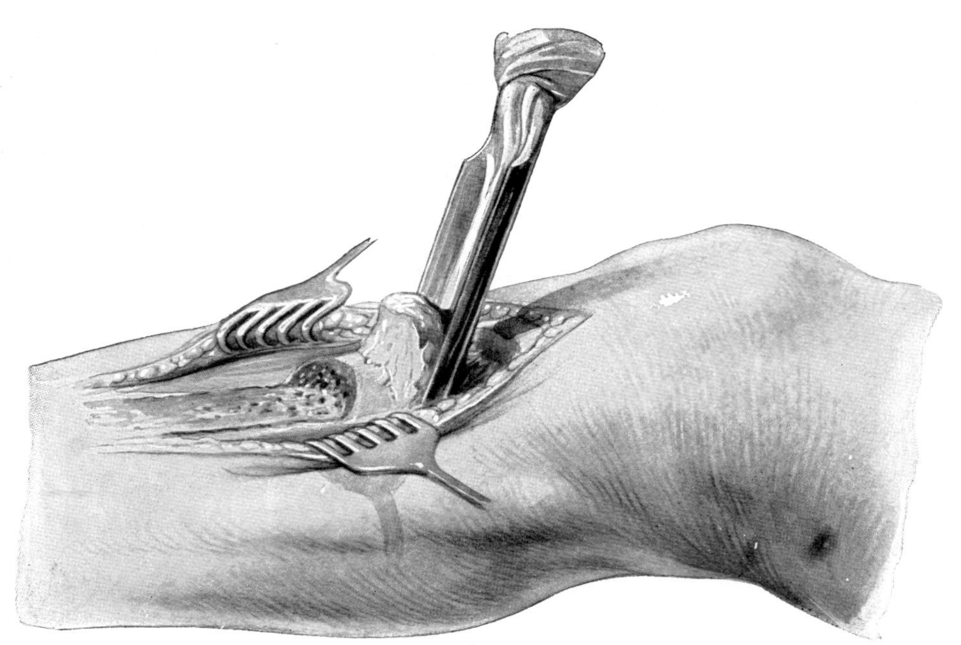

FIG. 578. Incorrect method of chiseling a bone. When the chisel is held nearly vertically the pieces of bone are thicker and are snapped off.

cut saw (Fig. 585 a), so that the blade will not jam in the cut. The blade should be stretched in the bow so that the teeth will cut when the saw is

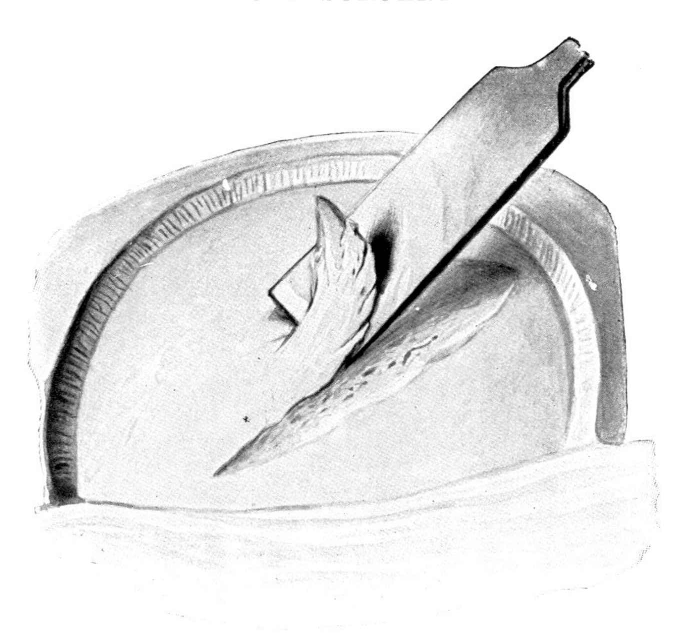

Fig. 579. Cutting through the skull. A trough is made which is gradually deepened.

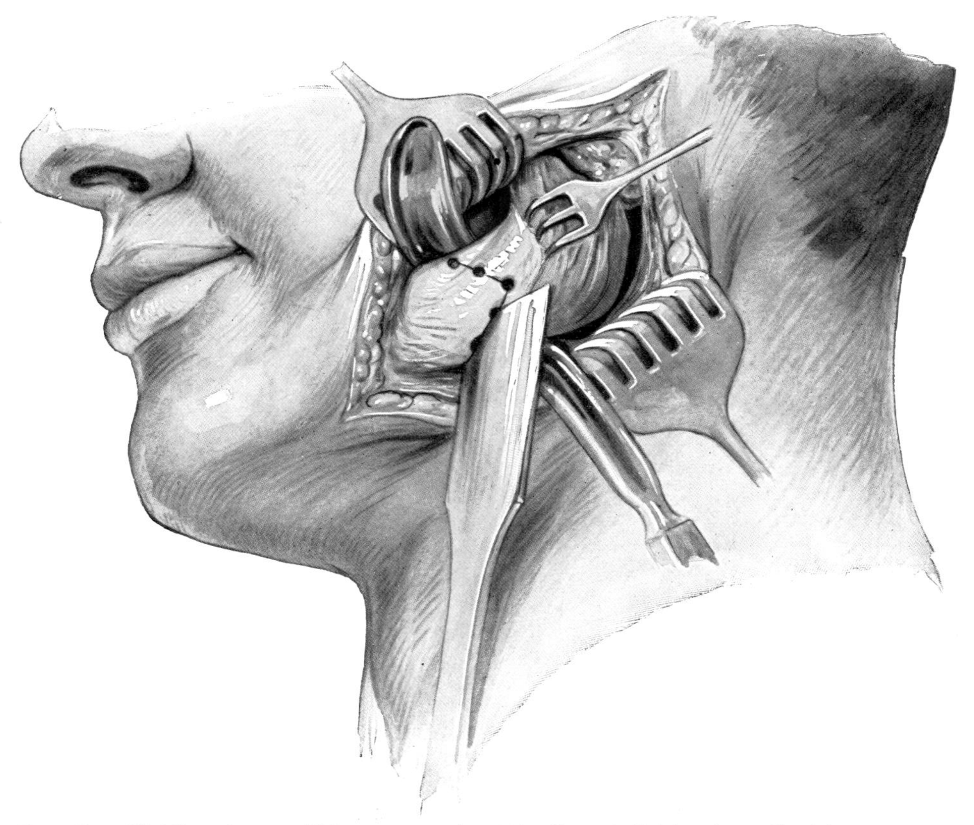

Fig. 580. Dividing the mandible at an angle. The line of division is outlined by a series of drill-holes.

pushed away from the operator (Fig. 583) and there will be no interference from the bow in sawing. The saw should be moved evenly forward and backward, avoiding any pressure. A curved line can be followed only with a narrow blade (Fig. 585 b). Wide blades (Fig. 585 a) cut in one direc-

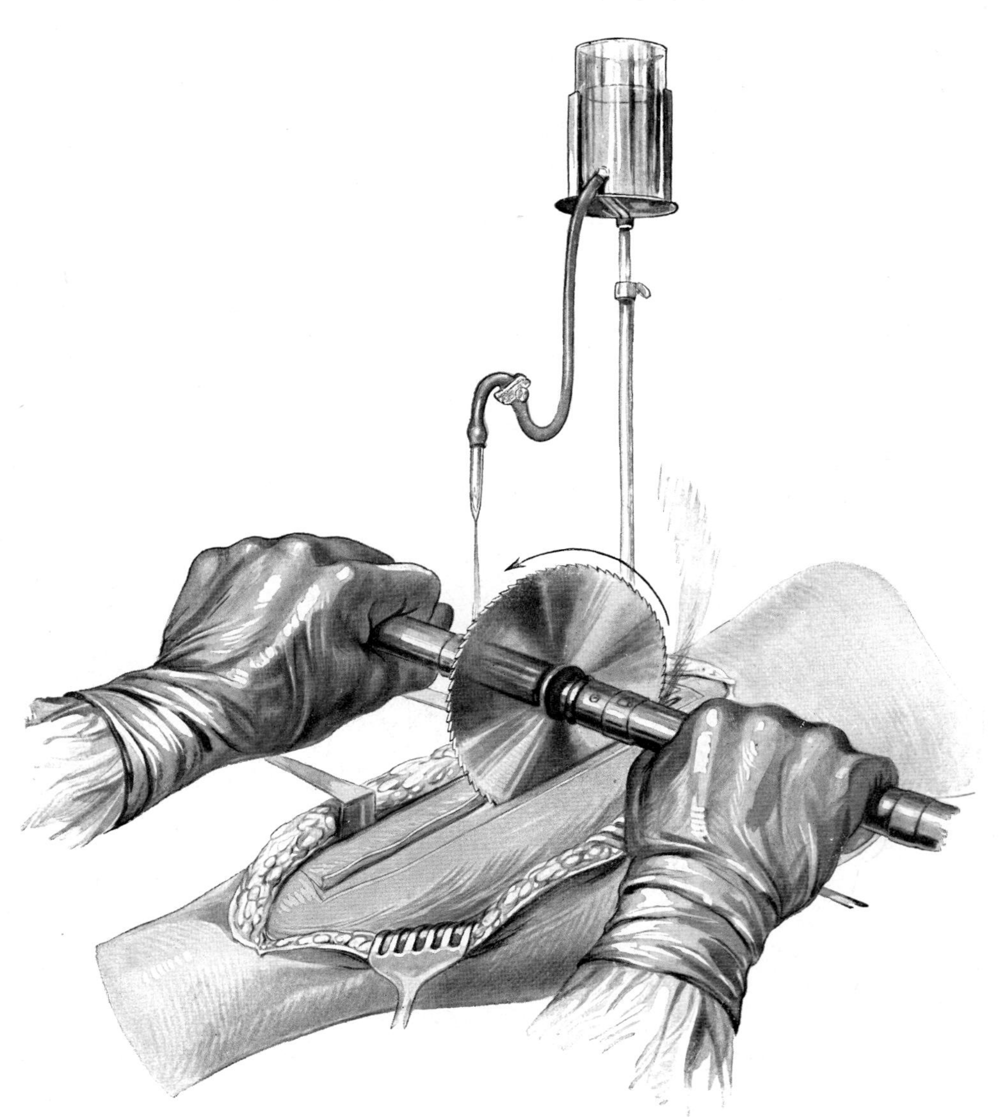

Fig. 581. Method for cooling circular saw, with salt solution.

tion only. To cut a sharp angle a double-edged blade must be used (Fig. 585 c. Kirschner, Brun's Beitr. z. Klin. Chir., Vol. 71), so that at the corner the opposite set of teeth can be employed (Fig. 586). I often use the wire (Gigli) saw (Fig. 587) for more delicate bone work.

When a wire saw is to be used, the wire must first be drawn under the bone that is to be divided, either directly or with the aid of a silk thread, one end of which is fastened to the saw and the other carried under the bone with a Deschamp needle, a special guide, a Bellocq cannula, a catheter, etc. After the two rings at the ends of the wire are hooked to the handles, the saw is drawn backward and forward in the desired direction, being held as nearly straight as possible (Fig. 587). Although the soft parts are adequately retracted, they still interfere with a completely straight position of the wire, so that it must be bent more or less at an angle at the site of sawing. The saw may be pulled backward and forward by one or by two

FIG. 582 a and b. Marginal sequestrum around a bored hole, the result of overheating the bone while drilling.

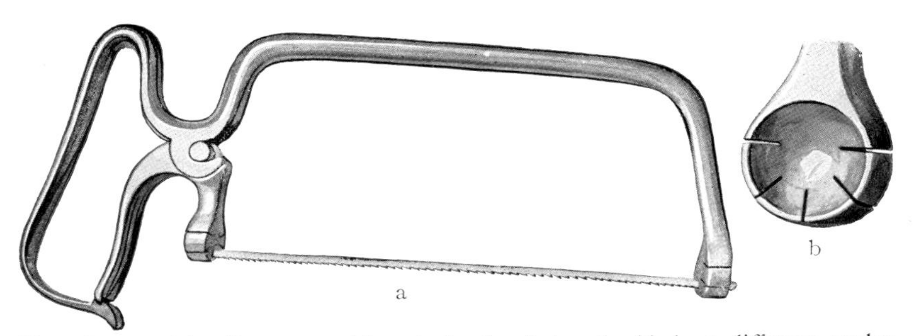

FIG. 583 a and b. Bow saw with a device for fixing the blade at different angles.

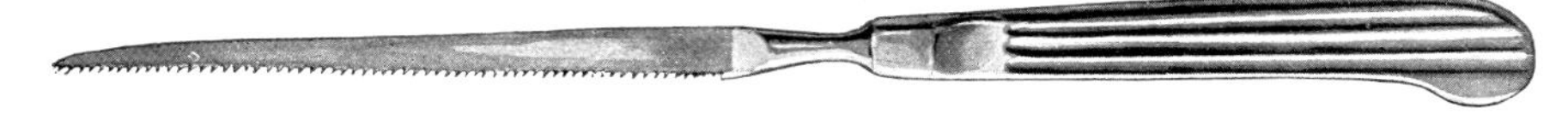

FIG. 584. Metacarpal saw.

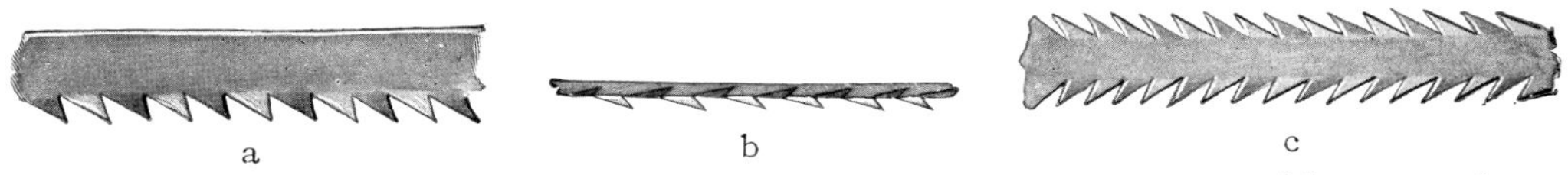

FIG. 585 a–c. Saw-blades with various teeth, (a) wide for straight cuts, (b) narrow for curved cuts, (c) double-cutting for angles.

persons. Salt solution is used continuously for cooling. If the wire breaks and the separation can not be completed with a chisel, a new wire must be used. Careful sawing is necessary just before the bone is finally divided, for it is at this point that the wire breaks most easily. The skull may also be sawed through with the wire saw. A number of holes are drilled, the wire saw is drawn under the bone between two adjacent openings and the bridge is sawed through.

A bone may be cut through with the electrically-driven circular saw

(Fig. 588) in less time and with less effort than by any other means. The teeth of this saw must also be set for cross-cutting. Besides the already mentioned overheating of the tissues, the circular saw has the disadvantage of scattering blood, marrow and bone chips, and the slightest carelessness in guiding it may result in serious injury. The circular saw must therefore be used with discretion. The saw provided with two handles is the safest to handle. (Fig. 581.) The greater the diameter of the circular blade, the thicker the bone layers that can be cut through and the more convenient the approach to a bone which lies deep. For parallel incisions, such as are necessary for the removal of a bone graft and for the preparation of bone canals, I use Martel's double-bladed saw, the distance between the blades being adjustable (Fig. 589).

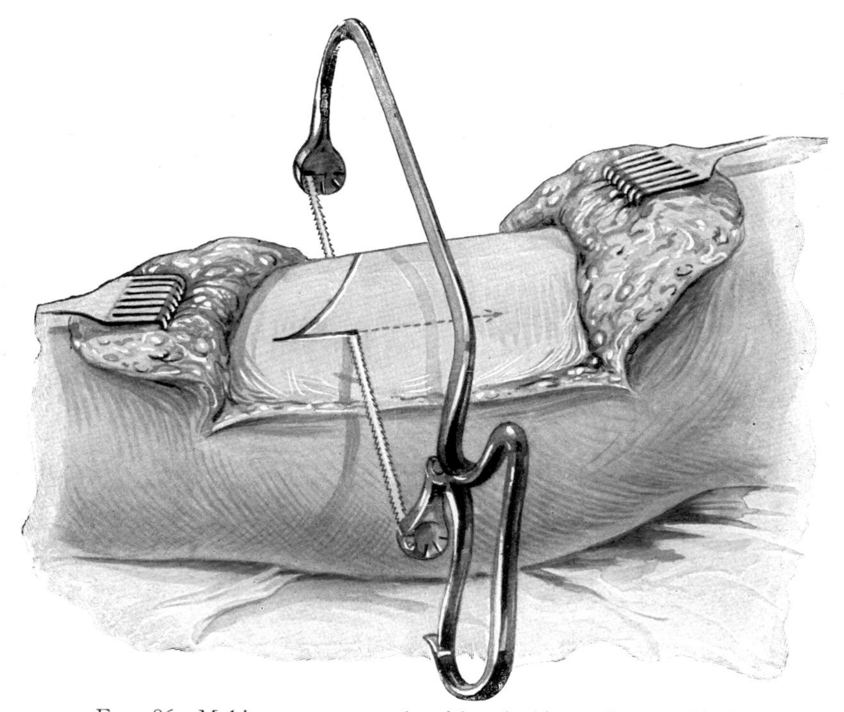

Fig. 586. Making an acute angle with a double cutting saw blade.

The bones of the skull can be cut through rapidly and easily with an electric drill. As a protection to the dura mater, the drills are either adjusted for a certain depth (Fig. 590), in which case they do not break entirely through the bone, or, they may have a button-shaped dural protector at their lower end, and divide the bone through its entire thickness (Fig. 591), as for example, Borchardt's skull drill. Gaylord's (Fig. 592) and Martel's drills are provided with a special handle to be manipulated with the left hand; this makes them easier to guide and to regulate the pressure of the drill on the bone. They are a distinct addition to the surgeon's equipment. To change the direction of the line of division, the handle only is moved in another direction, which does not change the position of the shaft of the drill enough to be noticed.

Dahlgreen's bone punch (Fig. 593) is an excellent, dependable instrument for trephination. It can be adjusted by a screw for various thick-

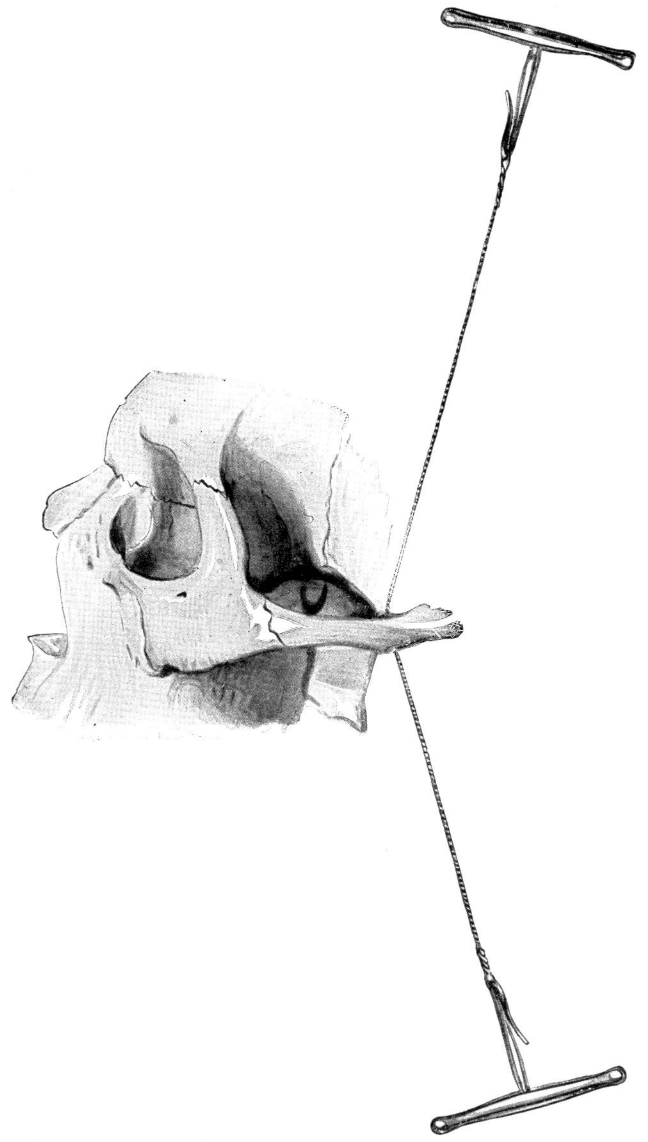

Fig. 587. Separating the zygomatic process with a wire-saw (Gigli). The saw, held taut and slightly angulated, is drawn back and forth.

nesses of the skull, and its cutting arm serves also as a dura protector. In cutting through thick bone it is necessary to use great force, and the cutting tooth occasionally breaks, so that it is well to have a second instrument always in readiness. Because Dahlgreen's punch is pulled out of the bone with each cut and has to be reinserted, De Quervain has fitted it with a special guiding tip, which does away with this inconvenience, but makes the instrument more clumsy (Fig. 594).

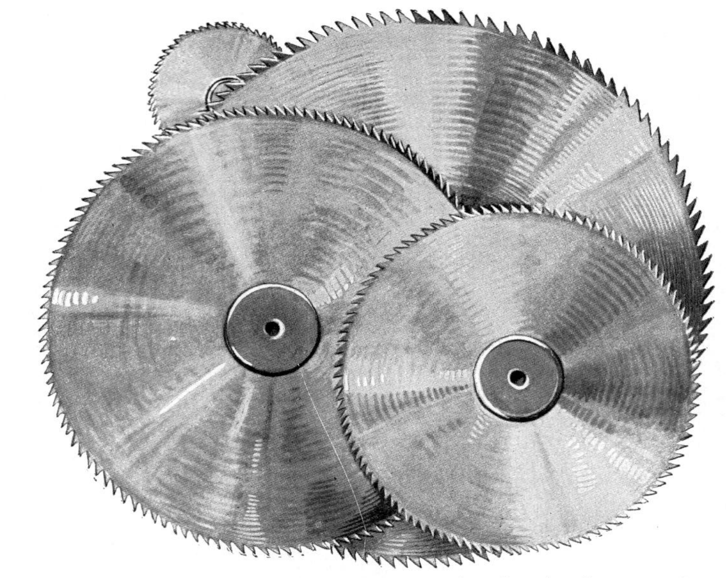

FIG. 588. Blades of different sizes for the circular saw.

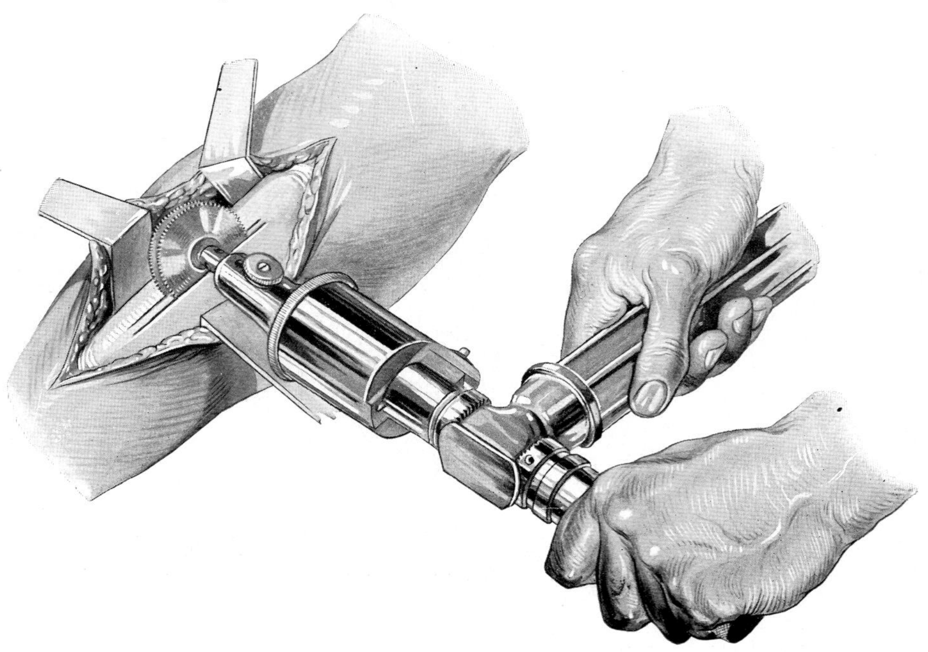

FIG. 589. Removal of a bone graft with a double bladed electric saw.

The old trephine has been modified and reintroduced recently by Jentzer. It affords a rapid, easy method for trephining the skull with the least trauma. A small hole is drilled at the center of the intended opening and the center screw of a small trephine is inserted in this hole. The small

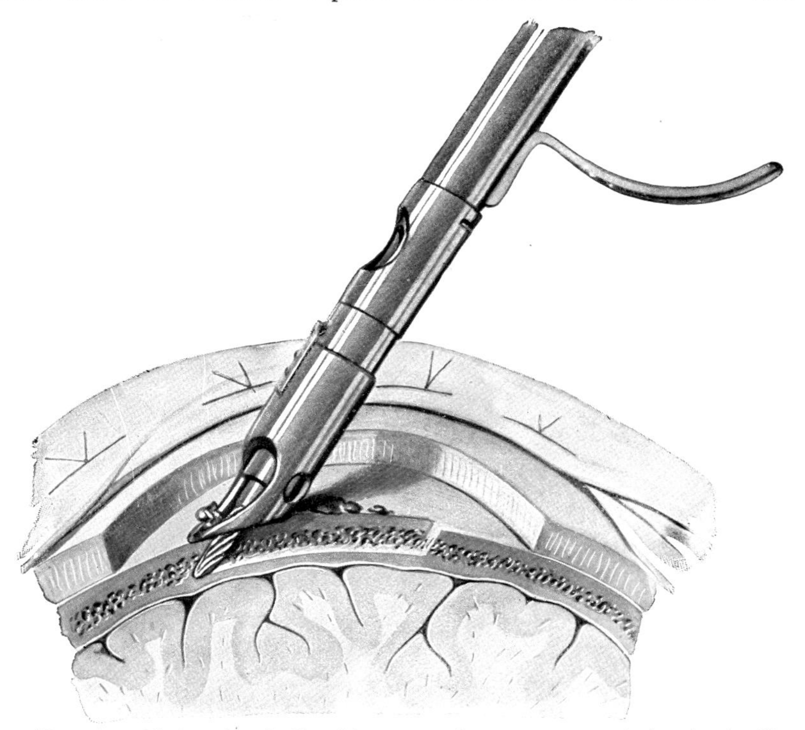

FIG. 590. Electric drill for the skull, with an attachment to control the depth (Borchardt).

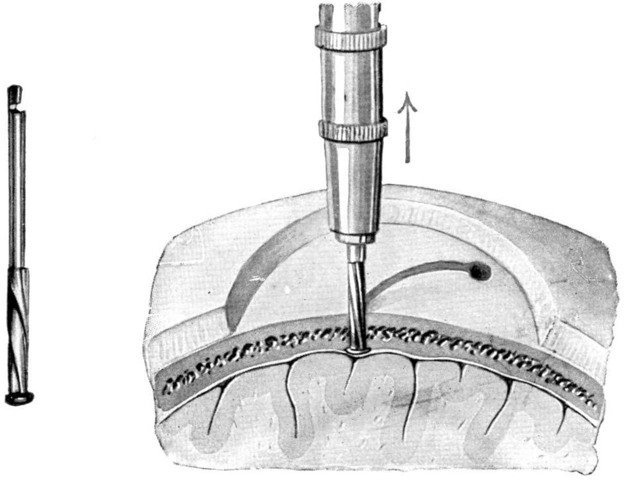

FIG. 591. Electric drill (Borchardt) for the cranium, with button-shaped dura protector, which permits the drill to slide along the inside of the skull when held close against it.

trephine (Fig. 595) is provided with two detachable handles. As it is screwed deeper it cuts out a bone disk of 2.8 cm. in diameter. A T-shaped guide is introduced into this opening which lies in such a way that its wings extend between the dura and internal table and its shaft projects beyond the skull. The directing instrument is fastened on the skull. A trephine of either 4 or 6 cm. diameter (Fig. 596) is screwed on the stationary shaft of the guide, and as the two handles are turned the trephine gradually pene-

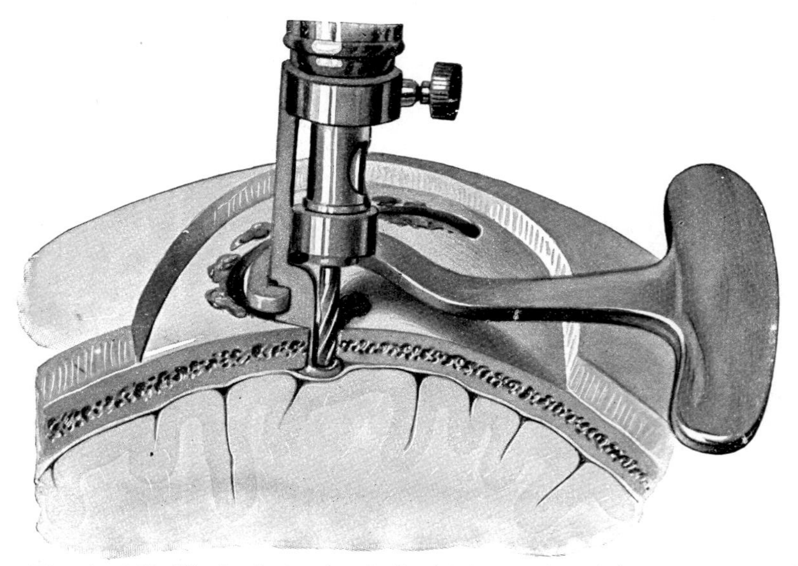

FIG. 592. Electric drill (Gaylord) for the skull with button-shaped dura protector and handle. By means of the handle the direction of sawing may be changed.

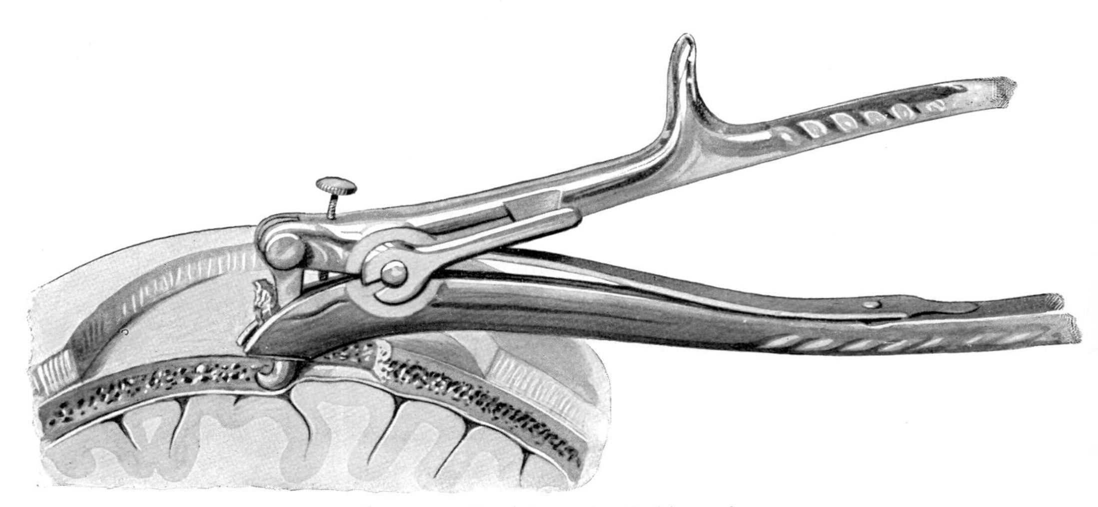

FIG. 593. Cranial punch (Dahlgreen).

trates the bone which is easily divided. It is impossible to injure the dura because the cutting teeth, after the bone is divided, are automatically protected by projecting springs. Several openings can be placed side by side. The disks of bone can be replanted in the holes after the intracranial operation is completed.

A bone can be given any form desired with the various chisels, forceps,

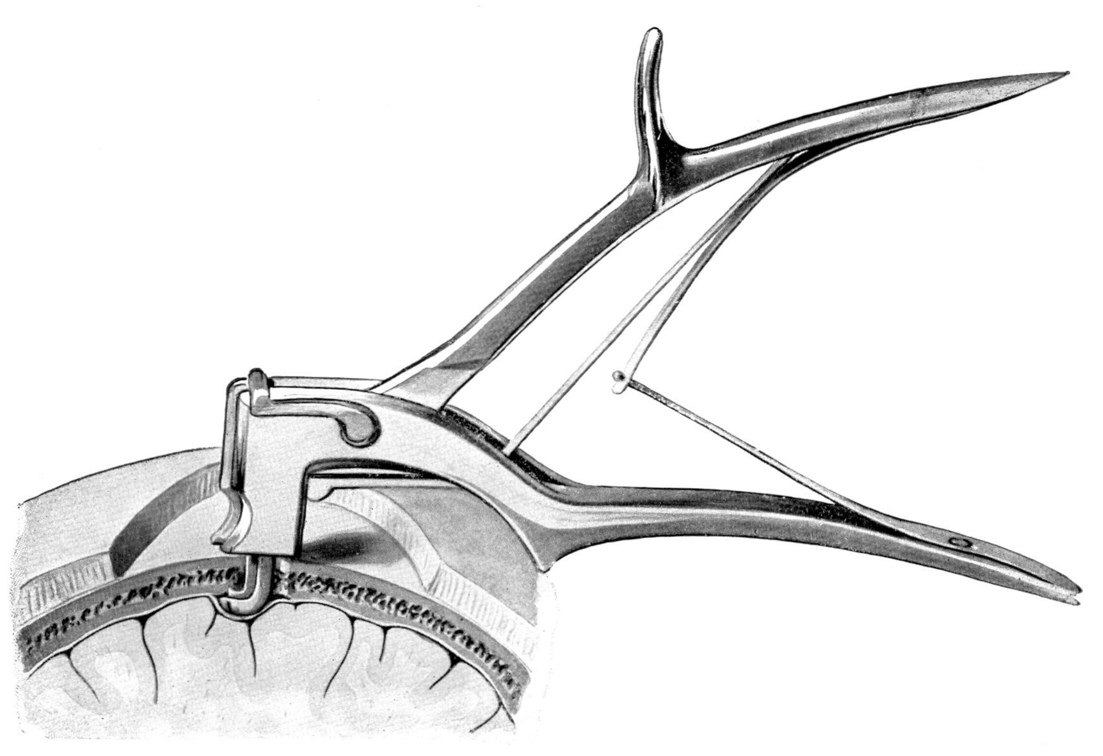

Fig. 594. Cranial punch with directing tip (DeQuervain).

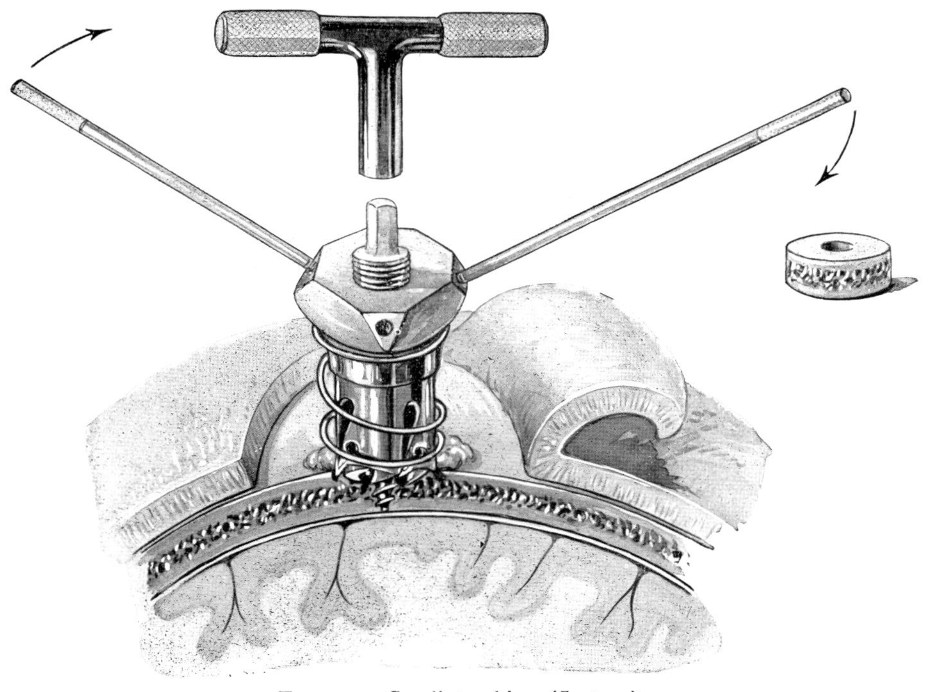

Fig. 595. Small trephine (Jentzer).

saws and drills. To smooth rough surfaces, to make slight changes in shape, rasps and files of various sizes and shapes (Figs. 597 and 598) are used. Chips, bone dust, and filings should be removed with wet sponges, or if necessary by flushing out the wound, before suturing.

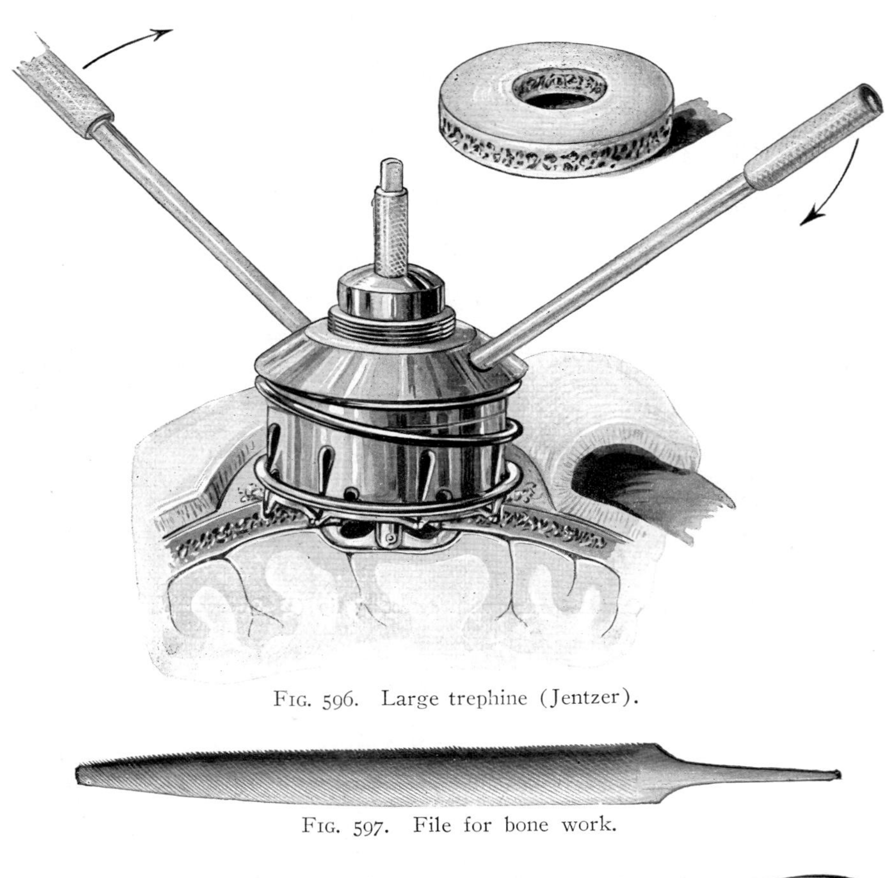

FIG. 596. Large trephine (Jentzer).

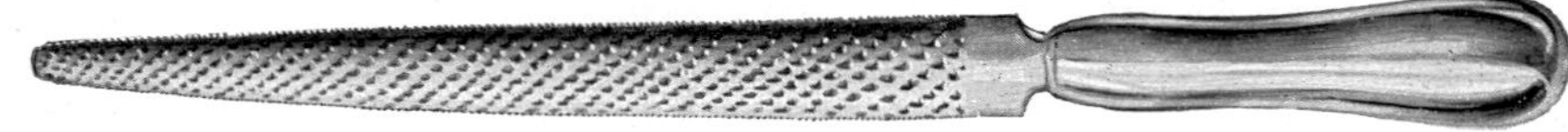

FIG. 597. File for bone work.

FIG. 598. Rasp for bone work.

C. OPEN OPERATIONS FOR FRACTURES AND PSEUDARTHROSIS (NON-UNION)

When there is displacement of the fragments after fracture, which can not be overcome by conservative measures, open reduction is necessary. In these days of modern aseptic surgery crippling deformity should never follow a fracture. The reduction of a fracture is easier if done soon after its occurrence.

Nevertheless, for open reduction, the seventh or eighth day after injury is the time for election, because by this time the bone is in its most favorable condition for rapid bone regeneration, and the tissues have recovered from the effects of the primary injury. Every operative division of bone should terminate in bone union.

Open reduction attempts first, approximation of the fragments, and second, their retention in the correct position.

The fractured bone should be clearly exposed, but the periosteum must be carefully protected, whether the exposure is extra-, or superiosteal. The insertion of muscles should be divided only if it is absolutely necessary for clear exposure and sufficient mobility of the fragments. In attempting to approximate the fractured surfaces the bones are manipulated by longitudinal traction, angulation, lateral pressure and rotation. To aid in this there are numerous instruments, such as pointed and dull bone hooks (Fig. 606), variously shaped elevators, bone holding forceps, and Lambotte's bone elevator (Fig. 599). Satisfactory approximation can frequently be obtained

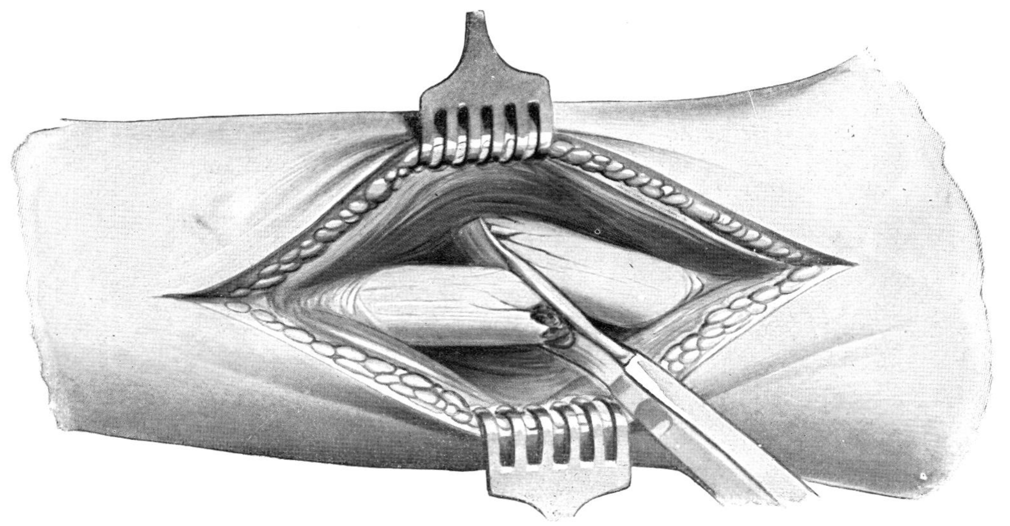

Fig. 599. Lambotte's bone elevator for use in the open reduction of fractures.

by elevating the fragments from the wound at an acute angle and gradually lowering them again in the proper position (Fig. 614). If the fractured surface can not be brought together in this manner, some of the bone must be removed, first rongeuring away any obstructing edges, and then, if necessary, shortening one or both fragments as little as can be done to obtain satisfactory results. In shortening the bone, provision for future suturing should be made, as for example, by a bayonet form of the ends of the bone.

In a fracture of both bones of the forearm or leg, it is necessary, as a rule, for proper reduction to expose and free both bones. It is advisable to make separate incisions for the exposure of each bone. In recent fractures of the leg no attention need be paid to the position of the fibular fragments, but in long-standing fractures the fibula is chiseled apart through a special incision, or a piece may be removed, the position of the fragments not demanding any particular attention.

Only rarely, and then only when the ends of the bone can be joined firmly so that subsequent displacement is unlikely, is open reduction done without fastening the fragments to each other. As a rule, an effort should be made to secure the fragments in place so that, even with early motion, they will keep the correct position until bony union occurs. This is done by some form of permanent mechanical union, bone suture in a broad sense.

Fixation of fragments may be done either (1) directly, or (2) indirectly, by various means.

1. Direct fixation may be done by nails, screws, or wires (Fig. 600). Materials made entirely of metal, with the exception of wire, should be chromatized, so that they will not be weakened in the body. Wires are not chromatized because they could not be soldered. Nails and screws are most

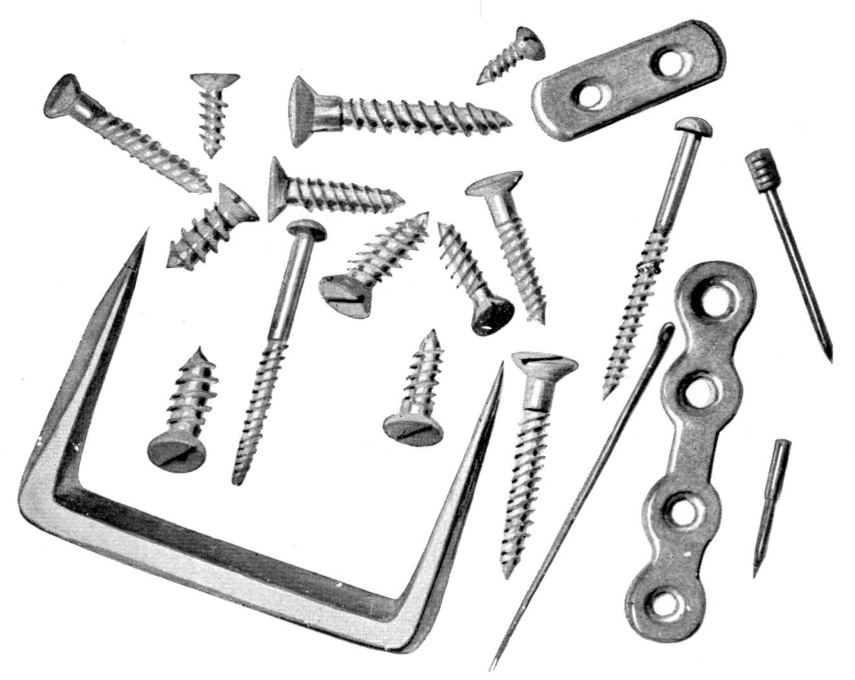

Fig. 600. Steel screws, pins, needles, plates, etc., used for the retention of fragments after open reduction of fractures.

suitable for fastening small fragments to the end of a bone in the region of cancellous substance, where there is no particular force acting to separate the parts. They are less suitable for fastening fragments on the shaft. Displaced fragments must be placed in the proper position and held in that position while being fastened with nails or screws.

(a) Steel nails of various lengths and strength are used. Fine steel needles 3¼ cm. long are well suited for this purpose, also, sewing needles, phonograph needles, and ivory pegs have been used (Fig. 600). Nails are used when the separating force acts parallel to the fracture surface, the nails taking up the force. They are driven in as far as necessary with small hammers (Fig. 601) or with a plain forceps (Fig. 602), more easily if small holes have been previously drilled. The projecting portion is cut off with cutting pliers and the soft parts are closed in the usual manner. Only in exceptional cases are nails driven through the skin (percutaneous nailing) and left to project from the surface of the limb. Many operators after resecting the knee joint fasten the femur and the tibia in this manner (Fig. 603). Subsequent infection may occur after nailing through the skin, and for this reason it is seldom used.

(b) Screws with broad threads stay more firmly in bone than screws with fine threads (Fig. 600). I purchase the necessary assortment of screws

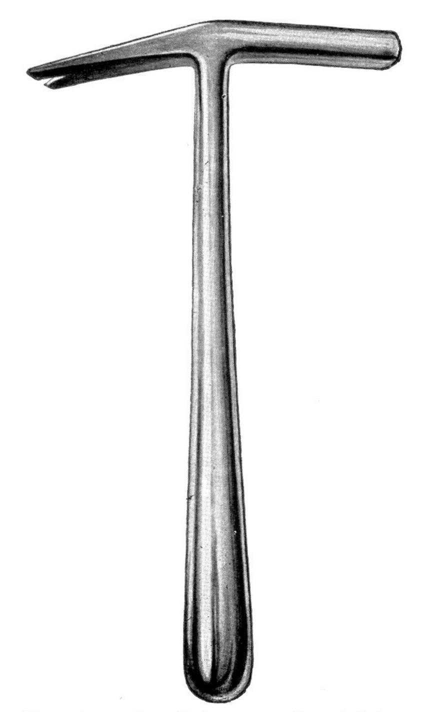

FIG. 601. Small hammer for driving bone nails.

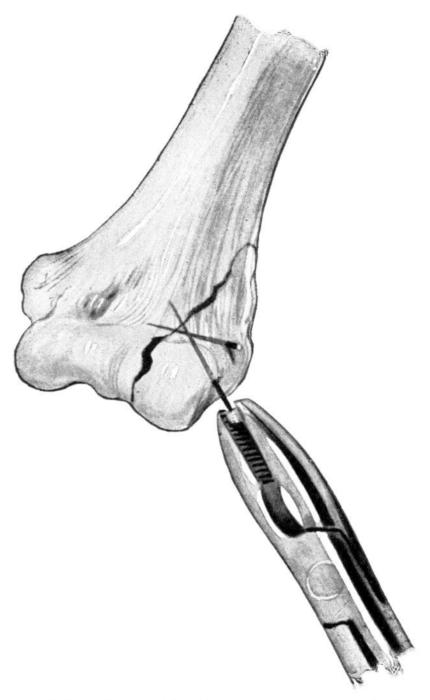

FIG. 602. Nailing a fracture of the external condyle of the humerus. The steel nails are forced in with a pliers, and the projecting ends are then cut off.

in the hardware store, and have them nickel plated, zinc plated, or better, chromium plated before using them. I also occasionally use for special cases ivory screws. In using screws, care must be taken that the holes previously drilled are not too large. Screws are used when the separating force acts perpendicular to the fracture surface, the traction being borne by the screws (Fig. 604).

(c) Wire is without a doubt the most widely used and dependable material for uniting bones. It is either looped around the ends of the bone (annular wire suture Fig. 605), or it is carried through previously bored holes (Figs. 606 and 607) (suture in a limited sense). The wire can be prevented from slipping by making a groove around the bone with a chisel or a rasp (Fig. 611).

Every wire suture consists finally in a closed ring. If such a ring suture is to fulfil its purpose completely, it, first, must surround the structure with great strength, and, second, it must maintain this firm hold until the bone has united. The wire sutures commonly used until a short time ago were fastened by simply twisting the ends together with a plain forceps, but this

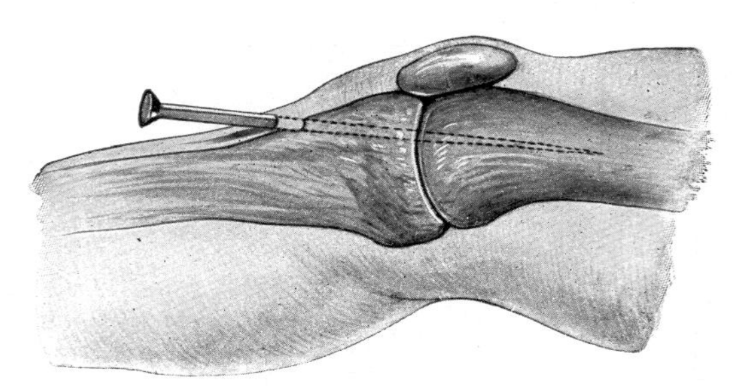

FIG. 603. Percutaneous nailing of the bones of the knee joint. After the joint surfaces have been resected the nail is driven through for immobilization of the tibia and femur. This method often invites infection.

does not suffice. At the present time, the two conditions are fulfilled in the following manner: the wire used for bone suture is extremely durable, so that it does not break even when subjected to severe strain. The stronger the wire is, the thinner it can be, which is of importance when considering the size of a foreign body left in the tissue. With regard to the method of closure, the wire must stand soldering. Both these requisites are best fulfilled by steel piano strings, which are cautiously heated to remove

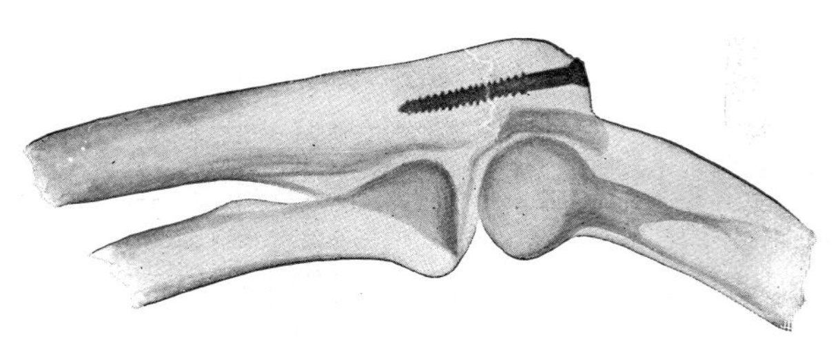

FIG. 604. Retention of a bony fragment with a screw after fracture of the olecranon.

their awkward inflexibility. Wires of 0.5, 0.7, 0.85 and 1.0 mm. are employed, according to the strength desired. The rust-free steel wire frequently used is not as strong and solders poorly.

The wire can not be stretched tightly enough around the bone nor fastened with the hands. Leverage is needed for this work, and this may be obtained by the use of Kirschner's wire stretching forceps (Fig. 605). I believe it is superior to other similar instruments, in that the ends of the wire can be soldered, as well as twisted together. After the wire is carried around the bone or through the drill holes, its ends are looped once around

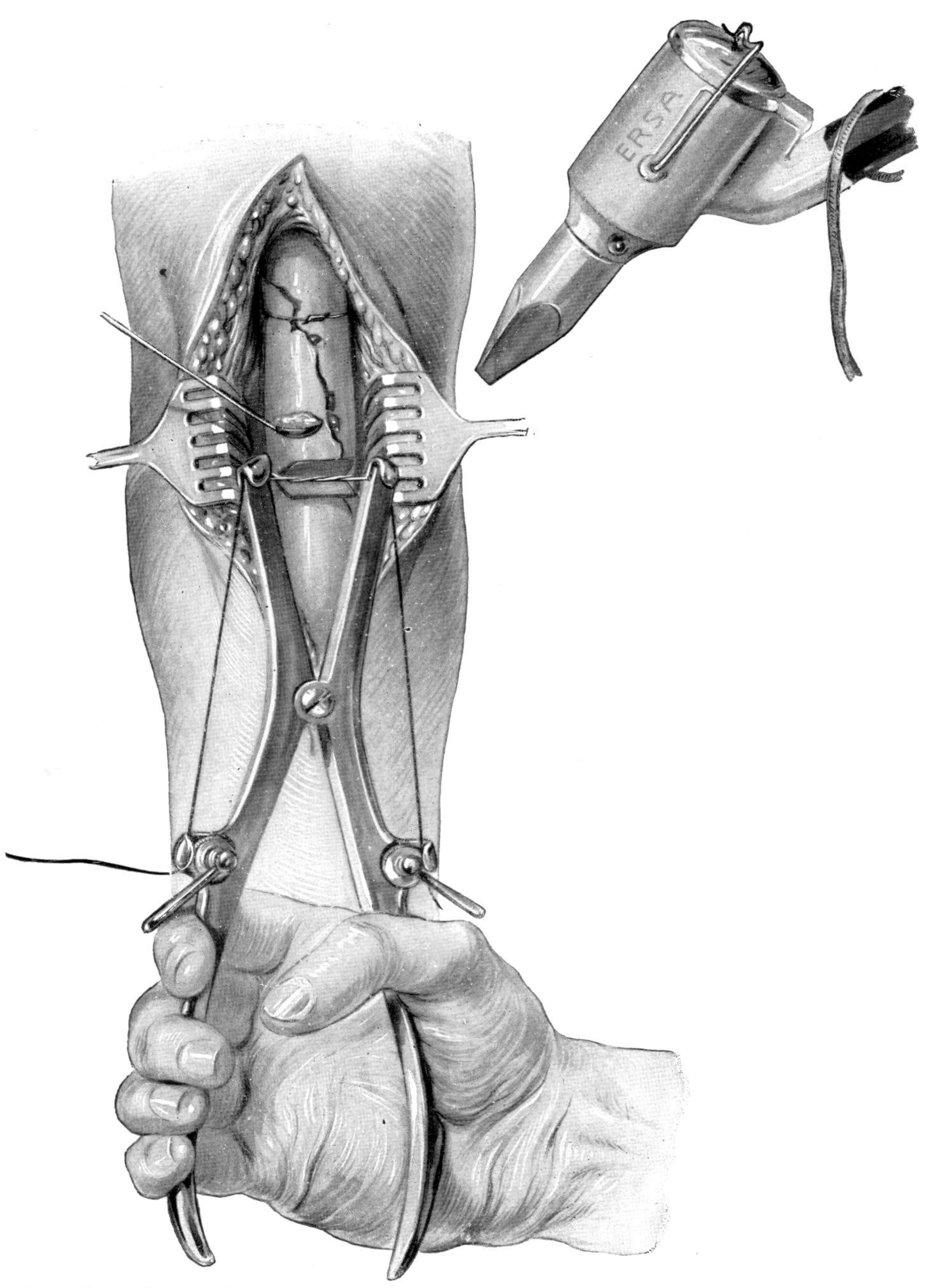

FIG. 605. Immobilization of an oblique fracture of a long bone with the use of wire sutures which are made taut with Kirschner's tension forceps. The upper wire has been completed; the lower wire is about to be soldered. A small fiber pad temporarily protects the bone.

each other, introduced in the corresponding slit of the wire stretcher, and tightened under tension by drawing the handles together. The degree of tension on the wire can be regulated by the pressure used to bring the handles together so that the parts of bone fastened by the wire can be held firmly together.

The wire stretched around the bone in this manner can be fastened in two ways. The ends may be twisted around each other several times, by turning the tension forceps several times in one direction about its longitudinal axis. The stiffness of the piano wires offer considerable resistance

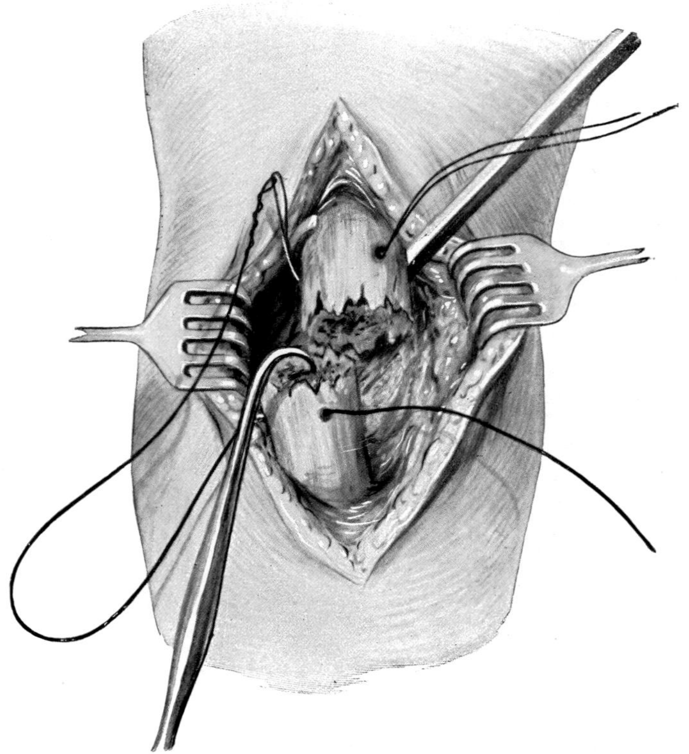

FIG. 606. Retention of a transverse fracture of a long bone with wire sutures passed through the fragments.

to the untwisting and loosening of this simple closure. It is sufficient in many cases.

The most dependable and durable means of fastening the wire in all cases is by soldering. It is done as follows (Fig. 605): before the wire is drawn taut a rectangular fiber pad about 0.1 mm. thick, boiled and dried, is placed under the twisted wire and is bent like a trough at the sides. When the handles of the wire stretcher are brought together, the little fiber pad is clasped tight. It is surrounded on all sides with moist, but not wet, sponges. After removing all tissue, blood, and moisture from the wire over the pad, and placing the area as nearly horizontal as possible, the wire is covered with a little soldering paste which has been boiled in the original box, care being taken to avoid spilling any on the surrounding tissue. A

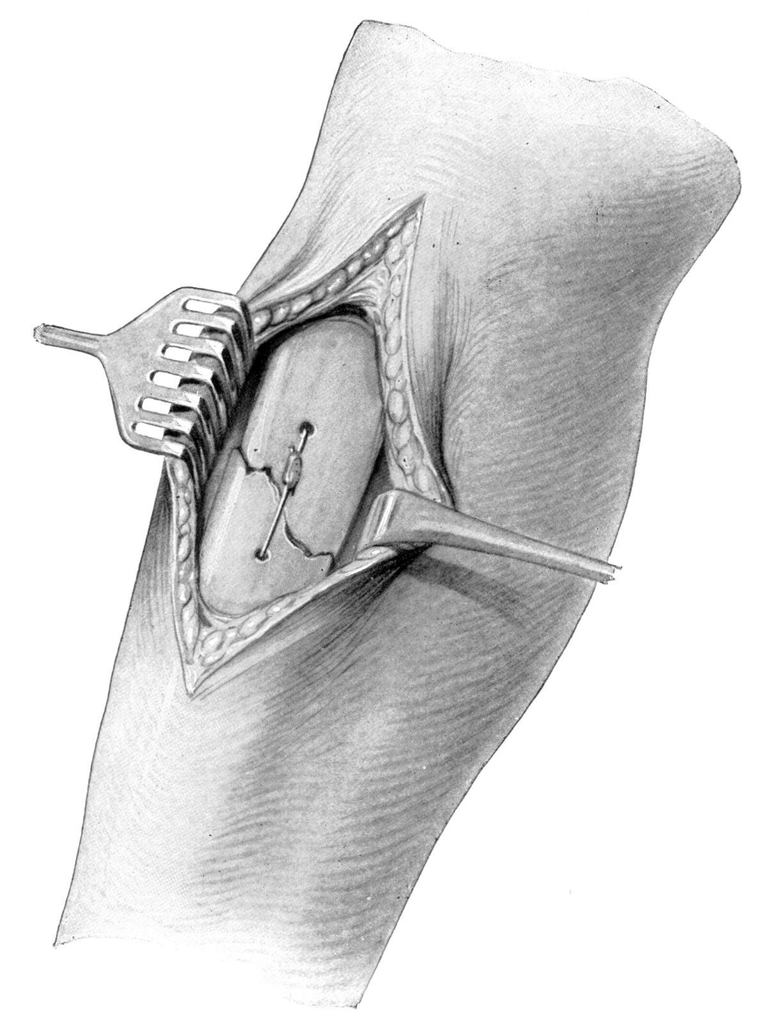

Fig. 607. Wire suture of transverse fracture completed.

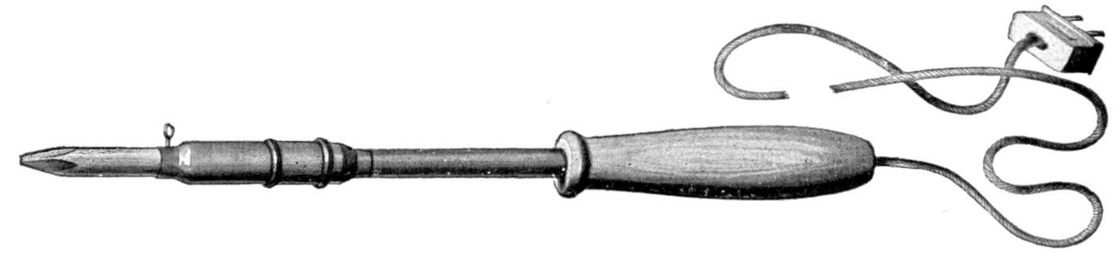

Fig. 608. Electric soldering iron.

soldering iron that has not been heated to red heat is touched to the point to be soldered, while the tension of the wire is maintained, so that the iron comes in contact only with the solder and the wire. An electric soldering iron is best suited for this work (Fig. 608). As soon as the solder melts the metal is distributed with the soldering iron over the entire length of the twisted wire, and allowed to harden (Fig. 607). Only when the wire has cooled, which can be hastened by placing sponges wet with salt solution over it, should the tension of the wire stretcher be released. Care must be taken to make sure that the wire is well soldered. If that should not be the case, the soldering must be repeated with fresh soldering paste. The ends of the wire which project from the solder are cut short with wire-cutting pliers. The small fiber pad is wiped off with wet cotton to remove any soldering paste or metal, and is removed by cutting or tearing it along the wire. The area is cleansed with wet sponges.

The superstition that a soldered wire may produce electrical current and thereby injure the tissue, need hardly be refuted. To produce electrical currents it is necessary to have two different metals separated by a salt solution. Two touching metals can never produce an electrical current.

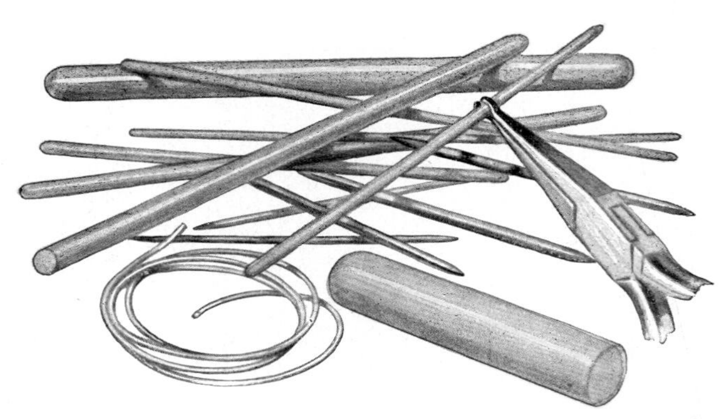

Fig. 609. Ivory pegs of various thicknesses for use in bone pegging; forceps for handling pegs; and silver wire.

It is not advisable to unite the wire ends by welding, because the wire melts as soon as it is welded and loses its tension.

2. In indirect fixation of fractures the connection is established by plating. The splints or plates consist either of inert or living material. The inert material is either unabsorbable or absorbable.

Unabsorbable plates consist of metal, such as iron, rustless steel, aluminum, nickel, alloys of silver and gold. It is well to have on hand rectangular bars of aluminum of various thickness and widths, from which suitable pieces may be cut when needed. Although the disadvantages of leaving foreign bodies on the rigid bone are less than in the movable soft parts, the use of metal plates should be avoided as much as possible. In my experience the union of bones by metal plates is not entirely dependable, for the plates, unless they are massive, often break or become loose.

As absorbable material for plating, ivory should be mentioned first, because it is easily procured, it can be boiled, and because it surpasses other material, especially horn, in its readiness of healing and of absorption. For these reasons I use ivory, especially for pegging. I keep on hand round ivory pegs, about 20 cm. long, and from 2 to 8 mm. in diameter, the gradations in thickness being about 0.25 mm. (Fig. 609), from which I cut suitable pieces with a fret saw and a hand vice (Fig. 610). The sawed surfaces are rounded by filing. In addition, I occasionally use rectangular ivory pegs of various widths, that are cut the same way for individual cases.

Bone plates from animals or other humans may be considered as inert absorbable material, for whether they are living or dead when they are used, they perish immediately, and from a practical standpoint they should be considered as lifeless. In view of this fact, they should always be sterilized by boiling, which may be a deciding factor against their use. They may be obtained from individuals who have just died, from amputated limbs,

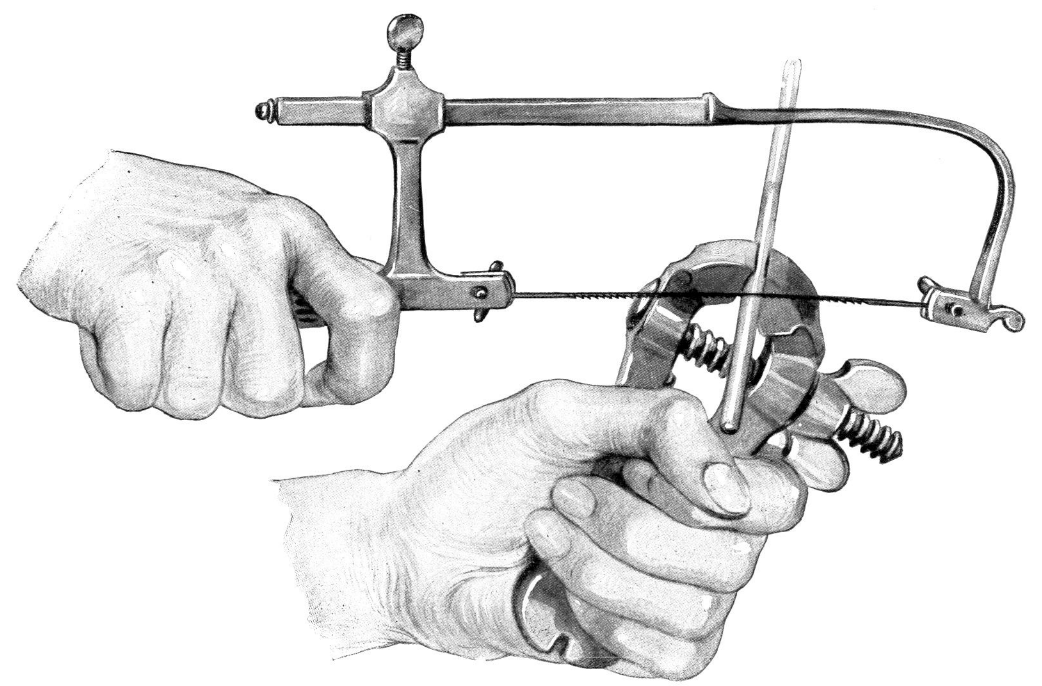

FIG. 610. Method of cutting ivory pegs to desired length.

and from animals of all kinds such as monkeys, dogs, cattle, etc., among which there is no choice on biological grounds.

Living autoplastic material has the disadvantage of being difficult to procure, since a special operation is required. The great advantage of autoplastic transplants is the certainty of a smooth and lasting healing. According to the investigations of Ollier, Marchand, Barth, Axhausen, and others, the autoplastic bone graft breaks down, as does other "living" tissue, and is gradually replaced, yet its periosteum and endosteum share actively in the reconstruction of the bone. Autoplastic grafts in general, should be used only for special indications, as when the healing power of a bone is diminished (non-union), and for bridging a bone gap, but never for ordinary fixation. Material for bone grafts is plentiful, for it can be obtained from the anterior parts of the tibia and fibula, from the ribs, part of the sternum, and the crest of the ilium. Bone grafts should be transferred with the greatest care. It is important that the bone retain on one side at least its attached periosteum. If the bone is not transplanted in its entire thickness, as are the ribs and the fibula, it is advisable to include the endosteum also.

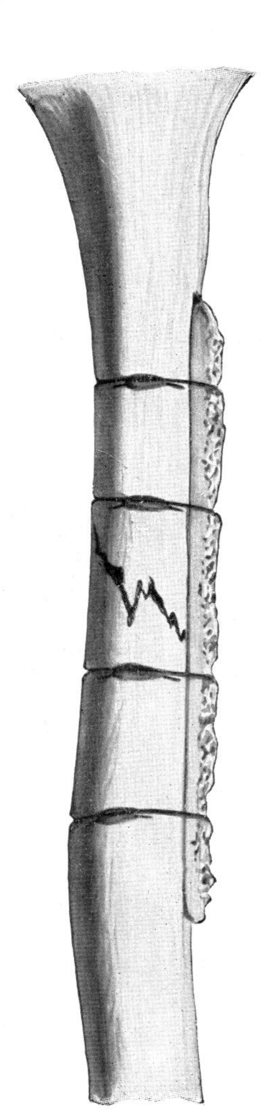

FIG. 611. A piece of bone taken from the opposite tibia is fastened to the fractured bone with wire sutures.

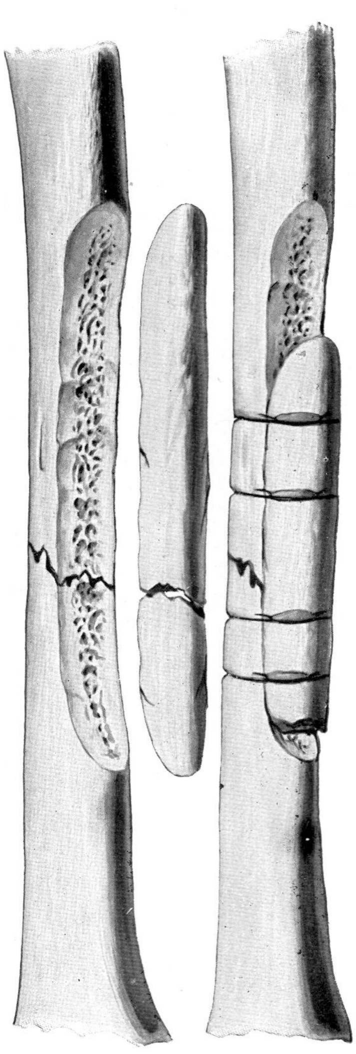

FIG. 612. A piece of bone is taken from the fractured bone and is fastened to the bone over the line of fracture with wire sutures.

The fixation splints are fastened either along the bone (Figs. 611, 612, 631), placed in a bone groove (Fig. 613), or introduced into the medullary cavity as pegs (Figs. 615 and 617). The splints must be fastened to both bones so firmly that they will not move but will retain their position, regardless of the direction of the force exerted on them. These conditions can be fulfilled easily as far as pressure and traction affect the fixation, the difficulty lies in successfully withstanding force acting in a transverse direction. The most favorable method of fixation is pegging; fixation by splints placed along the bone is more difficult. For firmness, every splint should be held to the bone at at least two points on each fragment, at least four points in all. They are fastened by screws or wires. Since screws easily become loose,

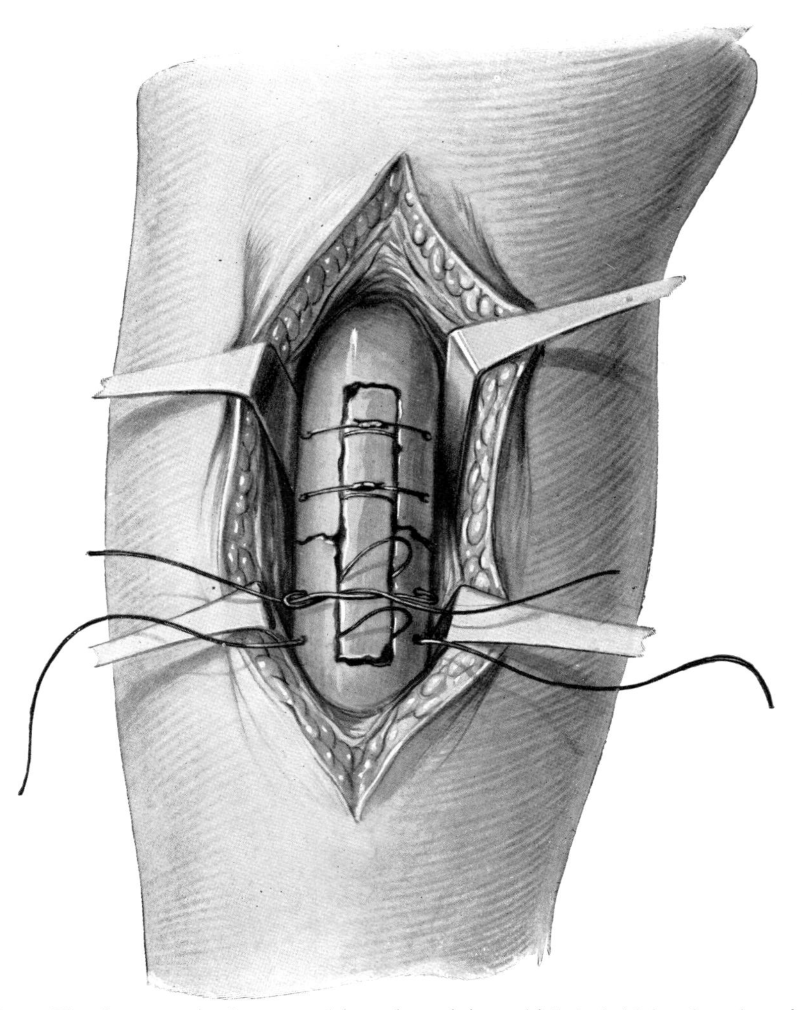

FIG. 613. The fracture site is spanned by a bone inlay which is held in place by wires passed through holes drilled in the fracture fragments. (The graft is somewhat short.)

wire is preferable. Fixation by a large metal staple (Gussenbauer Fig. 600), which penetrates each bone in one place only, is not satisfactory.

(a) An external bone splint is applied after reduction of the fracture by fitting it accurately in position across the site of fracture so that the splint lies close to the bone at all points. If it is to be fastened with screws, which is the rule for metal plates, and occasionally used for ivory plates and autoplastic bone grafts, at least two holes are drilled at each end of the splint, if the plate has not been made with holes. The holes should be just large enough to catch the thread of the screws. Holes are then drilled at corresponding places on the bones with a finer drill. The splint is fastened with screws first to the end which is more inaccessible and then to the other fragment in the same way.

My experience with metal plates has not been good, because the splints break easily and the screws frequently pull out. (This experience is not universal and in our own clinic we frequently use the metal plate. We have not had the difficulty which the author has encountered of screws becoming loose. Because of this we have prepared an illustration of this method [Fig. 618] I.S.R.). When I do use an external splint, as I may in pseudarthrosis or non-union, I prefer to use autoplastic bone, or at least ivory. These splints should also be fastened in at least four places (Figs. 611, 612, and 631). For retention wire is used principally (wire ring suture). It is applied with a stretching forceps and soldered in the manner previously described. The wire can be prevented from slipping by chiselling narrow grooves around the bone. It is not necessary that the wire should entirely surround the bone, which is the most convenient method, but it can be carried through holes drilled in the bone (Figs. 630 and 631). A splint of the proper size and shape is fastened by two wires to the less accessible fragment. After the ends of the fracture are readjusted, the splint is fastened by two more wires to the other fragment.

(b) For a lateral inlay, an outline of the bone splint in the position which it is to occupy is made on the fractured bone. The fractured bone is chiselled or sawed out with a double circular saw within these lines to a depth equal to the thickness of the inlay. The inlay should lie so deep, that its surface is just level with the surface of the fractured bone (Fig. 613). The inlay is held in place either with screws, which are preferable for metal splints, or with wire sutures, when autoplastic bone and ivory inlays are used. The wire sutures either entirely surround the fragments (Fig. 612) or are carried through holes drilled lateral to the bed of the inlay (Fig. 613).

If the splints connecting the ends of the fractured bone are placed in the medullary canal (internal splinting) they either fill it completely (pegging) or incompletely. When the splint fills it incompletely, it must be fastened to the bone with wire, but since the cylindrical shape of the medullary space prevents lateral displacement, one suture to each fragment is sufficient. The fixation is done as follows: an ivory peg or a bone graft is introduced as an internal splint in the medullary canal of each fragment. In case the introduction of the peg is difficult, the cavity of the bone is enlarged with a burr or drill of suitable size. The longer the splint and the further it penetrates into each fragment, the more successful is the union apt to be. At some distance from the line of fracture, but a little less than half of the length of the splint to be introduced, a hole is drilled through each fragment close to the site chosen for placing the splint. A wire is passed through the drilled holes and a loop of the wire is drawn out of the medullary cavity with the aid of a small nerve hook. The splint is placed through the loops and in the medullary cavity of each fragment in the proper position. When the wire is drawn taut and the ends soldered, the splint is fixed against the side of the fragments.

I use pegs almost exclusively for internal fixation, the peg filling the entire medullary space and being driven tightly into both fragments. For

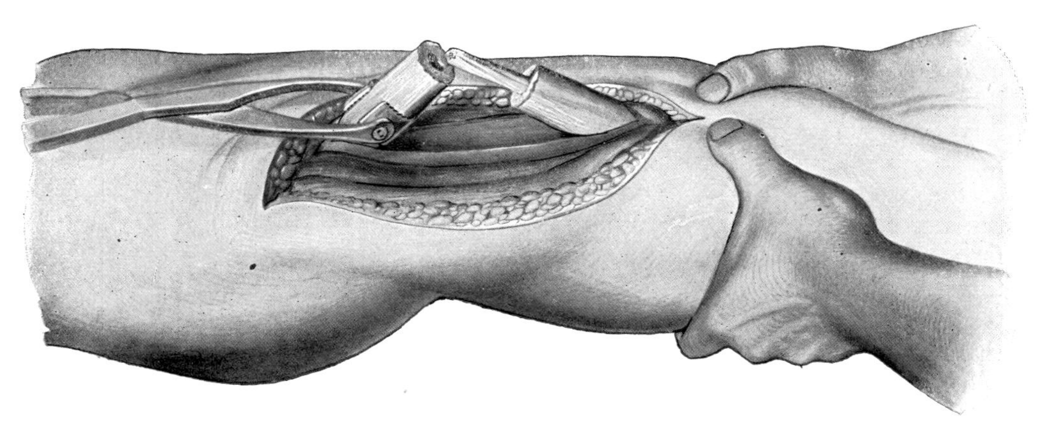

FIG. 614. Immobilization of a fracture with a medullary peg. The fragments are angulated so that the peg can be inserted into the upper canal.

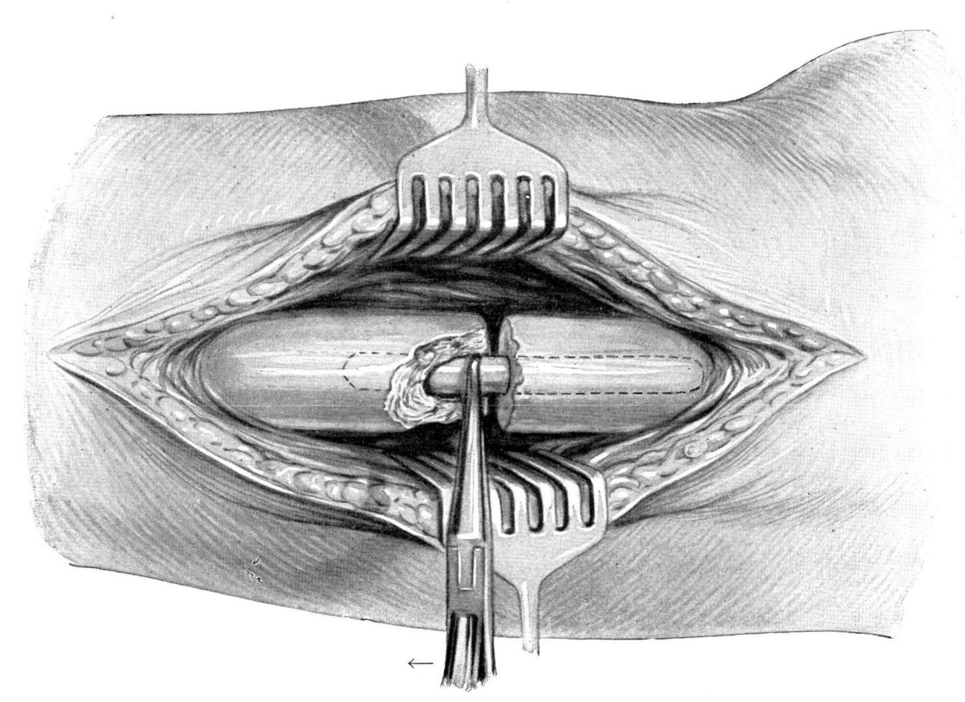

FIG. 615. Immobilization of a fracture with a medullary ivory peg.

pegs, I use either ivory or living grafts from the tibia, or, for pegging the femur, the fibula. The deeper and tighter the peg lies in the cavities of both ends of the bone, the more dependable is the fixation. The possible length of the peg is, however, limited by the difficulty of its introduction into the second fragment. An attempt to overcome this difficulty may be made through one of several procedures. The following descriptions are for the use of ivory pegs, but bone pegs are introduced in much the same manner.

(a) Insertion of Peg by Angulation of Fragments (Fig. 614). The ivory peg chosen should be of such a size that it can be inserted with difficulty into the wider of the medullary cavities, which is, as a rule, the medullary cavity of the proximal fragment. It is introduced, for a trial, as far as it will finally remain. The point at which it emerges from the bone is marked on the peg with a blue dye. The peg is withdrawn and the length of the part previously inserted is measured. The peg is then hammered in the narrower medullary cavity of the other fragment until it is perfectly firm. The projecting part is shortened with the fret saw until, by angulating the fragments, it can be inserted into the medullary cavity of the other fragment. The length of the projecting part of the peg must not be greater than the length which was previously introduced in the trial. The sawed end of the peg is rounded with a rasp and file. By removing a little of the bone from around the medullary cavity of the fragment to receive the peg, the peg is introduced into the cavity, so that the fragments can be brought into alignment as the peg is snapped into place. If this does not succeed, the peg is gradually shortened, with repeated attempts to insert it. The length must not be reduced beyond the limits that are necessary for firm fixation. When the peg has been shortened as much as it can safely be, and yet can not be inserted, the pegging must be done by a different method. There are two other methods for this.

(b) Partial Transfer of Peg (Fig. 615). The ivory peg which was driven into the narrower fragment, as described above, is withdrawn and replaced by the next smaller peg. This peg is inserted in each fragment to make certain that it can be moved in and out without much difficulty. It is then trimmed to the desired length, and the point marked that should later lie at the line of fracture. The peg is now inserted so deeply into the larger medullary cavity that only a small piece of it projects into the medullary space of the second fragment, after the long axis of the bone has been accurately brought into alignment. A special forceps is inserted between the ends of the bone, and the peg is shoved gradually into the second medullary cavity (Fig. 615), until the mark made on the peg appears in the space between the fractured ends. The narrow space in which the forceps must be used can be widened temporarily by pushing the ends apart lengthwise with an elevator or rasp. When the room thus obtained is not enough, the bone is rongeured away little by little at one side of the line of fracture, until the forceps can be manipulated.

(c) Osteoplastic Insertion of Peg (Fig. 617). Instead of the peg being inserted as previously described, it can be inserted into the second fragment with a driver. This requires a longitudinal opening in one fragment through which the peg can be inserted into the medullary cavity. The opening is best made with a two-bladed circular saw. When the peg has been introduced and the fragments reduced, the peg is driven into the marrow cavity of the other end with the driver which is hammered in the direction the peg is to be driven, until the peg lies equally in both fragments.

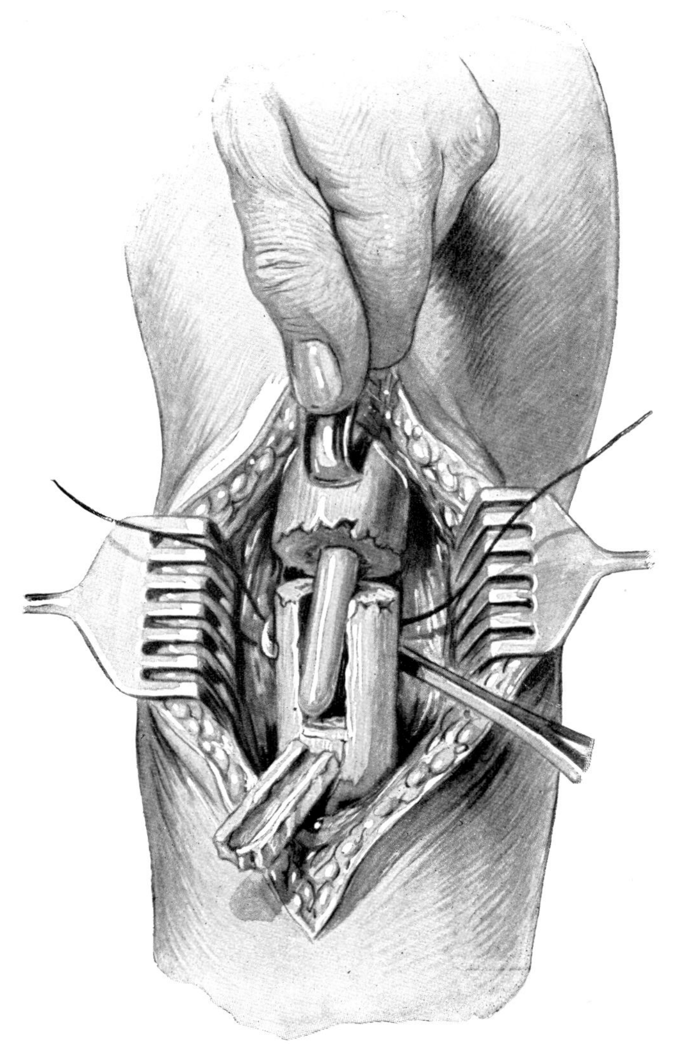

FIG. 616. Insertion of a bone peg in one fragment by removing a section of the bone which is later replaced and held in position by a wire suture.

(d) Osteoplastic Insertion of Peg, Second Method (Fig. 616). If the end still can not be attained by this method as well, nothing remains but to open laterally the medullary cavity of one of the ends, by chiselling out a piece of bone. The ivory peg is driven firmly into the other fragment and is then introduced into the chiselled out opening. The piece of bone removed should correspond to about the length of the projecting portion of the peg. It should, if possible, remain connected with the rest of the bone by a periosteal pedicle, and after the peg is in position, it should be replaced and fastened with wire rings which are applied with the wire stretching forceps and closed by soldering.

An autoplastic bone peg may be cut from one fragment and inserted as

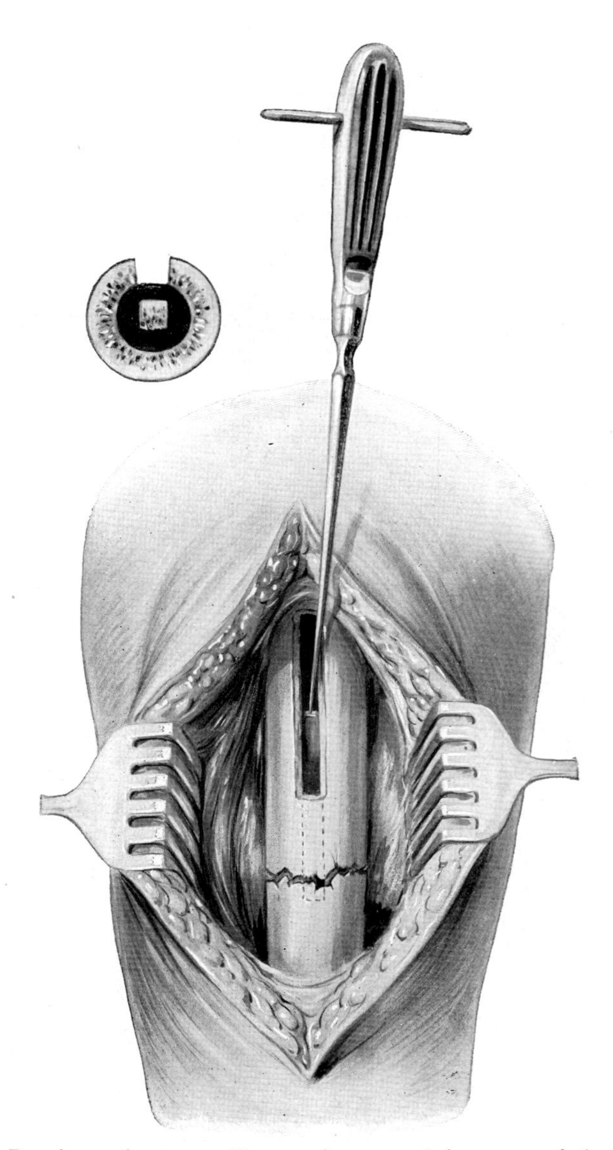

FIG. 617. Pegging a fracture. The peg is removed from one of the fragments.

follows: one fragment is exposed for a distance which is at the least one and one-half times the length of the desired peg. At a distance of one-half the length of the peg from the line of fracture the bone is cut longitudinally with a two-bladed circular saw, so that two parallel cuts are made the length of the peg to be used. The bone splint so cut is freed completely at both ends with a chisel. It is then dropped into the medullary canal and pushed forward with an instrument into the other fragment so that one half lies on each side of the line of fracture (Fig. 617).

Operations for Pseudarthrosis (Fig. 619). These consist, in most cases, of fixation of the ends of the bone by suture. The periosteum must be carefully protected during exposure of the area. To prevent injuring the bone by heat, it is preferable to work with a chisel and gouge forceps rather than with saws. The healthy medullary cavity of both bones must always be opened.

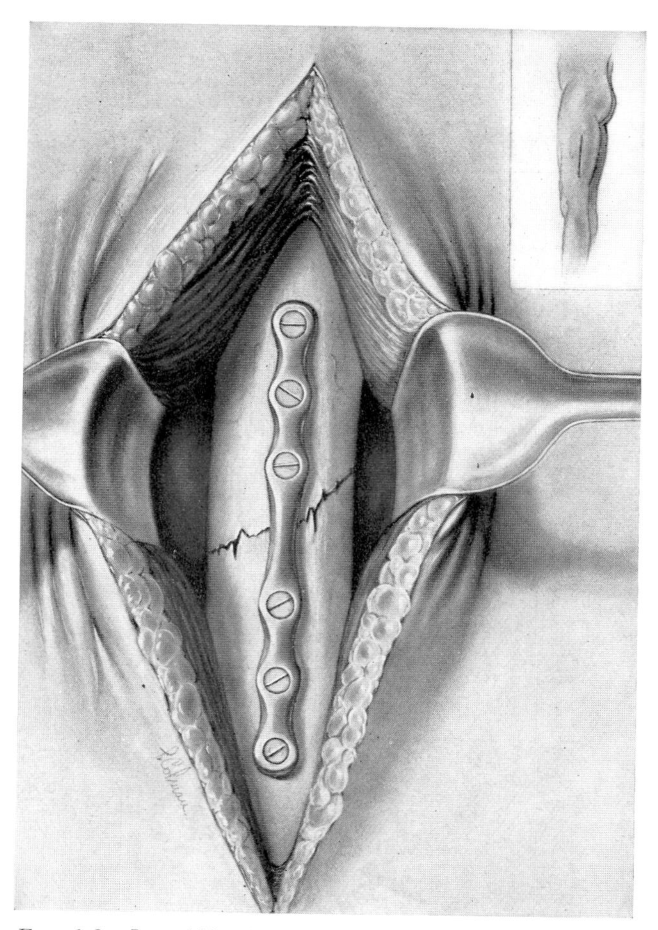

FIG. 618. Immobilization of a fracture with a steel plate.

The simplest procedure, but one which causes some shortening, a serious matter when it affects the leg, is the excision of the affected bone and the union of healthy bone (Fig. 619, 1). The sclerotic ends of the bone, which may be covered with cartilage and are always surrounded with fibrous tissue, should be removed, and the medullary canal of each end opened. I prefer the method of excision which leaves the ends bayonet shaped (Fig. 619, 2). The ends so shaped can be brought in contact with one another over the widest possible surface. They are fastened together by two wire rings. When the fragments have been freshened transversely it is best to use a bone peg (Fig. 619, 1c), rather than attempt to retain the fragments with wire (Fig. 619, 1b).

If shortening must be avoided, the false joint is excised only in so far as it forms part of the bed for the insertion of a bone inlay (Fig. 619, 3a). An autoplastic bone splint is placed in the bed made for it and fastened with four wires (Fig. 619, 3b), as described previously for fixation with external and

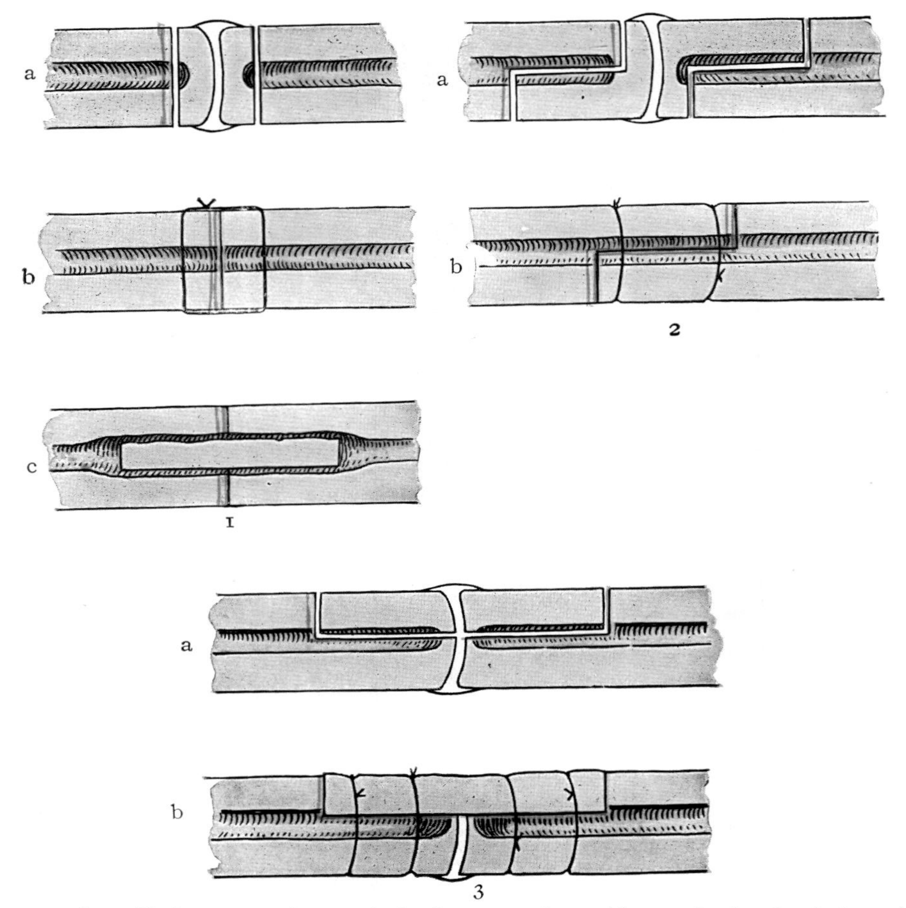

FIG. 619. Various operative methods for non-union with pseudarthrosis (schematic). 1. (a) Excision of the pseudarthrosis by transverse resection. (b) Immobilization with wire sutures. (c) Immobilization with a bone peg. 2. (a) Excision of pseudarthrosis by osteoplastic resection. (b) Immobilization by wire suture. 3. (a) Lateral resection of pseudarthrosis. (b) Immobilization with a bone graft.

lateral inlay splints. This procedure is not as sure as the complete removal of a false joint. The fixation of the bayonet-shaped ends can be reinforced by the lateral application of a bone splint, which makes it doubly secure. Even if union follows the operation, the graft may subsequently break in the region of the old pseudarthrosis and a second false joint may form.

A further possibility in the management of pseudarthrosis consists in splintering the eburnated bone well into healthy bone tissue (Kirschner).

This method is described in the next section, where the straightening of bone curvatures is discussed. This procedure may also be combined with an autoplastic inlay or splint.

Injections of blood into the site of fracture (Bier) constitute one of the most excellent means for promoting repair in the delayed union of fractures and in the prevention of non-union (Fig. 620). Several large needles, through which citrate ointment has been squirted, are inserted under local anæsthesia from different positions to the site of fracture. When the needles are properly

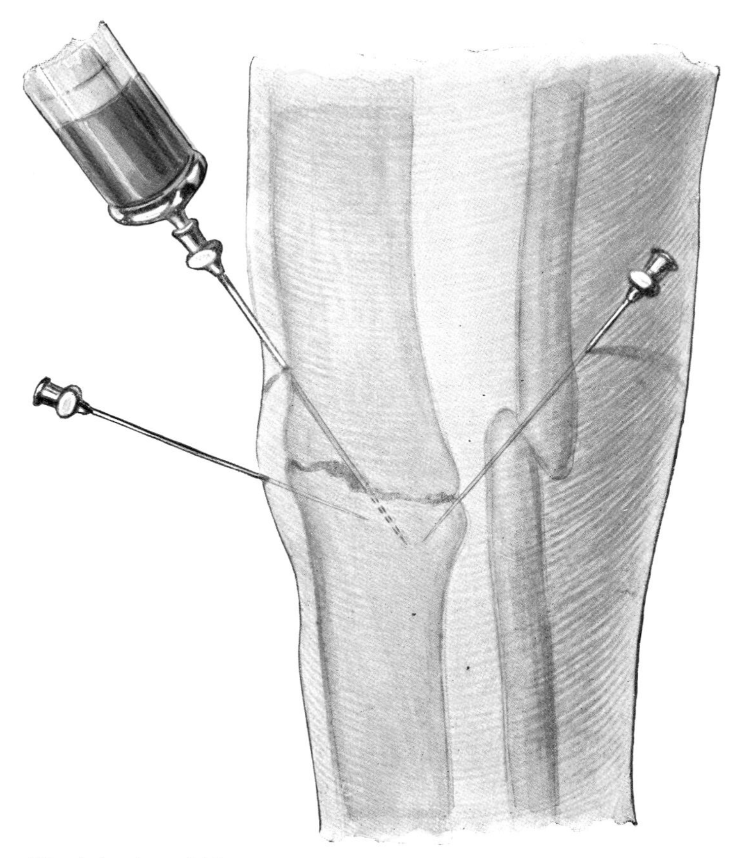

FIG. 620. The injection of blood at a fracture site to promote callus in delayed union.

placed, 10 cc. of blood are withdrawn from a vein at the elbow into a syringe lubricated with citrate ointment, and the blood is injected forcibly through the needles into the tissues. The depth of the needle is changed during the injection to obtain better distribution of the blood. As soon as the injection through one needle is finished, the needle is withdrawn, and the puncture opening is closed with a finger to prevent leakage.

Of the various methods just discussed I consider the following to be excellent in practice: when a small piece of bone has been broken off, and the muscle pull which displaces it acts parallel to the fracture surface, as for example in a fracture of the condyle of the humerus, the fragment is nailed on.

If the displacing force acts perpendicular to the line of fracture of a small fragment, as for example, in a transverse fracture of the olecranon, the fragment is screwed on. Oblique fractures of a shaft, as for example, a spiral fracture of the humerus, are fastened with two wire rings. Transverse fractures are preferably pegged, when there is good approximation of the ends, for example, in a fracture of the forearm, or, occasionally, a suture is carried through holes drilled through the bone. For pegs and splints I use under ordinary conditions ivory, or, if there is evident devitalization of the osteogenic tissues, autoplastic bone grafts. In the treatment of non-union if marked shortening is unimportant, I prefer to excise the affected site, shaping the ends of the bone like bayonets, and to fasten them together with two wire rings. If the shortening is of some importance, I prefer to freshen the ends transversely and join them with an autoplastic peg. If it is essential that no shortening result, I then use an autoplastic bone graft, either as an inlay, or placed laterally on the bone and fastened with four wire rings.

Every fixation of bone should be as firm and dependable as possible. Fixation by the soldered wire ring and by means of pegs is highly dependable, provided the proper technic is followed. It is of such strength in many cases that the union of the fragments may be considered so firm directly after applying the suture that active and passive motion can be begun as soon as the soft parts have healed, which is in about a week. A fracture treated by the open method may thus have the advantage of early motion of the adjoining joints.

The Time for Operative Treatment of Recent Fractures. Closed reduction of a fracture should be attempted as soon as possible after its occurrence, since it becomes increasingly difficult to reduce it. Stromeyer's classic rule for strangulated hernia should be applied to the treatment of fractures. "Should you find a fracture during the day, reduce it before sunset; should you find it at night, reduce it before sunrise!" This rule does not apply to open reduction of recent fractures. Generally speaking, I operate after eight days, when the preliminary healing of the tissue is in full swing and the chances for infection are considerably lessened. An immediate operation is performed only when a fragment endangers the nutrition of the skin, when it presses on an important structure, as for example: a nerve; or when dealing with a compound fracture, when, of course, bone fixation and immediate primary wound toilet are combined.

Preoperative Care of the Patient. The eight days of waiting must not be wasted. If open operation is not inevitable, the intervening time should be employed in an attempt to reduce the fracture by closed methods. If an operation must be done, the fracture is placed in the best possible position for rest. The skin over the injury is covered with zinc ointment. It is very important to see that the site of fracture is well elevated, so that edema and hematomata may be relieved as much as possible. A fractured arm is suspended in a splint, the angle of the elbow-joint being about 130°. The leg is fastened on a splint, so that the thigh is approximately vertical and the leg forms an angle of about 45° with the horizontal plane (Fig. 284).

D. MANAGEMENT OF DEFECTS OF BONE

Bone and Cartilage Transplantation

A bone defect must be corrected when it interrupts the continuity of long, tubular bones, when it occurs in the skull, or for cosmetic reasons, if it is in a bone of the face. On the other hand, hollows, holes, or defects of insignificant size resulting from operations may be neglected, or they may be handled according to the procedures described in Chapter IX, H, 2: "Chronic Osteomyelitis".

Defects which occur in the shaft of a long bone are most easily corrected by direct approximation of the ends of the bone, though this involves shorten-

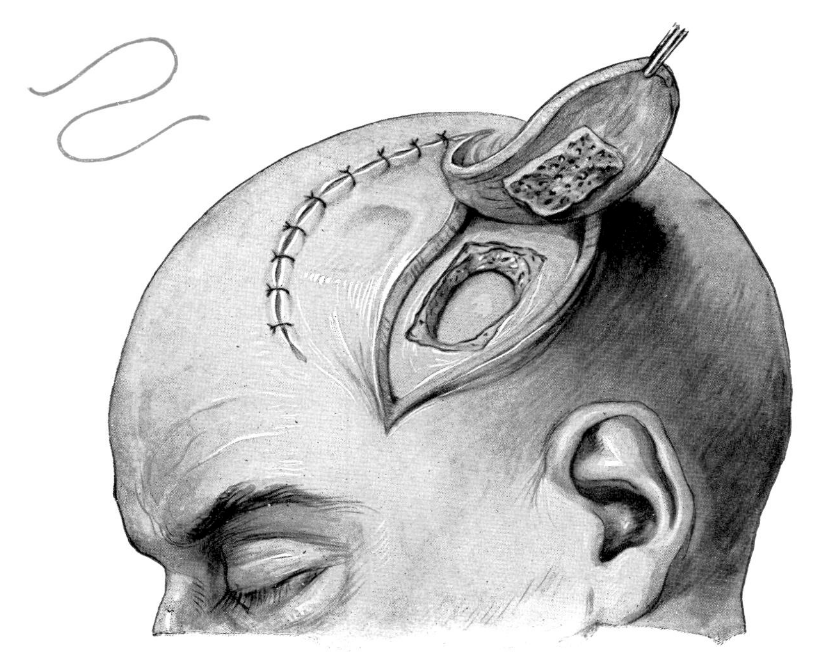

FIG. 621. Pedunculated skin and osteoperiosteal flap for covering a cranial defect (Müller-König).

ing of the extremity. The methods for uniting ends of bone were discussed in the previous section.

To avoid shortening, a substitute must be obtained for the section of bone lost. The problem of the substitute is two-fold: it should hold the bone straight, in the proper position, as a purely mechanical internal splint, until new bone is formed around it from the osteogenic tissues, and it should enter into a lasting organic union with the bone, or at least be replaced by organic tissue.

The best material for repair of a bone defect is an autograft, either pedunculated or free. Since the pedunculated graft is much more apt to survive than a free transplant, it is preferable. It is, however, seldom possible to obtain a suitable pedunculated flap containing bone near the site of a defect.

If the connection between the bone graft and the overlying soft parts can be preserved (pedunculated bone graft), a pedunculated flap is formed over bone which lies adjacent to the defect, leaving on the under side of the flap

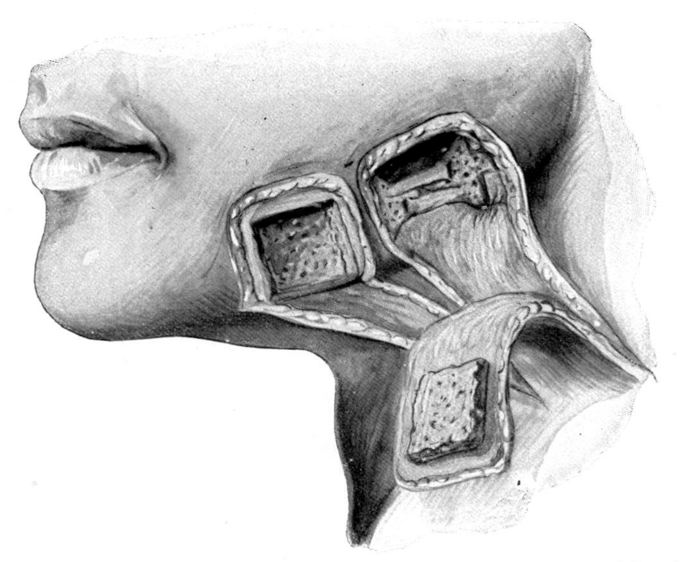

FIG. 622. Skin and osteoperiosteal flap for bridging a defect of the mandible after freshening its edges.

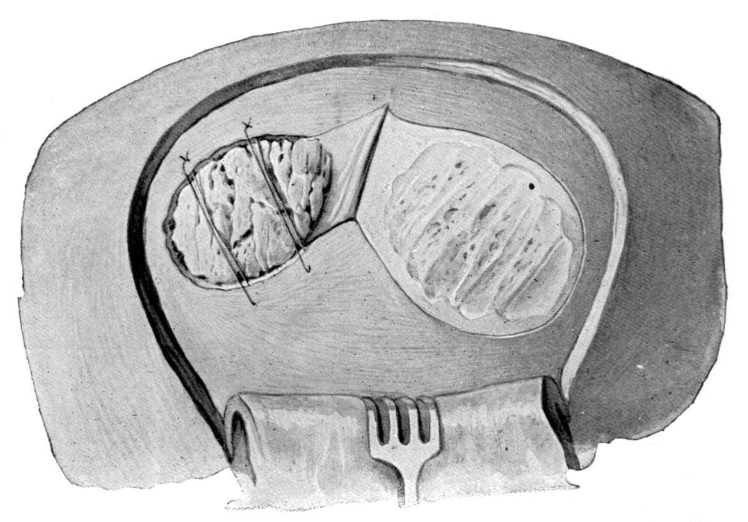

FIG. 623. Osteoperiosteal flap for covering a cranial defect (v. Hacker-Durante).

a piece of bone corresponding in size to the defect. The pedicle may include the skin (Figs. 621 and 622) or it may be a periosteal flap (Fig. 623). In the former case, after transplantation the skin covering the defect can be excised if it is not transferred to the site from which the pedicle was removed. Pedunculated bone grafts are used for closing skull defects (Müller-Koenig), and occasionally for replacing missing bone in the mandible (Fig. 428). They are also used for defects of the tibia, in the Indian rhinoplasty, and plastic operations on the larynx with cartilage from the sternum. Pedunculation without skin requires either a muscle flap or the periosteum alone, as for example in Hacker-Durante's cranioplasty (Fig. 623). After the periosteum is cut around, like a flap, a sharp knife-chisel is placed nearly parallel to the bone surface and the outer table of bone is chiseled off so that it remains attached to the periosteum in the form of a thin scale. This periosteal bone flap is laid over the defect and sutured in place with catgut. It forms, as a rule, new bone of sufficient thickness. This procedure is admirably adapted for filling defects of the skull. Such bone flaps can be used to advantage in other places as well, for example, as an osteoplastic covering of the end of the bone after amputation, as a substitute for Bier's plastic. In exceptionally favorable cases, the connection of the transplant with the original bone can to a great extent be preserved, as when the fibula is transplanted into the tibia to replace lost bone (Fig. 624).

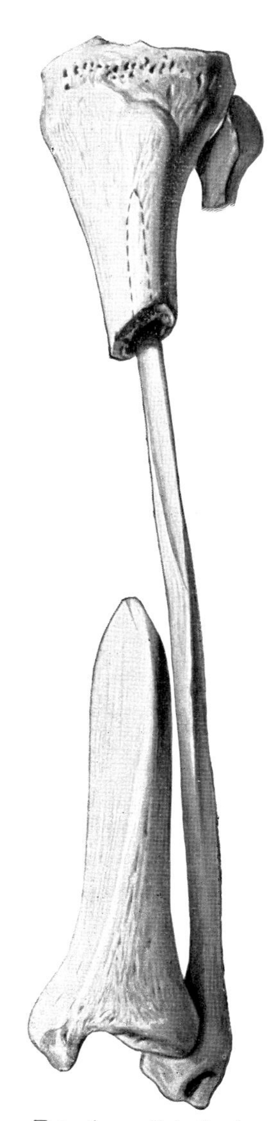

Fig. 624. Substitution of an adjacent bone for bridging a defect. (A defect of the tibia is compensated by substitution of the fibula.)

Foreign material is used to bridge defects only when autoplastic grafts can not be removed, as in replacing a joint. Absorbable material is always preferable. As already mentioned, homogeneous bone, the bones of animals, ivory, and horn must all be considered in transplanting as dead and absorbable, and of about equal value, for even if alive when transferred, they die immediately. They are, also, always boiled before being used. I prefer ivory. I rarely use metal for bridging a defect, and only when in an infected wound I do not expect final healing but wish to retain the bone in its proper position until new bone formation occurs, at which time the metal is removed.

After complete preparation of the new bed, the size of the piece of bone that is to be transplanted is measured exactly, or, in difficult cases, as in a cranioplasty, a rubber model is used. The bone from which the transplant is to be taken is exposed, as a rule, by a longitudinal incision directly over it. In excising a graft from the tibia (Fig. 625) the longitudinal incision is made about 1 cm. lateral to the anterior border of the tibia, so that the resulting scar does not lie directly over the bone. The skin is freed from the anterior surface, and the muscles are retracted from the anterior part of the lateral surface. After the periosteum is incised on the antero-lateral surface a few millimeters larger than the size of the proposed graft, it is pushed back slightly to expose the line along which the bone is to be cut. The graft that is to be removed is then outlined with a chisel held perpendicular to the bone surface. The chisel grooves are deepened until the bone splint is detached from the base and can be lifted out. The chiseling must be done with caution, for force may break not only the bone graft, but the tibia as well. The splint may be loosened more easily by drilling holes a few centimeters apart along the line of division, and dividing the bone between the holes with the chisel (Fig. 580). This procedure has the same disadvantage as the technically simple method of cutting out the transplant with a circular saw, which is of injuring the bone by heat. The common peroneal nerve must be kept in mind when removing the fibula. To prevent injury to the pleura when removing a rib, the periosteum is left attached to the costal pleura.

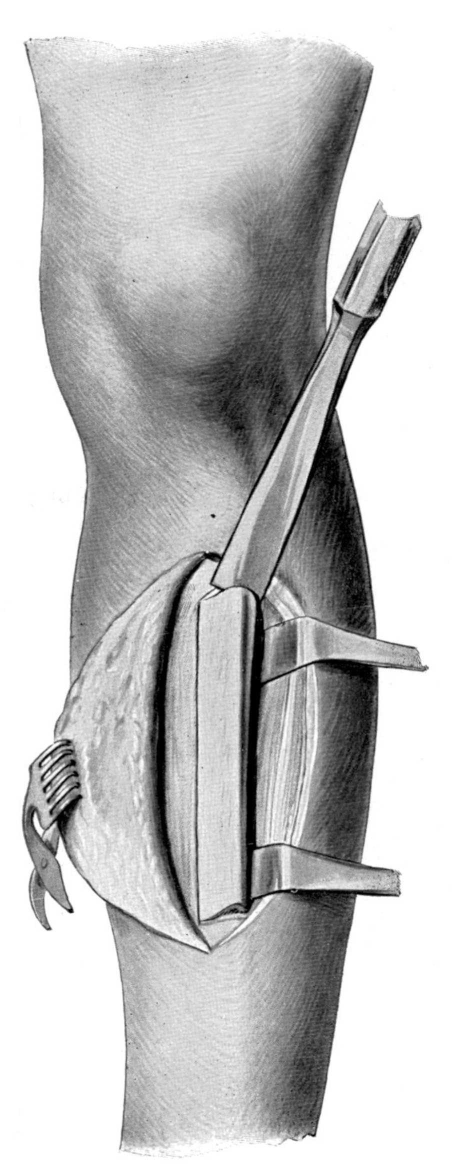

FIG. 625. Taking a bone graft from the anterior surface of the tibia. The periosteum is retained on the graft.

The lower portion of the scapula is an excellent source of bone for repair of a defect of a thin bone. The scapula is exposed by a longitudinal incision, the muscles are detached and a suitable part of the bone is excised. The entire infraspinous fossa of the scapula can be removed without resulting functional disturbances. The detached muscles, however, should be carefully united. The crest of the ilium can be used as a remarkably good substitute for the mandible. In removing it, the line which offers attachment to the muscles should if possible be preserved.

After the bone is taken out, in order to lose no time in transplanting the graft, the wound is either closed temporarily or by another operator. When the graft has been taken from the leg, the leg is later placed on a splint, or if the tibia has been weakened too much, it is placed in a plaster cast.

The bone graft so obtained may be properly shaped with Luer's forceps, chisels, fret saws, rasps and files. When it is difficult to work on the bone, it may be held in a hand vise or a small screw vise. The bone can be curved in a longitudinal direction by the use of a pair of wrenches (Fig. 626). Flexible bones, such as the ribs, can be considerably curved without fracturing them. A splint from a compact bone must have several transverse incisions on the side intended to be convex before attempts to bend it are made (Fig. 626).

No matter what material is chosen, a most important requisite of a bridge over a bone defect is that it should be held firmly and immovably to the ends

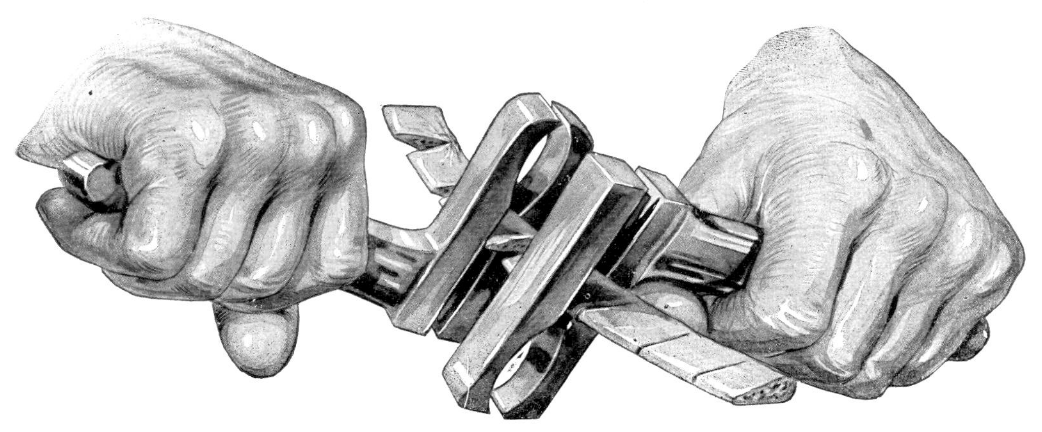

FIG. 626. When a curved bone transplant is needed the rib can be used. The curve can be increased by sawing the bone in numerous places and then using wrenches as illustrated.

of the bone to which it is transplanted. The rules previously given for fixation of bone (Chap. IX, page 510) should be followed, whether the structures are joined by pegs, screws, inlays or lateral splints which are held by wires or

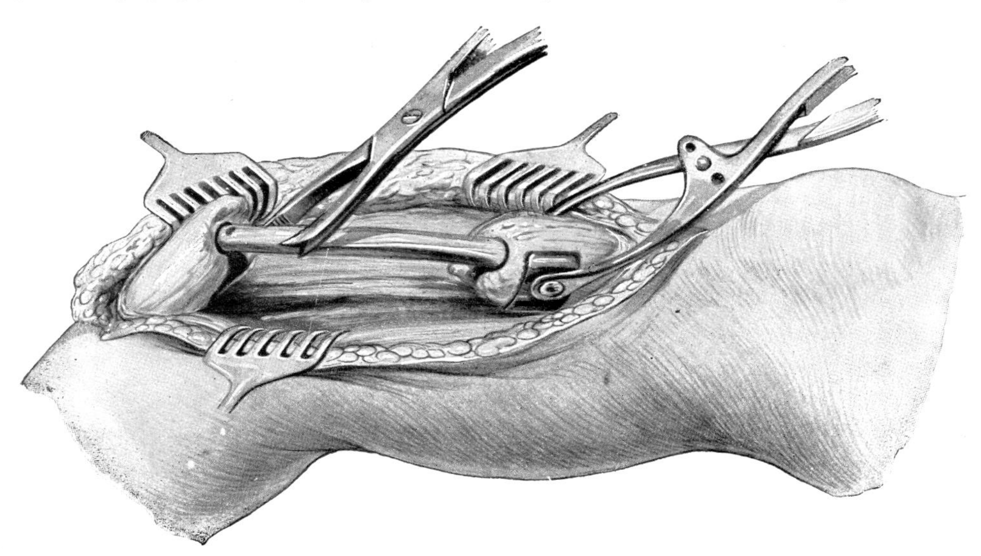

FIG. 627. Bridging a defect in a long bone with a bone transplant. A defect of the femur is bridged with a portion of the shaft of the fibula.

screws. The best methods of joining two ends are pegging (Figs. 627 and 628), and the lateral splint which is fastened to each end of the bone by two wire rings (Figs. 629, 630, and 631).

When the bone transplant is used to replace the end of a bone which forms part of a joint, only one end of the transplant can, of course, be attached to the bone, the other end being free to form the joint and being brought into contact with the end of the other bone which forms the joint. This end must be shaped exactly like the bone removed, if it is not possible to find a bone which is naturally of the proper shape. The head of the fibula is well adapted to serve as a substitute for the head of the humerus, the phalanges and metatarsal bones as substitutes for the long bones of the hand.

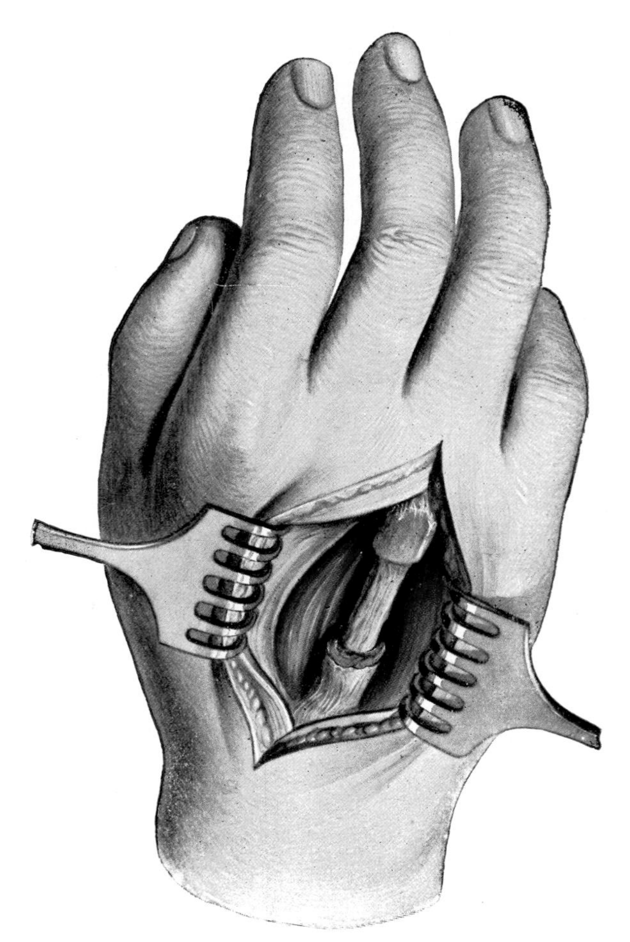

Fig. 628. Bridging a defect of the fourth metacarpal with a transplant removed from the tibia.

A long bone can be replaced by another bone in its entire length from one joint to the other. It is doubly important here to choose as a transplant a bone that approaches in form, length, and cartilaginous covering the bone to be replaced. The bones of the fingers are best replaced by the corresponding bones of the toes.

It is possible to transplant freely not only one bone of a joint, but both bones composing the joint, and they may even be transplanted with the capsule and ligaments, as an entire joint (Lexer). To do this, the diseased joint is exposed and removed by dividing its proximal and distal bones. A closed joint of corresponding size is then fitted into the gap and the ends of the bones are fastened firmly together. Only postmortem or fresh accident material should be considered for large joints. This procedure, however, has very little practical significance. On the contrary, autoplastic transplantation of the interphalangeal joint of the great toe has repeatedly proved successful as a substitute for a stiff elbow joint (Fig. 632).

The soft parts must be carefully sutured over a bone plastic, to give the transplanted bone increased support and to prevent later infection. The extremity should be immobilized. Motion should be begun as soon as possible, but it must be deferred somewhat longer and handled with greater caution than in simple fractures. Some authors recommend prolonged immobilization.

Free transplants of bone live in a new site not only when they are in contact with bone, but also when they are imbedded in the soft parts. Use is made of this to correct facial disfigurement, such as saddle-nose, absence of the zygomatic arch, or absence of the orbital margins. The piece of bone is inserted through a small incision made at a short distance from the defect and is pushed under the skin to the intended site (Fig. 633). Ivory is also useful for this purpose.

A piece of bone transplanted to the subcutaneous tissues may after it is shown to be viable be included in a pedunculated skin flap. In this way a pedunculated skin flap can be provided with bone or cartilage. This is used, for instance, in rhinoplasties and laryngoplasties. A piece of bone or cartilage is transplanted to the site of the future flap where it is given sufficient time to prove that it is viable, after which, it may be included in a pedunculated skin flap, which is transferred to the nasal or laryngeal defect. In this way even fingers may be reconstructed by first transplanting a bone under the skin of the chest wall or abdomen and later transplanting the pedunculated skin flap and bone to its new location (Fig. 429).

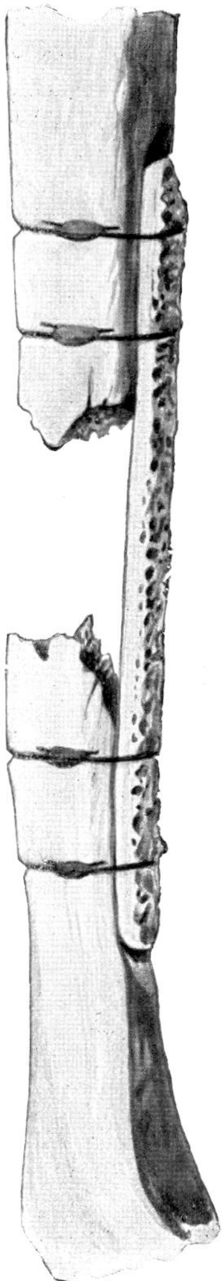

FIG. 629. Bridging a bone defect with a free transplant from the tibia. The transplant is retained by four wire sutures passed around both the transplant and the fragments.

In the correction of cosmetic defects, cartilage is used as well as bone. It has the advantage that it can be easily cut and shaped with a knife. The costal cartilages offer a convenient, almost inexhaustible supply. To remove cartilage an incision is begun along the lateral margin of the sternum a few fingers' breadth above the ensiform process and the incision is continued along the costal cartilages. The cartilage is easily reached after dividing the soft parts, and large pieces of it can be removed with the knife (Fig. 634). In my experience, though this is not universally confirmed, the viability of transplanted cartilage is not as great as that of bone. Suppuration and subsequent extrusion of the graft occurs more frequently. I prefer, therefore, the bone transplants. Free

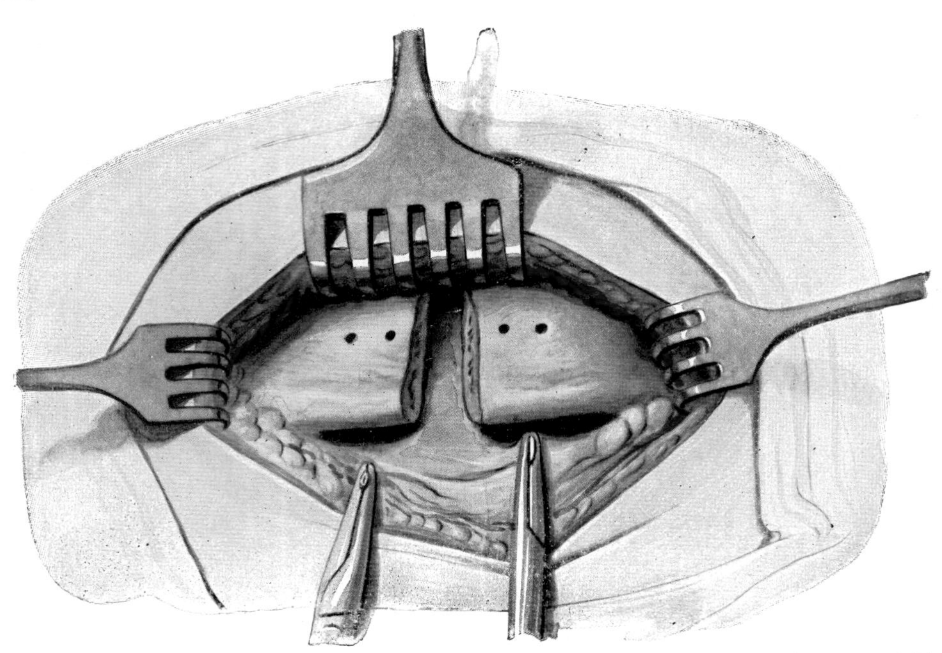

Fig. 630. Bridging a bony defect of mandible with a free bone transplant. Two holes are drilled through each fragment through which the sutures pass for retention of the transplant.

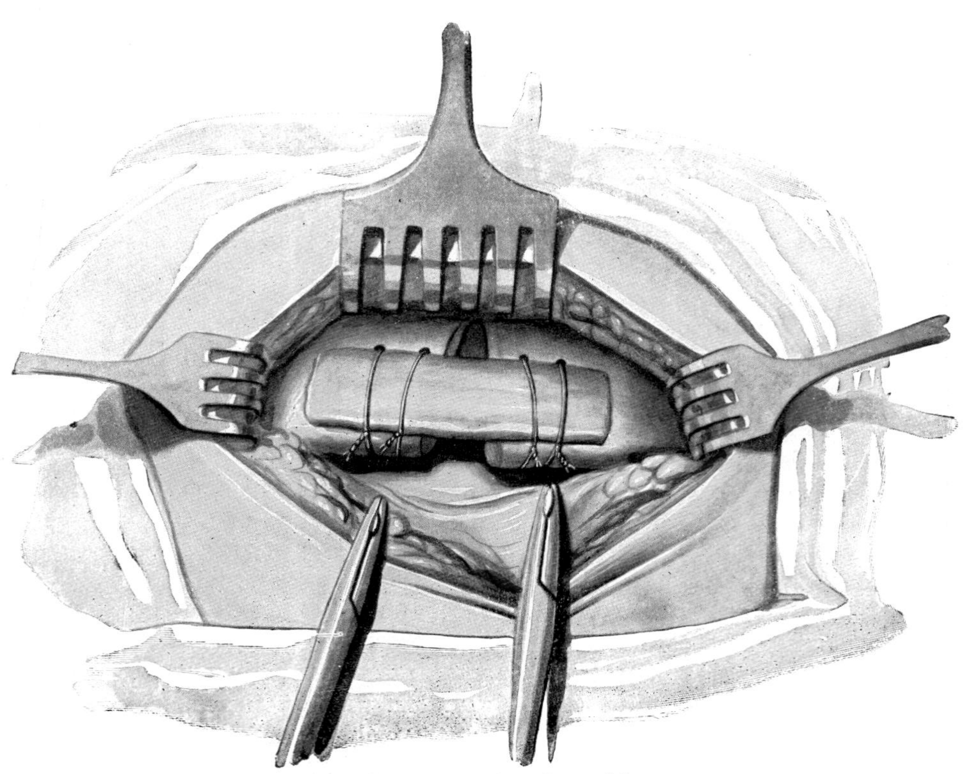

Fig. 631. Transplant in position.

cartilaginous transplants of the entire thickness of the helix of the ear have been used with some success to replace defects of the alæ nasi (Fig. 433). After the edges of the nasal defect have been freshened, a wedge is removed from the ear, properly shaped, and sutured in place. In order to increase the denuded surface, steps may be cut in the graft. Too much should not be expected from this procedure. The wedge-shaped defect in the ear should be closed by suture.

Osteoplastic Bone Resection. When a bone is to be divided temporarily, as for the exposure of underlying structures, the division should be so made as to facilitate mechanical and organic reunion. I prefer, therefore, an oblique, angular or Z-shaped line of division to the simple transverse division. The plane of division should, if possible, be planned so that the muscles attached to the bone splint the line of reunion. In this way, for instance, the mandible is divided from above downward, from within out, and from behind forward. If the bone is to be reunited later by wire, the drill holes should be placed before the bone is cut, in order to have the holes in alignment. When a Z-shaped division is made the bone is best reunited with wire rings.

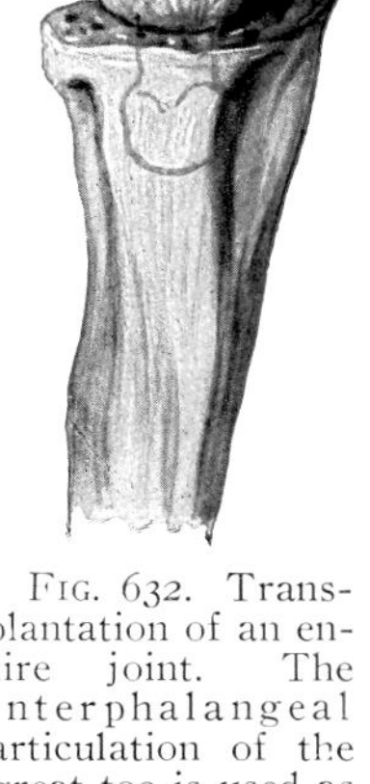

Fig. 632. Transplantation of an entire joint. The interphalangeal articulation of the great toe is used as a substitute for the elbow joint.

If the division of a bone at one place does not afford adequate exposure of the operative area, a section of the bone should be removed temporarily. The bone should remain attached, if possible, to the overlying soft parts. When the bone is replaced it is actually nothing but a pedunculated bone graft. In such cases there are formed extensive skin, muscle and bone flaps, which are temporarily turned back on their soft-part base, and later replaced after the operation is finished. The retention of the bone by special bone sutures is as a rule unnecessary.

This type of procedure is used in exposures under the zygomatic arch, the superior maxilla, and in cranial operations where a bone flap is temporarily laid back.

Occasionally, the osteoplastic bone resection can be done so that the detached piece of bone can be removed in one direction, but will not yield to forces acting upon it in other directions. This occurs, for example, in the temporary detachment of the tibial tuberosity when it is excised in the form of a trapezoid, for the purpose of opening the knee-joint (Kirschner, Fig. 586). The trapezoid of bone with the connecting patellar ligament may be pushed laterally from its bed, but can not be displaced by the longitudinal pull of the quadriceps. The knee-joint is thus closed after the operation.

E. THE CORRECTION OF BONY DEFORMITIES

The majority of operations which have as their purpose a change in the shape of the bone are necessitated by deformities, which are either the result of viciously united fractures, or the result of constitutional diseases such as rickets. It is but seldom that the form of a normally developed bone needs correction, but an alteration in shape may be necessary to relieve a deformity which is the result of faulty position of a neighboring joint or of an abnormal condition in another place, as for example, subtrochanteric osteotomy in contracture of the hip. The correction depends principally on changes of position

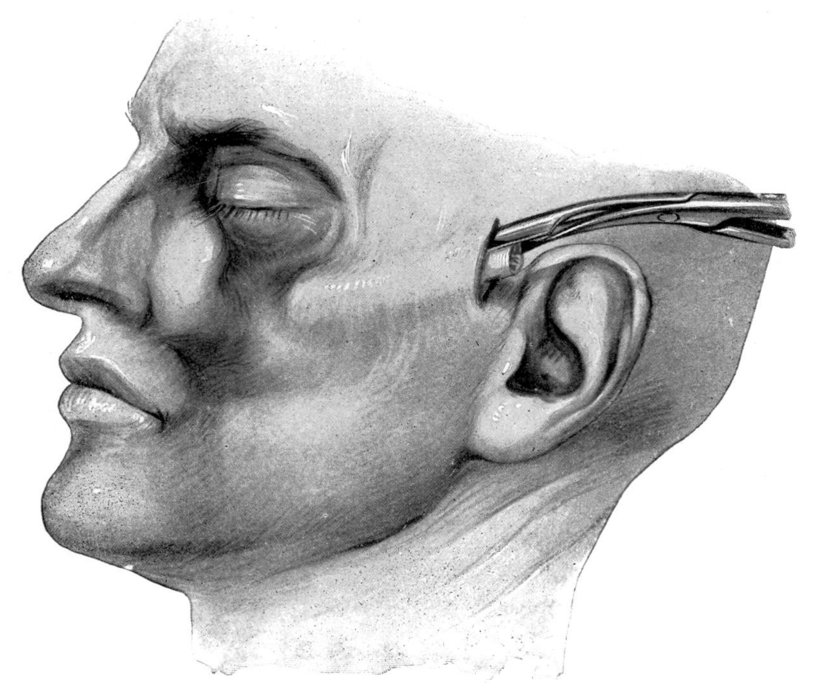

FIG. 633. Subcutaneous bone transplantation. Transplantation of a portion of a rib for correcting a defect of the zygomatic arch.

of the axis (angular correction), and on changes of length (correction of length). Lateral adjustment is seldom necessary.

1. ADJUSTMENT OF THE ANGLE

The bone is divided, as a rule, only after it has been adequately exposed by slitting the periosteum and separating it from the bone with elevators, subperiosteal division. The periosteal cylinder prevents to a certain extent an undesirable lateral displacement of the fragments. A bone is rarely divided with the periosteum intact, extraperiosteal division. When it is, the danger of lateral displacement is greater. In subcutaneous osteotomy (Fig. 635), which is extraperiosteal, a longitudinal incision is made over the bone, corresponding exactly in length to the width of the chisel. The edge of the chisel is carried in a longitudinal direction down to the bone, turned transversely to the long axis of the bone and the bone is divided without being exposed.

1. The simplest form of angular correction is transverse division of a bone at the highest point of the angulation and subsequent adjustment of the angle, linear osteotomy (Fig. 636). The bone is divided with a chisel or saw. It is best to leave a small bridge of bone on the convex side, and to

break this forcibly after the wound is closed. Or the bone may be first divided except for a thin bridge, immobilized in a cast in the original position until there is some callous formation, the cast then removed and the curvature straightened by breaking through the bridge of bone. The callus then prevents displacement of the fragments.

After linear osteotomy, there is naturally a separation of the divided ends on the previously concave side, and the ends are in apposition only on

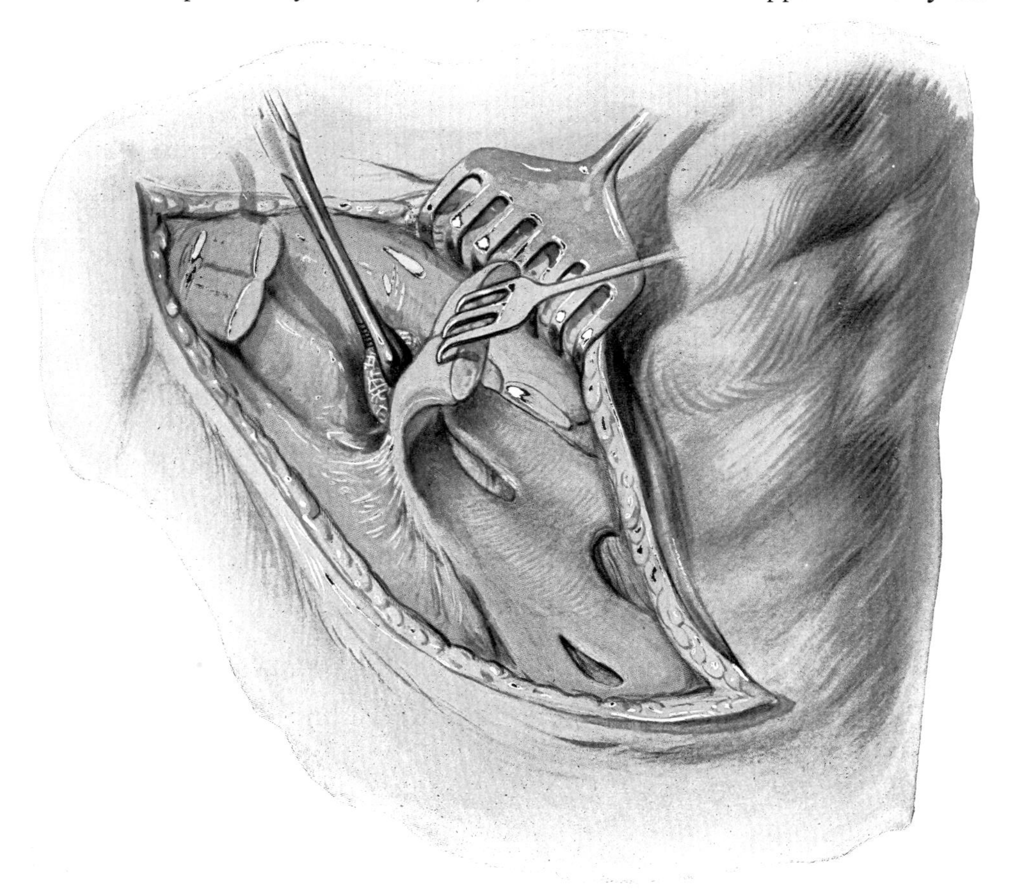

FIG. 634. Resection of a piece of cartilage for free grafting. Pericardium and pleura are carefully detached from the inner side of the cartilage.

the convex side. Practically, the gap is unimportant, since it rapidly fills in under normal conditions. If the bone is thick and the angulation considerable, linear osteotomy may cause so much lengthening of the limb that the skin, vessels, and nerves can not be stretched to the extent necessary for correction of the deformity.

2. These disadvantages can be avoided by removing a wedge of bone at the point of division of the bone, cuneiform osteotomy (Fig. 637). It is better to measure the size of the wedge that is to be removed, than to depend on the eye. I use a cardboard model of the bone made from an x-ray picture taken perpendicular to the surface of greatest curvature. I cut through this

model, as for a linear osteotomy, and then bring the ends together in the correct position (Fig. 638). The size of the angular end which overlaps the other end corresponds to the size of the wedge to be removed. In particularly difficult cases, as for instance in the correction of club-feet, I prepare plaster-of-Paris casts (Fig. 639) of the malformed limb, and remove wedges from them until I have determined precisely the necessary size and position of the wedge to be removed.

To lessen the shortening of the limb after removal of a wedge, Perthes suggests for the operation for flat feet to take a bone wedge from the convex side and re-implant it in a slit made on the concave side. This principle can

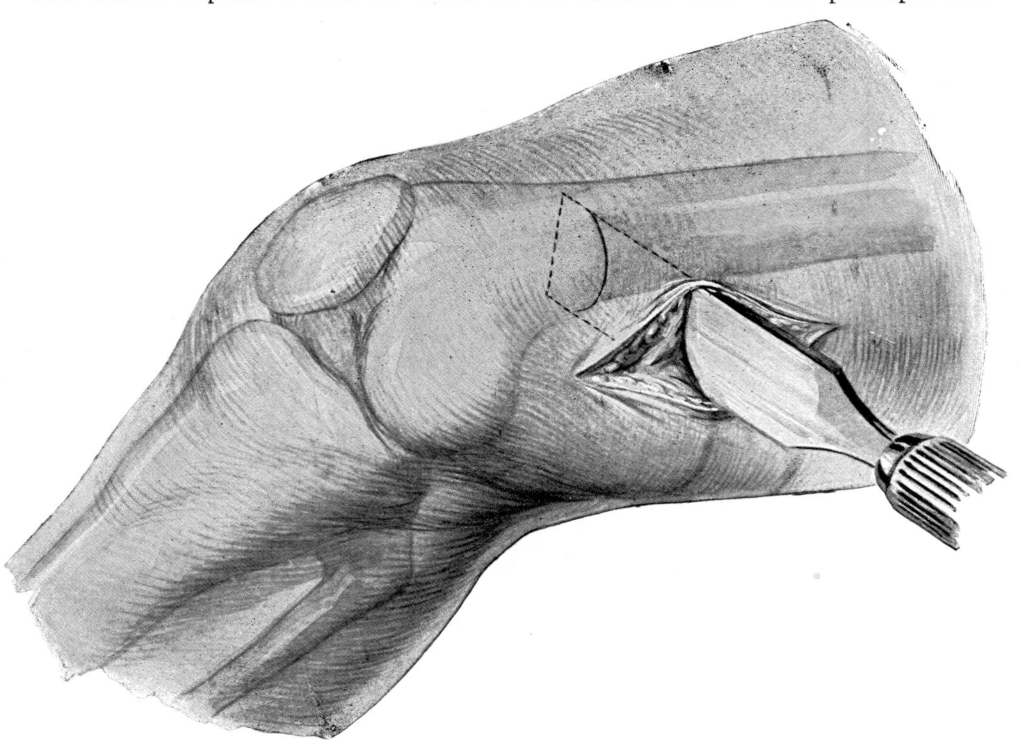

Fig. 635. Subcutaneous osteotomy of the femur proximal to the condyles. The sharp edge of the chisel is inserted in the long axis of the bone. It is then turned to a right angle with the long axis and driven through the bone.

be extended successfully to the correction of many malformations of bones (Fig. 640).

3. While elongation results from linear osteotomy, shortening of the limb occurs after cuneiform osteotomy. To bring about surface contact of the planes of separation without too pronounced shortening, one may use curved osteotomy (Fig. 641). The division of the bone is curved in the form of a semicircle. In practice, it is almost impossible to divide the bone so accurately that the concave and convex surfaces will lie intimately together throughout, when the angulation has been corrected. The curved division requires also very free exposure of the bone. It is, therefore, a theoretical rather than a practical procedure. This is also true of several other forms of osteotomy, as

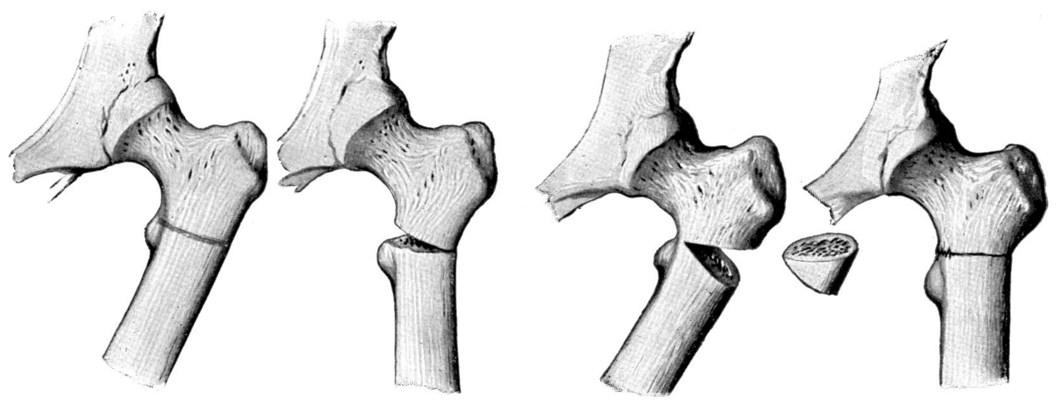

FIG. 636. Linear osteotomy for correction of bowing. A wedge-shaped defect on the concave side of the deformity results.

FIG. 637. Cuneiform osteotomy for correction of bowing. A wedge of bone is removed.

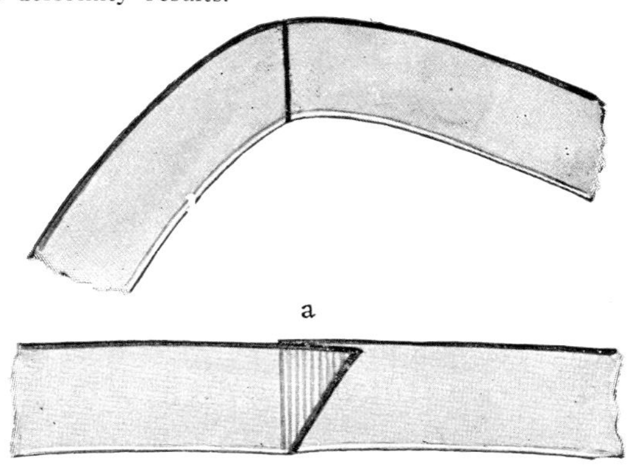

FIG. 638. Cardboard model for determining the size of the wedge to be removed in an osteotomy; (a) before, (b) after straightening.

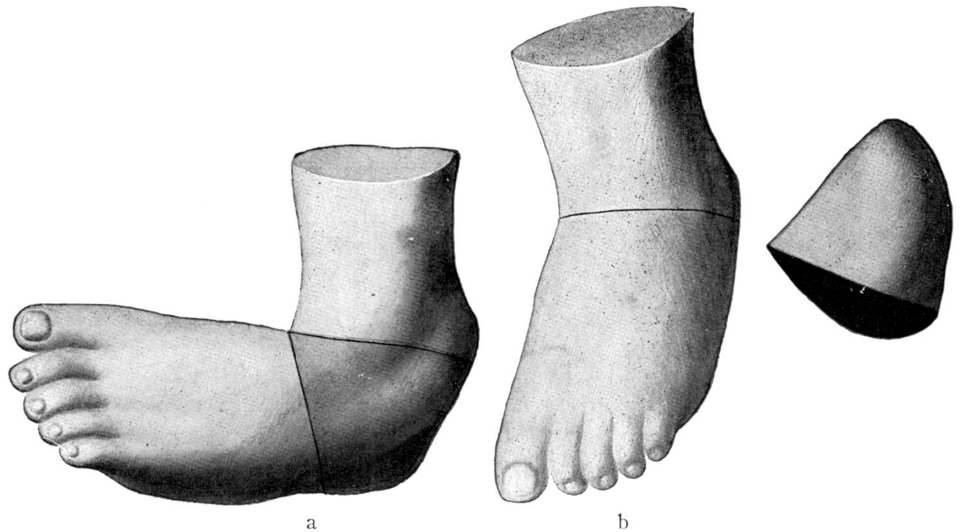

FIG. 639. Plaster model for determining the size and position of the wedge to be removed in an osteotomy; (a) before, (b) after straightening.

for example, the oblique linear osteotomy, in which the bone is divided diagonally. Many of the procedures which theoretically might be useful have been found in practice to be useless. Because of the variation of results after linear, cuneiform, curved, and oblique osteotomies, I prefer in certain cases

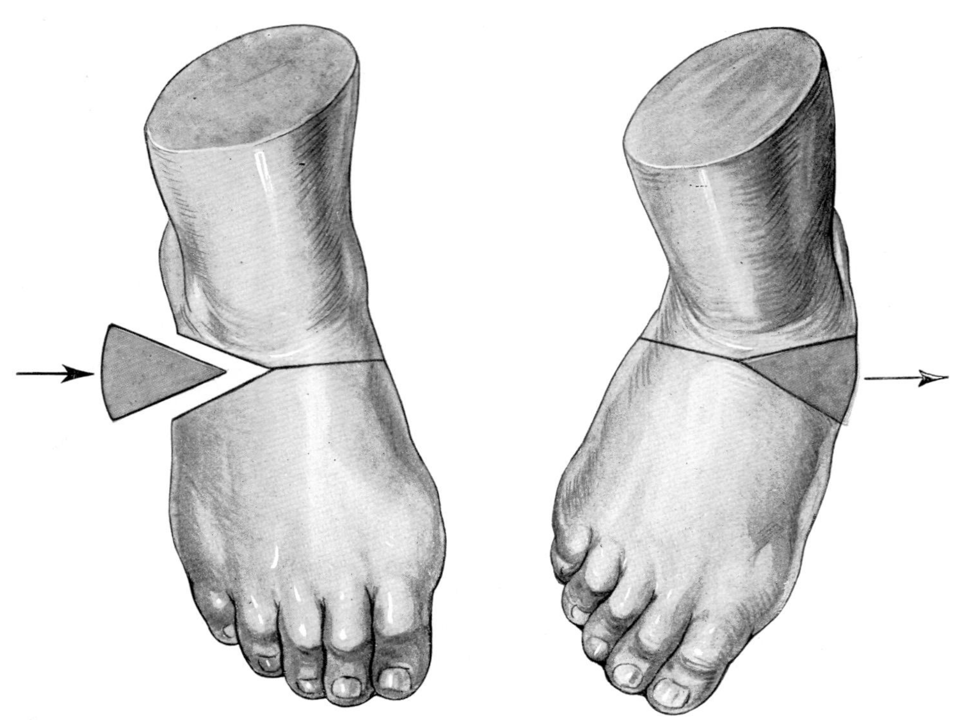

FIG. 640. Plastic wedge osteotomy with free transplant of a bone wedge.

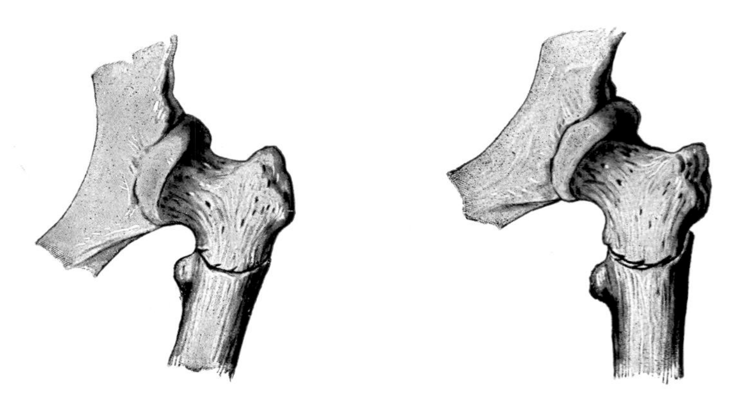

FIG. 641. Curved osteotomy for correction of bowing.

destructive osteotomy, described below, by which every type of correction, even longitudinal, is possible, without sacrificing the continuity of the bone, and in which the individual bone fragments align themselves in a most practical way.

Complete correction of a deformity by the methods described thus far is impossible in many cases, because the deformity extends over a long portion of the bone, while division of the bone affects only the transverse plane. However, the incomplete adjustment often suffices as far as the posture of the patient is concerned. In children, the remaining curvatures will often be compensated for to a considerable degree in the course of time. Notwithstanding this, in severe deformities involving a long section of bone, it is better to distribute the correction over a greater area than is usually done. The following procedures are to be considered for this purpose.

4. The entire deformed section of bone is removed subperiosteally. The periosteum is split longitudinally and elevated, the bone is divided with a wire saw proximal and distal to the affected section, and this part of the bone is then removed. The periosteal tube may then be sutured and left in place. As a rule sufficient new bone forms after a time in the corrected position so that function can be resumed. Springer saws the bone taken out of the periosteal tube in disks about 1 cm. thick, the bone being held in a sterile vise (Fig. 642), and puts back into the periosteal tube as many of these disks as possible (Fig. 643). Löffler and Voelcker crush the bone into a "bone salad", a term that expresses at the same time the ill treatment of living tissue, and refill the periosteal tube with this mass (Fig. 644). Rohde places in the empty periosteal tube the medullary material removed from the compact bone, adding some small pieces of the crushed bone.

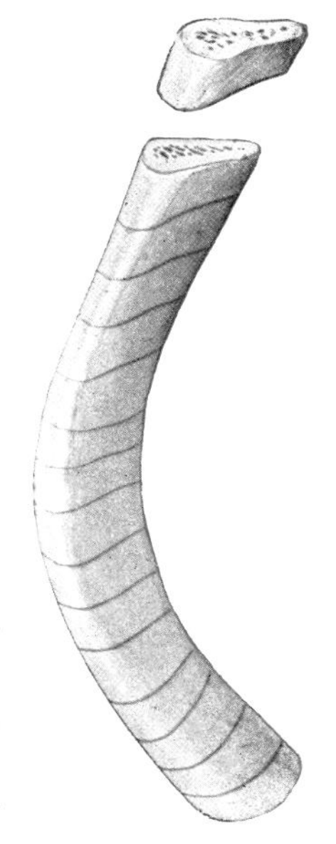

Fig. 642. Correcting extensive bowing by dividing the bone into disks after separating the periosteum from the bone (Springer).

5. These procedures involve to a large extent free transplants, which carry certain risks, and their prospects are not enhanced by the rough handling of the tissue that takes place. Tissue necrosis, infection and absence of ossification are constant dangers of such procedures. Furthermore, when the fragments are widely separated and without support, there is the possibility of undesirable displacement. A procedure which I have suggested is free of these disadvantages. It consists in exposing the bone, splintering it over the entire length of the deformity, and then correcting its position, but without removing any part of it from the body (Fig. 645). The tissue becomes plastic but there is a minimum of interference with its nutrition. Another advantage of this procedure is the rapidity with which it regains its firmness, an observation that coincides with experience in extensive comminuted fractures. The dangers of fat embolism and infection are not increased by this procedure.

The technic is as follows (Kirschner: Arch. f. Klin. Chir., Vol. 126; Ger. Congress report 1923; and Med. Klinik., 1926): the bone is exposed through a long longitudinal incision along the entire length of the deformity on the side easiest of access. Elevation of the periosteum need not follow this exposure, but may be done for the retraction and safety of nerves and vessels lying directly on the bone. The bone is then splintered by numerous chisel strokes, which are not made transversely, but principally in the longitudinal and oblique directions (Fig. 646). The splintering should cover the entire area of deformity, yet it should not be carried so far as to cause complete division of the bone. When working in the vicinity of important joints, care must be taken that the bone is not split into the joint. This risk is not great, because long cracks do not result except in hard compact bones, the soft

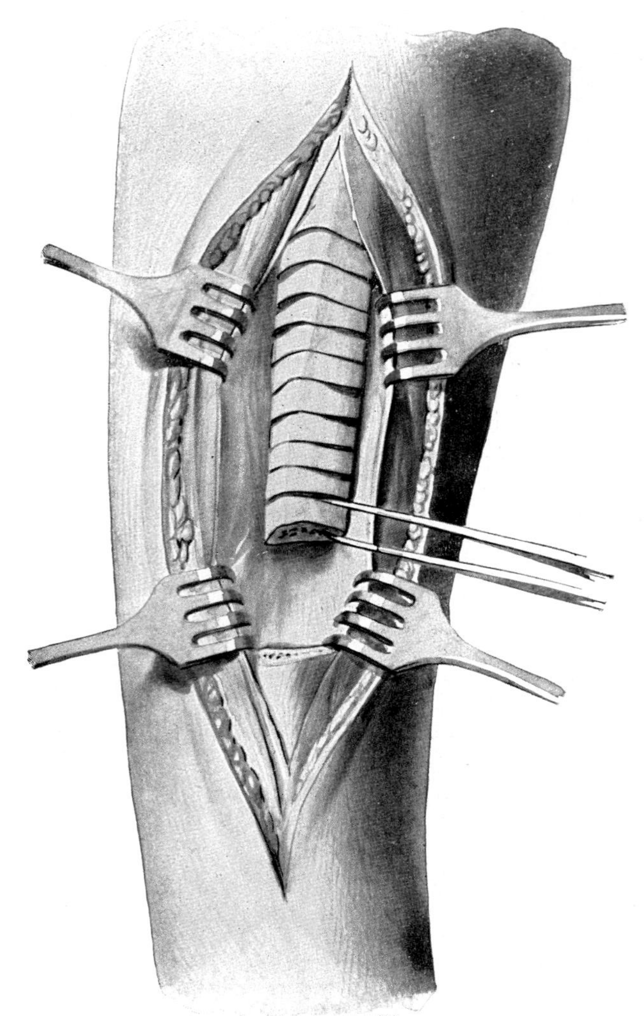

FIG. 643. Correcting extensive bowing by dividing the bone into disks (Springer). The disks are replaced in the periosteal sheath.

epiphyses adjacent to the joint not being apt to splinter. When it is difficult to splinter a bone because of its firmness, the individual splints can be completed by turning the inserted chisel in its longitudinal axis by means of a wrench. Bone treated in this way gradually loses its firmness. Attempts are made from time to time, by applying gentle force to the bone, to determine whether the bone begins to give way and whether it permits of adjustment in the desired direction. As soon as the bone becomes plastic enough for correction of the deformity, nothing more is done to the bone. The wound is carefully closed in layers and is covered by a small dressing that does not conceal the shape of the limb. The deformity is then corrected. It may be done simply with the hands, over the edge of the table, over a little bench, or with

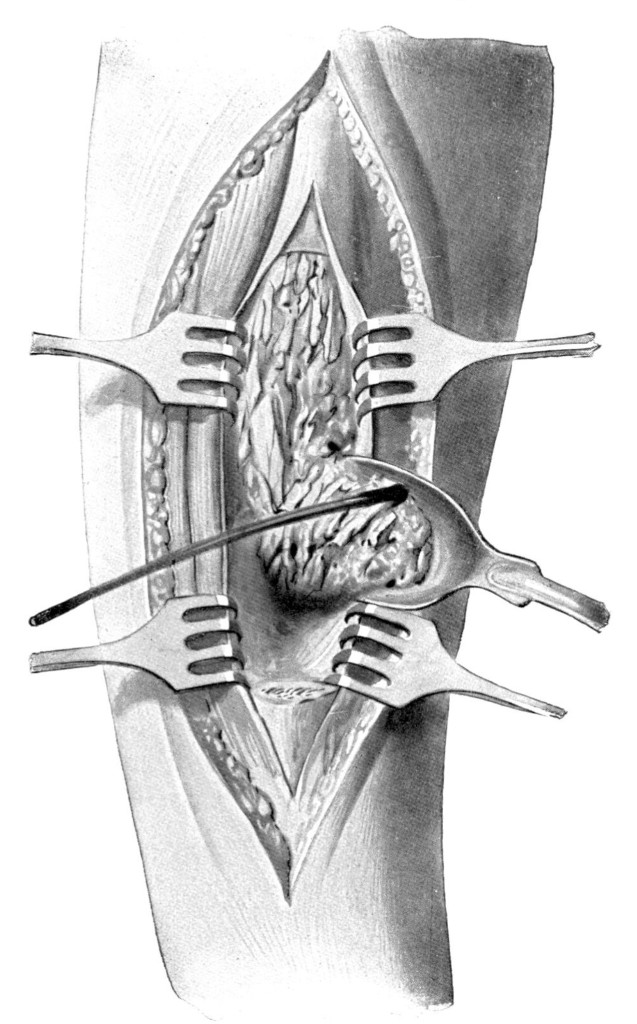

FIG. 644. Correction of extensive bowing by removing, crushing and replacing the bone (Löffler and Voelker). The "bone salad" is placed in the periosteal sheath.

the aid of one of the usual reduction apparatus, as for instance, the Lorenz apparatus.

In this procedure, an attempt should be made not to make the correction of an extensive curvature by breaking the bone at a circumscribed place, but to extend the correction over the whole length of the curvature. The bone should not be fractured in a narrow limited place, but rather the numerous fragments of bone should be displaced imperceptibly, the continuity of the bone being maintained (Fig. 647).

In the case of bones of less firmness, as the bones of children and rachitic bones, the necessary straightening can be accomplished by pressing them forcibly together and crushing the bone in several directions with a crushing tool or a hand vise, instead of splintering it with the chisel in the manner described. This procedure has an advantage over the chisel-splinter method,

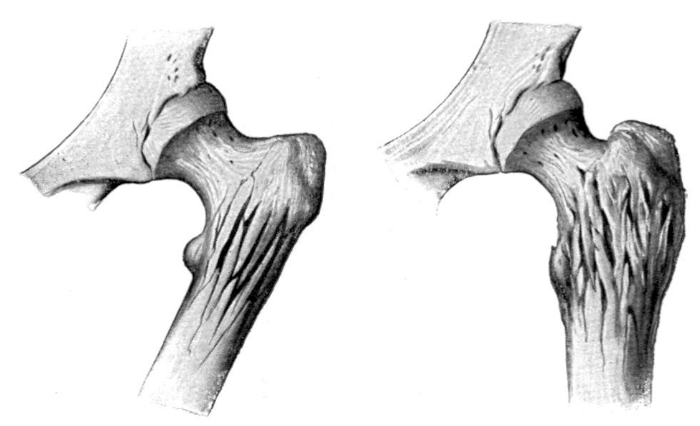

FIG. 645. Correction of a deformity by splintering the bone (Kirschner's Crushing Osteotomy). The straightening is accomplished by imperceptible displacement of the separate fragments, against one another.

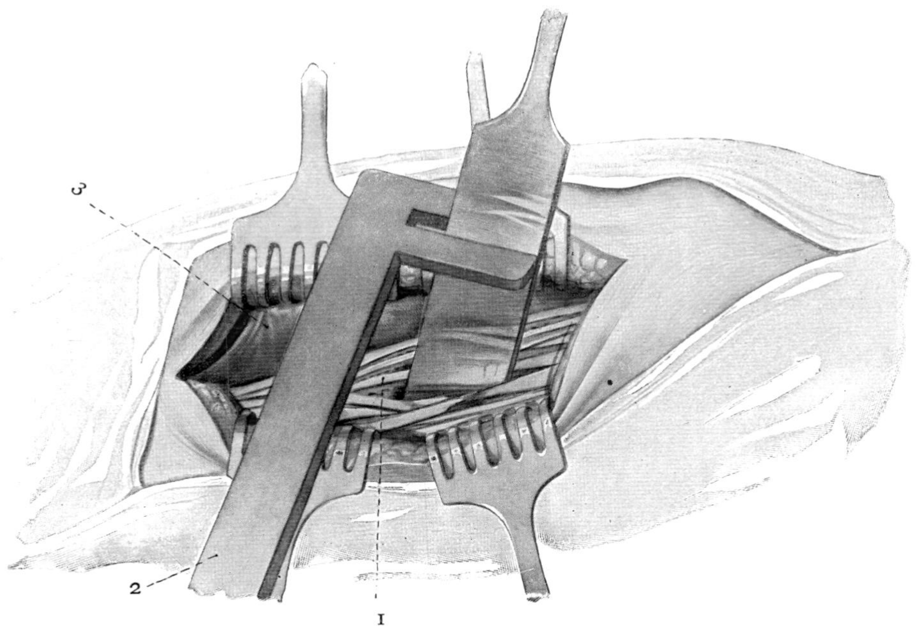

FIG. 646. Splintering the deformed bone with the chisel (Kirschner). The splinters are formed with the aid of a wrench (2) placed on the chisel. (1) Bone splinter. (3) Muscles.

in that the bone may be flattened somewhat (as may be desirable, for example, in the sabre-shaped tibia) by pressing it together, thus restoring to a certain degree its natural roundness.

It is not fundamentally important that the curvature be completely straightened until after the operative wound has been closed. Occasionally, however, it is more practical to correct the deformity under the guidance of the eye while the wound is open. If this is done, the symmetry of the correction can certainly be made uniformly over the entire length of the deformity by grasping the bone at either end of the section to be straightened with two adjustable wrenches and bending it gradually to a proper angle. I have had made for this purpose two adjustable wrenches, the English, or universal screw-wrenches.

After the bone is brought to the desired position by any of the procedures above described, it is immobilized in a plaster cast, or occasionally by an extension dressing. In case lateral displacement of the fragments is feared, when the bone has been completely divided, a cast may be applied without correction and this done only after a period of about 14 days. By this time the healed wound and the beginning of callous formation impart a certain protection against displacement. After crushing the bone may be drawn longitudinally by means of nail, wire, or tong extension.

The first plaster cast dressing is removed as soon as callus is sufficient to prevent displacement, but before it is complete, so that there is still a possibility of making subsequent adjustments guided by the eye and fluoroscope while the limb is fully exposed. The time for the removal of the first cast is usually from 1 to 3 weeks, depending upon the thickness of the bone involved, the patient's age, the degree of crushing, and the extent of the previous correction. After manipulation for improving the position, a plaster cast or an extension dressing is reapplied. The extension dressing should be applied as soon as possible so that motion can be begun.

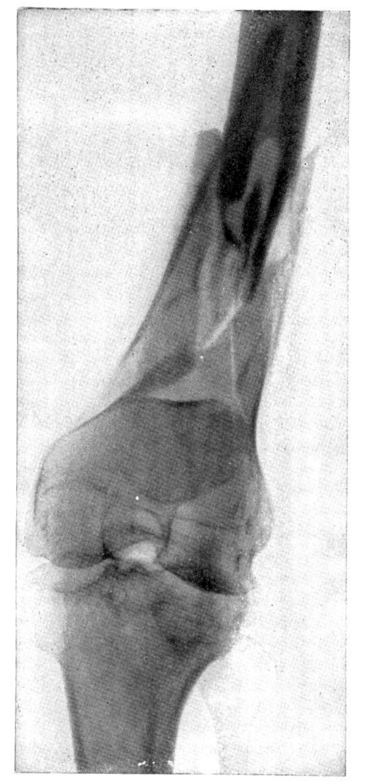

Fig. 647. Roentgenogram of a corrected curvature of the distal end of the shaft of the femur after a splintering osteotomy.

2. Longitudinal Adjustment

1. **Bone Shortening.** It is only seldom that the problem of shortening a bone arises. It may be necessary when one of the bones of the forearm or leg is already shortened and its lengthening is not feasible, or when it is impossible to try any other method to bring together important nerves or vessels that have been divided. The shortening of a healthy bone may be considered when its adjacent bone is already shortened and its elongation involves greater dangers and difficulties. To shorten it, the bone is either divided obliquely and the two fragments overlapped somewhat without being fastened, or still better, the bone divided transversally or in a Z-shape is shortened as much as necessary, and the ends retained by a method of bone suture.

In most cases, the removal of a section of bone from the continuity (continuity resection) of the bone and the resulting shortening of the limb is not desired in itself, but is an undesirable result of the removal of a diseased section of bone. When a section of bone is affected by a tumor with a tendency to malignancy, the amputation of the limb or the complete removal of the bone may be avoided now and then in favorable cases by resection in con-

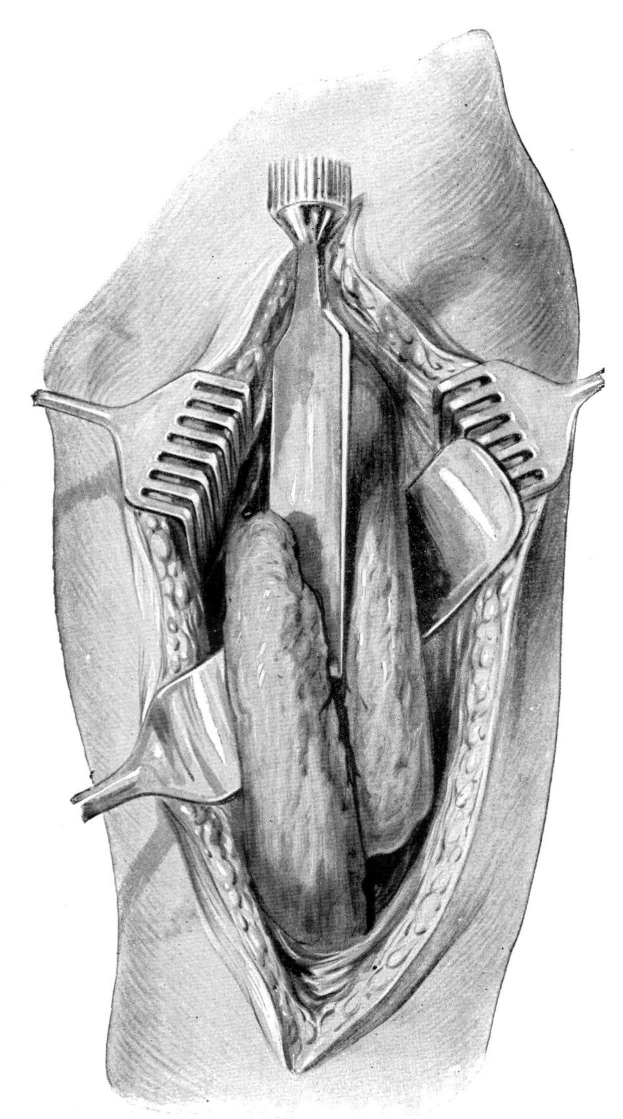

FIG. 648. Chiseling apart the fragments of a fracture of the femur from the surrounding callus, when the fragments have united in malposition.

tinuity. In such cases, the periosteum must be removed at the same time, consequently, an extraperiosteal resection is done. The diseased section is freed on all sides from the attached muscles by sharp dissection, protecting the neighboring nerves and vessels. The bone is divided above and below the diseased area. Should the disease extend to a joint, the bone is separated at this place. The resulting bone defect should be taken care of according to the procedure described in Chapter IX, D: "Management of Bone Defects."

2. **Elongation of a bone** is necessary most frequently after the bone has been fractured and has healed with marked shortening, occasionally in unilateral disturbances of growth. I have performed, for the first time, the elongation of both lower extremities in a case of stunted growth. The site of elongation in such cases is usually the thigh. In a viciously united fracture the correction should be made preferably at the site of fracture instead of in the virgin bone, except in cases where latent infection is suspected, or where the site of fracture is difficult of approach or important structures are endan-

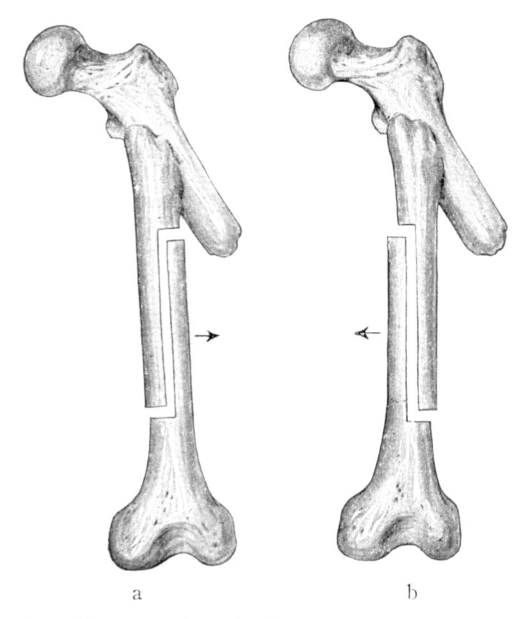

FIG. 649 a and b. Step-like separation of a femur, at some distance from the united fracture, for the purpose of elongation (schematic); (a) the proper form, the new distal fragment lies under the old proximal fragment. (b) Wrong form, the new distal fragment lies on the opposite side to the old proximal fragment.

gered (paracallous osteotomy) (Fig. 649). When the operation involves the old fracture site, the fragments are freed roughly by dividing the intercellular substance (Fig. 648). The free exposure of the fracture fragments from the firm soft-part cicatrix facilitates the subsequent reduction. The fragments are separated with a chisel, saw, or with both instruments.

Paracallous Osteotomy. In dividing the bone for the purpose of elongation at a site where it was not injured, I prefer the step method (Fig. 649). Since I have shown that a femur completely divided and elongated by several centimeters can be rendered firm again by a bone bridge, it can be assumed that the bayonet-shaped division, assuring direct contact of the fragments is safer from the standpoint of union. It is advisable to prepare a diagram before the operation on which one may quickly find the necessary data during the operation. This diagram must show: 1. the direction of the lateral displacement of the old fragments; 2. the position, form and length of the intended step-like division: the length of the step should be 2 to 3 cm. more than the desired elongation; 3. the direction of the step-like division; the step should be planned so that in case of lateral displacement the new distal fragment is placed vertically under the old proximal fragment (Fig. 649).

The technic of bone lengthening when the shortening is not the result of vicious union of a fracture is somewhat different. (Kirschner, Beitr. z. Klin. Chir., 100, 3). The bone should be adequately exposed and the soft tissues protected with metal spatulæ. The bone is bisected longitudinally with a circular saw according to the plans previously decided upon and laid out in the diagram. Various sizes of circular blades must be available so that the

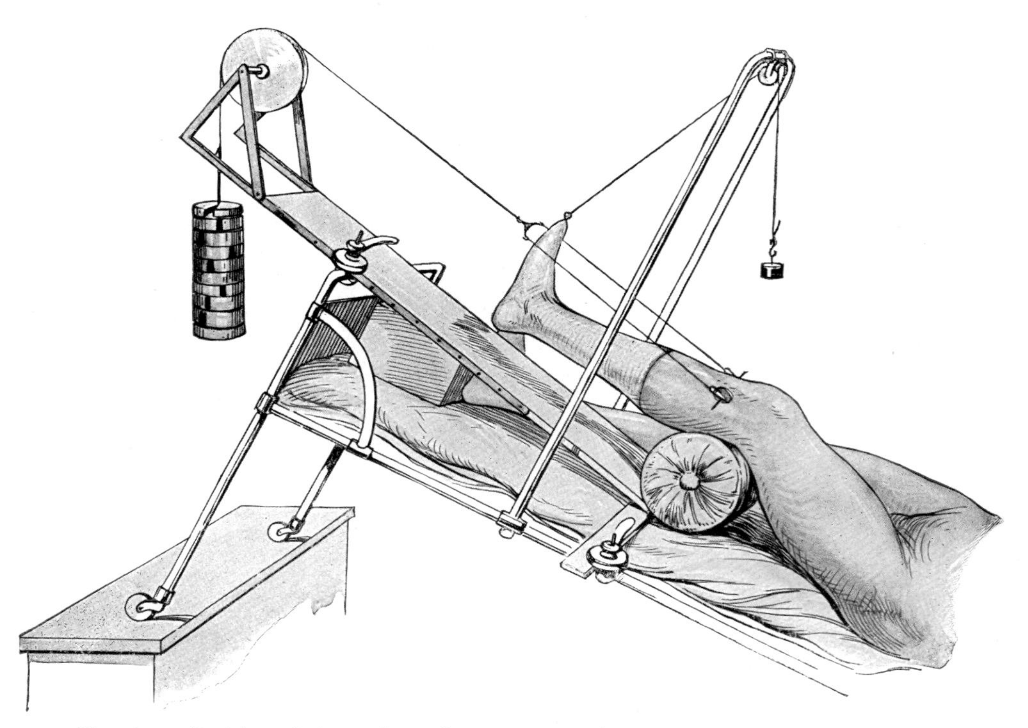

Fig. 650. Position of the patient after osteotomy for elongation of the thigh. The foot of the bed is elevated. The sound leg is prevented from moving toward the foot of the bed by a block. Traction is obtained by a nail through the tibia. The foot of the affected extremity is kept at a right angle to the leg by extension attached to the tip of a stocking.

surgeon is able to work comfortably in the depths of the wound. The blades of larger diameter are preferable. At the ends of the longitudinal line of division the two halves of the bone are divided in opposite directions with the chisel. The chiselling is done alternately at each end so that the final division is simultaneous at both ends, the last spicules of bone being broken. Although it requires more care, complete division with a chisel results in less trauma. If the chisel is used throughout the two transverse incisions are made first and their ends joined by a longitudinal division of the bone. Great care is necessary to avoid breaking the bayonet-shaped processes. The formation of small splinters, however, does no harm. When the fragments are freely movable it is certain that they have been completely separated.

It is impossible to elongate a limb to any extent immediately after the bone is separated. Immediate elongation by force with powerful traction will injure the vessels and nerves. The elongation should be distributed over a period of days or even weeks. Nail extension is indispensable in obtaining the desired effect. The nail is run through the condyles of the tibia directly after the operation. The limb is placed in the usual extension frame with the knee slightly flexed (Fig. 650) and the foot held at a right angle to the leg by a counter weight. The rope which passes from the points of the nail to the extension weights is carried over a large pulley (15 cm. in diameter). At first the weights should be quite light. Only after healing of the soft parts, which takes 8 to 10 days, is the elongation proper begun by increasing the weight for extension. I have gradually increased this up to 80 pounds. The foot of the bed is raised more and more to act as counter-traction, so that the bed finally forms an angle of 45° with the floor. It is necessary to observe constantly the degree of elongation by measurements and x-ray pictures, and to adjust the weights correspondingly.

F. NAIL AND WIRE TRACTION

I consider nail traction as one of the greatest advances in the treatment of shortened limbs. Nails, screws, steel bars, tongs or wires can be fastened through the skin directly to the bone and can then be connected to a weight. Although I have discussed double nail traction before (Kirschner: Brun's Beitr. Vol. 64), in which two nails are driven through a bone and extension is made in opposite directions on each, I believe that this apparatus and those which have been developed since, as the result of my suggestions, are too complicated.

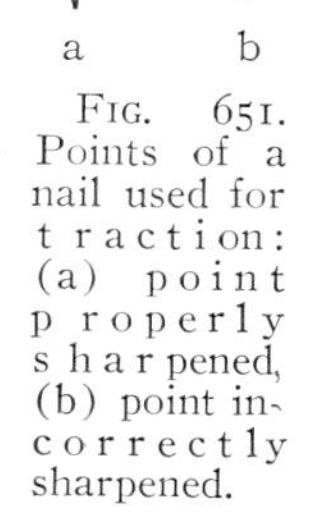

Fig. 651. Points of a nail used for traction: (a) point properly sharpened, (b) point incorrectly sharpened.

1. General Principles

(a) TRACTION BY MEANS OF NAILS

The best form of nail extension is that in which traction is exerted uniformly on the bone by means of a nail or wire driven entirely through the bone. Formerly, when nails were inserted for a short distance on each side of a bone there was danger of their turning, becoming loose, and pulling out, but now those dangers have been eliminated by an ingenious apparatus which holds the nail at an angle so that it can not move, and which by its action forces the nail constantly deeper. However, the short steel points which are only partially driven into the bone, have relatively little resistance from the bony tissue so that, after prolonged traction, they may move forward, forming a groove in the bone, as well as in the soft parts. Nails and wire that are inserted through the bone, on the other hand, have such a large surface of the bone resisting the pull on them that they are almost fixed, even after prolonged heavy traction. This has been found true both clinically and experimentally. When the wires can not be carried through both longitudinal margins of the bone (as in the calcaneous) in the direction of traction a special arrangement must be used for traction.

For nails that are inserted through the bone I use pieces of chromium plated steel wire, 3 to 6 mm. in diameter and 12 to 20 cm. long. At one end there is an arrangement for fastening the nail to the borer. The other end is sharpened to a four angled point. The nail must be of the same thickness throughout (Fig. 651). Mechanics frequently flatten the nail point incorrectly, so that it is broader than the shaft, to avoid "jamming" when it is bored in. However, this "jamming" is essential if the nail is to remain firm. An electric boring apparatus is best for insertion of the nail, though they can be driven in by a hand borer, and the latter apparatus can be used in private homes. Boring through the bone itself is painless, so that local anæsthesia of the soft parts is enough. Reduction of the fracture, however, often requires a general anæsthetic. Nerves and vessels should naturally be avoided, as should the neighborhood of a joint capsule or bursa. The bored canal should never come in direct contact with the place of fracture or with an effusion of blood, because

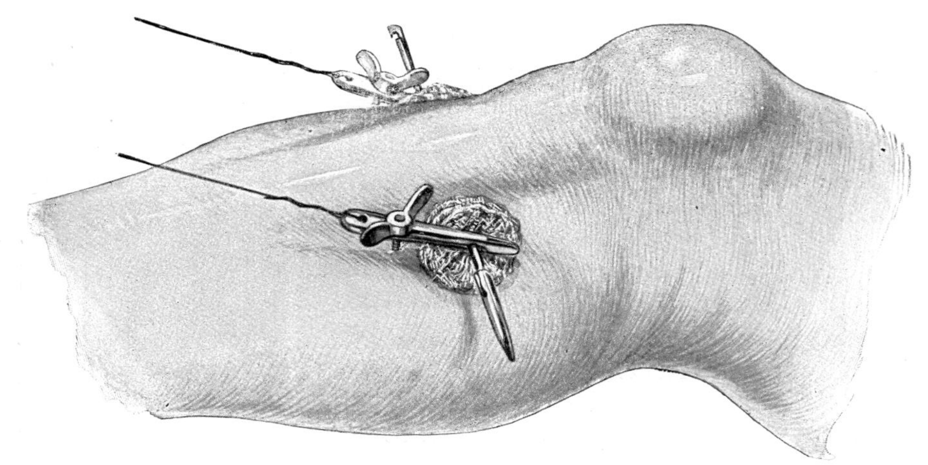

FIG. 652. Nail Traction. The skin at the entrance and exit of the nail is protected by gauze pledgets, pasted on with mastic. The traction clamps are attached to the nail close to these gauze pledgets. The point of the nail has a guard over it.

of the possibility of contamination of these structures. The epiphyseal cartilage should be avoided in young patients.

A chromacized steel pin is inserted through an extremity in the following manner: the desired points of entrance and exit of the borer are marked on the skin. The bone is then bored through from the side where the skin lies nearest to the bone or where there are structures such as nerves and vessels to be avoided. The operator assumes the same position to the borer as he would to the rifle barrel in aiming. The proper direction may be more easily maintained if a sight is fastened at the desired point of exit which can be seen above the surface of the limb. The skin must not be incised with a knife, but pierced with the borer itself. In this way only can infection from the skin be most limited in its penetration with the borer. The skin is drawn proximally before setting the borer and during the boring. As soon as the center of the nail lies at the center of the bone, the boring is discontinued and the handle used for boring is removed. The skin surrounding the nail or pin is covered with little mastic pledgets. A small clamp provided with a screw for fixation and hooks is pushed over each end of the nail, and is fastened close to the mastic pledgets (Fig. 652). The point is protected with a guard or a cork. The ends of a wire of suitable length are fastened to the clamp. The wire is provided in the center with a central hook, to which is attached the line for weight extension. This passes over a pulley having a minimum diameter of

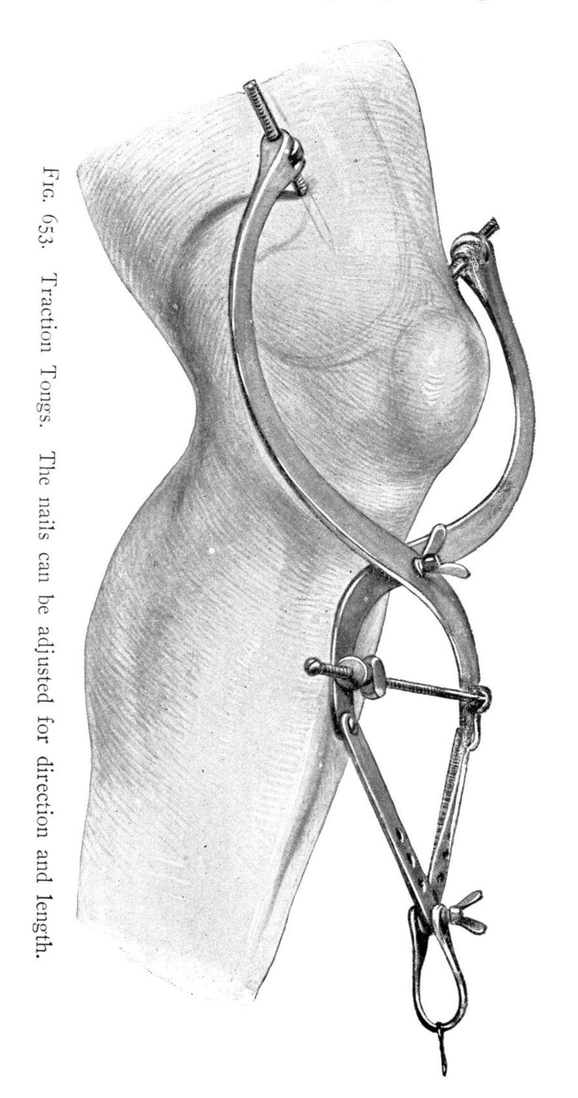

Fig. 653. Traction Tongs. The nails can be adjusted for direction and length.

15 cm. Extension should never be applied to the leg unless the foot is suspended vertically (stocking traction) (Fig. 650).

To remove the nail, its projecting parts and the surrounding skin are freed of all connections and dressings, the skin is thoroughly cleaned and the point of the nail is painted repeatedly with tincture of iodine. The base of the nail is seized with a smooth forceps and the nail pulled out. The openings in the skin are dressed aseptically. They heal rapidly as a rule. Should they suppurate for some time, the wound should be washed out repeatedly with an antiseptic solution. In obstinate cases the canal should be scraped out with a sharp curette or enlarged. It is very seldom that operative exposure is necessary for extensive osteomyelitis following this procedure. An x-ray will show in such case the extent of a subsequent sequestrum. (The Steinmann pin which has been used considerably in the United States can be screwed apart at its middle so that it is not necessary to pull one of the projecting ends through the bone when it is to be removed. I. S. R.).

The principle of the mechanism of two steel pins which penetrate the bone only superficially consists in the following: two steel nails are driven

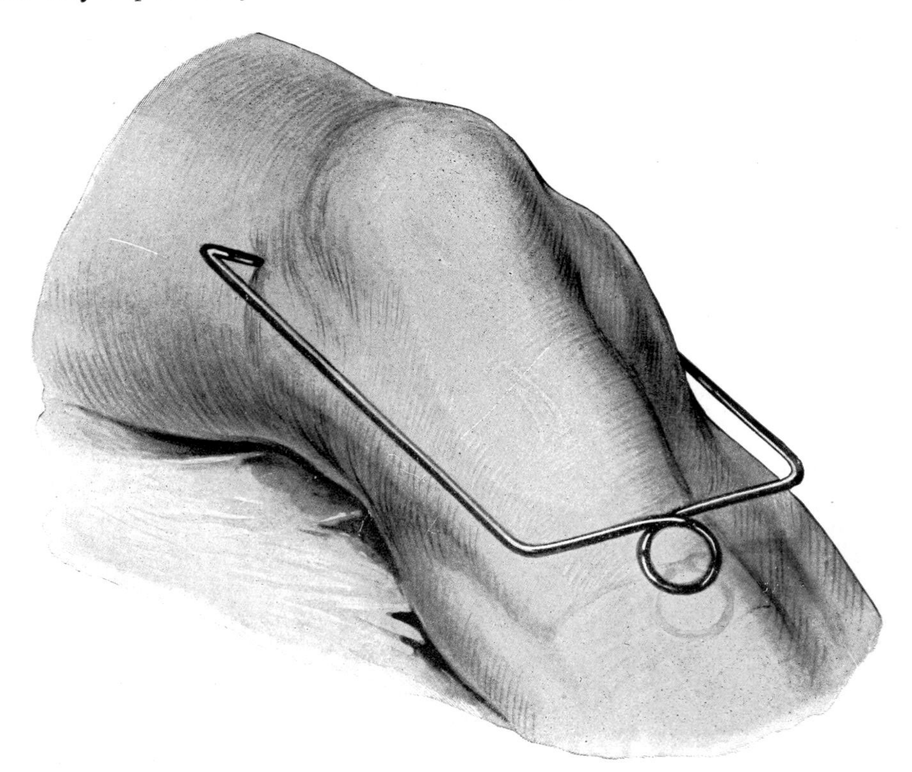

FIG. 654. Steel wire spring traction clamp (Schmerz).

superficially into the bone at an angle so that the inner end is more distal than the outer end. The angular position of the steel pins is maintained by a rigid bar, but the traction exerted on the tongs in the longitudinal axis of the limb or the spring presses the pegs more deeply into the bone. Fixation of the tongs can prevent their deeper penetration. The apparatus is applied, in order to prevent slipping, in places in which the bone below is broader, as for instance, above the condyles of the femur. The tongs most widely used are Steinmann's extension tongs (Fig. 653); while of the wire spring apparatus, Schmerz's clamp is used more frequently than is any other. Both of these can be obtained in several sizes.

The Schmerz clamp (Fig. 654) is applied as follows: the two points which the tips of the clamp should pierce, are marked on the skin with a dye. The skin of the limb is drawn proximally. After the clamp is well spread, the two tips are placed on the skin points, pushed through the soft parts down to the bone, and driven with a few light strokes of a hammer into the bone. The clamp is then weighted.

The tips of the apparatus are inserted into the points marked on the skin in an oblique direction, the inner end being distal, the outer end proximal. The attached weight causes further penetration of the tips into the bone.

(b) TRACTION BY MEANS OF WIRE

Wire traction has surpassed all the procedures described thus far. For wire traction chromium plated steel piano wire is best, since simple steel wire is not so resistant to rust. The wire is drawn through the bone, made taught by means of a bow and connected with a traction apparatus, or a wire may be carried through the soft parts proximal to a projection of bone, such as the tuberosity of os calcis, so that when traction is exerted in a distal direction, it holds firmly against the projection, without slipping off. The points of entrance and exit of the wire are protected with mastic pledgets.

Wire traction had until recently two drawbacks. One of these was that the wire could not be inserted directly through the bone, but had to be drawn through a previously bored canal, so that there was increased danger of infection, regardless of the care taken. The second drawback was due to insufficient resistance of the wire, so that the wire bent considerably when heavily weighted, the soft parts were injured and the danger of infection increased. I have eliminated both of these drawbacks by a special procedure. (Kirschner, Surgic. Congress, 1927). The wire which is drawn to a point at one end is stretched in a harmonica-like supporting apparatus (Fig. 655) and is bored directly through the soft parts and the bone by means of an electrically driven boring machine. The supporting apparatus draws together as the wire advances, allowing the necessary length of wire to come out. Care must be exercised in boring through a bone, to use only moderate pressure and to push the wire forward slowly. When the wire is in place, the support and the borer are removed. The wire is fastened to one end of my extension bow (Fig. 656) by tightening the screw clamp; it is inserted loosely in the other clamp and fastened in the set extension key by tightening its screw clamp. By screwing the extension key the wire is made taut and is then fastened to the second end of the extension bow by tightening the screw clamp. The extension key is then removed. The wire is now very tightly drawn in the extension bow and fastened so that there is no noticeable bending of the stretched wire, even when heavily weighted and after a long period of time. The ends of the wire which project laterally from the extension bow are fastened to it. Such extension bows may be had in all sizes. A specially long bow is used for the wire extension above the condyles of the femur, which allows a complete extension of the knee-joint; an exceptionally small bow is used for extension of the olecranon.

I use wire traction in preference to steel pin traction, since the development of this new form of insertion, stretching and fastening of the

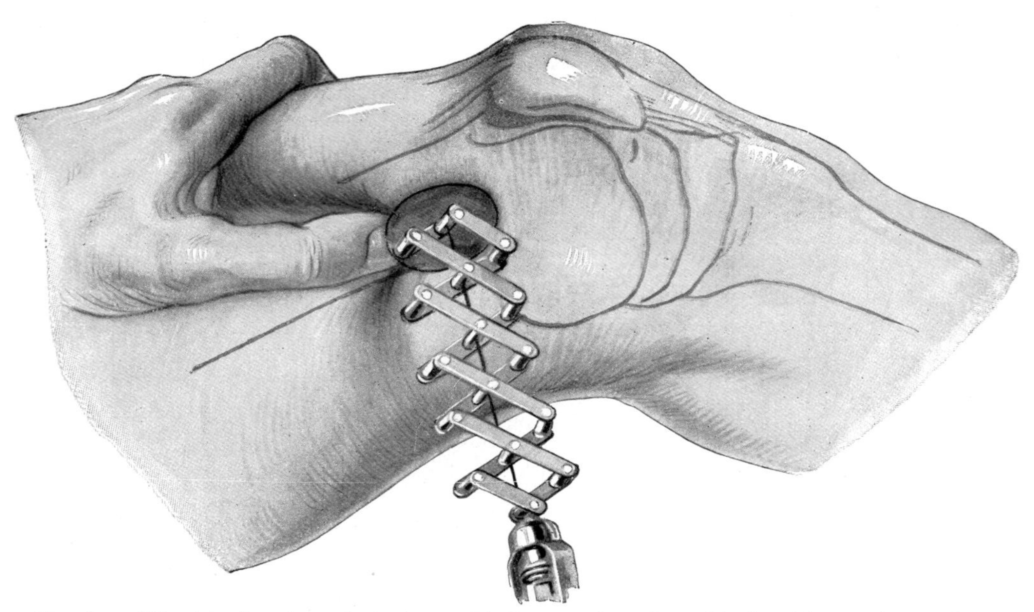

FIG. 655. Direct boring through the bone with fine traction wire, with the aid of an harmonica-like supporting apparatus (Kirschner).

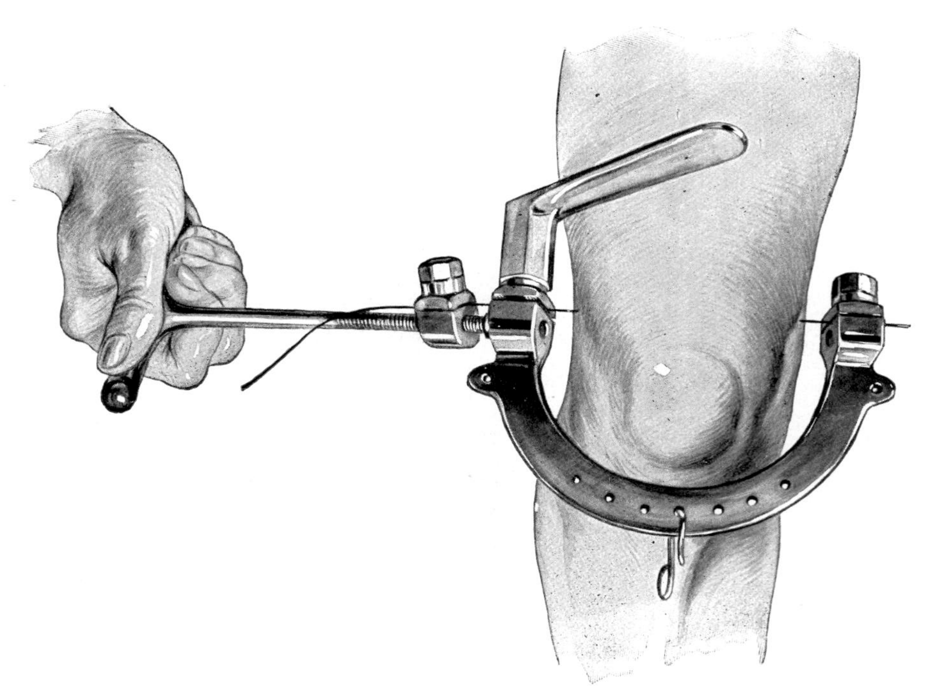

FIG. 656. Stretching the traction wire in an extension clamp (Kirschner), with the help of a screw device. The screw, in which the setting key is placed, is not tightened until the wire is taut.

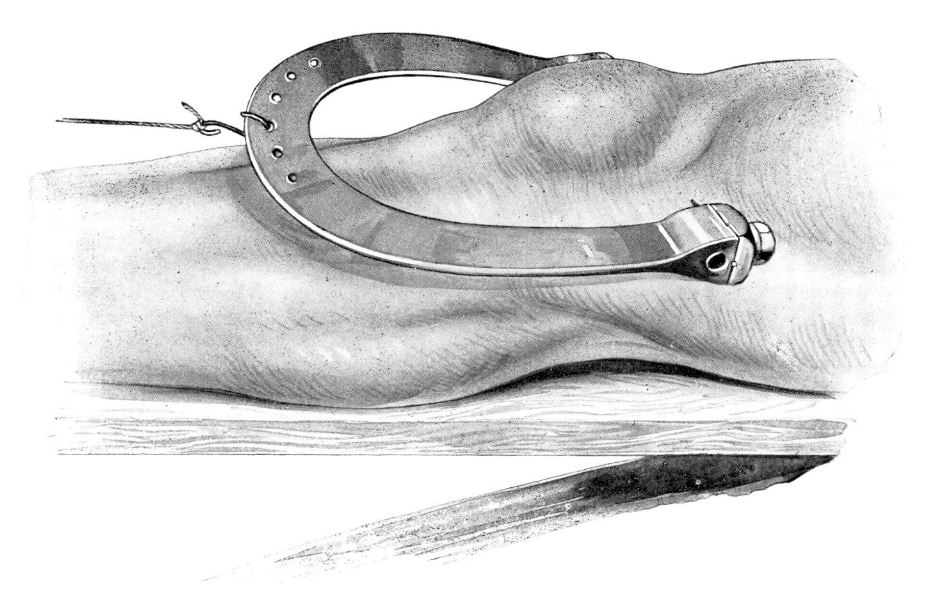

Fig. 657. Wire extension (Kirschner) through the condyles of the femur.

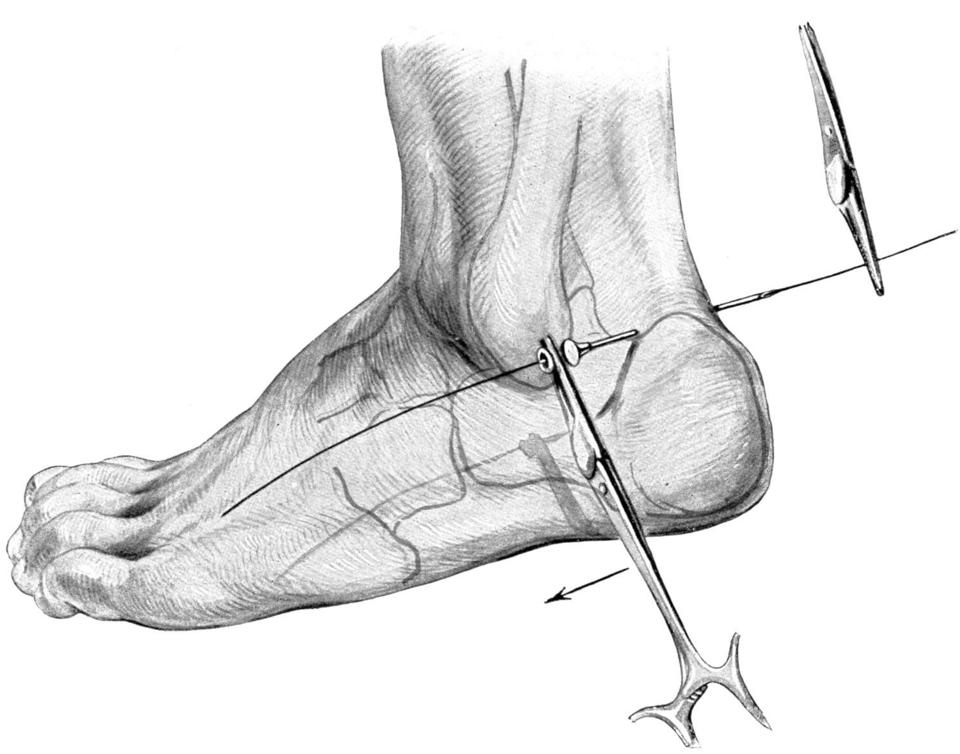

Fig. 658. Simple method for carrying the wire through the soft parts, for wire traction over the os calcis.

wire. Moving of the wire in the bone does not occur even when heavy weights are used.

If the apparatus for insertion of the wire is not available, the wire may be carried through the limb in other ways. If the wire need only be inserted through the soft parts, a hollow needle of suitable diameter is first inserted (Fig. 658), and the lubricated wire pushed through it. The needle is withdrawn, leaving the wire in place. If the wire must be carried through a bone,

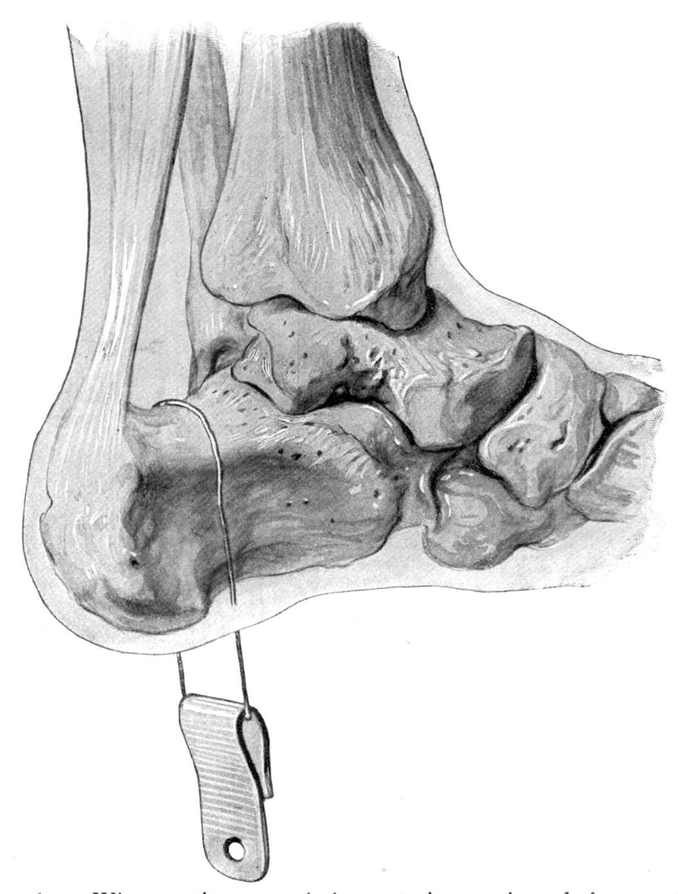

Fig. 659. Wire traction around the posterior portion of the os calcis.

the soft parts and bone are bored through with a fine borer, which has at its tip an eye, the wire is fastened in the eye and is drawn through the canal as the borer is withdrawn.

I use chromium plated steel piano wires 0.7 to 1.2 mm. in diameter.

In removing the wire it is cut close to its exit from the skin and is drawn out at the other end.

2. Traction at Particular Locations

There are certain anatomical locations particularly suitable for traction with wire or nails.

Calcaneus (Fig. 660). The wire or the nail is inserted about 4 cm. distal and somewhat posterior to the tip of the lateral malleolus directly through the os calcis from the medial to the lateral side.

Instead of inserting the wire through the calcaneus, and making it taut by stretching it in a bow, traction may be applied to this bone by carrying a loop of wire around its posterior process (Fig. 659), in such a way that the wire runs in direct contact with the lateral surfaces of the bone and the ends emerge through the plantar skin at a distance apart which corresponds to the

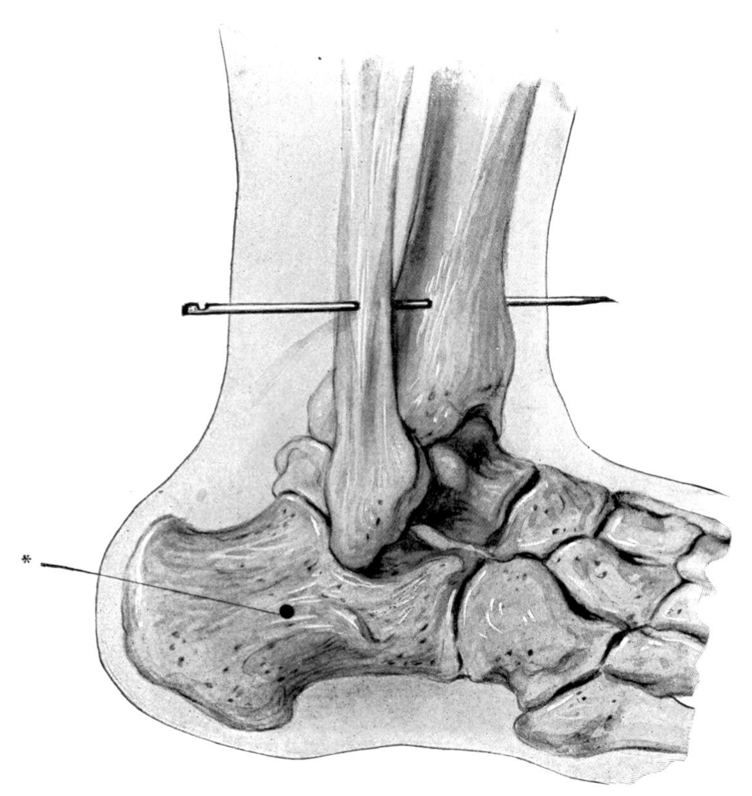

Fig. 660. Wire extension of the distal part of the leg. The black point designated by * indicates the place of wire extension on the calcaneous.

width of the calcaneus. The wire is carried through a hollow needle which has been inserted transversely along the proximal surface of the calcaneus, between the tendon of Achillis and the bones of the leg (Fig. 658). Both ends of the wire are threaded in large curved needles, the hollow needle is inserted in the exit place of the wire on each side and carried out the sole of the foot, touching the bone. When the ends of the wire on the sole of the foot are quickly pulled, both slings disappear in the lateral openings, and the wire forms a loop around the posterior process of the calcaneus. Since I possess the efficient extension bow for wire, I have not found it necessary to resort to this complicated method of forming a sling.

The Leg (Fig. 660). Since the proximal part of the ankle-joint extends

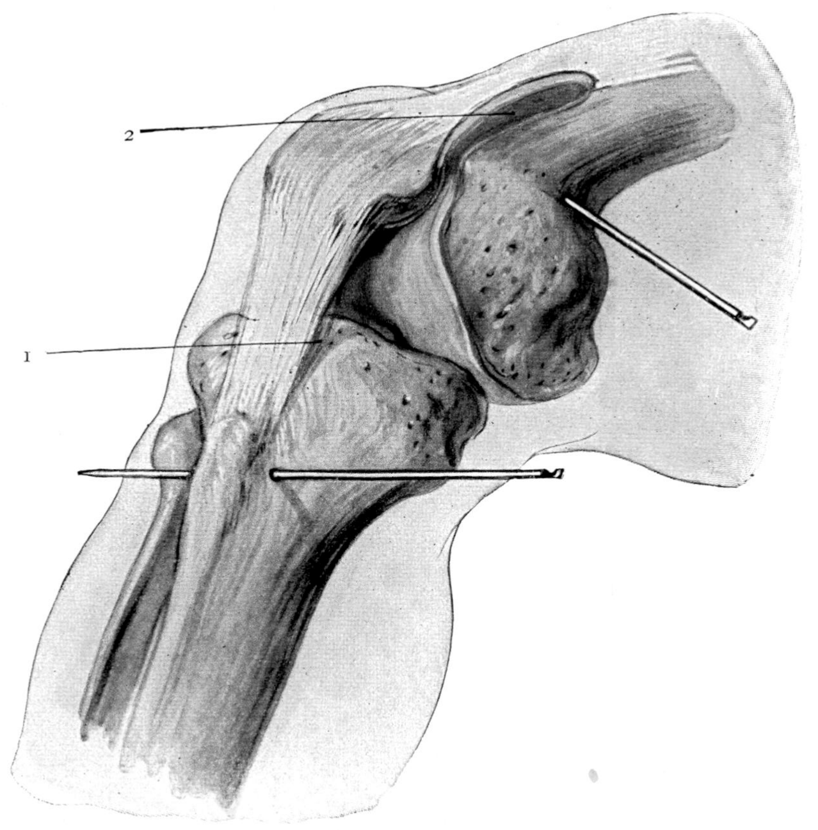

Fig. 661. Nail traction through the tibial tuberosity. Nail traction through the condyles of the femur. 1. Infrapatellar bursa. 2. Suprapatellar bursa of the knee-joint.

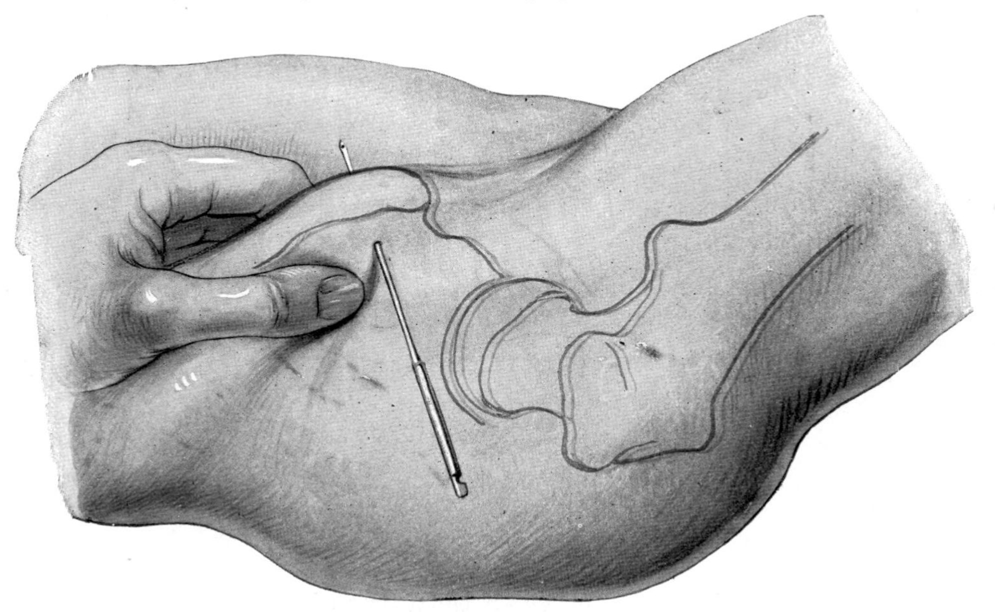

Fig. 662. Nail traction through the crest of the ilium.

upward between the tibia and fibula for several centimeters above the distal tibial end, and this must be absolutely avoided in placing a nail for traction, the nail should be inserted about 7 cm. proximal to the tip of the medial condyle. The fibula is first bored in a transverse direction, then the tibia.

Tibia (Fig. 661). At the level of the tuberosity, the tibia lies directly under the skin and can be bored through from the medial to the lateral side, perpendicular to the axis of the bone, so that the anterior bridge of bone is from 1 to 2.5 cm. thick.

Thigh (Fig. 661). The nail is inserted from the medial side. With the knee extended, the operator presses forward, at the level of the proximal patellar margin, the thickness of the vastus medialis of the left thigh with his left thumb (Fig. 665), so that he feels the femur directly under the skin at

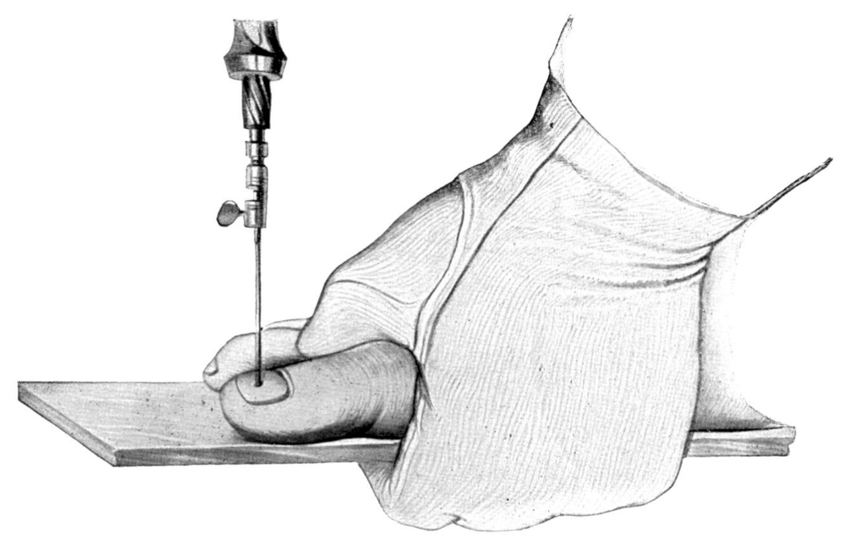

FIG. 663. Drilling a hole for wire extension through a terminal phalanx.

the place where it begins to project into the medial condyle. The nail is placed here and is driven perpendicular to the axis of the bone. When working on the right limb, it is better to hold the nail in the left hand and to push aside the muscles with the right thumb.

Iliac Crest (Fig. 662). If it is desired to make counter-traction on the crest of the ilium, which is rarely used, the region of the anterior superior iliac spine is grasped with the left hand and the soft parts of the abdominal walls are pressed vigorously back from the bone. The bone is bored through perpendicular to the crest of the ilium from without inward, about 2 cm. proximal and 2 cm. dorsal to the end of the spine. It must be done with care to avoid injury to the peritoneum. This method of counter-traction is simpler than one which uses the great trochanter, which is covered by heavy layers of muscle but which may be bored from the anterior to the posterior side.

Fingers and Toes (Fig. 663). The drill is placed over the center of the

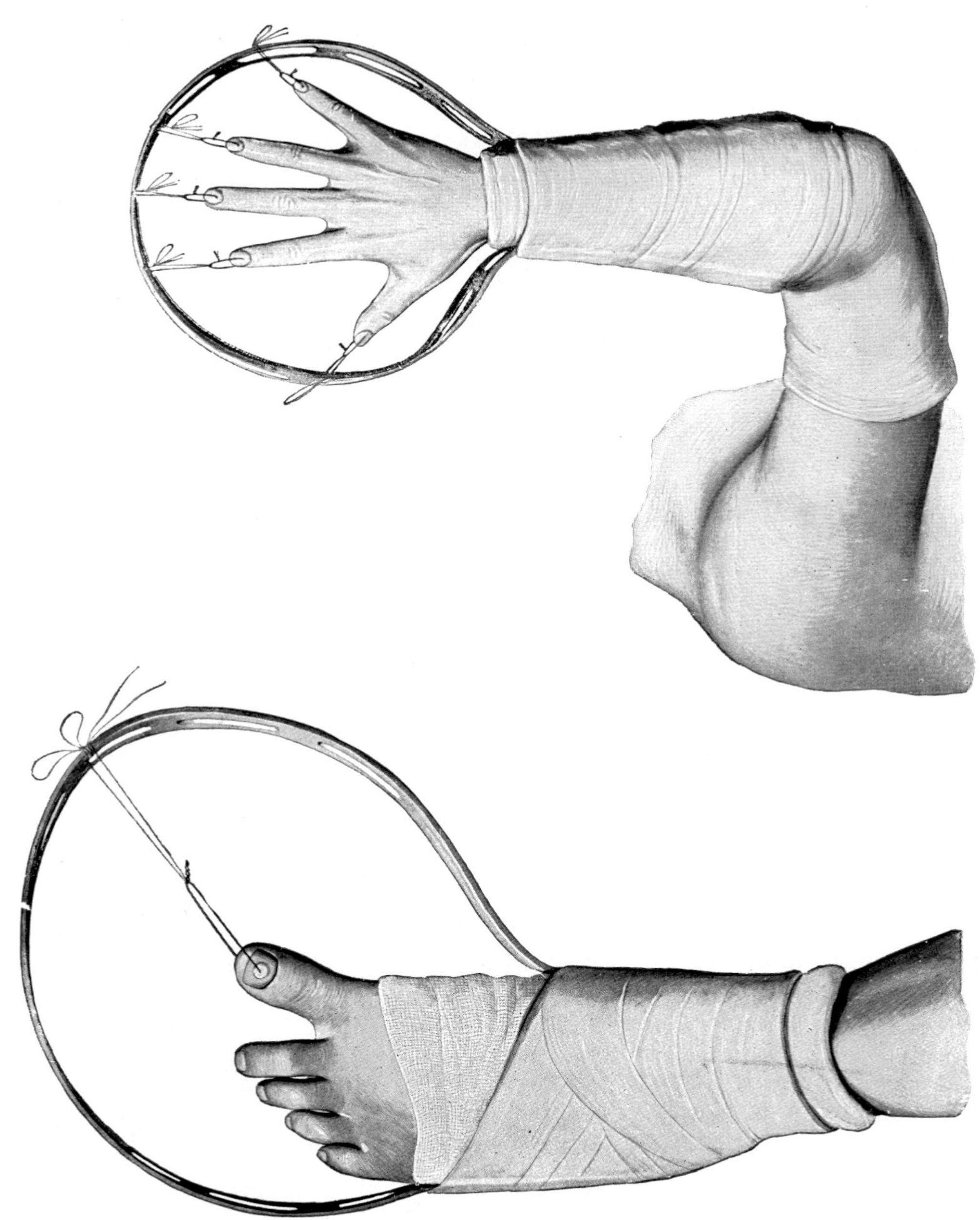

Fig. 664. Wire traction dressing through great toe.

Fig. 665. Wire traction through the terminal phalanges of the fingers.

nail and the canal drilled vertically, as the extremity is supported by a plank. Fine wire is drawn through the canal and knotted in a loop. The traction wires are carried as a rule to a metal hoop, that is fastened over the fingers or toes by a plaster of paris dressing which includes the leg (Fig. 664), or the forearm (Fig. 665).

When the fingers are used for extension of the forearm or of the entire arm, such loops are placed through the terminal phalanges of the 3rd and 4th fingers and the extension is fastened to a wire connecting both slings.

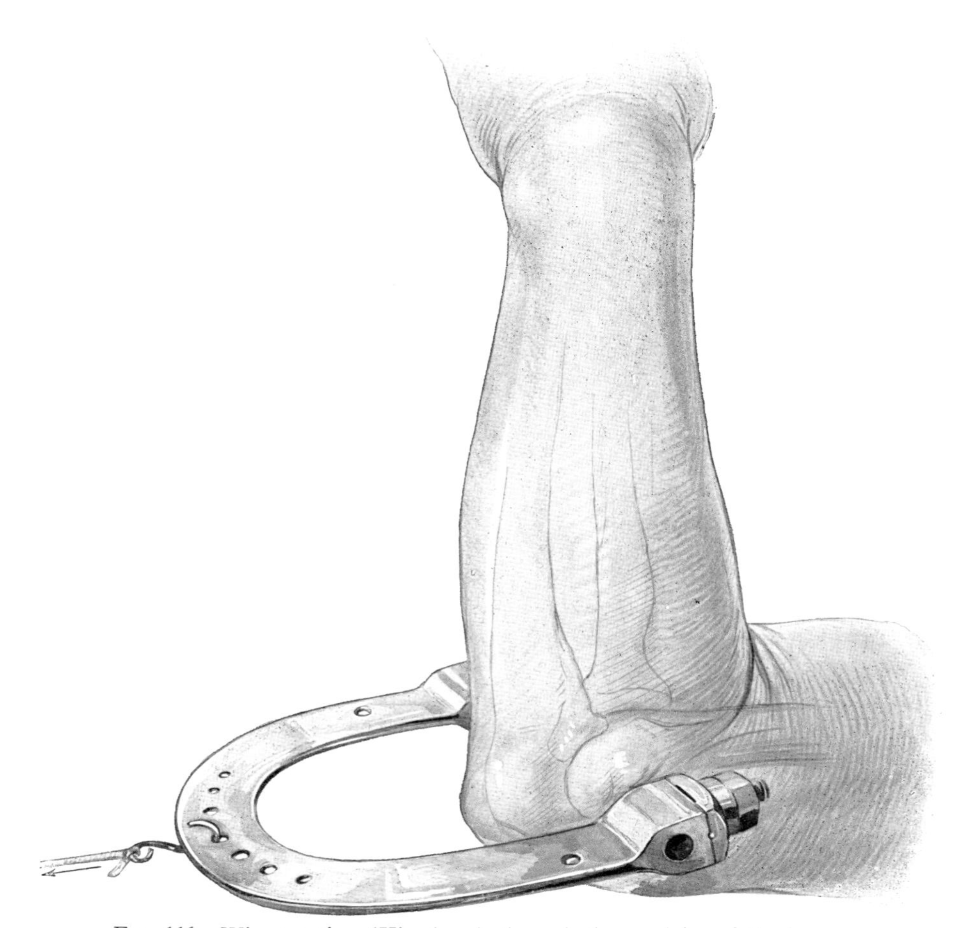

FIG. 666. Wire traction (Kirschner) through the condyles of the humerus.

Arm (Fig. 666). The wire is inserted transversely through the bone from without inwards, just above the elbow joint.

Ulna (Fig. 667). The arm is bent to a right angle at the elbow and the forearm is rotated so that the thumb points to the corresponding shoulder. About 5 cm. distal to the tip of the olecranon, the ulnar edge is bored through from the lateral to the medial side in a direction perpendicular to the axis of the forearm, and in such a way that the bridge of bone has a thickness of from 1 to 2 cm. The wire is stretched in a small special bow.

G. MANAGEMENT OF BONE TUMORS

A cartilaginous exostosis should be exposed down to its base by an incision made over the top of the tumor, and then with the aid of good retraction the tumor is fully exposed by sharp dissection. The tumor is removed with

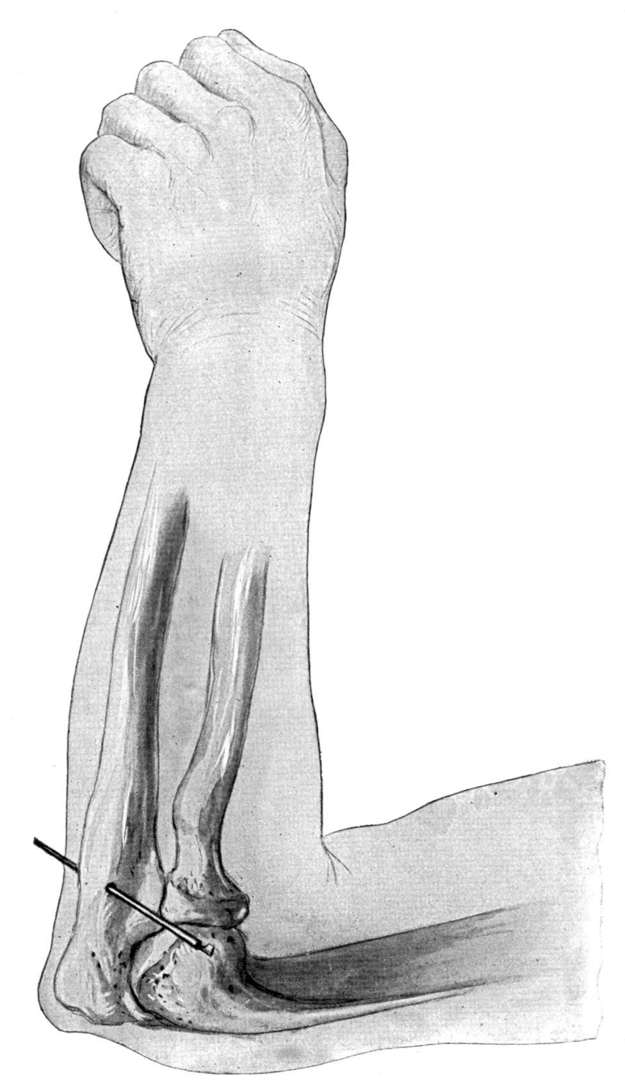

FIG. 667. Nail traction through the ulna, distal to the olecranon.

a Luer forceps or a chisel in such a way that the base which lies in the bone is removed with the main tumor mass (Fig. 668). Its removal can be completed by a sharp curette. If a mucous bursa lies over the tumor it should be excised. If important structures lie directly on the exostoses, as for example, the subclavian vein in exostosis of the first rib, caution should be exercised in detaching the soft parts and in removing the tumor.

In all **benign tumors,** whether solid or cystic, particularly the enchondromata, it is sufficient, as in osteitis fibrosa, to remove entirely the altered tissue, in order to prevent a recurrence. Usually the bone may be easily exposed in the region of the tumor, but sometimes the size of the tumor may make exposure difficult, or, as for instance in the pelvis, it may make it impossible. Whenever possible operation is done from the side on which the tumor has caused the greatest destruction of bone. The diseased tissue is freely removed with a sharp curette, chisel, gouge, and scissors, and, if possible, a portion of the adjacent healthy bone is also removed. An effort should be made not to break the continuity of the bone by retaining a sufficiently wide bridge of healthy bone if this is obtainable (Fig. 669). The defect

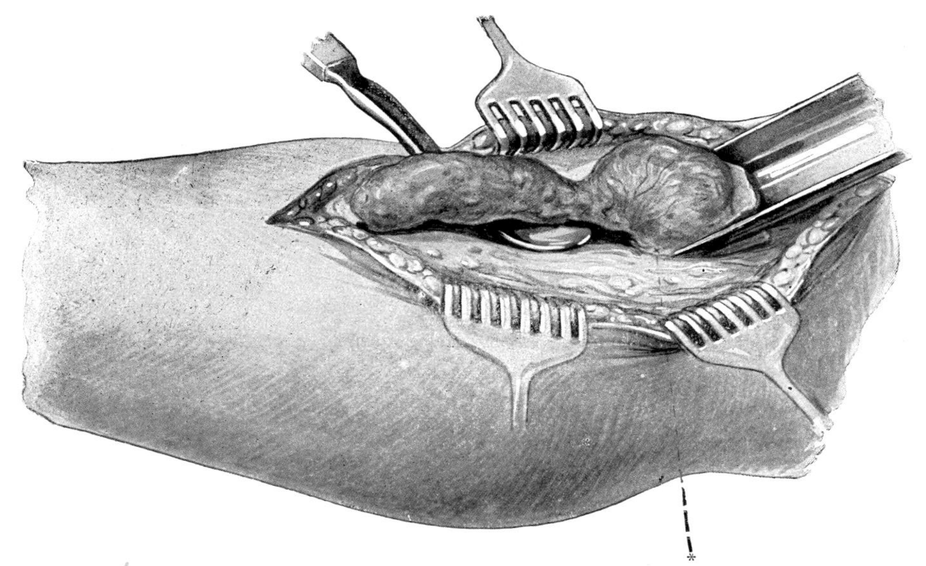

FIG. 668. Removal of a benign pedunculated bone tumor (cartilaginous exostosis) by chiseling it from the bone. * Peduncle of the tumor.

remaining in the bone after the tumor is removed, is taken care of as described previously under bony defects. When the tumor involves the entire cross section of a bone, the bone should be removed in its entire thickness or, when such a tumor is located on the fingers or toes, the digit involved should be disarticulated. This mutilating procedure is necessary also, when a recurrence follows the removal of a benign tumor.

Complete extirpation is the first rule in the treatment of **malignant bone tumors** (Fig. 670). Giant cell tumors, which can frequently be recognized by their brown-red color, slow growth, smooth borders, and limitation to the bone itself, are in the main benign, and conservative treatment should be attempted. True sarcomata, particularly the periosteal sarcomata, are especially malignant. Therefore, only in very favorable early cases where the tumor is still quite small and has not invaded the soft parts should one try to preserve the limb by removing the affected section of bone alone. Usually it is necessary to amputate the limb, so that the entire bone may be removed. Because sarcomata very early extend into the muscles adjacent to the diseased bone, the rule is to remove these muscles as well, in their entire extent. Therefore, high amputation of the arm is done for sarcomata of the forearm, and interscapulo-thoracic disarticulation for sarcomata of the arm. When the sar-

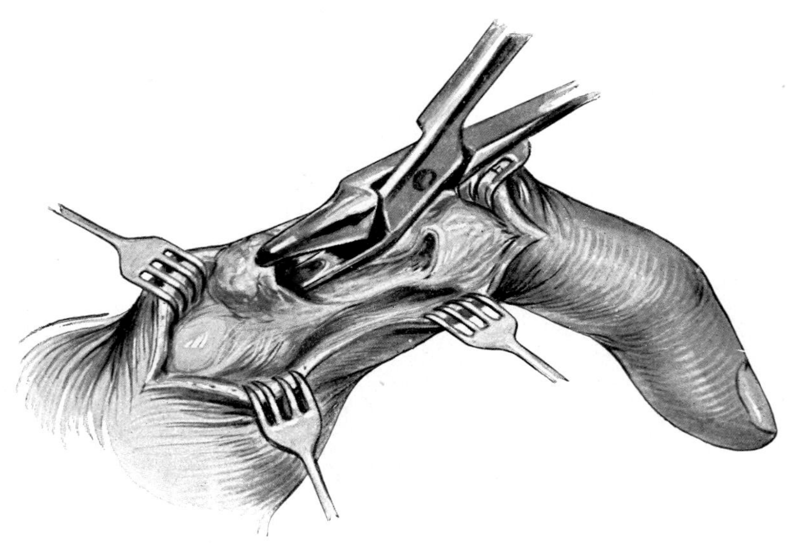

FIG. 669. Removal of a benign tumor lying within the bone of the proximal phalanx of the second finger. A small bone margin is preserved.

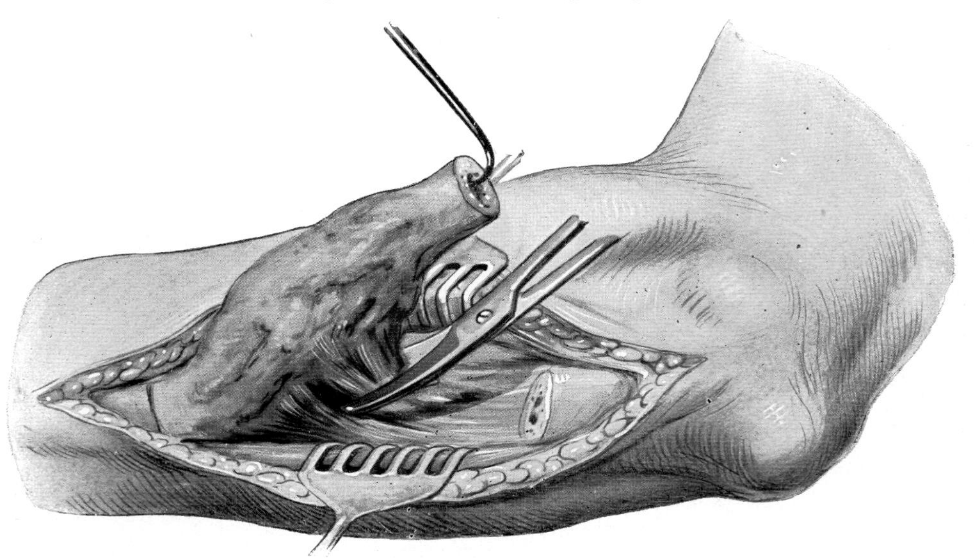

FIG. 670. Removal of a circumscribed malignant bone-tumor, that has not as yet invaded the soft parts; the affected bone with the adjacent soft parts are carefully excised.

coma originates in the leg, high amputation of the thigh is necessary. For sarcomata of the thigh, disarticulation at the hip, with excision of the pelvic muscles should be done, or, even better, interilio-abdominal disarticulation.

When the nature of the tumor can not be determined at the time of operation, a piece of tissue should be removed for microscopic examination by the frozen section method while the operation is being done. If the result of the histologic examination is uncertain, the operation should proceed as in proven benignancy. Should subsequent examination reveal malignancy of the tissue removed, an amputation should be performed immediately.

H. TREATMENT OF OSTEOMYELITIS

1. Acute Osteomyelitis

In operation for acute purulent osteomyelitis, the first concern is to stop the progress of the infection which threatens the life of the patient. This is accomplished by following the old surgical axiom, "ubi pus, ibi evacua". The operation is facilitated by Esmarch anemia since bleeding increases the danger of spreading the infection. The bone is exposed over a sufficient area by a longitudinal incision, in the region of the suspected inflammatory focus, avoiding vessels and nerves. Flap incisions are not advisable. Vessels should be avoided not only because of the danger of injuring them, but also to prevent hemorrhage from erosion. The periosteum is split and detached over a limited area only, so as not to endanger the nutrition of the bone. Frequently the periosteum is almost detached from the bone by a form of subperiosteal abscess, or drops of pus exude from the bone canaliculi, after its detachment. Many surgeons stop at this stage of the intervention.

I am of the opinion that it is essential to open the suppurative medullary cavity. When there is doubt as to where the pus is located, the bone should be drilled with a medium-size drill in several places and the contents of the medullary cavity examined (Fig. 671). When the area of suppuration is located, the bone is opened with a chisel, gouge, or trephine in the region of the infected marrow. The size of the opening should be in proportion to the severity of the infection. In many cases, it is sufficient to make a narrow longitudinal groove throughout the extent of the suppurative area. Only when extensive suppuration is present in the marrow cavity is it permissible to use a curette. In my opinion, opening of the medullary cavity is the best way to prevent a dangerous increase in pressure, an extension of the purulent process to a neighboring joint and its entrance into the blood stream.

The wound should not be sutured but should be kept wide open with drainage and temporary packing to allow the escape of pus. It will gradually become smaller as the infection subsides, but in many instances a fistula will remain, which continues to drain and which must later be operated upon. The affected limb requires absolute rest during the acute stage, but motion should be begun as soon as the acute symptoms have subsided. During the postoperative treatment the formation of intramuscular abscesses and suppurative arthritis must be kept in mind, as well as the possibility of metastatic invasion of other bones.

2. Chronic Osteomyelitis

Cases of chronic osteomyelitis are seldom without fistulous openings to the skin. The exciting causes are either the usual pyogenic organisms, especially the staphylococcus, or specific bacteria, such as the tubercle bacillus.

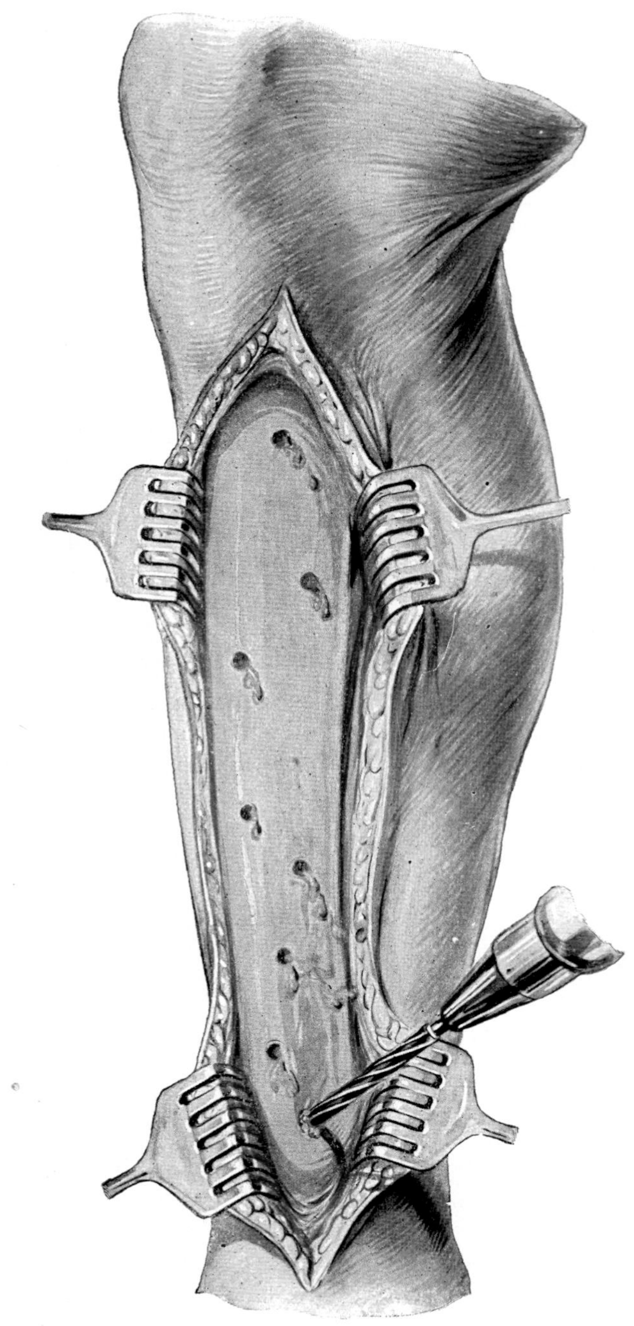

Fig. 671. Drilling holes in the tibia in acute osteomyelitis. The pus which comes from the distal holes indicates the location of the infection since blood and healthy bone marrow are coming from the proximal holes.

The suppurative cases may begin as a mild form of infection from the start, or are the result of a previous acute suppurative process of the bone.

At operation the closed cases may in general be regarded as practically bacteria free, and they may therefore be sutured immediately. The cases with fistulæ must be considered as infected and must therefore be left more or less open after operation. However, it should be noted that in mild suppurative inflammations, the wound occasionally closes by primary intention, because bone tissue is extraordinarily slow in its reaction. We may also attempt occasionally to close the wound completely in an infected area, a procedure that would be contra-indicated in other tissues. The results of such undertakings, however, remain constantly uncertain.

In most cases of chronic osteomyelitis with fistulæ suppuration is maintained by the sequestrum. Sequestrectomy should be performed only after the

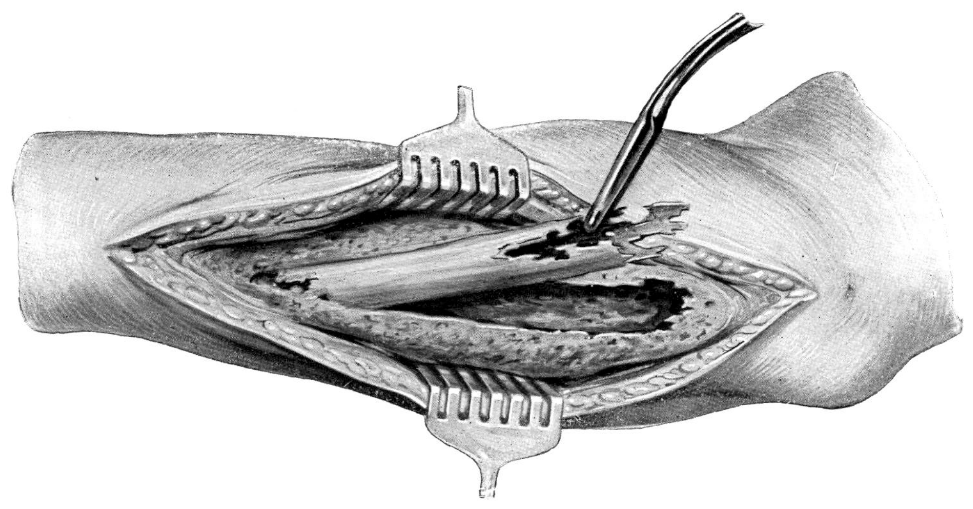

FIG. 672. Sequestrectomy in chronic osteomyelitis of the ulna. A wide opening is made in the involucrum and the sequestrum freed on all sides is removed with a sequestrum forceps. Behind it lies purulent granulation tissue.

building of a firm involucrum and after the sequestrum is completely detached. Within limits, the longer the operation is deferred, the easier it is to complete it. X-ray pictures taken during the interval are indispensable guides. Access to the sequestrum should if possible follow a straight course, in connection with which flap-shaped incisions may be made. Of the involucrum, which offers but little resistance during the first months of its formation, no more should be removed than is necessary for the extraction of the sequestrum (Fig. 672). Its removal may be facilitated by dividing it in two or more parts. Granulation tissue surrounding the sequestrum, which may contain elements important for subsequent regeneration, should be curetted only when it is probable that there are other sequestra or abscesses back of it. In such cases, the entire inflammatory area within the bone must be transformed into a uniform, smooth cavity.

Bone abscesses or chronic granulation foci within the bone should be opened widely by the shortest possible route by removing the overlying bone after elevating the periosteum. They should then be cleaned out with chisel, sharp curette and bone forceps down to healthy osseous tissue.

At the end of the operation for chronic suppurative bone disease, the field of operation should be cleansed with a copious saline irrigation. Other fistulous tracts in the soft parts should be curetted with a sharp curette; after the focus has been removed they heal of their own accord.

All these operations result in a more or less rigid bone cavity, which may be handled as follows:

In the cases closed primarily the soft parts are sutured in as thick a layer as possible over the cavity. The cavity fills up with blood and tissue fluids, which may become gradually organized; in unfavorable cases suppuration

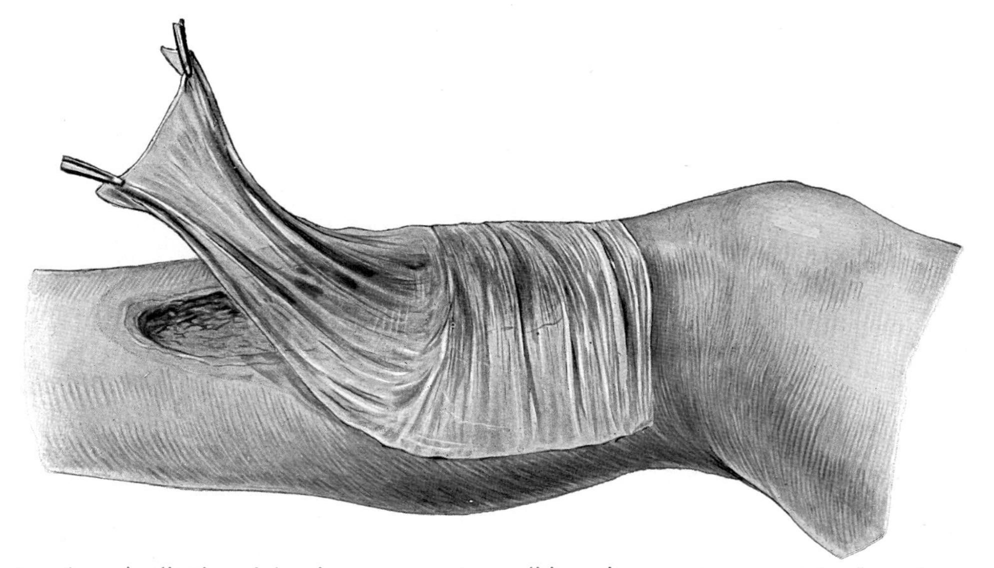

Fig. 673. Application of dressing over an osteomyelitic cavity so as to prevent the flow of pus.

occurs and the integrity of the suture line is destroyed. In these cases fistulæ result.

When a fistula has existed the cavity is loosely filled with a tampon. The cavity gradually fills more or less completely with granulation tissue, over which epithelium from the margins of the wound advances centralward. Deep cicatricial contractions may result from this slow process of healing, which may result in considerable and permanent disfigurement.

I do not agree with Bier, who believes that retaining the pus by covering the wound with gaudafil (Fig. 673) and attaching this around the wound margins accelerates the healing process or that it may lessen the remaining disfigurement. On the other hand, I believe that thorough removal of the wound secretions is a very effective therapeutic measure. Among other methods, I attempt to favor the removal of pus by changing the patient's position, having him lie on his abdomen, for example, in cavities of the tibia.

If the cavity is very extensive, the patient's strength may finally become taxed and healing of the bone may not take place even though the soft parts are united over the cavity. It is therefore advisable to lessen the depth of the cavity by partial removal of its walls. For safety and rapidity of healing, the cavity should be made as shallow as possible, regardless of appearance, but care should be taken to leave enough bone to retain continuity. Removal of bone to obliterate a cavity is limited in many cases by the vicinity of joints, which must naturally remain intact. It is therefore impossible to "saucerize" cavities in the articular ends of the tibia and lower thigh (Fig. 674).

Attempts have been made to diminish bone cavities by breaking in the walls without detaching the soft parts from them. To do this one wall, or two opposite walls, are cut through from within with a chisel until the periosteum is reached. They are then allowed to lie in the cavity with their attached soft parts, thus narrowing or obliterating it. The fragments are maintained in this position by sutures. This procedure possesses no particular advantage, since

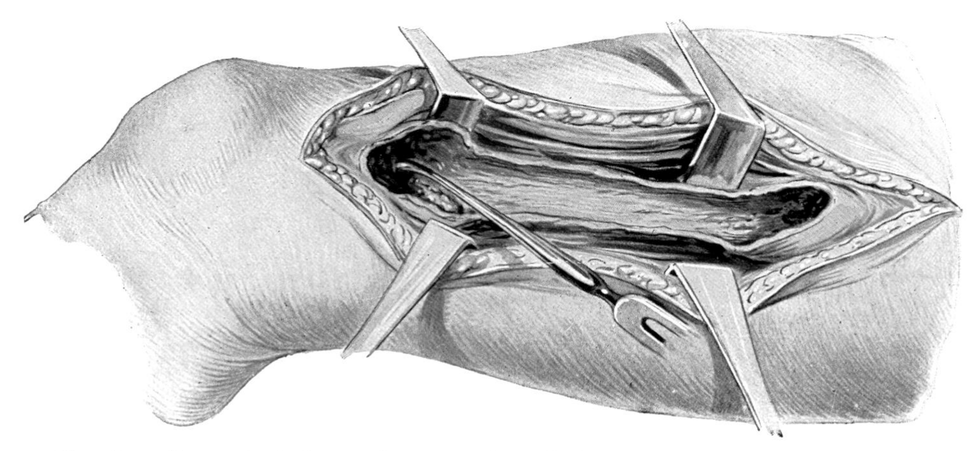

Fig. 674. Removal of the overhanging edges of the bone of a cavity remaining after a sequestrectomy. To avoid injury to the knee joint, a curette is used in the region of the epiphysis.

it results in weakening the bone. It has the disadvantage of endangering the life of the mobilized bone in case of severe infection.

In many cases, a cavity may be obliterated by filling it with some foreign material, a bone plug. The filling should be used chiefly in aseptic cavities, but it succeeds occasionally in the presence of mild infection. The eventual discharge of the filling is frequently followed by obliteration of the cavity with granulation tissue and final healing, without the necessity of further operation.

In other cases the filling must be removed and the healing of the remaining cavity brought about by any of the operative procedures described above. The cavity must be carefully prepared to receive the filling. All the diseased tissue must be cleaned out and the walls made smooth. Grooves and niches are not undesirable since they afford a good hold for the plug. The cavity must be thoroughly dry, so that the filling mass will lie in contact with the bone. Hemorrhage between the plug and the bone affords a medium for bacterial growth. Tampons, heat from a hot iron held free in the cavity, hot air from a fan or electric dryer, are not always successful in rapidly reducing the time necessary for the control of hemorrhage. A certain degree of disinfection may be obtained by wiping out the cavity with tincture of iodine.

The most frequently used material is the iodoform mixture of Mosetig (iodoform, 60; spermaceti, 40; oil of sesame, 40), best obtained already prepared in hermetically sealed tubes. It is warmed in a water bath before using, liquefied, shaken, and poured into the prepared cavity. It hardens within a few minutes. There are several proprietary preparations which have been used, among which is Dermatol. Personally, I have obtained satisfactory results from the use of ordinary sulphur, and from rosin, heated in a vessel

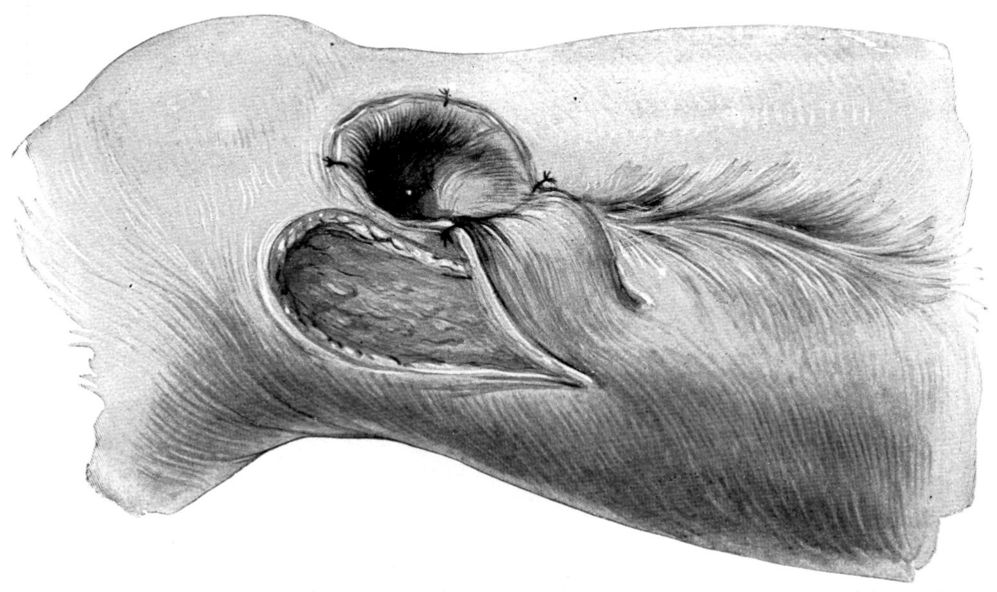

FIG. 675. Closure of an osteomyelitic cavity by a pedunculated skin flap taken from the vicinity.

to the point of liquefaction and poured into the cavity. I prefer these. Lately, plaster of paris has also been recommended.

A pedunculated flap is the only living material suitable for filling a bone cavity. Free transplants are destroyed because of the poor tissue of the bed. The use of a pedunculated flap is in many ways the most commendable procedure. Pedunculated muscle or skin flaps taken from the neighborhood are used (Fig. 675). They are fastened by sutures, or by pads, which are held firmly in place by tension sutures, or by nails which pass through small lead or rubber plates.

There are, unfortunately, cavities in the vicinity of the knee joint whose closure defies all modes of treatment.

CHAPTER X

OPERATIONS ON JOINTS

A. GENERAL CONSIDERATIONS

Joints are particularly susceptible to infection. In operations on joints meticulous asepsis is essential, as is the avoidance, as far as possible, of mechanical injury to the tissues. Aside from the evident insignificance of the resistance of the synovial membrane to bacteria, the seriousness of an infection is increased by the fact that an articular cavity, in contrast to the peritoneal cavity, shows no tendency towards encapsulation of an infection. For this reason, an infection of one area of a joint soon spreads to the entire joint cavity. This spread is still further encouraged by the breaking up of adhesions through movement of the joint, with the result that the contents of the joint cavity are moved about from one part to another.

Therefore, complete and prolonged immobilization of the joint might be considered the ideal method of treatment after operation or in the presence of infection, were there not serious disadvantages. Immobilization constantly predisposes to limitation of movement of a joint. It results in shrinking and adhesions of the capsule, formation of connective tissue within the articular cavity, degeneration of the articular cartilage, bony ankylosis, muscular atrophy and loss of mobility of adjacent tendons. The joints are so sensitive, that even when asepsis is maintained in an operation, there is always present a certain degree of danger.

Because of these conditions, there must be a conflict in the methods of treatment after an operation on a joint. For uncomplicated healing prolonged rest is indicated, but for restoration of function, motion must be instituted early. In practice, the following plan is adopted: the joint is immobilized for one week after an aseptic operation. If healing is uncomplicated, motion is then begun and is rapidly increased. In the presence of infection, the joint must be immobilized as long as acute symptoms are present. When the infection subsides, light exercise is cautiously begun. If symptoms of a recurrence of the infection should reappear, the joint is again placed at rest, but if there are no symptoms, the motion is increased.

Various operative procedures endanger the motion of the joint to different degrees. If there are several operative possibilities for combating a condition, the intervention least harmful to function is always preferable. Such considerations are especially important in the operative treatment of purulent articular disease. The operations worthy of consideration may be graded according to their effect on function of the joint as follows: puncture, irrigation, simple drainage, wide exposure of the joint, resection, and finally, amputation. This does not mean, of course, that an infection can not be treated at once by any method mentioned, for the method chosen depends upon the severity of the infection. The main difficulty in treating an infection of a joint is to determine the simplest method for the degree of infection present. If too little is done the infection may continue and cause sufficient damage so that a more extensive operation is necessary than would have been required in the first place, or life itself may be endangered. Too conservative treatment, perhaps postponement of a necessary amputation, has cost, especially during the war, the life of many wounded. It is better, when a mistake has already been made, to proceed promptly. The maintenance of life is then the principal object.

Immobilization is best accomplished by plaster dressings; on the arm, in the form of a plaster splint, on the leg, a cast. Starch dressings reinforced with wood and pasteboard may also be used. The extremity should always be placed in the position which will later be the most favorable for function. If it is necessary to change the dressings often, the fenestrated or interrupted plaster dressings are as a rule, but a poor make-shift; plaster or wire splints are better. In severe articular suppuration the splint should be applied so that the wound dressing can be changed without removing the immobilizing dressing. Otherwise the inevitable movement during the dressing causes the patient great pain. All dressings intended for immobilization of a joint should completely invest at least the limb on either side of the joint. It is frequently advisable to extend them still further.

As soon as motion can be instituted, a traction dressing should be applied. It is used also when a plaster cast would cause great inconvenience to the patient, as for example, in operations on the hip-joint. The traction dressing has the advantage not only of immobilizing the joint, but also of separating the diseased surfaces of the joint.

Exercise of a type may be started almost immediately after the operation, even before the joint can be moved. As soon as the patient is free of pain, but before he is permitted to use his muscles, the muscles may be gently tapped and massaged, without changing the position of the joint. Active movements are to be instituted after the wound has healed or after subsidence of the infection, the results depending less upon the degree of motion than on the persistence of the attempt over many hours. The constant sending in of impulse to the adjacent muscles is of the greatest value. Passive movements also may be carried out in part, by patients who are cooperative, by the use, for instance, of pulleys attached to the limb (Fig. 696). The force of gravity, aided by a weight, can be used to overcome articular resistance. In a knee-joint which has become fixed in extension the leg may be allowed to hang over the edge of a table (Fig. 698), or when the stiffened knee is in a flexed position the leg may be supported on the heel only and the knee weighted with sand bags (Fig 697). Heussner's elastic splints and Schepelmann's traction splints act in a like manner. Later, a pendulum apparatus may be applied. The pendulum apparatus is not used so much to bring about extensive movements of the joint, but it is used to continue flexion and extension as gravity shifts from point to point.

B. ARTHROTOMY—MANAGEMENT OF WOUNDS OF JOINTS

A joint is opened either for the purpose of viewing the interior of the joint for diagnostic purposes, exploratory arthrotomy, or for removing foreign bodies or movable bodies within the joint, circumscribed portions of the capsule which are diseased, or injured, or diseased portions of the cartilage. It may also be opened for the purpose of adjusting a dislocation which can not be reduced by conservative means, of mobilizing a stiff joint, or of causing a joint to become fixed. Since the cicatrix of the capsule left after every operation produces a more or less prolonged irritation, evidenced usually by effusion, the incision is made as small as possible, and yet not so small as to endanger by this economy the view, the accessibility, or the rapid execution of the operative procedure. The joint should be opened whenever possible at a place where the articular capsule lies nearest the skin and where it is not covered by nerves, large vessels or muscles. Longitudinal incisions are recommended in most cases. Should muscles have to be detached, they should be cut through in the direction of their fibers, if possible. If it is necessary to displace an important muscle, its division can sometimes be avoided by removing a piece of bone with the insertion of the muscle and later fastening it in its old place. In this way, the elbow-joint may be opened by temporarily removing the olecranon; the knee-joint, by removing the tuberosity of the tibia. It is occasionally more expedient and the visualization is better if the joint is opened by two incisions instead of one (Fig. 695).

Since joints can usually be approached from more than one side, since the operation within the joint is often limited to a circumscribed area, and since extensive search over a large part of the joint is more difficult and injurious in many ways, it is desirable to establish exactly the site of disease prior to the operation. It is possible then to place the incision near the focus of disease and to attack it directly. However, a loose body in a joint changes its position within the joint. Thus, after determining the location of the joint body by the x-ray and palpation, we may be disappointed in finding upon opening the joint that it has changed its site and can not be located except after a great deal of trouble and considerable trauma to the joint. When the body does not appear upon opening the joint, one may try to bring it out by milking and massaging the individual joint-pockets and attempt to get it out by various movements. These attempts can be aided by irrigations of the joint with physiologic salt solution, allowing the stream to reach the deepest recesses and then suddenly forcing the fluid out by joint motion.

This search can be avoided if one succeeds in fixing the position of the loose body before operation and cutting directly down on it. Loose bodies that are only occasionally palpable, may require days of waiting. If the body can be grasped by the patient or an assistant, the operation should be undertaken at once and, if possible, without a change of position. In such case, the bone body may be speared, without releasing it from the hand, with a large sterile pin, after disinfecting the skin and injecting the overlying soft parts with novocain (Fig. 676). It is then removed through an incision made directly over it. Or the field of operation and the fingers holding the body may be painted with the disinfectant, covered with sterile covers, and after a local anæsthetic has been injected, the incision is made. The loose body is held by the fingers until removed.

Open reduction of a dislocation (Fig. 677) also begins with the opening of the joint. The dislocated limb is wrapped entirely at the operation with sterile cloths, so that all attempts at reduction may be made unhindered while the wound is open. Both displaced ends are exposed and surveyed after the joint has been opened. In some cases, the hindrance to reduction may at once be seen to be a tendon or contraction of a capsular tear. An obstructing tendon should be pushed aside, or if necessary it should be detached temporar-

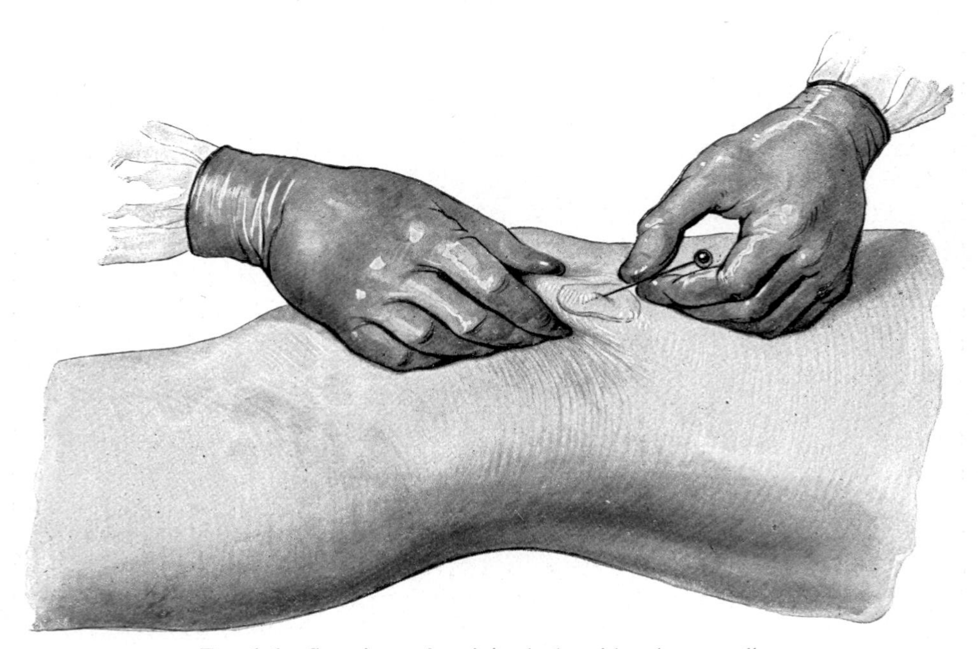

FIG. 676. Spearing a free joint body with a long needle.

ily; a capsular tear should be enlarged. In other cases, an elevator is carried between the two ends of the bones, with which they are pried apart so that they may be snapped in place. Muscles, whose tension can not be overcome, should be nicked or temporarily detached. In old cases the ends of the bones are involved in callous and the joint cavity is filled by cicatricial tissue. Here, the joint cavity must be reamed out and reconstructed. The articular ends of the bones must be excised from the cicatricial tissue and made movable, even if this involves excision of the ends of the bones, and to this end muscular insertions must be sacrificed as a rule. In most cases the bones can finally be brought to their proper position in this way. In addition, in order to prevent ankylosis, soft parts, fascia or fat, may be interposed.

After a successful adjustment, difficulties may be met with in maintaining the proper position. One may try to prevent slipping by deepening the articular cavity, by suitable suturing together of the soft parts, or by fastening the bones with catgut or bands of fascia. While the sutures are being placed an assistant holds the bones in the correct position and this position is maintained until the fixation bandage is applied. The position of the bones should be watched by frequent x-ray examinations in the after treatment.

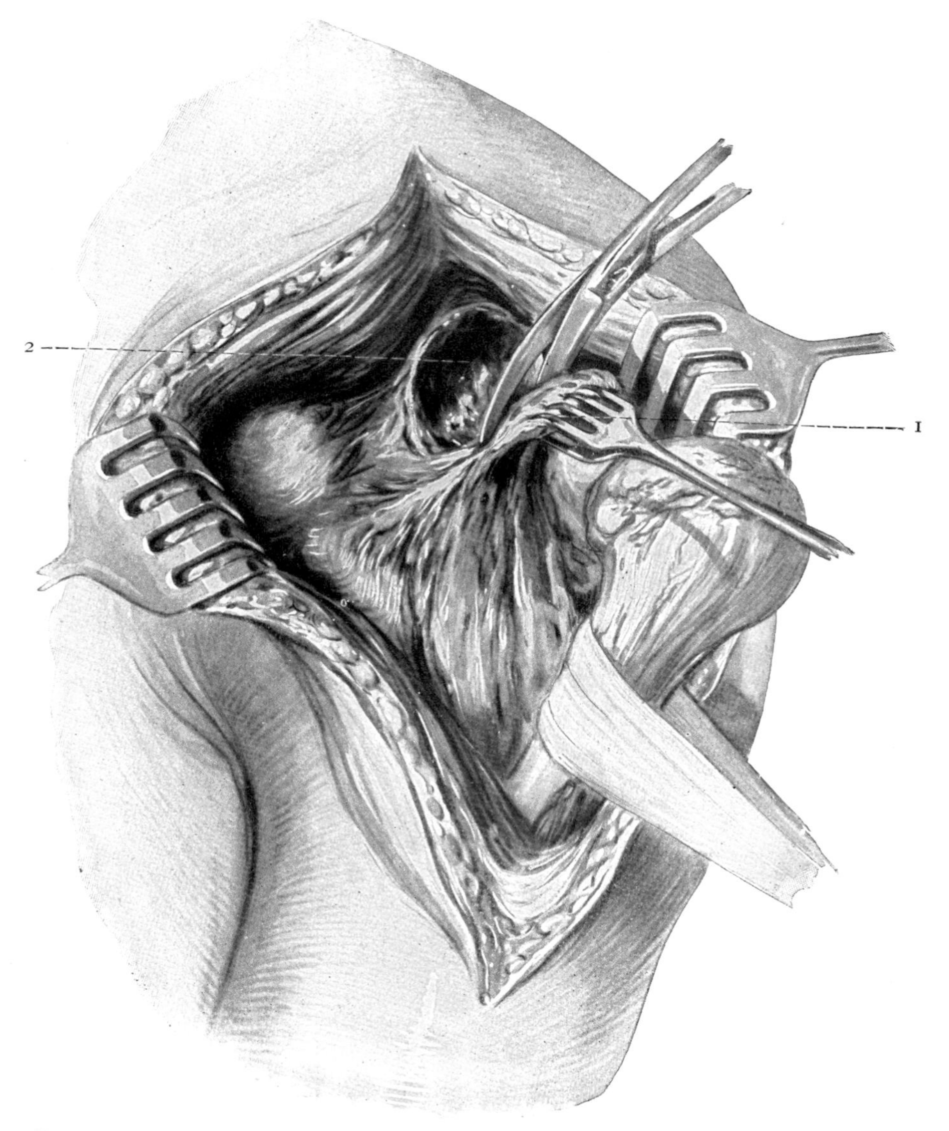

Fig. 677. Open reduction of an old dislocation of the shoulder. The head of the humerus and the glenoid are exposed; the cicatricial tissue filling the joint cavity is excised. 1. Cicatricial tissue. 2. Glenoid cavity.

In treating a fresh open joint injury the first indication is protection against infection. If an infection has not already begun in the joint, the only chance of preventing it is to close the joint cavity immediately. This is done by freshening the wound and closing it in layers. The synovial membrane should be sutured with extra fine catgut, the capsule with stronger catgut, the skin with silk (Fig. 678). If the injury has resulted in a skin defect which can not be covered by drawing the skin margins together, a pedunculated skin flap must be used to cover it. When a wound into a joint remains open for any length of time it inevitably becomes infected.

Whether the joint should be washed out, prior to closing the joint cavity, with an antiseptic solution, or whether this should be done by puncture, de-

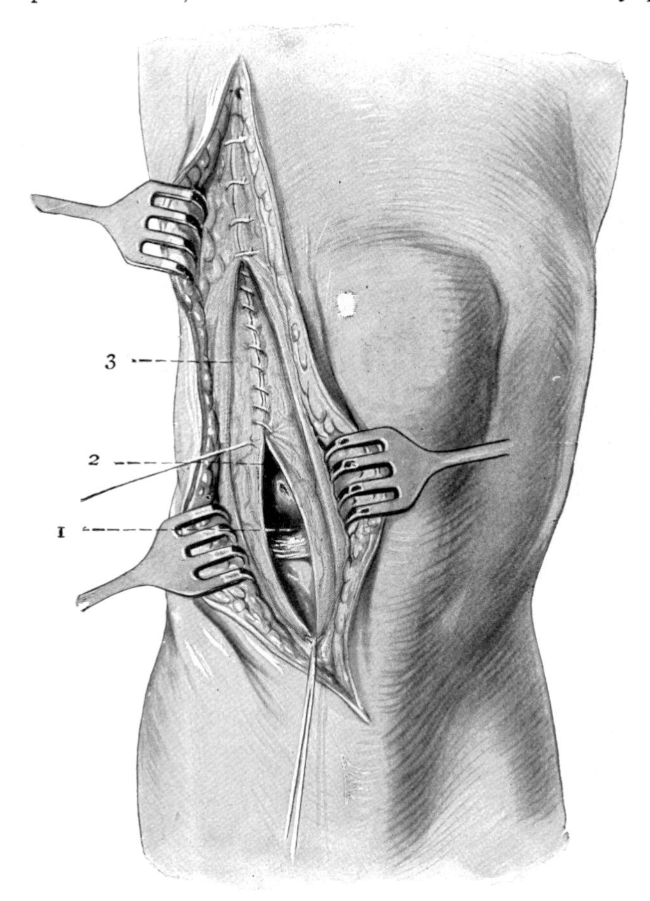

Fig. 678. Suturing a wound of the knee-joint in layers. The synovial membrane is sewed with fine catgut, the capsule with heavy catgut, the skin with silk. 1. Joint cavity. 2. Synovial membrane. 3. Fibrous capsule.

pends upon the degree of contamination, the presence of inflammatory symptoms, and the operator's point of view. As a prophylactic against the development of suppuration the introduction of a few cubic centimeters of Chlumsky's solution (phenol, 30; camphor, 60; alcohol, 10) proves effectual.

Careful hemostasis is of the greatest importance in all joint operations, because hemorrhage does not stop of itself until the joint is completely filled with blood. An effusion of blood in a joint encourages infection and subsequent ankylosis.

A wound into a joint is always sutured in several layers, as previously described (Fig. 678). Drainage of a joint after an aseptic operation is to be avoided, because it is apt to lead to secondary infection. If an infection occurs after complete closure it should be handled in the usual method for treating suppuration in joints. A pressure dressing should be applied after every operation on a joint, and the joint should be immobilized for about a week, after which motion is begun if there are no adverse symptoms.

C. ASPIRATION OF JOINTS

The joint capsule, which consists of an external connective tissue layer and an internal synovial membrane, possesses, especially in inflammatory conditions, but an insignificant absorptive power, though it has considerable secretory ability. Most diseases of joints are accompanied, therefore, by an increased accumulation of fluid. Because the joint cavity forms a complete unit, in which the most remote parts are connected with the main joint, such an effusion fills the entire joint in most instances because of the previously mentioned slight power of the synovial membrane to wall off an inflammatory process. It is very seldom that there is walling off of any of the normal channels of communication with the various recesses or bursæ around a joint, for example, of the superior recess of the knee-joint. If this should occur a bursa alone may be affected, or it may remain unaffected when the main joint is diseased.

A joint may be aspirated, as is any collection of fluid, for diagnostic or therapeutic purposes, or for both.

Diagnostically, aspiration is often done to determine whether there is a collection of fluid in a given joint. This can not always be determined by external examination, especially in poorly accessible joints or in the presence of a thickened capsule, or hypertrophy of the villi. If aspiration elicits the presence of fluid, it is important to determine its nature, whether it is simply an increase of the joint fluid, a serous, fibrinous, purulent or ichorous effusion; whether the effusion contains blood or is blood; whether the fluid is yellowish or has a greenish tinge; whether it has a particular odor. The microscopic examination of the precipitate after centrifugation will show the content of white and red blood corpuscles, fat, or tumor constituents, and often permit of the recognition of bacteria. Bacteriologic cultures and animal inoculation determine the individual types of bacteria. The aspirated fluid is frequently useful for a Wassermann examination. Therapeutically, aspiration serves chiefly for removal of fluid. The absorption of a joint effusion, in the presence of an inflamed capsule with a low absorbing capacity, takes a long time or may never take place. The evacuation by puncture may be repeated if need be, and the withdrawal of the fluid may induce or hasten healing under favorable circumstances. In a purulent effusion, the increased pressure, which favors the infection, is decreased by aspiration.

A puncture serves further as a therapeutic measure by making possible irrigation of the joint, or the introduction of an antiseptic solution. For irrigation saline solution is used, or an antiseptic solution, such as a 3 percent solution of phenol, 2 percent sagrotan, rivanol, or a host of other solutions may be used. The solution is allowed to flow in from an irrigator placed not over a 0.5 meter above the insertion of the needle till the joint is completely filled. The tubing is then removed and the fluid permitted to flow out of the needle, finally emptying the joint by gentle milking of the capsule or by aspiration. Irrigation is repeated until the solution returns clear. At the final irrigation the joint may be completely emptied, or, in order to obtain prolonged action of the antiseptic, part of the fluid may be left in.

If a more concentrated solution is to be used, the joint is irrigated, and then completely filled with 5 to 20 cc. of the stronger solution by means of a syringe. The solution is distributed throughout the joint by gentle stroking. In tuberculosis a 10 percent solution of iodoform in glycerin is useful. In purulent infections Chlumsky's solution, vucin, or rivanol 1 to 500, may be used, and in gonorrheal arthritis a 2.5 percent solution of protargol.

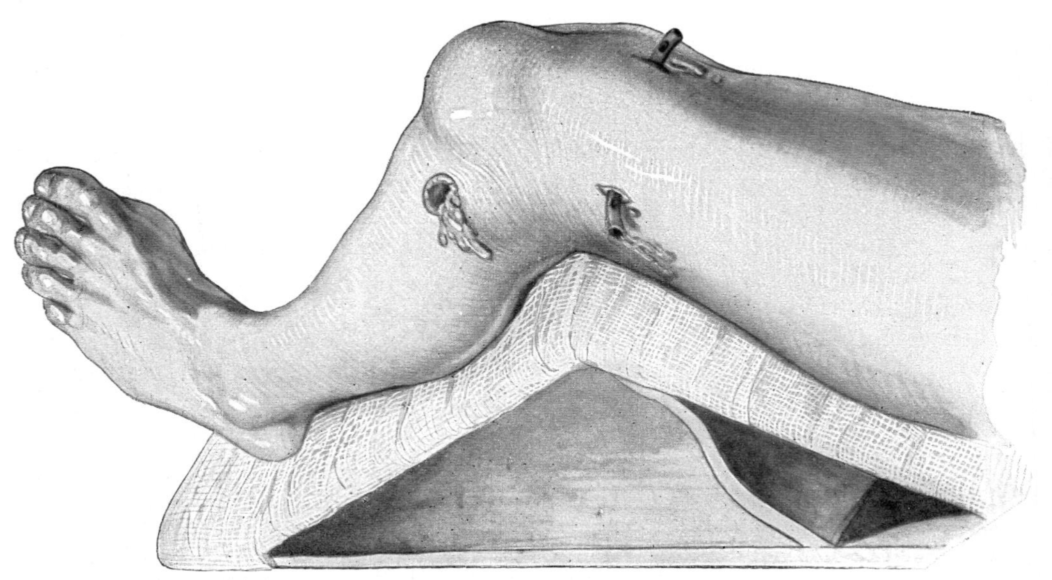

Fig. 679. Drainage of the knee-joint. Dependent drainage is established by the distal incisions. A rubber drain is pulled across the upper recess of the joint.

According to Payr, if the capsular space of a dislocated joint is filled with a solution of novocain, reduction is facilitated and rendered painless.

To obtain a better roentgenologic exhibition of foci of disease within a joint, especially of free joint bodies or roughness over the joint surfaces, the joint may be filled with air before the picture is taken. A rubber bulb is attached to a fine needle inserted in the joint, and air is carefully injected until the joint cavity is well filled and the patient experiences the sensation of slight tension. The needle is then withdrawn and the roentgenogram taken. Stereoscopic plates are most useful. As soon as this is done, the air is released by a second puncture, for if left in the joint it would take some time for it to be absorbed.

The technic of aspiration is the same as that used for the aspiration of abscesses, which has been previously described in Chapter III. It is a mistake to use too fine a needle for aspiration of a joint. However, a needle should be used whenever possible, and a trocar and cannula only when necessary. If a cannula has to be used, one should not forget to suture immediately the small skin incision made before its insertion, because of the susceptibility of the joint to infection.

D. DRAINAGE OF JOINTS

In severe infection, continuous drainage must be provided for the pus which is continually forming within the joint. Drainage should be established at the most accessible sites which drain the most dependent part of the infection with the patient in the customary position (Fig. 679). Sometimes it is necessary to adopt a more radical method of treatment to establish good drainage, as the partial chiseling off of the condyles of the femur for the drainage of the posterior recess of the knee-joint. In most cases one point of drainage is not sufficient but 2, 4, or even 6 openings may be necessary.

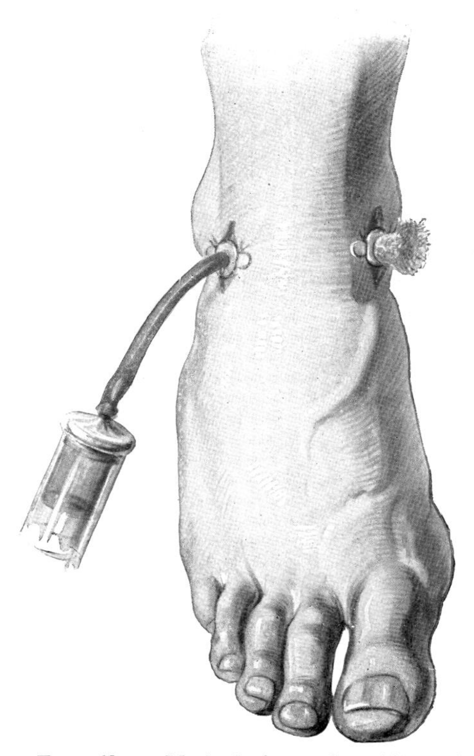

Fig. 680. Method for using bilateral glass drains in the ankle-joint (Payr). The solution to be used is injected through one drain while the opposite one is plugged with gauze.

For small joints, situated just beneath the skin, as for example, an interphalangeal joint, a simple incision through the overlying layers, arthrostomy, is frequently sufficient. When the walls of such an incision have a tendency to close, they may be kept open by rubber tissue or by drains which have been cut in half. In cases where the covering layers are much thicker (Fig. 679), drainage is best obtained through cutting out a hole. The insertion of drains is essential for large joints and severe suppuration. I prefer the rubber drains for this, since they best protect the tissues. The incisions required for the insertion of the drains should not be larger than necessary for easy passage. The drains should not project into the joint cavity itself, but they should merely hold apart the soft parts between skin and synovial membrane. Only in severe suppuration, and then for the shortest possible time, are the drains carried through the joint cavity itself, so that they project from two places.

A properly placed drain forms an outlet for any purulent fluid forming in the joint cavity. As a result of the joint being emptied, the inflamed walls of the capsule come in contact, and there is an excellent opportunity for them to become adherent. Ankylosis of the joint is unfortunately favored by this. For this reason, Payr recommends a middle path between drainage and pus retention (Fig. 680). Short glass drains are sutured into incisions which lead into the joint so that there is no leakage around them. Through the drains a phenol-camphor solution is injected by means of a syringe and fine Nelaton catheter, after which the opening is closed with a gauze plug. The joint capsule is extended by the phenol-camphor introduced and the pus which collects in it. The contents of the joint are drained off from time to time by removing the gauze plugs, fresh phenol-camphor is injected and the drainage opening is again closed.

As soon as the infection subsides, the drainage is removed and early motion is instituted.

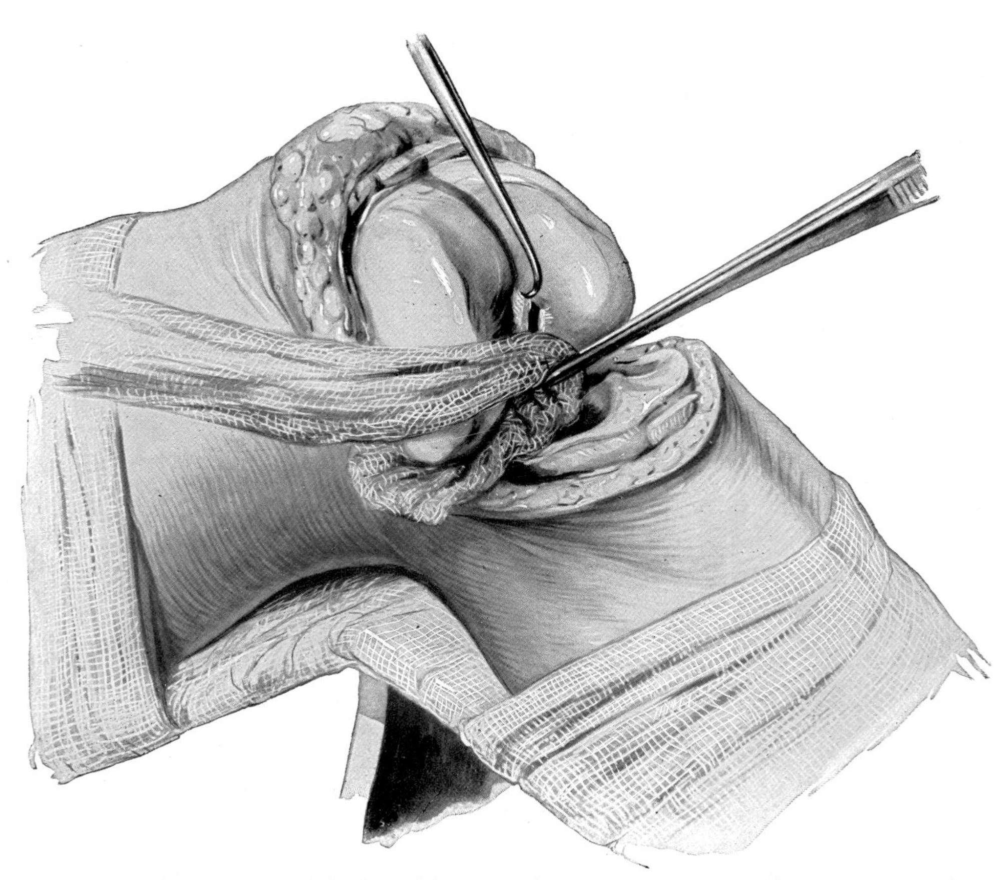

FIG. 681. Wide exposure of the knee-joint. The important structures which prevent complete exposure are severed and the joint is loosely packed with iodoform gauze.

When the openings made for the drains do not suffice to drain the pus, they may be enlarged or joined; or the joint may be freely opened by large incisions or wide exposure. In wide exposure of a joint (Fig. 681) the insertions of muscles which are in the way must be ruthlessly divided. After the joint cavity is opened, it is either loosely packed with gauze and the wound placed in a position favorable to drainage, or the articular extremities are dislocated and fixed outside the wound, in extreme angulation. When the infection subsides as a result of these measures, the joint is then placed in the position most favorable for ankylosis, for which it is frequently necessary to remove the articular surfaces. In my experience, opening the joint in this way seldom accomplishes the desired result and I believe resection or amputation is preferable.

E. EXCISION OF JOINTS

In complete excision (resection), the entire joint, articular ends of the bones and the capsule, are removed from the body. The extent of the removal depends upon the type and severity of the disease, and may include only the

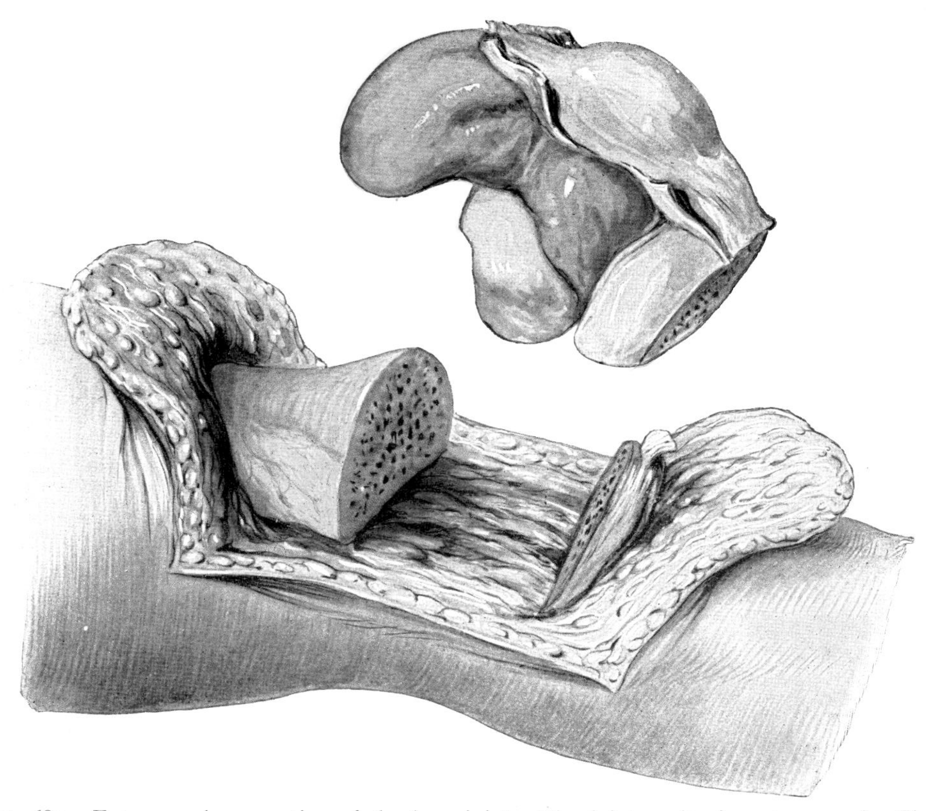

FIG. 682. Extracapsular resection of the knee-joint. The joint cavity is not exposed. The procedure is employed in the excision of malignant tumors.

synovial membrane, or also the connective tissue portion of the capsule as well. It may include only the cartilage covering the ends of the bone or also portions of the bones. The joint should be widely opened by an adequate incision and thoroughly examined from the inside, so that the extent of the operation can be gauged by the extent and severity of the disease. It is very seldom that extracapsular resection is done, in which the unopened joint is exposed from all sides and is removed closed after the ends of the bones are divided (Fig. 682).

A classic excision consists in opening the joint, resecting the articular surfaces, excising the capsule, and suturing the wound.

Every excision may result in severe derangement of function of the joint, which can not, as a rule, be avoided. Ankylosis is the most disturbing result. This is undesirable for any joint, but it is of different importance for the various joints. It is more annoying in the arm than in the leg, for in the leg a painless ankylosis in a favorable position is preferable to the insecurity of a weak joint. In excision of a tuberculous joint, with regard to the extent of the operation, we know for certain that muscular fixation can hardly be counted on. The prospect of healing of tuberculosis of a joint is much more favorable in ankylosis than when the joint is movable. We therefore always attempt to obtain ankylosis after a joint excision for tuberculosis. If, however, some motion occurs it may be of some advantage in certain joints, but this is not true in the knee.

Whether an attempt is made to obtain a movable or a stiff joint, the muscles adjacent to the joint should always be protected. For this reason the incisions are made, whenever possible, in muscular interspaces. Since, however, good exposure and thoroughness are essential for the success of an excision, the transverse division of important muscles can be avoided less often than in arthrotomy. It is better to avoid complicated operations, such as the temporary displacement of the insertions of muscles. As a rule, I prefer the incisions described by v. Langenbeck for excisions, for they provide excellent exposure and easy access. After division of the overlying soft parts, considerable protection for the adjacent muscles is gained by freeing them as far as possible without separating them at this time from the capsule. To do this longitudinal incisions are made close together and perpendicular to the bone so that the muscles can finally be stripped off the articular ends as a single covering. This is particularly adapted to the elbow-joint. In other cases, certain muscles must be transversely divided, as for example, in excision of the knee-joint. In spite of all precautions to protect the muscles surrounding the joint, the influence of the detached muscles on the joint leaves much to be desired. Thus, flail joints often develop when there is motion, or contractures and curvatures occur during growth in stiffened joints, particularly in young patients.

Shortening of the extremity, which always accompanies resection, is an undesirable complication in the leg, but is of less importance in the arm. In order that shortening be minimized, as little as possible of the bone ends is removed. This may be accomplished through freshening the articular ends (Fig. 683), by excising a disk a few millimeters thick from each bone end, but retaining the natural contour of the articular surfaces. I use a bow saw with the narrowest saw blade. The sawing is done as soon as the joint surfaces are exposed, because inspection and further intervention is facilitated by the excision. If on the surfaces, after this excision, additional foci of disease are found, they may be removed with a sharp curette if they are small, or if they are extensive, further bone may be removed by the saw. After the excision the bone surfaces are examined to make sure that they are properly shaped and that when brought into position the axis of the limb will be correct. The surfaces must be reshaped if they are not correct.

In joint excision for acute suppurative disease the operative procedure terminates with the opening of the joint and the removal of articular cartilage. The cavity is filled loosely with drains and gauze, without suturing, bandaged and placed at rest, keeping the articular space open as much as possible. In nonsuppurative disease, including tuberculosis, the capsule is also removed (Fig. 683). Beginning at one angle, the capsule is removed with scissors and knife in one piece, making strong traction on it during the dissection. Infected sinuses are explored, excised, or scraped out with a sharp curette. After the excision is finished, the wound should be surrounded by nothing but healthy tissue.

I use Esmarch's anemia in all excisions of the leg, with the exception of those of the hip-joint; Momburg's anemia can not be considered harmless. In

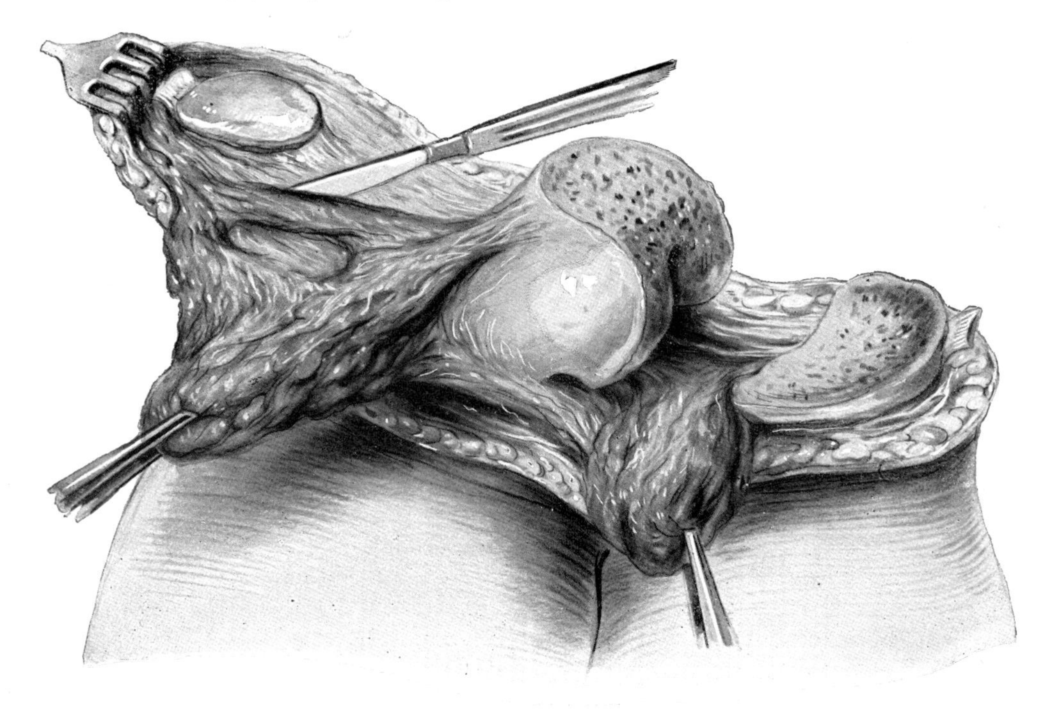

Fig. 683. Resection of the knee-joint after wide exposure of the joint. The joint surfaces are removed but the contour of the joint surface is maintained. The joint capsule is removed as one piece.

the arm, because of danger of nerve injury, anemia by the use of a tourniquet is used only for excisions of the wrist joint and of the articulations of the fingers, in which case the tourniquet is placed on the forearm. Hemostasis is carried out carefully. At the end of the operation in tuberculous joints, the cavity may be impregnated with iodoform powder or phenol-camphor mixture. The bone surfaces are brought together in the proper position and held so until the bandage is applied. Fixation by nails driven through the skin, is not only superfluous but dangerous because of the possibility of infection. The position of the ends of the bones to one another is maintained to a certain extent through careful suturing of the soft parts and skin. In extensive wound cavities I insert, under aseptic conditions, one or two drains for a few days. Should the joint become ankylosed, which is the rule, the correct apposition of the sawed-off surfaces is maintained by a plaster cast. When occasionally a movable joint is desired, the bone surfaces are held apart by a traction dressing.

The indications for excision of a joint vary. In malignant disease one must decide between excision and amputation. Excision is indicated only when the malignancy is very early and there is great probability that it will be completely removed by this procedure. In acute purulent infection, after failure of drainage or of wide exposure, resection is again the last resort before amputation. Here its principal benefit does not depend upon the elimination of the infected focus, since new freshly infected surfaces result from the excision, but upon the elimination of sinuses and recesses and the establishment of uniform conditions. This is particularly true in the hip and shoulder joints. The suction action of the narrow articular spaces is done away with; favorable drainage is established, and the cartilage which prolongs suppuration removed.

In tuberculosis of joints, excision has passed beyond the stage of extravagant recommendation and complete condemnation to the point where each case must be decided on its own merits. Personally, I believe there are several important considerations which affect the choice of treatment. Conservative treatment is often impractical for social reasons. The results in excision for tuberculosis vary greatly at present. The individual joints do not respond in the same way, and the results are unfavorable at the shoulder, wrist, and hip, because at these sites there may be great difficulty in doing a thorough operation. Because of this, excision of these joints is rarely undertaken. On the other hand, excision of the knee-joint gives very satisfactory results, even in the presence of extensive fistulæ. Age is also of great importance in the result. Aside from the fact that the conditions for conservative healing are more favorable in children, there is danger of epiphyseal trauma in every excision of a joint in growing bones, resulting in disturbance of growth which may lead to shortening, lengthening, and deformity. For this reason, no doubt, excision of tuberculous joints in children is but very seldom employed. In old persons, or those whose resistance is weakened by pulmonary tuberculosis or some other disease, excision is inadvisable, because in my experience there is not enough resistance to bring about healing. Amputation is here the proper procedure.

Arthritis deformans or other painful joint diseases justify excision of the diseased joints, when the pain is a greater handicap than a stiff joint and when every conservative measure has failed to give relief.

Excision is also indicated to correct the position of a joint which is ankylosed in bad position. These excisions are atypical as a rule, for only enough is removed from the articular ends of the bones to make it possible to place them in the proper position. In other cases, a cuneiform, or crushing, or splintering osteotomy is performed in the region of the joint to correct the deformity.

F. ARTHRODESIS—ARTIFICIAL PRODUCTION OF ANKYLOSIS

Arthrodesis is indicated when the muscles controlling a joint are deficient; when as a result of the development of a flail joint, voluntary movements in the joint can not be executed with the necessary surety; when it is

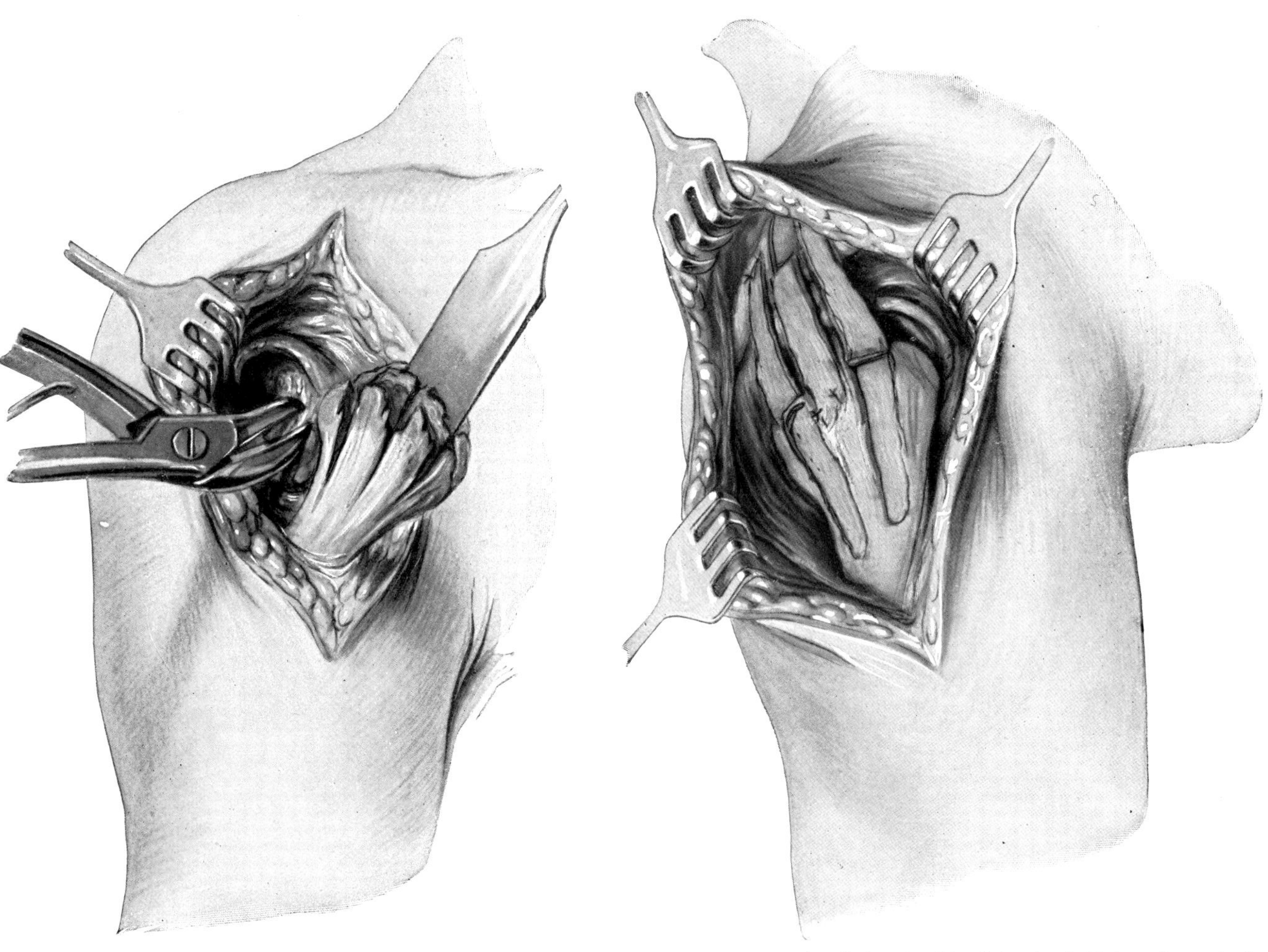

Fig. 684. Arthrodesis of the shoulder-joint by freshening the joint surfaces; excision of the cartilage and splintering of the head of the humerus.

Fig. 685. Arthrodesis of the shoulder-joint by bridging the articular cleft with narrow pedunculated osteoperiosteal bone grafts.

impossible to substitute for the deficient muscles or to strengthen the joint, and when the usefulness of the affected limb will be greater with a stiff joint than in the present condition.

The most useful procedure in producing ankylosis is moderate freshening of the articular surfaces, so that there will be bony union between the surfaces of the opposed bones. The joints are exposed by the usual incisions for excision. If the synovial membrane can not be completely removed, it is advisable to remove large sections of it, because the rapidity of ankylosis is increased when the joint is surrounded with considerable cicatricial tissue. Even so, rapid ankylosis in good position does not always occur. There have been a number of methods suggested for increasing the safety of this procedure, and for causing ankylosis in other ways.

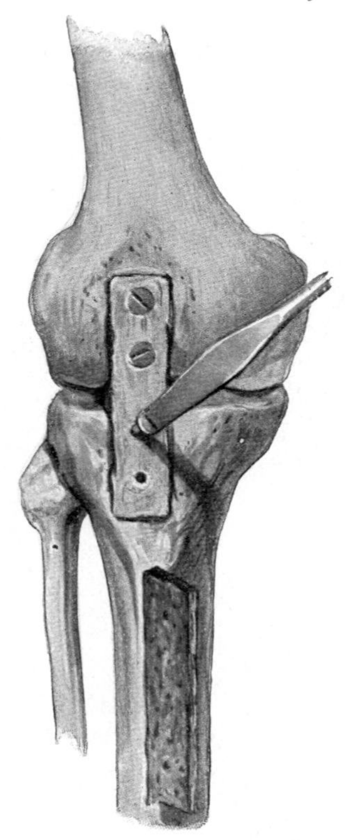

Fig. 686. Arthrodesis of the knee-joint by bridging the joint with a free bone transplant that lies in a groove and is screwed to both bones. (The transplant in the illustration is too short.)

After excision, the bone surface from which the cartilage has been removed may be splintered as has been described under crushing osteotomy, so that instead of smooth surfaces, roughened ends of bone oppose each other (Fig. 684). By enlarging and roughening the opposing surfaces, callus formation is hastened and strengthened. For the same purpose, splinters of bone on periosteal flaps may be chiselled off the end of one bone (Fig. 685) and thrown back over the end of the other bone to form a bridge over the line of separation. These little expedients are simpler, easier, and more dependable than trying to join the ends by mortise and tenon such as is used in carpentry.

Another method for producing ankylosis is the use of a bone splint to hold the bones together. The splint may be applied in any one of the three methods described for bone fixation; lateral inlay, central pegging, or external splinting (Fig. 686). (See Chapter IX.)

A lateral inlay of bone is placed in a groove chiselled longitudinally out of both bones after they are brought in the proper position to one another. The bone splint thus bridges the line between the bones. It is fastened in its groove by wires or screws, in the manner previously described.

The external splint of bone (Kappis) is laid laterally on the bone, bridging the articular space and extending beyond it. The splint is brought into the closest possible contact with the bone, and whenever possible the periosteum is sutured over it after the bone is freshened, or it is fastened in place with wires.

In pegging (Lexer) (Fig. 687), the joint is placed in the correct position and a hole is drilled through both bones with a large wimble or long ball-drill. The holes should extend several centimeters into each bone and should be so

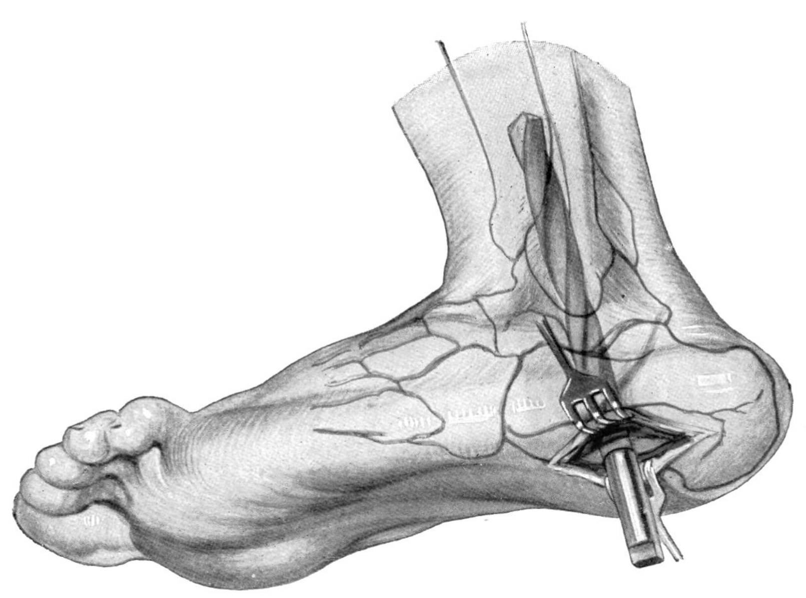

FIG. 687. Arthrodesis of the ankle-joint, by pegging with a free bone transplant. The tunnel for the bone peg is made with a wimble.

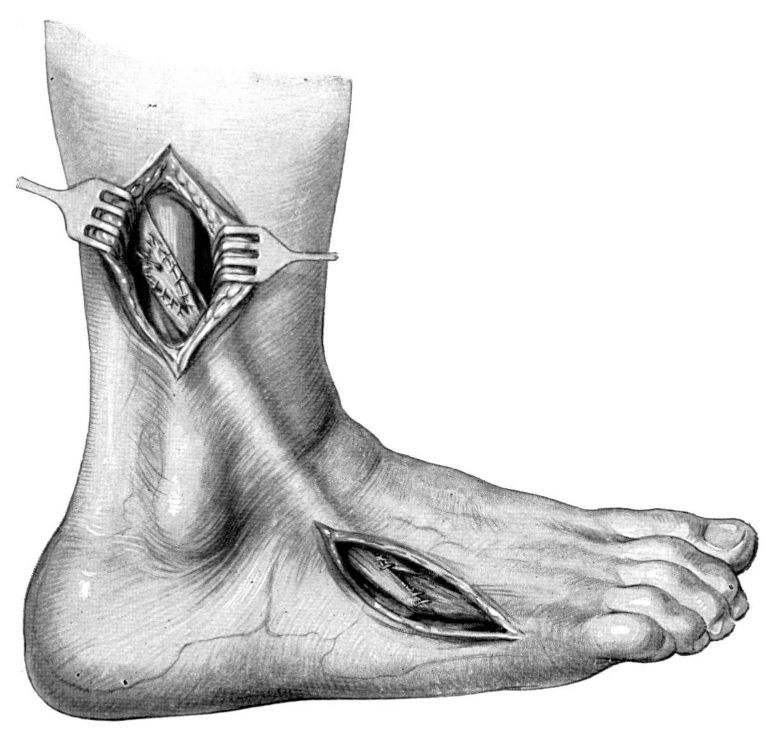

FIG. 688. Partial stiffening of the ankle-joint, by fasciodesis in peroneal paralysis. A sling from the fascia lata is fastened under tension between the fibula and the 5th metacarpal.

placed that there is no danger of the walls breaking. It is best when the drill can be used in the central longitudinal axis of the limb, as is possible for instance, in the ankle-joint, where the drill can be inserted from the plantar surface through the calcaneus, astragalus, and ankle-joint into the tibia. A piece of the fibula, a graft from the tibia, or an ivory peg is hammered firmly into the canal, so that the peg lies entirely within the bone.

The relatively short splints are as a rule not equal to the powerful forces of the long bones. They are also apt to be broken at the level of the joint through the gradual formation of a false joint. For these reasons attempts to ankylose a joint with the use of bone splints alone, without freshening the ends

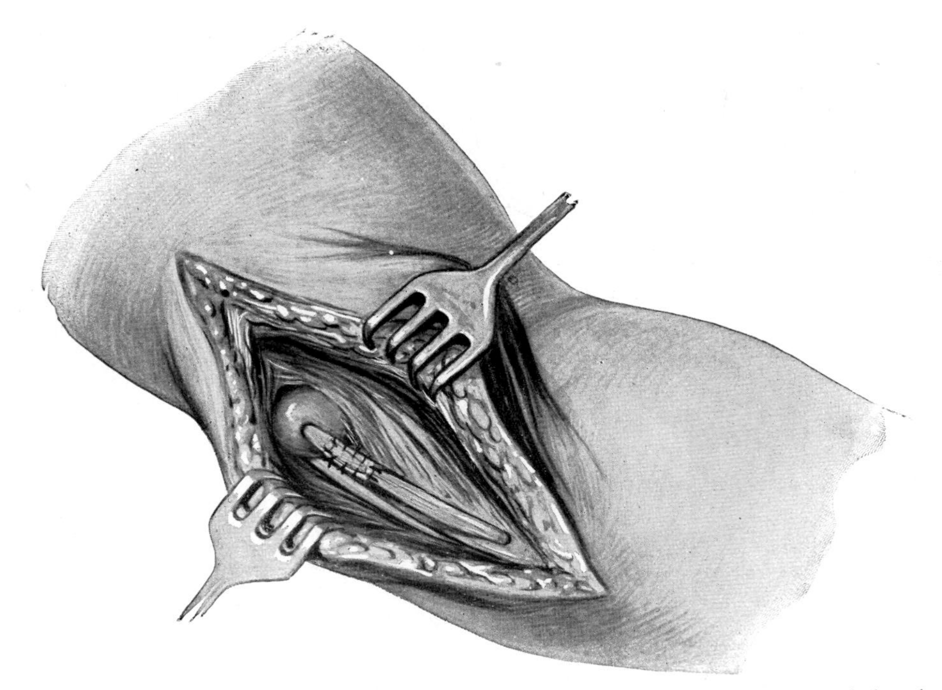

FIG. 689. An extra-capsular band between the medial epicondyle of the humerus and the ulna is formed from a free graft from the fascia lata.

of the bones, have not been satisfactory. Freshening the articular ends remains the procedure of choice. Only the splinting of the almost inaccessible and slightly movable vertebral joints by a bone splint laid in the split spinous processes (Albee's operation) has been satisfactory in my experience.

Joint fixation through operations on the soft parts alone, are incomplete and can not compare with the results obtained from operations on the bones as to excellence and durability. Fixation is attempted by shortening of the tendons that lie over the joint, or by transplanting tendons. Free fascial transplants may be stretched over the joint, and then either drawn through holes drilled in the bone or fastened by sutures to the periosteum (fasciodesis) (Fig. 688).

Partial fixation of a joint for the elimination of abnormal weakness and repeated dislocations (habitual luxations) should be attempted by placing bands within and without the joint. Free transplants of fascia only should be used for these bands. For extracapsular bands the fascia is quilted on, fastened with nails or drawn through canals drilled in the bone and united in a ring (Fig. 689). New lateral ligaments in hinge joints are best passed through canals drilled transversely through each bone and sutured together in a loop. For the substitution of intra-articular ligaments a strip of fascia is fastened to the points of insertion of the ligaments to be replaced, after

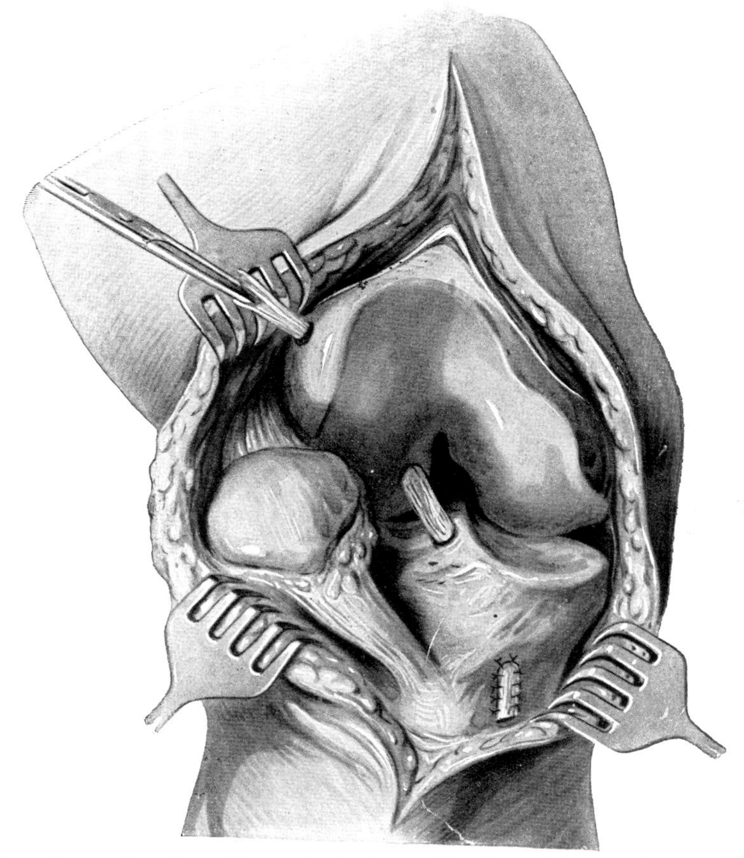

FIG. 690. Formation of an intra-articular band (Perthes) (the anterior crucial ligament) of the knee-joint, by a free strip from the fascia lata. The fascial strip is fastened in canals drilled in the bones.

the joint has been opened to afford a clear view of the whole interior. Their retention should be made as firm as possible with silk sutures. It is possible, sometimes, to anchor the strips of fascia in the holes drilled into the articular surfaces of the bones (Fig. 690).

G. ARTHROPLASTY—OPERATIVE MOBILIZATION OF A JOINT

1. INDICATIONS

Operative mobilization is attempted only when corrective procedures have failed after prolonged trial, or when, because of bony ankylosis, there is no possibility of success with them. Helferich presented a patient in 1894 with a temporomaxillary articulation which he had mobilized. This led to all the subsequent work in this field. Decision to operate can not be made haphazardly, since the results are always uncertain and since, particularly in the case of large joints, operation is not without danger. The dangers of operation must be weighed, particularly infection which by causing suppuration and ankylosis is not trifling (war wounds!). It must be remembered that after an unsuccessful operation, the joint does not always return to its previous condition, but may be left in a worse condition. The advantages to the individual patient resulting from the usual or the most favorable outcome of the operation must be weighed against these considerations. A workman, for instance a smith, will fare better with a painless ankylosed knee, than with a joint which has been made too freely movable; a young girl will prefer a movable though less dependable knee, to a stiff joint. The joint involved, as well as the economic status of the patient, should be considered. The patient's cooperation is essential, particularly in the after-treatment, and success or failure frequently depends on obtaining this.

For the success of the operation it is necessary that the articular ends are large enough. When small ends of bones are opposed, flail joints result. The condition of the muscles is of great importance. When they can no longer be depended upon to control the joint, the prospects of a good result are lessened. In 1913 Helferich said that muscles which have become atrophied through ankylosis of the joint will even after many years recover and become strong if they are again used. This has been confirmed many times. On the other hand, complete paralysis of important groups of muscles in general contra-indicates mobilization of a joint. Heavy cicatricial overgrowths or defects of important groups of muscles, as are frequently found after grenade injuries, are contra-indications, when muscle and tendon plastic operations have not been successful. Payr has succeeded in making movable knee-joints, in which the lost ligamentum patellæ was replaced by a free tendon transplant, or a fascial graft. Extensive scar tissue adherent to the bone must be freed before proceeding with the arthroplasty, and thin cicatricial skin should be replaced by skin padded with fat.

Special caution is required when there is danger of latent infection. Mobilization itself may cause an infection to recur through the formation of large recessed wounds, and through the transplantation of free or pedunculated tissue grafts. Uncomplicated healing is one of the most important conditions for success. The development of infection may cause the patient to lose either limb or life. Operation, therefore, should never be considered in the presence of an existing infection, however mild this may be. Even though good results are occasionally obtained, they are but chance results, and the patient has been exposed to unjustifiable risk. A period of time should elapse between the last inflammatory symptoms and the arthroplasty, the duration being in proportion to the size of the joint and the severity of the previous infection. This may be as long as one year in large joints when the infection was severe. It is never "too late" to undertake the operation. Large foreign bodies in the form of fragments of projectiles, or sequestra, which may harbor living organisms for years, should be removed by a preliminary operation. Tetanus antitoxin is indicated in certain cases.

2. Technic

In spite of the fact that occasionally bony prominences which definitely hinder motion must be removed, a warning should be sounded against partial operations on joints. From experience it has been shown that the classic, complete arthroplasty gives the best results.

Esmarch anemia should be avoided because of the frequency with which secondary bleeding occurs. There must be complete hemostasis before the wound is closed, and if a tourniquet has been used it should be removed before wound closure so that every bleeding point can be ligated.

Exposure of Articular Surfaces. Because it is necessary, in every case, to examine and have access to every part of the joint, the ends of the bones, as well as the entire capsule and the adjacent ligaments, the division of important muscles is frequently unavoidable. Occasionally it is better to expose the joint by two longitudinal incisions than by one transverse incision. The skin incision should if possible not lie directly over the incision for the opening of the capsule.

In ankylosis due to connective tissue overgrowth the knife, after division of the skin and the underlying soft parts, will penetrate the more or less contracted articular space. With gentle force an attempt is made gradually to bend the joint, but care must be used in applying too great force because it may result in fracture of the atrophic ends of the bones, tearing out pieces of bone, and detaching the periosteum. The connections existing between the bones, the capsular ligament, the accessory ligaments and all cicatricial bands are divided to such an extent, and the ends of the bones so exposed, that the joint can be sharply bent and thoroughly exposed.

In bony ankylosis the bone is completely exposed at the joint site by detaching the soft parts and elevators are then passed between the bone and the soft parts. The bone is then sawed through in the direction of the former axis of the joint. The scattering of bone dust should be prevented as much as possible by covering the area with moist compresses, since scattered bone particles may give rise to new bone formation.

Removal of the Diseased Tissues. The success of the operation depends to a great extent upon the radical removal of the altered soft parts and the periosteum lying between the two ends of the bones, or surrounding them. From cicatricial tissue which is left new connective tissue may develop. Shreds of periosteum which remain may form new bone to restrict motion. Therefore all pathological cicatricial bands and pieces of periosteum should be thoroughly excised. The surgeon must consider the fact, that the success of the operation depends to a considerable extent on the completeness of this step, and he must not be influenced by hemorrhage from the superficial soft parts. Although complete removal of the capsule would make subsequent motion of the joint comparatively painless because the associated nerve endings are removed with it, most surgeons prefer to preserve every part of the capsule which is normal, or nearly so, since from this a new capsule may be formed. Degenerated articular ligaments are completely removed.

At this stage of the operation, the bones forming the articulation should be surrounded by a girdle free of cicatricial tissue and periosteum, and united only by healthy or freshly incised soft parts.

Formation of the New Joint Surfaces. The articular surfaces are, in general, made to resemble their natural shapes, so that the efficiency of the new joint will be as nearly as possible that of the original joint. Reconstructing the natural form of the articular surfaces is especially important for the avoidance of unstable and loose joints. The new surfaces are, however, rougher and simpler than the original forms. Aside from the impossibility of copying the fine modeling of nature in the limited time available, an exact imitation after the previous loss of bone is often impossible and in addition is frequently unnecessary, since subsequent use will of itself shape the surfaces to their

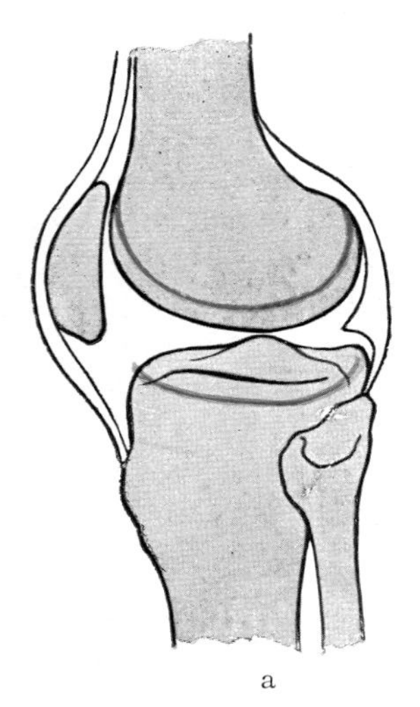

a

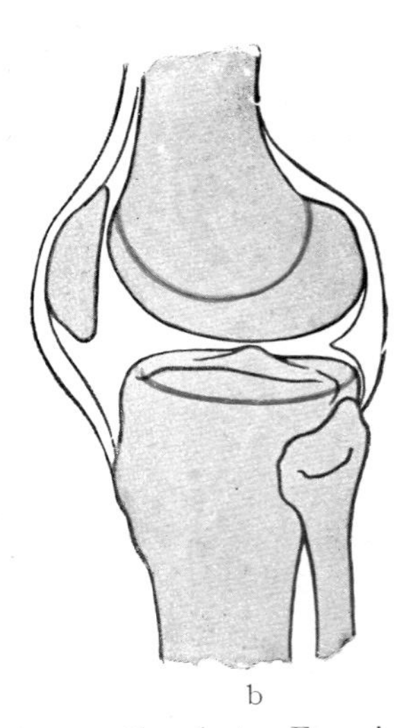

b

Fig. 691. Excision of the surfaces of the knee-joint, in an arthroplasty. Experience proves that excision in imitation of the natural form (a) is not as favorable as is reshaping of the ends of the tibia and femur (b).

finer form. Certain deviations from the natural form have even proved to be desirable. For example, the posterior sections of the condyles of the femur may be less projecting in restoration of the knee-joint than they are normally (Fig. 691), since practically the resistance to flexion appears usually in this area. Also in other joints it is frequently better to make the diameter of the arch greater than normal on the concave surface and smaller on the convex surface. Particular attention should be paid to the removal of bony projections at the periphery of the joint surfaces which may interfere with motion. Hass recently advised that true reproduction of the articular surfaces should be disregarded and suggested the formation of see-saw, or tilt joints, instead of hinge joints (Fig. 692). For this type of joint the concave surface is excised as a shallow concavity, the convex end as a wedge. The principle of this idea is to reduce to a minimum the contact of the bones and in this manner to prevent reformation of the ankylosis. When this method is used soft parts are interposed as in other methods.

For the shaping of the articular surfaces I use bow saws with narrow blades, chisels, strong knives, sharp curettes, rasps and files. Schmerz, for his "polishing" method employs in the shaping of the surfaces special burrs and cupped drills.

Diseased cartilage should be entirely removed. The question as to whether healthy cartilage should be retained, has been variously answered. Bier thinks the cartilage may spread over the wound surfaces as epithelium does. I am of the opinion that it is not good practice to retain healthy islands of cartilage, and I remove the entire cartilaginous covering in one piece.

Prevention of Union Between the New Articular Surfaces. If the new joint is to maintain its mobility, the surfaces must be prevented from adhering to one another. It is most important to keep the surfaces adequately separated, and to maintain a sufficient space between them. The question of the development of a flail joint must have less consideration. The formation of a joint requires the removal of sufficient bone to provide an interspace of from 1 to 3 cm. In the body, however, there is always a tendency to close every defect with cicatricial connective tissue and through its contraction to make the defect smaller. It is therefore necessary to use special means to prevent adhesions which will restrict motion. These measures are the interposition of soft parts, continuous separation of the ends of the bones by means of traction, and active and passive motion.

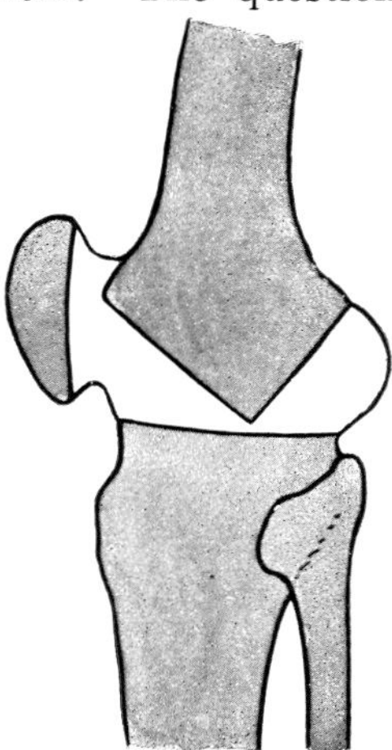

Fig. 692. Excision of the ends of the femur and tibia in arthroplasty of the knee in the form of a "see-saw" joint (Hass).

Although amnion hardened with formalin, or the sac of a hernia or hydrocele, may still be recommended occasionally, the interposition of foreign material or dead tissue between the ends of the bones has today but a historic interest. An autoplastic transplant is generally preferred. It is employed either as a pedunculated flap or as a free graft. Muscle, tendon, fascia, fat, skin, or periosteum, may be used. Muscle tissue (Helferich) is used exclusively in the form of pedunculated flaps, in which a section of tendon may be included, as in the use of flaps from the triceps brachii or triceps suræ. Fascia (Kirschner), fat (Lexer), fascia with adherent fat (Kirschner), and periosteum (Hofmann) may be placed between the bones either as pedunculated flaps or as free transplants. There seems to be no essential difference in results whether pedunculated flaps or free transplants are used. Free transplants of fascia from the fascia lata are used by most surgeons. Some fat should be left on the fascia, the amount depending on the space between the articular surfaces. I always use a single piece of fascia, making a pouch which entirely envelops the end of one bone, suturing it in place with catgut sutures (Fig. 693). In this case, the fascia alone withstands the demands for firmness placed upon it, while the fat is cut through. The pouch is formed in the following manner: both longitudinal sides of a rectangular flap of fascia are sutured together with catgut to within a few centimeters of the narrow side. The pouch thus formed is drawn over the articular surfaces. The margins of the sac are firmly sutured in place with catgut, then completely

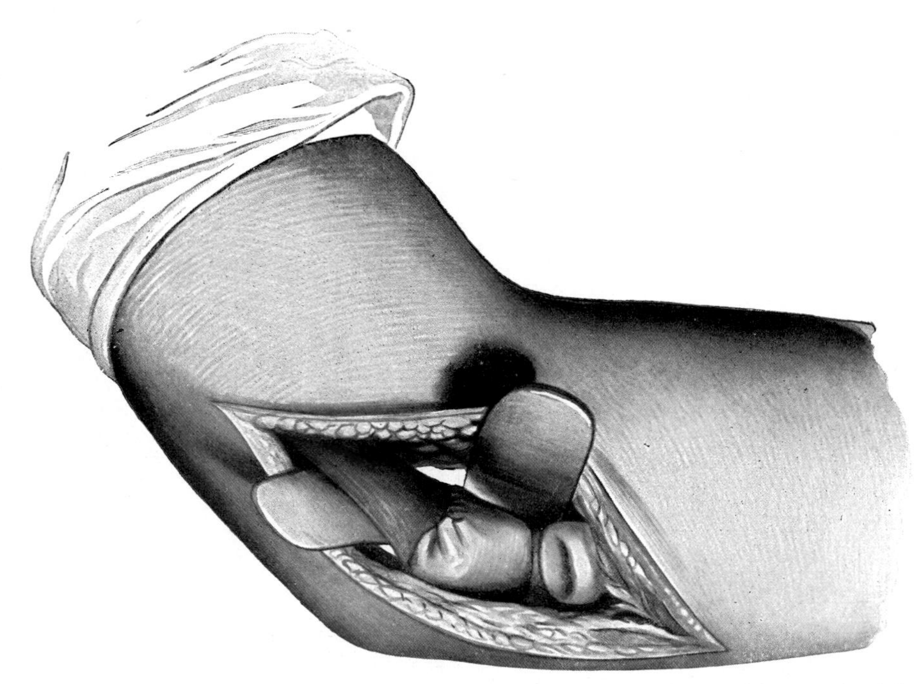

Fig. 693. Covering the condyles of the humerus, during an arthroplasty, with a pouch of fascia. The fascia is drawn into a tight pouch by catgut sutures.

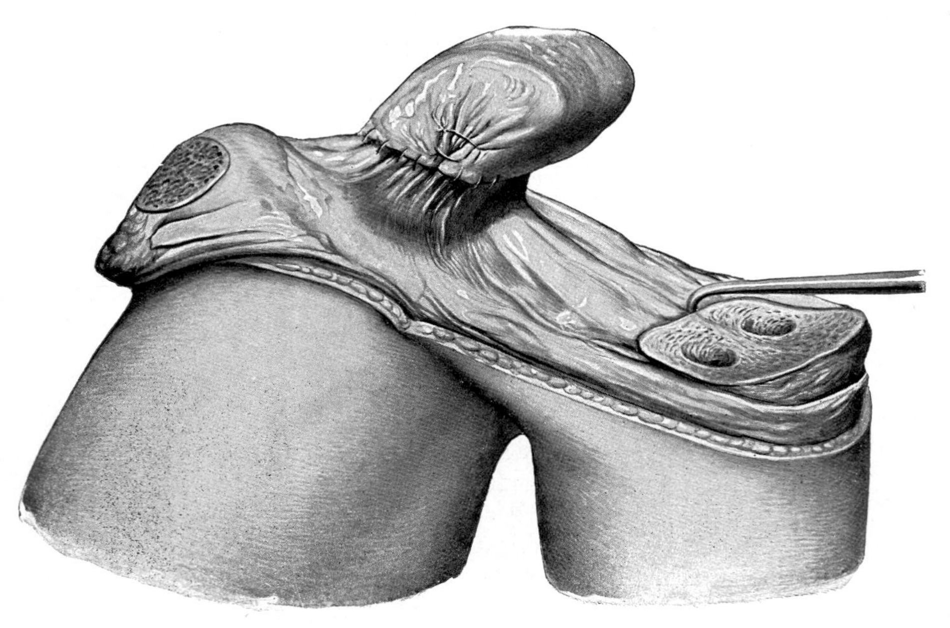

Fig. 694. Covering the condyles of the humerus, during an arthroplasty, with a fat flap. The fat flap is fastened to the humerus by catgut sutures and fills the gap between the humerus and ulna.

closed around the bone by additional sutures. If this method is used it is unnecessary to cover the end of the other bone.

When fat is used for interposition, a fat flap of at least 1 to 2 cm. in thickness is fastened by catgut sutures (Fig. 694) over the sawed surface of one of the bones.

If a pedunculated muscle flap is used, one should cut a sufficiently wide and long muscle flap, about 1 to 2 cm. thick, which should if possible be pedunculated very near the joint. The flap is drawn through between the ends of the bones, or it is fastened like a cap over one end (Fig. 695).

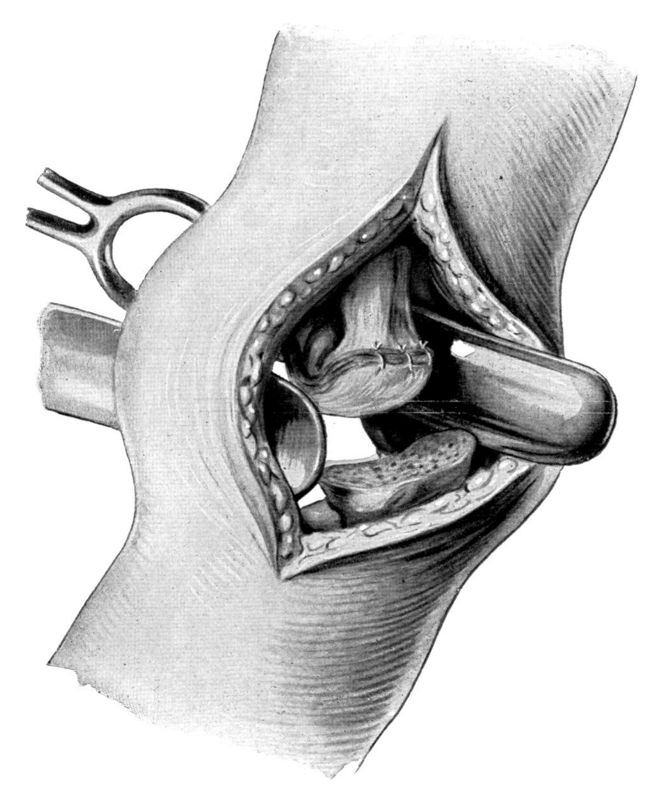

FIG. 695. Covering one of the bones of the elbow-joint, in arthroplasty, with a pedunculated muscle-flap.

The use of skin, tendons and periosteum has not proved successful.

Lexer has used entire joints of amputated limbs and from cadavers for interposition, but his results are not encouraging. I have repeatedly obtained satisfactory results from the use of free autoplastic transplants of toe joints (Buchmann) for the mobilization of elbow- and finger-joints.

In arthroplasty of the hip-joint, I have succeeded in firmly closing the sawed-off shaft of the femur by pegging it with a piece of bone from the excised neck. The result was good. The purpose of such pegging is to strengthen a much atrophied end of bone, to stop bleeding from the shaft, and to counteract the formation of bony outgrowths which interfere with motion.

Schmerz and Schepelmann have pointed out that the results of joint mobilization are evidently not dependent upon the use of interposed tissues, but that equally useful new joints may be obtained without interposition. While Schepelmann does not advocate any particular preparation of the articular surfaces, Schmerz finishes them according to his "polishing" method. The sawed surfaces are first smoothed off with coarse files, then with fine, flat, curved, or round files, so that the ends of the bone assume a silky, slippery appearance. Even when the possibility of obtaining a good movable joint without interposition seems unquestionable, the procedure obviously does not possess the certainty of result that follows interposition. I prefer therefore the interposition of autoplastic fascial grafts with fat attached to the fascia.

After completing the joint, the soft parts are carefully closed, layer by layer, with catgut, to prevent a later infection and to insure a certain primary firmness to the new joint. The articular space must not be encroached upon by the sutures. Muscles and tendons that were divided should be carefully sutured together. In large joints, after a prolonged operation, or when there has been imperfect hemostasis, one or two drains may be placed at suitable points, and left in place for 1 to 2 days. The joint is surrounded with an aseptic, light pressure dressing, which may be reinforced with wood, plaster, or cardboard splints, and by starch-bandages, to prevent lateral motion.

3. After-treatment

At first, the main object of after-treatment, besides rest, is the maintenance of the space between the ends of the bones. Contraction of the surrounding muscles tends to draw the ends together and this tendency is increased by contraction of the wound during healing. The intra-articular space is preserved by the application of traction. For the arm, an adhesive traction dressing suffices, while for the leg it is necessary to use wire traction. The weight used for traction varies from 3 to 10 kg. The best traction dressing for the fingers is a wire inserted through the terminal phalanx and carried to a lyre-shaped splint (Fig. 665). Traction is an effective method for relieving pain.

The amount of space between the bones should be frequently observed by x-ray examinations. The size of the gap, which should be from ½ to 2 cm., according to the size of the joint, is regulated by adjusting the weight. If the dressings do not become saturated, if there is no constant fever, pain, or other inflammatory symptoms that would compel an early change of dressing, the original dressing should be left on for at least eight days, though drains must be promptly removed if these have been used. Any demonstrable hematoma should be aspirated by puncturing through the skin at some distance from the operative site. If pus accumulates in the joint, it should be aspirated. Only in case of severe symptoms should the joint be drained or reopened.

Functional after-treatment is probably the most important and most difficult part of the postoperative care in arthroplasty. It is carried out as early as possible (Figs. 696 to 698). It should be cautiously begun and faithfully continued. Of the greatest importance are active exercises, and in these the will and the perseverance of the patient prove to be deciding factors in the result. Attempts to obtain any degree of motion of the new joint should not be made before the tenth day, and pendulum exercises should not be started before the second or third week after the operation. They must be used carefully at first, and for only a short period of time. Later the oscillations must be carried out for several hours daily. The use of the pendulum is an important therapeutic measure but it should be constantly

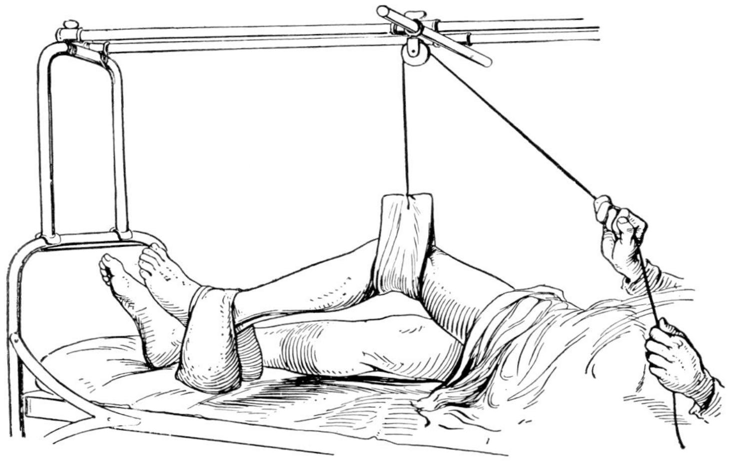

Fig. 696. Flexion of a stiff knee by traction over a pulley. The ankle is weighted.

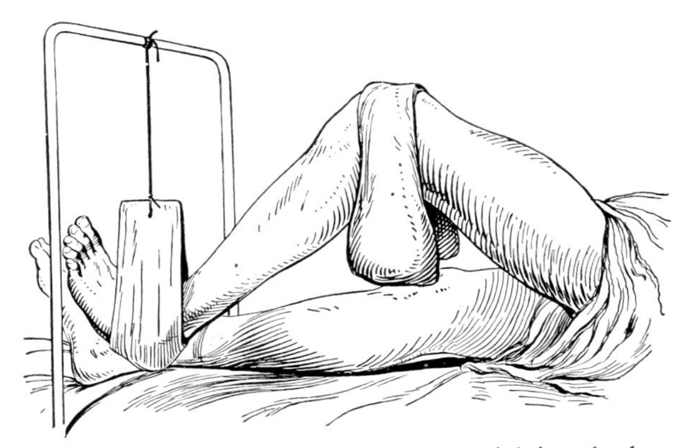

Fig. 697. Extension of a stiff knee by weighting the knee.

supervised. Its main value is the active motion of the pendulum exerting its action against resistance. As soon as feasible, the joint motions should be those by which it will function in every day life. In mobilization of a joint in the arm, the patient may be compelled to use the arm operated upon and to move the new joint by temporarily bandaging the healthy arm to the side. The first functional movements, especially in the hinge joints of the elbow and the knee, may be advantageously made under the safeguard of plaster splints which will prevent lateral motion. These will at the same time act as a support and thus should prevent undue strain and a diminution of the articular space.

Pain which occurs during motion is often the cause of the difficulty experienced in making patients use an exercise apparatus and to attempt or assist in motion. Thus pain is frequently responsible for the reformation of ankyloses. Every painful passive motion should therefore be discontinued. Bier's constriction has been recommended to allay pain. When more extensive motions are necessary the pain may be controlled by repeated injections of a local anæsthetic. I have often had good results from injections of human fat (humanol) into the joint. When, in spite of all these measures, the movements of the newly formed joint are insufficient, one may resort to "brisement forcé," under anæsthesia. After such forcible mobilization, the joint should be surrounded for a few days with an elastic bandage, to prevent an effusion. As a rule, but very little is gained through the use of force.

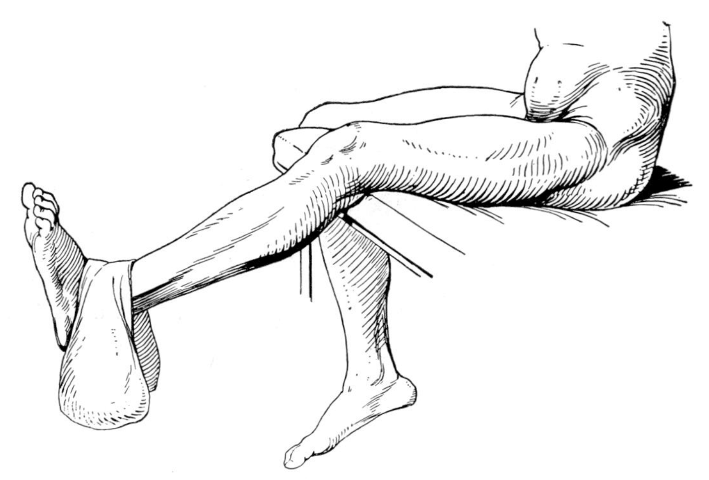

FIG. 698. Flexion of a stiff knee by weighting the ankle.

When the newly formed joint has insufficient motion, or when the degree of motion gradually diminishes, an investigation should be made for localized and accessible obstructions. Stereoscopic roentgenograms often give valuable information. Bony prominences or bony outgrowths interfering with motion (Fig. 699) should be removed surgically. The results of these secondary operations are often unsatisfactory, even though the newly developed tissue has been thoroughly removed.

When there is a considerable excess motion in a reconstructed joint, which occurs particularly in the elbow and knee, a special brace may improve the condition, and if worn for a long period may prevent the development of abnormal positions. Since the formation of a new joint depends to a certain degree for its results upon the movements carried out, so certain joint movements may be prevented in such a way that they become impossible. Should this measure prove futile or should we wish to free the patient of the burdensome brace, the only thing left is to try to strengthen the joint by operation. Two procedures were previously described. The joint may either be strengthened by reinforcing it with fascial bands (page 592 and Figs. 688

to 690), by the shortening of muscles or tendons around the joint, or by the transplantation of muscle insertions. The type of operation must be chosen to fit the individual case.

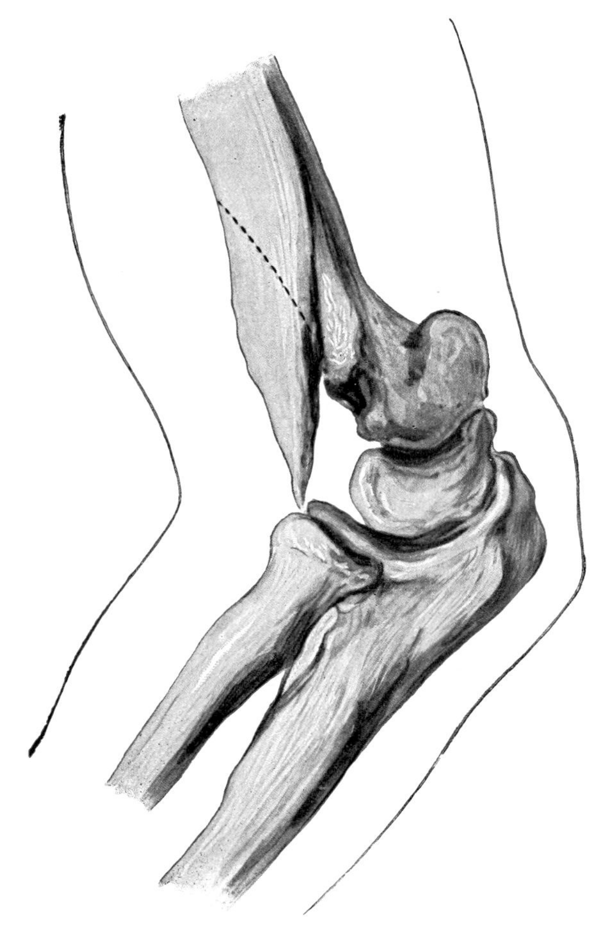

FIG. 699. Spur on humerus which limits flexion of the elbow. The dotted line is the level at which it should be removed.

The new joint is subject, also, to certain subsequent gradual changes. Changes in the bones, capsule, muscles, and therefore changes of motility toward the normal or toward the abnormal may drag along for years. Generally, it takes about two years to get a stationary condition of the joint.

CHAPTER XI

AMPUTATION AND DISARTICULATION

A. INTRODUCTION

The removal of part of an extremity is an operation of the greatest seriousness because of the resulting mutilation. It is always a last resort in a losing battle. The modern surgeon has great repugnance for this operation. However, in spite of the modern advances in surgery he must still resort to it frequently. When it is a question of saving a life or saving an extremity, the latter should be sacrificed so that the opportunity of saving the life may not be lost by too great delay. "It is no triumph, to preserve an extremity and to lose thereby a human life." "It is more profitable for thee that one of thy members should perish and not that thy whole body should be cast into hell." The decision to amputate is often made easier by the fact that conservative treatment, involving risk, pain, and loss of time is not always rewarded, even when a favorable course is run, by as good a functional result as the patient would have with an artificial limb. Experience in the World War showed that frequently amputations were performed too late to save life, and that after endless suffering and danger, extremities were preserved that were useless after the wound healed. These useless appendages cause permanent hardship, and make it nearly impossible later to fit a good artificial extremity.

Amputation is the removal of a part of or an entire extremity with transverse section of the bone. **Disarticulation** is the removal of an extremity or of a portion of it at a joint. Disarticulation has the advantage over amputation, in that the end of the bone is a natural stump and for the most part is well able to carry weight; furthermore, the removal can be carried out with ease and rapidity; soft parts only need to be separated and these are present to a lesser degree here than in the middle of the long bones. These advantages however are offset by many disadvantages that preclude the use of disarticulation as a routine procedure.

The bone after disarticulation presents a club-like end which requires large pedunculated flaps of the soft parts to cover it adequately. Material for extensive flaps is often deficient and the tendinous structures in these areas are more liable to necrosis. Should this occur, infection and necrosis of the cartilaginous surfaces together with infection in the bursæ around the joint are unavoidable. Infection in this area is extremely refractive to treatment and nearly always requires secondary amputation. Disarticulation should be performed only when large, well-nourished flaps are available and when primary healing is almost a certainty.

Disarticulation stumps have the further disadvantage of providing poor sites for the attachment of artificial limbs. Since prosthetic material of a certain thickness must be inserted between the end of the stump and the axis of the joint of the artificial limb, the new joint is several centimeters more distal than the natural joint. The result of this is that the two joints are at different levels, so that, for instance, in knee-joint disarticulation, the new knee-joint projects conspicuously when bent. These latter disadvantages are to an extent as true of the distal amputation stumps (Stokes-Gritti), as for actual disarticulation stumps. The experience with disarticulation during the war was unfavorable; a good functional stump after disarticulation was the exception. Consequently, in importance disarticulations are by far inferior to amputations. This is not, of course, the case at the shoulder- and hip-joints, when proximal extension of the disease will no longer permit of amputation, with soft parts for a useful stump.

There are two aspects of particular importance in the present day technic of removal of a limb: first, the fact that there is no need for great haste during the operation since the introduction of hemostasis. The operation can be performed as any other classic procedure, with the same care and orderliness. The removal of a limb is undertaken after applying Esmarch's bandage or any other suitable tourniquet or under the safeguard of compression of the great vessels to the part. In disarticulation of the shoulder joint manual compression or the previous ligation of the subclavian artery are alone available unless the hæmorrhage can be controlled by a special technic, during the operation. Digital compression of the main trunk of a vessel may be the only satisfactory method in advanced arterial disease, where there is danger of causing permanent injury to the sclerotic vessels if constricted by a tourniquet. In such cases, every incision is followed by careful arrest of hæmorrhage and the principal vessels are ligated doubly as soon as they are exposed. Occasionally, the main vessels are ligated at a point of election proximal to the site of amputation.

Secondly, the site of operation is now governed by consideration of the level at which the most efficient stump for prosthesis can be obtained. The knowledge of this has been enhanced by the experiences gained during the last war. The first question in connection with this, is whether or not the stump surface will be able to carry the entire body weight, or at least a part of it. The experiences of the war have shown that we can never obtain stumps capable of complete weight bearing in the leg except Pirogoff stumps and occasionally Stokes-Gritti stumps. On the other hand, by suitable measures one may obtain a stump capable of partial weight bearing. The greater the weight bearing capacity of the stump the more favorable it is for the later use of an artificial limb. When, however, in the following procedures, the consideration of the weight bearing capacity of the stump is constantly kept in mind, we become aware of the fact, that the ideal weight bearing capacity can not be attained in the majority of instances.

The conditions for a useful stump should be fulfilled if possible, in the operative interference. One of the most essential requisites is primary healing of the wound. The flaps made during amputation should be sutured primarily whenever possible. Muscles used for the elimination of dead spaces and for padding the bone-stump should be united in layers over the end of the bone, with catgut sutures; the skin should be sutured with silk. Only in the presence of infection should consideration for ultimate usefulness be subordinated to that of combating the suppuration. In such cases the wound should remain partially or entirely open, and the stump closed by secondary suture after control of the infection.

I always outline the skin incision with a colored solution before amputation. This enables one to use care and precision in shaping the flaps in each individual case. Proximal and distal to this site, the limb is enveloped in sterile covers held securely by clamps, safety pins or sutures. The limb is elevated by an assistant up to the moment of its separation. The operator stands so that the amputated limb, falls to his right (Fig. 666). Proximal to the place of removal, with their backs turned towards the patient, stand two assistants. One of these makes proximal traction on the skin, when it is incised. As soon as the limb is removed, one assistant takes hold of the stump, so as to direct it obliquely towards the ceiling which is the position best suited for the surgeon.

It is possible to carry out all amputations, excepting hip-joint disarticulation, under local, or block, or spinal anæsthesia. Spinal anæsthesia is extremely useful in arteriosclerotic patients. On the other hand the conscious patient is subjected to considerable psychic shock during the sawing through of the bone in a major amputation, even though the ears are plugged or artificial sounds are made. It may be, therefore, often preferable to use general anæsthesia.

B. THE SITE OF REMOVAL

The site of amputation of a limb is designated according to the place at which the bony skeleton is divided. A mid-thigh amputation is one in which the femur is divided through its middle, although the skin and other soft parts are frequently divided more distally. The mistake is easily made, when one plans to amputate in the middle of a limb, of placing the knife for the skin incision in the center of the limb, resulting, unfortunately for the patient, in the subsequent division of the bone at a higher level than was planned.

The extent and the kind of disease present determines how much of the limb must be removed, so that, including the flaps, only healthy tissue is left behind. We should endeavor to proceed as conservatively as possible, since in general, the usefulness of the remaining portion of the limb is greater with every joint that is preserved and the longer the distal diaphysis stump. In spite of this the older viewpoint is no longer held that the usefulness and the length of the stump are in direct proportion to one another, so that every centimeter should be conserved. A diaphysis stump is valuable only when it is long enough, measured from the proximal joint, to control adequately the artificial limb. Otherwise, it makes it difficult to apply the artificial limb and lessens the weight bearing capacity. In choosing the height of amputation there are excellent, good, fair and poor sites for functional results. A view concerning this is given in Zur Verth's schematic drawings (Figs. 700 and 701).

One can not always state with any degree of certainty where healthy tissue begins especially in malignant tumors, infections or disturbances of nutrition. In the presence of an infection one may occasionally make concessions in order to obtain a useful extremity. The decision as to at what level

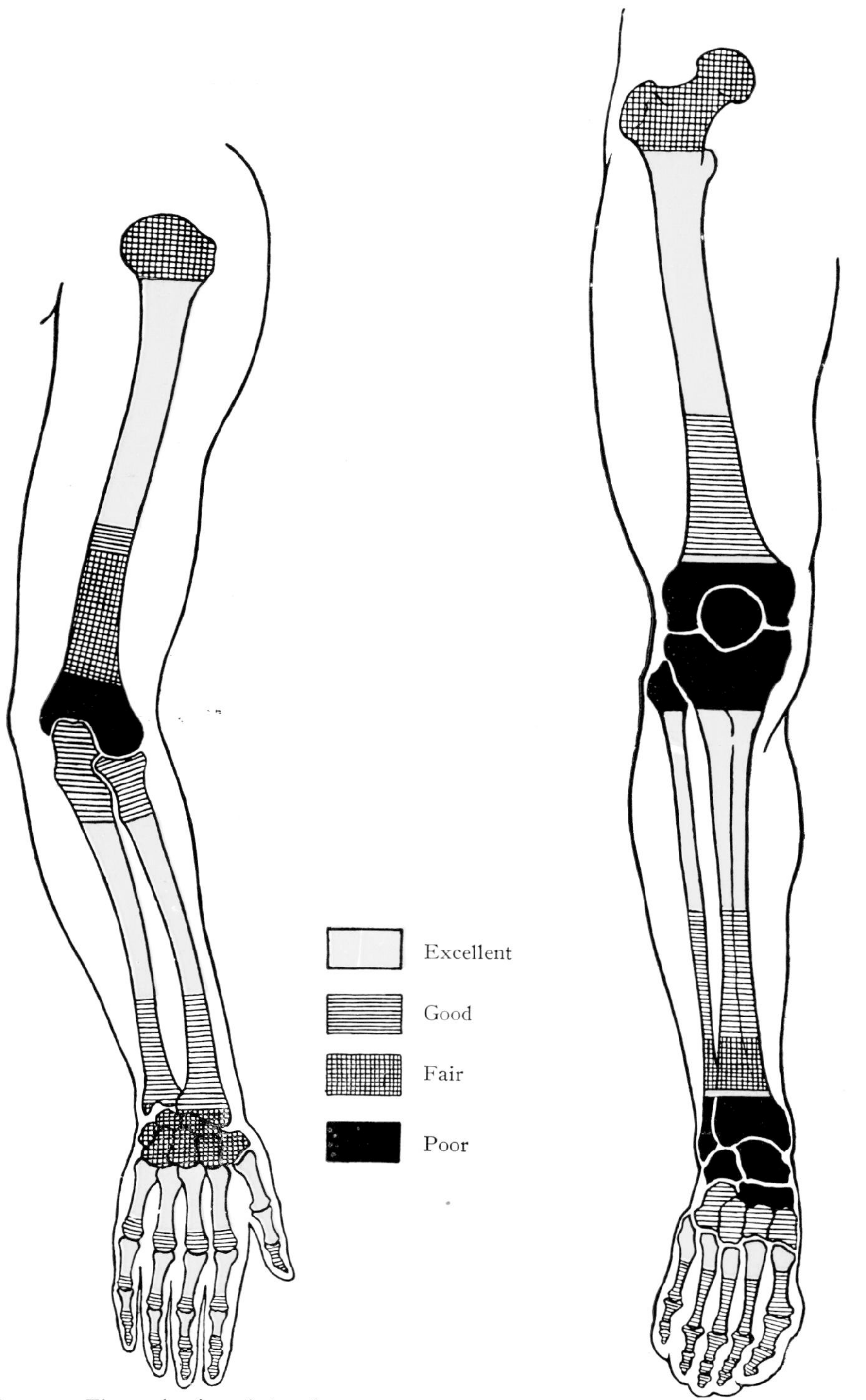

FIG. 700. The evaluation of sites for amputation of the upper extremity (Zur Verth).

FIG. 701. The evaluation of sites for amputation of the lower extremity (Zur Verth).

the tissues may be considered viable in arteriosclerotic gangrene is often difficult, and depends partly upon axiomatic considerations. The site most favorable for the healing of an amputation wound of the lower extremity, in the presence of circulatory disease, is the middle of the thigh. This is therefore the safest site to operate. Based upon an experience obtained from many cases in recent years I am convinced that in arteriosclerotic gangrene, amputations in the middle of the thigh will result in good wound healing. Amputation below the knee is practicable, when the general condition of the patient is good, when circulatory disturbances of the skin and evidences of infection do not extend above the metatarsus, when the pulse in the popliteal artery is palpable and when the main arteries in the leg give evidence that they are not entirely thrombosed. Otherwise I amputate in the thigh. Moskowicz's sign (see Chapter VI. B: "Vessel-suturing," p. 437) is depended on for determining the height of amputation. In amputation of a limb for malignant tumors, all bones affected by the disease and all muscles adjacent to the tumor should be entirely removed. (See Chapter IX, G: "Management of Bone Tumors," p. 566.)

C. INCISION OF THE SOFT PARTS IN AMPUTATION AND DISARTICULATION

In order to shorten the time of wound-healing and prevent troublesome cicatrices, it is customary to shape the skin edges in such a way that the wound can be closed by primary union.

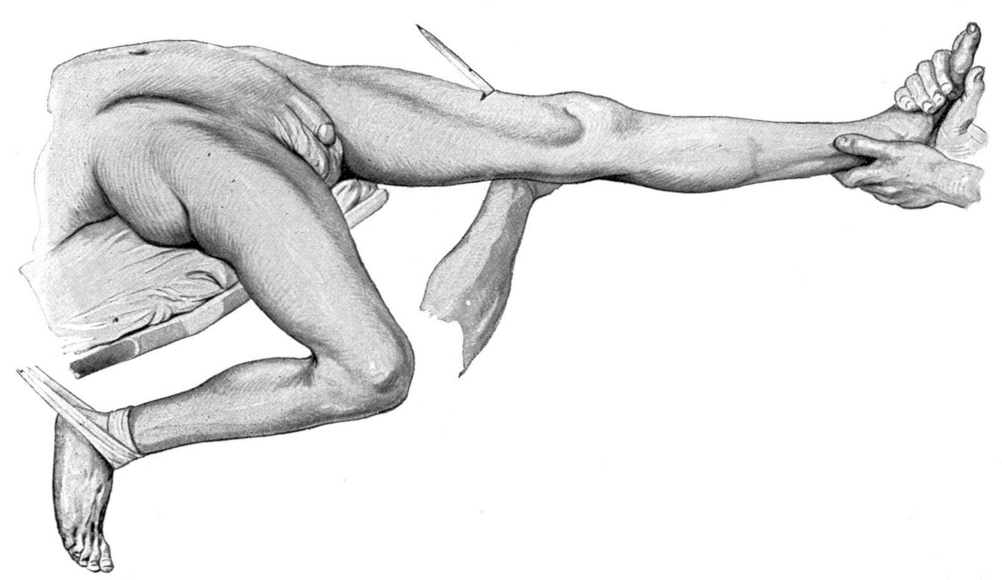

FIG. 702. Position of the patient for amputation of the left femur. The lower end of the table extends to the gluteal fold. The healthy limb is fastened with the knee bent towards the head, the limb to be amputated is held by the foot in extension by an assistant.

If, because of infection, primary closure can not be done, the skin is incised so that after the infection has subsided, secondary closure is possible, without too great cicatricial formation. Only in the presence of very severe infections, where the first consideration must be the conservation of life, is a guillotine amputation the proper procedure. Because of the rapidity with which this operation is done and the simplicity of the wound which does not provide primarily any covering for the stump, it is necessary later to perform a secondary amputation, or a plastic operation. It is desirable when an arti-

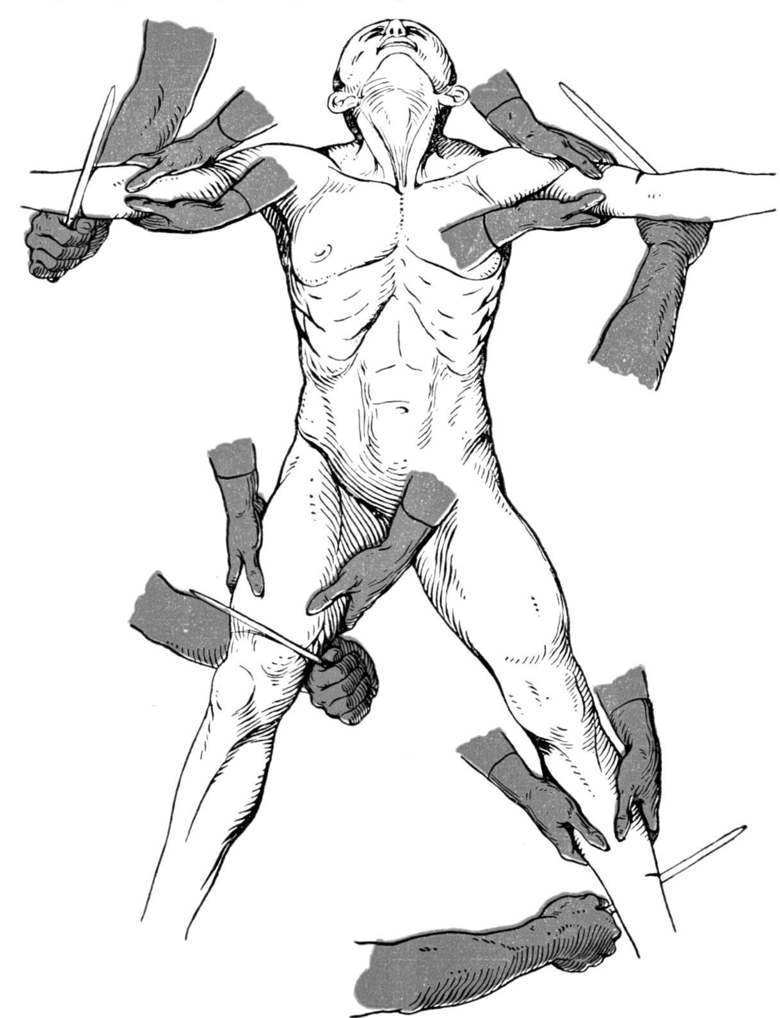

FIG. 703. Position of the surgeon and of the hands of the assistant who is retracting the skin proximally for circular amputations.

ficial limb is to be used, that the scar should not lie on the supporting surface, in order to avert chafing of the wound.

For the nutrition of the skin flaps it is advisable in many cases to leave intact the attachment of the skin to the deep fascia or use the muscle itself for a nutritional base. If the nutrition of a skin flap appears doubtful because of the shape of the flap or because of an existing disease, such as calcification of the arteries or diabetes, skin-muscle-flaps from half the thickness of the limb are made.

The hope has not been completely realized that by covering the end of the bone with thick layers of muscle an elastic cushion would be formed which would reduce the impact of the prosthesis and thus increase the weight-bearing capacity of the stump. Nevertheless, we generally try to cover the stump with muscle, in order to prevent pressure of the bone against the skin, with its associated injury.

Difficulties are often encountered in obtaining sufficient skin and muscle for flaps to cover the stump, if one does not want to sacrifice unnecessarily valuable parts of the limb, as for example after injuries. In practice, there-

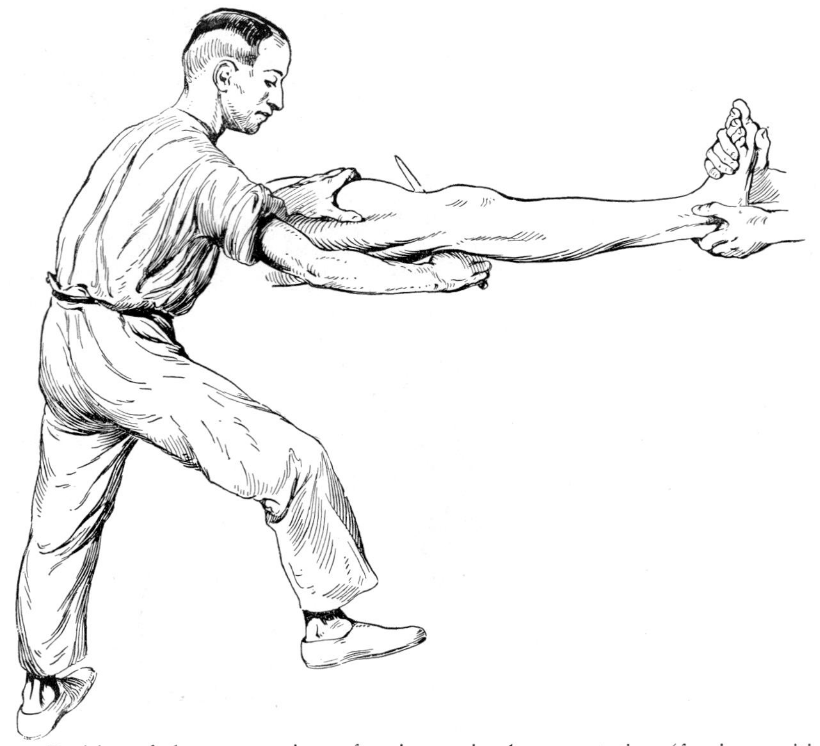

Fig. 704. Position of the surgeon in performing a circular amputation (fencing position).

fore, one method of amputation should not be depended upon, but a choice from a large number of various procedures must be made to meet the particular condition. The surgeon must be able to choose and apply the best procedure for the case at hand.

1. The Circular Amputation

The classic amputation is by the circular incision. The circular incision is performed as a single procedure, when the skin, soft parts and bone are divided at the same level (Fig. 710). A two-level circular operation is performed when the level of division of the muscles and bone is proximal to the level of division of the skin (Fig. 705). The procedure may be designated as a three-level circular amputation, where in addition the muscles are removed at two different levels (Fig. 711). (The single level operation de-

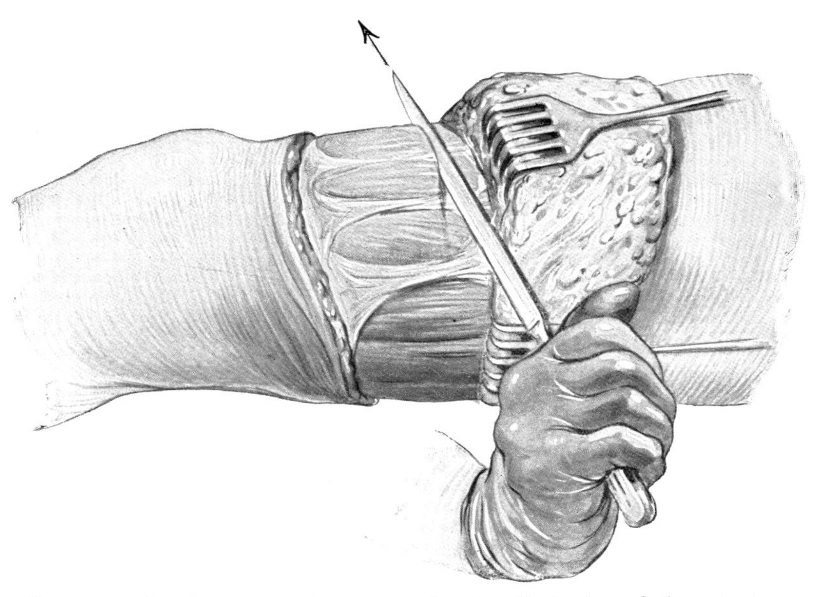

FIG. 705. Circular amputation at two levels. Beginning of the 1st step.

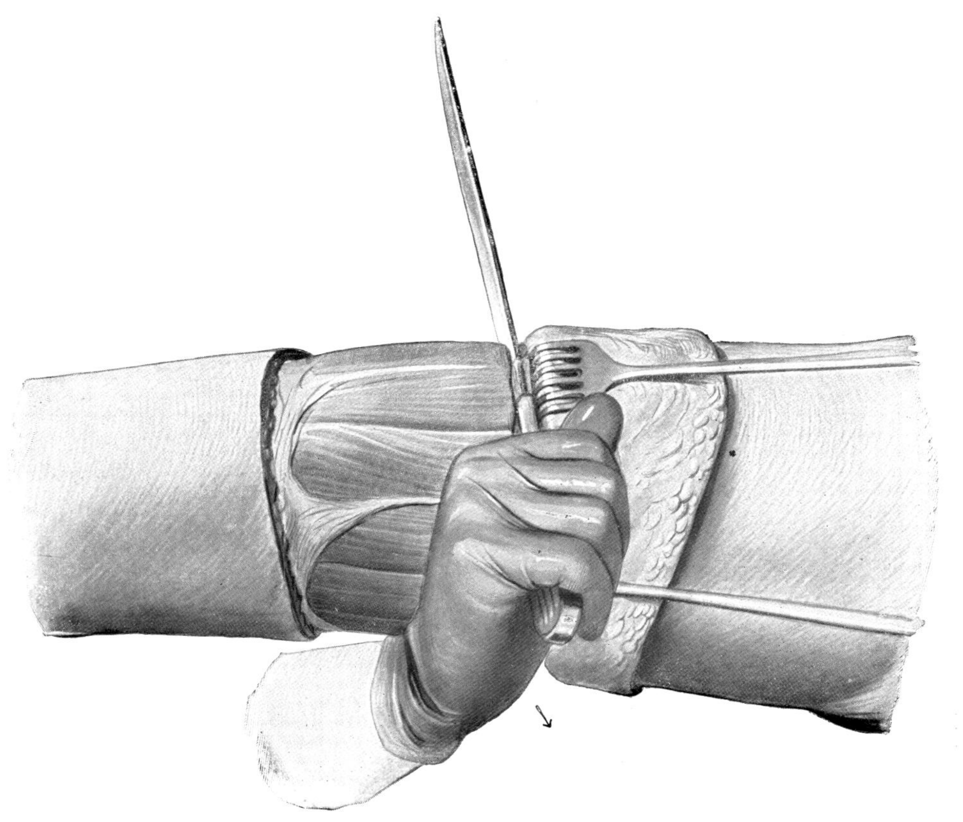

FIG. 706. Circular amputation at two levels. Beginning of the 2nd step.

scribed by Kirschner as a circular amputation is the one that we are accustomed to call the guillotine amputation. It is in fact the simplest or most primitive form of circular amputation. I.S.R.)

(a) THE TWO-LEVEL CIRCULAR AMPUTATION

To carry out the usual two-level circular amputation, the patient is placed in such a position that the limb to be amputated extends over the operating table. In an amputation of the arm, the patient lies close to the edge of the table, while an assistant holds the arm which hangs free. In amputation of the leg, the healthy leg may be fastened on the operating table with the knee flexed and hip extended, while the diseased leg which extends over the lower end of the table is supported by an assistant in any position

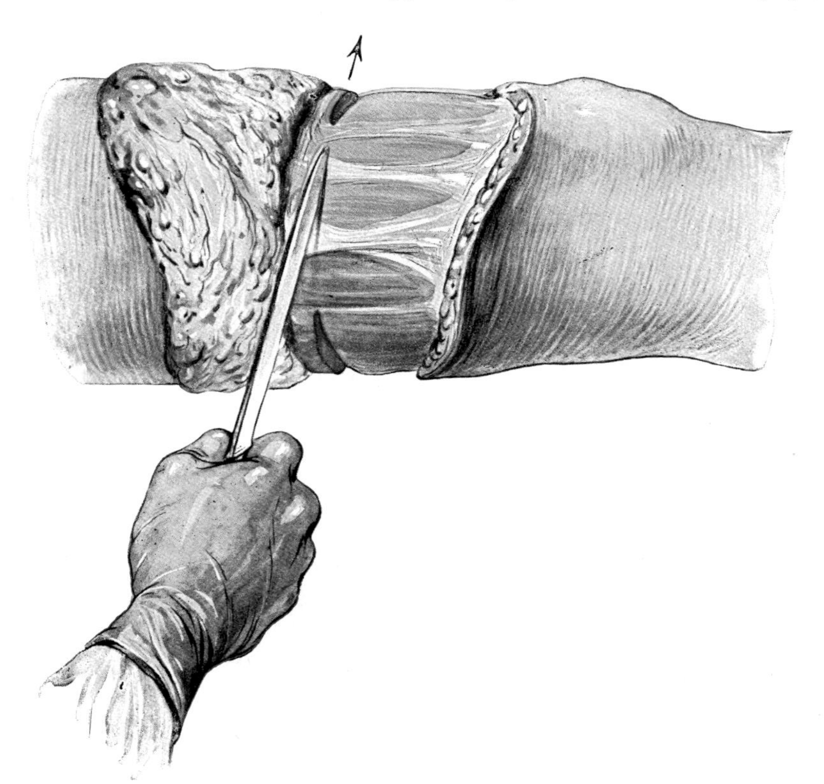

FIG. 707. Circular amputation at two levels. Beginning of the 3rd step.

the surgeon may wish (Fig. 702). The operator stands, as previously described, so that the amputated limb falls to his right (Fig. 703). When the right leg is to be amputated he stands to the right of the patient; when the left leg, between the legs; when the right arm, between the right arm and head; when the left arm, to the left side of the patient.

A circular incision is first made through the skin and superficial fascia, a circular incision is then made through the muscles and the remaining soft parts at a higher level. After the skin has been divided the assistants elevate and proximally retract the skin and superficial fascia, while the surgeon frees the cutaneous cuff by dividing the loose connective tissue between the underlayer of the cuff and the muscle fascia with long strokes of the knife made perpendicular to the underlayer, carefully protecting the subcutaneous

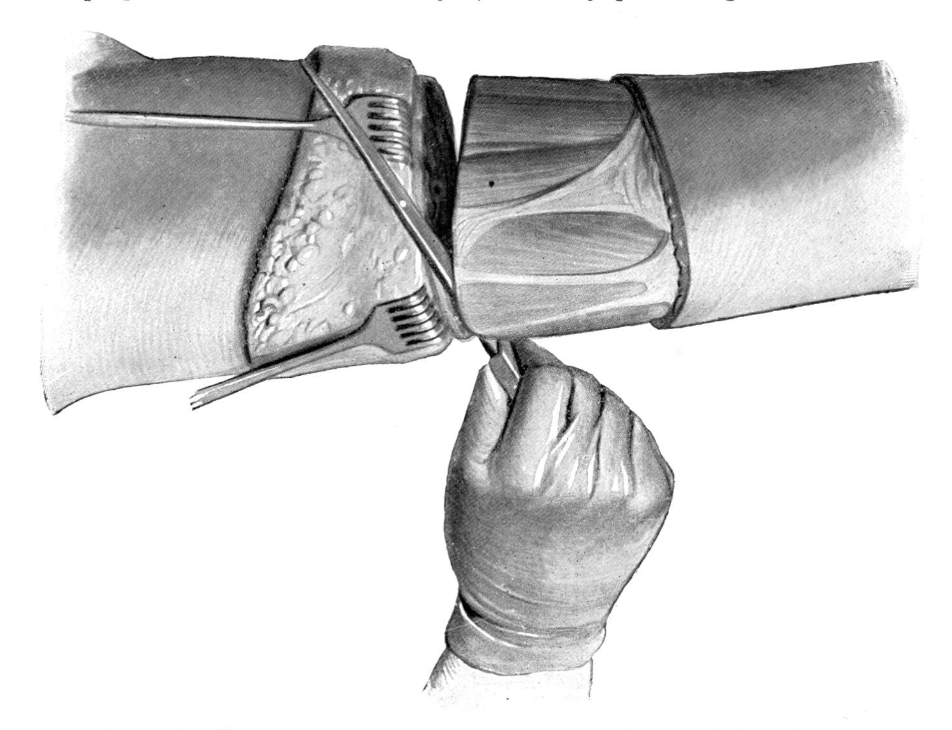

FIG. 708. Circular amputation at two levels. Beginning of the 4th step.

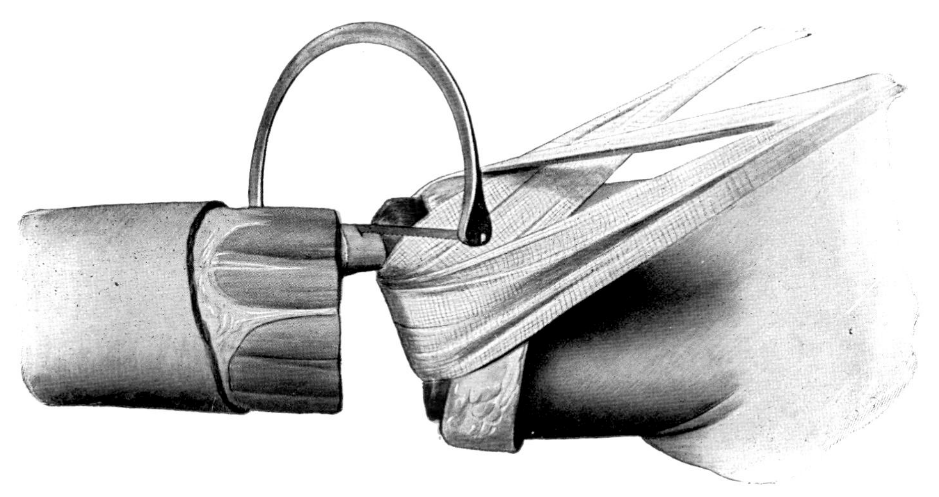

FIG. 709. Separation of the bone. Circular amputation of the thigh at two levels.

tissue remaining on the flaps. The length of the cuff should be equal to two-thirds of the diameter of the limb. This cuff is everted, and at its base another similar circular incision is made, which divides any subcutaneous tissue not already divided. At the base of the everted cuff the muscles are divided with a long amputation knife, in a circular incision which is made by two sweeps of the knife and which extends to the bone. The protruding muscles are retracted proximally with large hooked retractors, with tailed bandages (Fig. 709) or with a perforated disc, and the bone is sawed through in the same plane.

Method of Dividing the Muscle. The surgeon assumes a position with the right leg forward and bent (fencing position, Fig. 704). The division of the muscles takes four steps, but the knife is applied to the parts only twice. The art of the old surgeons, who incised the circumference of a limb in one stroke, is no longer practised. The operator grasps the long amputation knife in the palm of his hand, places the point on the side of the extremity opposite him, so that the limb is between the knife and the operator, and pushes it forward from the point to the handle (1st step, Fig. 705).

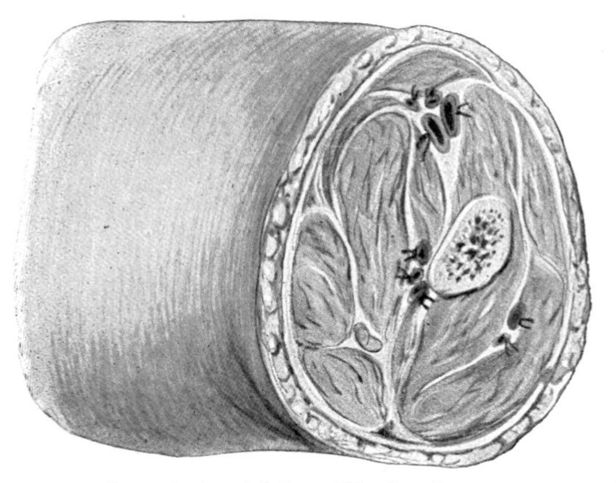

Fig. 710. Guillotine amputation of the thigh. All the tissues are cut through at one level.

The knife is then drawn back from the handle to the point through the adjacent second quadrant of the limb (2nd step, Fig. 706, end of the 1st stroke). If the incision is carried out properly, almost three-quarters of the circumference of the limb is now divided. The knife is now applied with the point in the center of the undivided section, on the side of the limb toward the operator, and is carried to the end of the first incision, by pushing it forward as far as the handle (3rd step, Fig. 707). It is then drawn back in the second incision from the handle to the point, separating the remaining soft parts (4th step, Fig. 708, end of the 2nd stroke). These four lines of incision are perpendicular to one another, thus justifying Larrey in characterizing this incision as the polygonal incision.

(b) THE SIMPLE CIRCULAR (GUILLOTINE) AMPUTATION

The circular amputation at one level (Fig. 710) combines the advantage of rapidity with the establishment of wound conditions affording good drainage. Because of the great disadvantage of the absence of skin covering, it is to be used only in the presence of severe infection (Kausch), when extreme rapidity is essential, or if the amputation must be done by an inexperienced person. Because of the absence of sufficient skin to cover the stump, it is frequently necessary to perform a subsequent reamputation or a plastic operation to cover the stump, though the skin margins may be considerably approximated by applying traction on the skin during healing (see page 631). The technic for the separation of soft parts is the same as in the two-level circular amputation, except that the skin and the muscles are separated in one plane at the same time without the formation of a skin cuff. The bone is sawed through at the same level.

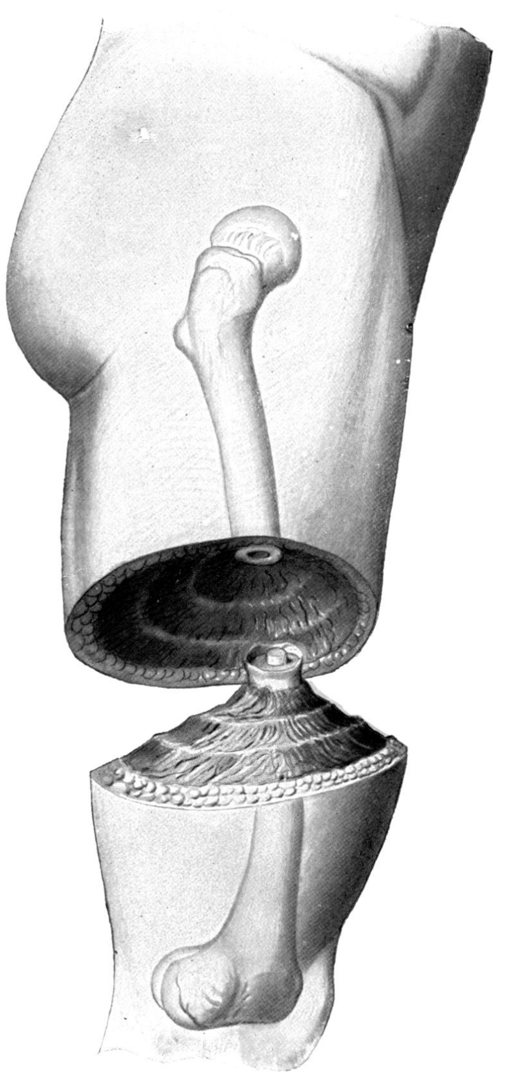

FIG. 711. Circular amputation of the thigh in five planes. The skin is removed in one plane, the muscles in three planes, and the bone in a fifth plane.

(c) VARIETIES OF CIRCULAR AMPUTATIONS

The classic method of circular amputation by two applications of the knife is subject in practice to many variations. Where the nutrition of the skin cuff is endangered, as for example, in amputations performed because of circulatory disturbances, the skin cuff may be so made as to contain the muscle fascia. This is practicable in the forearm or leg only when lateral incisions are made in the fascia to relieve tension. The division of the muscles and bone in one plane creates simple anatomical conditions, but it places the bone stump directly under the skin, which is disadvantageous in the femur. This disadvantage may be avoided either by dividing the bone a few centimeters proximal to the plane of division of the muscles, or by dividing the muscles at several different levels (Fig. 711). This may be done by retracting proximally the outer layer of muscles after they have been divided, and then separating the remainder of muscles at one or two higher levels. In this way a hollow cone is formed, which has at its apex the end of the bone. The muscles cover the deep end of the bone and are held in this position by a few catgut sutures.

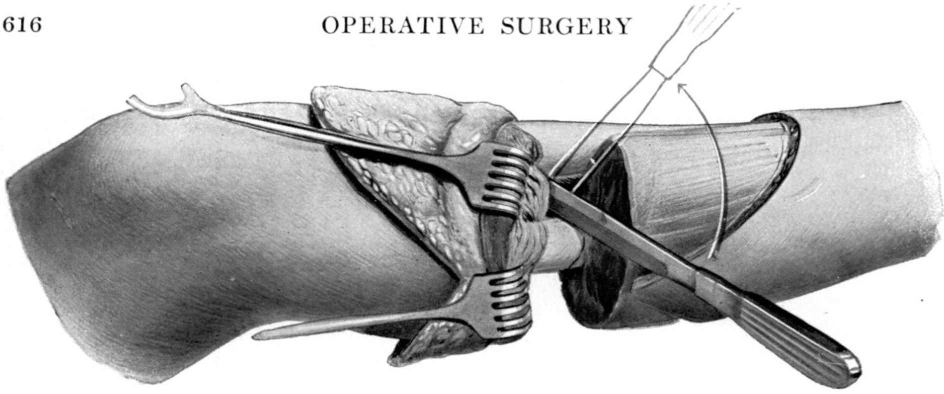

Fig. 712. Dividing the tissues in the interosseus space, in amputation of the leg. A double-edged knife is used.

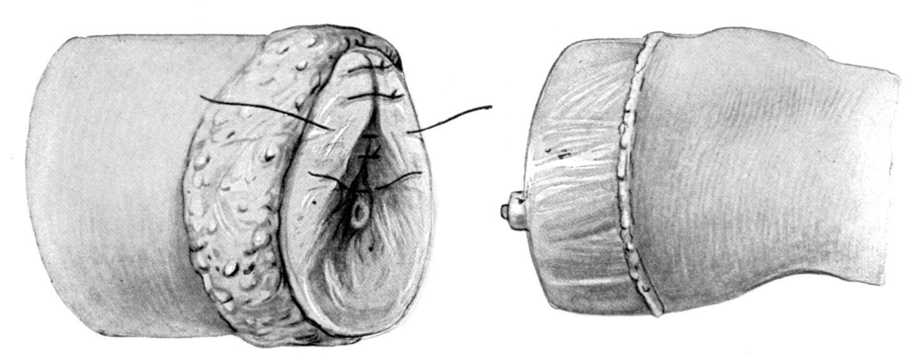

Fig. 713. Suturing the muscles in a two-layer circular amputation of the thigh.

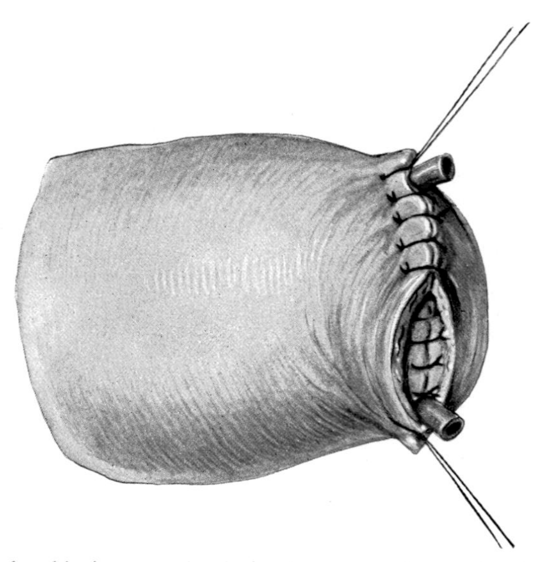

Fig. 714. Suturing the skin in a two-level circular amputation of the thigh. A drainage tube is placed at each end of the suture line.

When the skin cuff is considerably smaller at its distal margin, as occurs in conically shaped limbs (forearm, leg, in part also the thigh), it may be difficult to retract it and to evert it. To enlarge the skin cuff in such cases, it must be split longitudinally in one or more places.

In the forearm and the leg, where there are two bones, the soft parts lying between the bones can not be separated with the customary incisions. To divide them the knife must be carried between the two bones and all soft parts carefully separated. It is best to use for this purpose a double-edged knife (Fig. 712).

The suture of the wound after circular amputation is done in such a way that the muscles are sutured in layers (Fig. 713) and the skin cuff (Fig. 714) transversely. There arise at the end of the suture line two skin tips, which may be rounded, or, since they later contract, they really require no special correction. A short drain is, as a rule, inserted in each corner (Fig. 714).

2. Flap Amputations

There are single-flap and double-flap methods for amputation. The advantage of the flap method lies mainly in the fact that the flaps necessary for covering the stump may be shaped according to the material at hand, which often effects an economy of tissue, as compared to the circular amputation. The wound is more accessible and can be watched more easily, in most cases, than the wound after circular amputation, where the narrowness of the skin cuff may give rise to considerable trouble. In the single flap amputation the scar in the skin lies outside the supporting surface of the stump. When there are two flaps it may usually be placed at least beyond the region of the end of the bone. Because the skin of the extensor surfaces tends to be more resistant than that of the flexor surfaces, in a one-flap procedure the flap as a rule is taken from the extensor surface, and in a two-flap procedure the larger of the two flaps is taken from the extensor surface, if there is sufficient material on this side.

The flaps may consist merely of skin, or of skin and fascia, or of skin, fascia and muscle, depending upon the requirements of the individual case. The flaps may be rectangular, with rounded corners, or oval.

Since the nutrition of a flap depends principally upon the width of its pedicle, in a one-flap amputation the base of the flap should be wider than half the circumference of the limb that is to be amputated. The entire length of the flap should exceed the diameter of the limb at the level of amputation by one-fourth. When primary closure is not done there will be considerable shrinking of the flaps. They should therefore be cut considerably larger if they are to be used for secondary closure of the stump. It is better for the inexperienced surgeon to cut the flaps larger than necessary and then shorten them as desired. Flaps which were originally misshaped rapidly become smaller in wounds that remain open.

In a flap amputation, the soft parts not included in the flap and the bone are divided at the base of the flap at the same level (or the bone may be divided at a level slightly higher than the muscles. I.S.R.).

(a) AMPUTATION BY A SINGLE FLAP. OVAL, RACKET, AND LANCET INCISIONS

The oval, or oblique circular incision is one of the best methods for forming a single flap (Fig. 715). It is made in one plane, occasionally in two planes, which forms an angle of 45° with the long axis of the limb. The only disadvantage is that it requires the use of a great deal of material. However, this can be lessened if the muscles are strongly retracted and the bone sawed off at a slightly higher level. If the oval incision is performed at two levels, the skin is first divided, a cuff is everted, and the muscles are incised somewhat proximally.

The oval incision may be modified by making a longitudinal incision at the top of the oval, forming the racket incision, or by rounding the margins of the racket incision to form a lancet incision (Fig. 716).

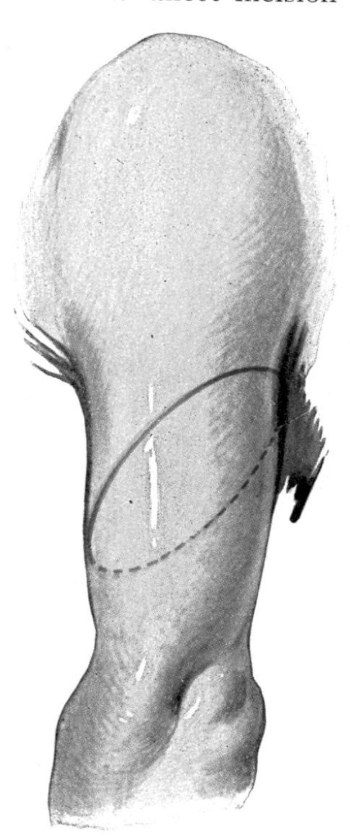

Fig. 715. Oval incision in amputation of the arm.

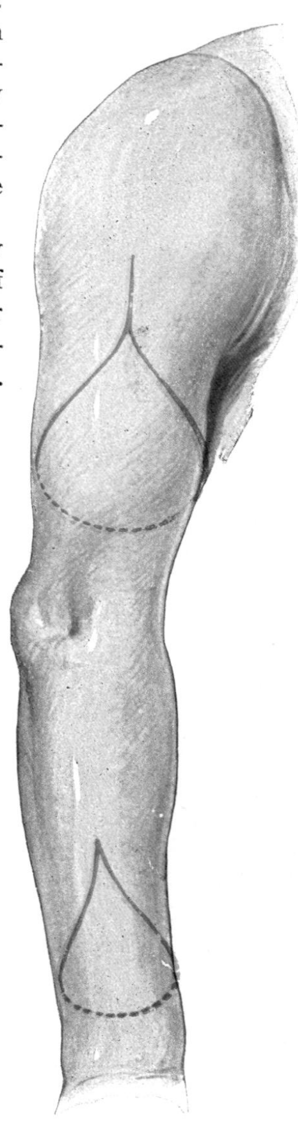

Fig. 716. Racket incision in amputation of the arm; lancet incision for forearm amputation.

(b) AMPUTATION BY DOUBLE FLAPS

The double-flap amputation is today the one most frequently used, because it combines economy of tissue with simplicity of technic. When the

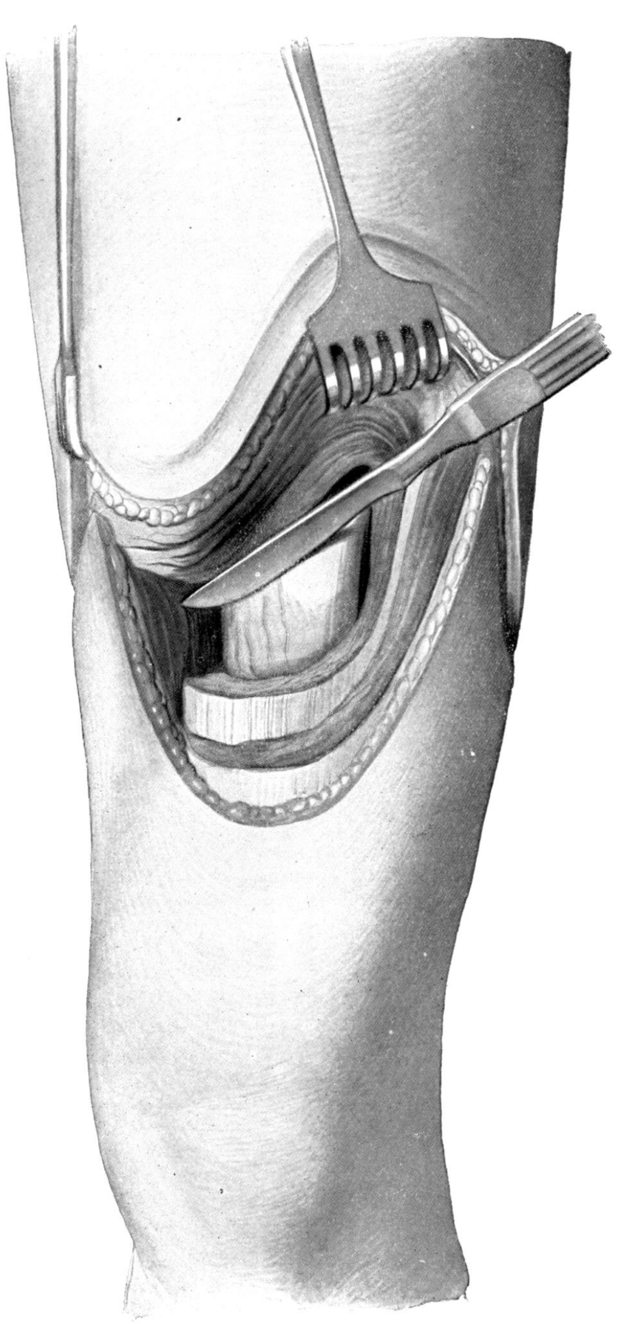

FIG. 717. Double-flap incision in amputation of the thigh. The knife divides the muscles in an oblique direction.

flaps consist only of skin, they are strongly retracted after the incision and gradually freed to the base with incisions directed perpendicular to the fascia. When the flaps contain skin, fascia and muscle, these three tissues are divided with an incision carried directly to the bone and the elevated flaps are detached from the bone by sharp dissection (Fig. 717). The muscles of the flap are divided in a plane perpendicular to their fibers,

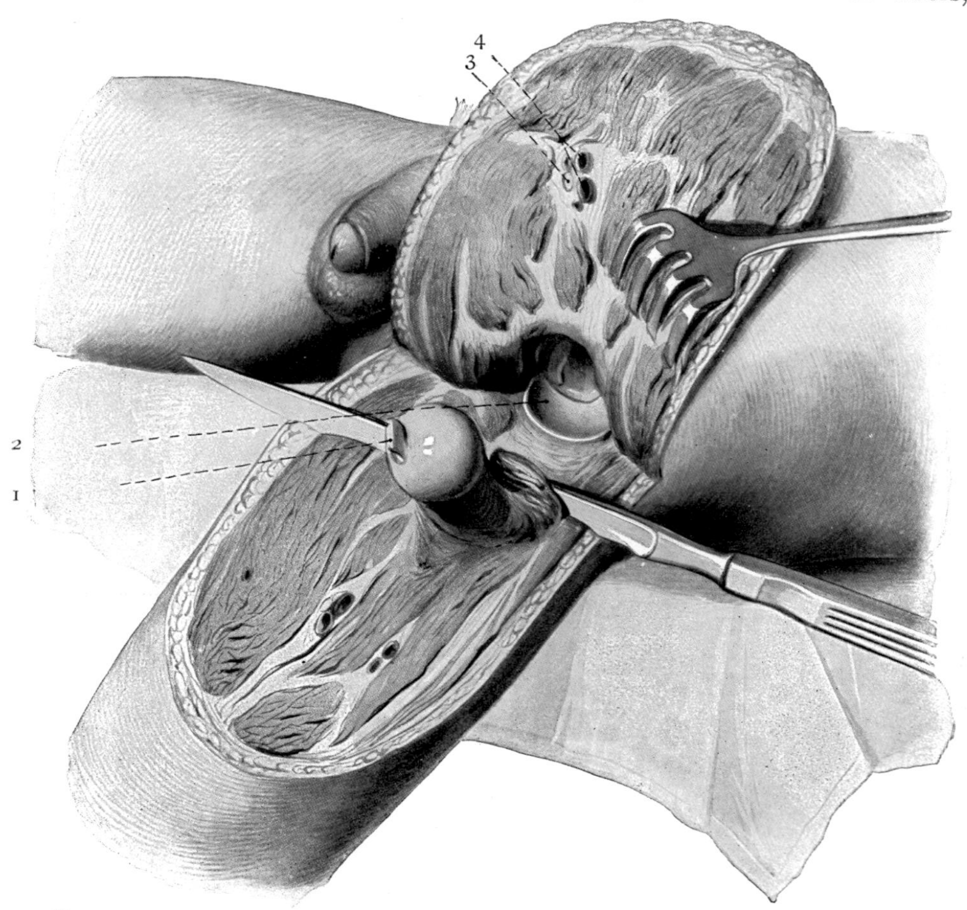

Fig. 718. Disarticulation of the hip-joint by transfixion. An anterior and posterior flap is outlined. 1. Incised surface of ligamentum teres. 2. Acetabulum of the hip-joint. 3. Femoral nerve. 4. Femoral artery and vein.

as far as possible, because it is easier to grasp vessels which are cut transversely, rather than obliquely. While the two flaps are retracted proximally with sharp hooked retractors, the bone is divided as high as possible. The bone may be divided after the formation of the first and before the formation of the second flap. The second flap is then cut from within with a large amputation knife (Fig. 718).

(c) AMPUTATION BY TRANSFIXION

Two varieties of flap amputation do not enjoy in my opinion the attention due them. The first is amputation by transfixion, also called the "French method." The performance of this method requires a long, slender and pointed amputation knife. The operation is simple and rapid. After marking on the skin the lines of incision, the knife with its cutting edge directed distally is inserted in the angle formed at the junction of the two lines of incision directly in front of the bone. The knife is thrust forward to the angle of the lines on the opposite side of the limb, being kept in contact with the anterior surface of the bone. The soft parts anterior to the bone are divided in the line of the incision previously drawn, by light sawing strokes, and the last bridge of skin is cut perpendicular to the surface if possible so that the edge of the skin is not too thin. In the same way, the knife is thrust through a second time from one angle to the other, but

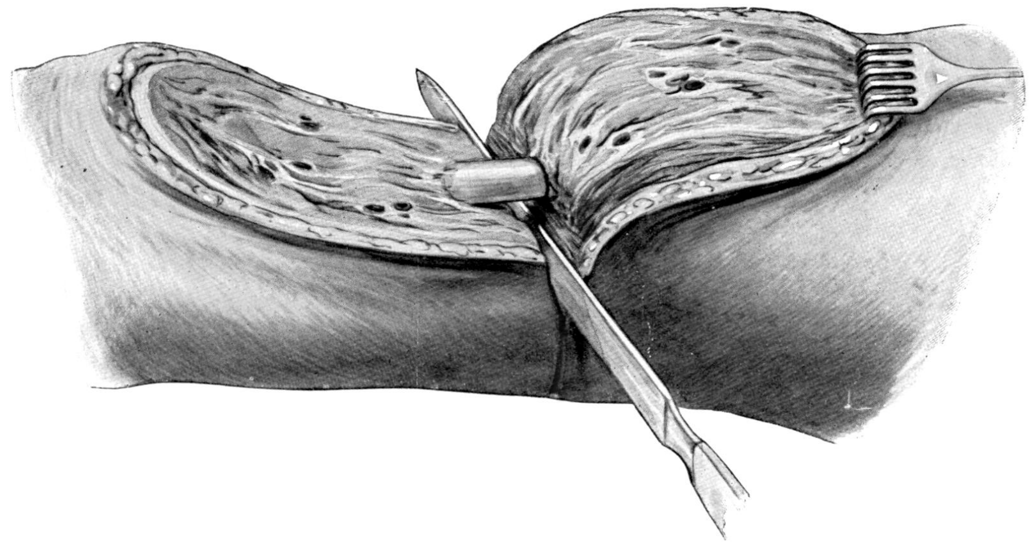

FIG. 719. Amputation of the arm with one flap by transfixion. The knife is inserted in front of the bone and the soft parts are cut through, making an anterior flap. The knife is then inserted behind the bone and the tissues are cut through at right angles to the direction of the bone.

this time posterior to the bone, and the posterior flap is made. While the assistants retract the two flaps, which gape like the mouth of a fish, with hooked retractors, the surgeon saws the exposed bone at the base of the flaps. This procedure was formerly popular particularly on account of its speed. While this advantage may be of subordinate importance at present, yet this procedure still possesses its remarkable advantages of economy, of a wide open simple wound, and of ease in covering the stump even when it is necessary to keep the wound open in a severe infection.

Transfixion may also be used in the formation of one flap. One flap is made in the manner described, but it is relatively larger, and the remaining soft parts are divided either by transfixion or from without with a semicircular incision perpendicular to the axis of the limb at the height of the base of the first flap (Fig. 719). The bone is sawed through at the base of the flap.

(d) AMPUTATION BY EQUAL FLAPS OF SKIN AND MUSCLE

The second method which deserves greater attention, especially in the amputation of infected limbs, is one which combines simple circular incision with the formation of two large skin-muscle flaps. In Germany this is

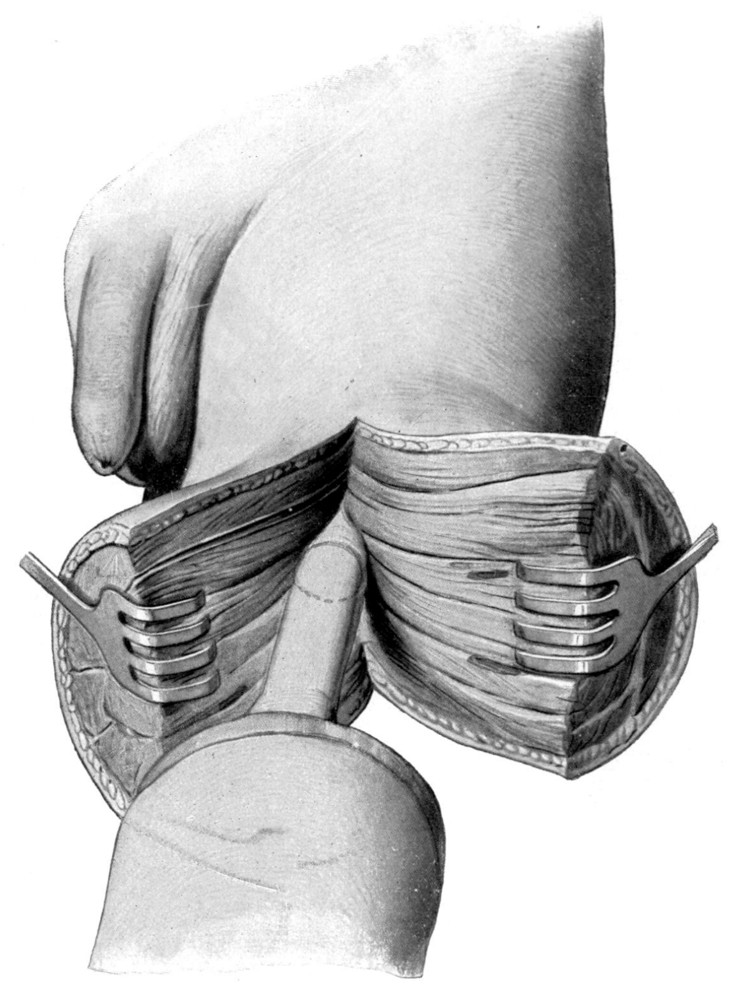

FIG. 720. "Double-door" procedure, in thigh amputation. A guillotine amputation is first performed. An incision is then made so as to outline two flaps, one on either side of the bone. At the base of the latter incision the bone is sawed through.

known as the "double-door" amputation. The principle of this operation can best be seen in the illustration (Fig. 720). The soft parts are divided to the bone at one level. Two incisions in the longitudinal axis of the limb are then made in a proximal direction from the point of amputation. These incisions also extend to the bone. In making them the vicinity of large vessels should be avoided so that no vessel will be slit longitudinally. The flaps can readily be made in such a way that the cleft will afford proper drainage for the wound when the stump is in its customary position. The two skin-muscle flaps held with large hook retractors are detached from the bone to their bases, at which level the bone is divided. The large flaps

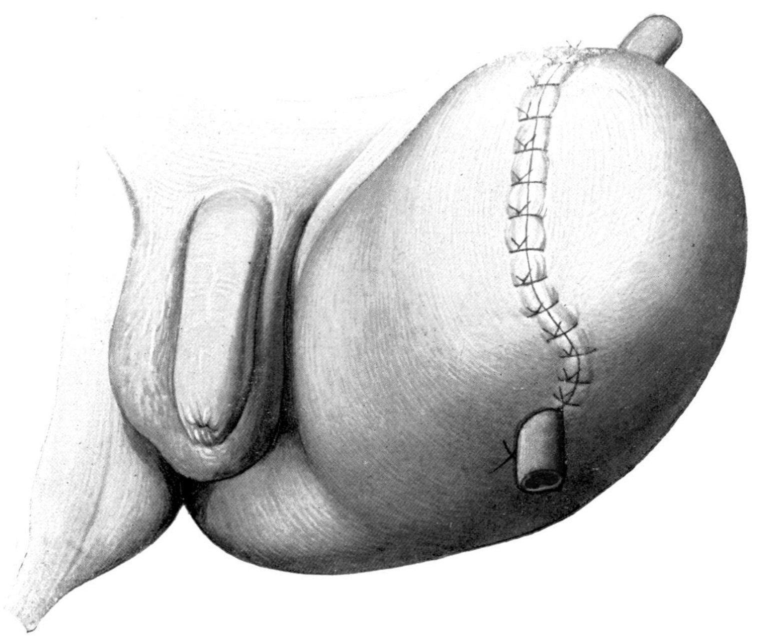

FIG. 721. "Double-door" amputation of the thigh after suturing. A rubber tube is inserted through the middle of the vertical incision.

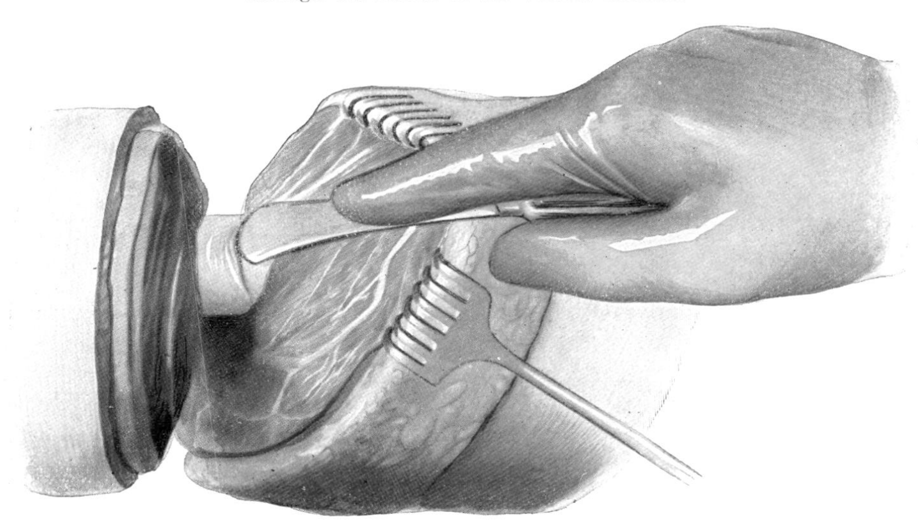

FIG. 722. Removing the periosteum from the bone stump in amputation of the thigh (Bunge).

lie together like the mouth of a fish. According to the degree of infection which may be present, the margins of the flaps are either united by sutures and the wound drained (Fig. 721), or the wound is kept open by gauze and rubber drains.

D. CARE OF THE BONE

The capacity for weight bearing of a stump depends to a considerable extent upon the condition of the end of the bone. The most unfavorable complication in this respect is the development of osteophytes (Fig. 735). The sawdust which results when the bone is sawed should be collected on wet sponges, and if any is accidentally scattered in the wound, it should be flushed out. The formation of bony proliferations on the end of the bone itself may be prevented by forming an "aperiosteal bone stump" (Bunge) (Figs. 722 and 723). In this method the end of the bone is freed for a short distance of its osteogenetic layers, the periosteum and the endosteum. This is accomplished by cutting the periosteum circularly around the exposed bone, about one centimeter proximal from the level at which it is to be sawed and pushing it distally with an elevator for a considerable distance before dividing the bone.

The bone is then sawed through at the desired level, while the muscles are carefully held back (Fig. 709). The marrow and endosteum are scooped out of the bone stump for a distance of about one centimeter. The end of the bone is thus free of all osteogenetic tissue for a distance of about one centimeter.

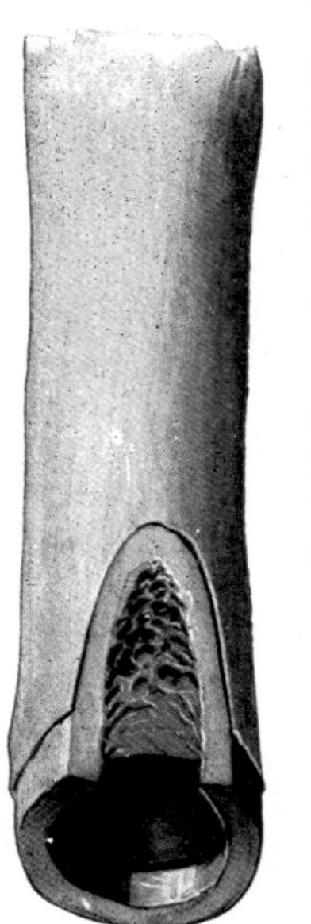

FIG. 723. Aperiosteal bone stump (Bunge) whose end is freed of periosteum and marrow, for about 1 cm.

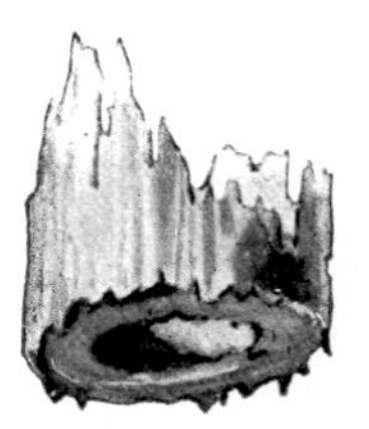

FIG. 724. Sequestrum from an aperiosteal thigh amputation stump, which became infected.

Stripping the bone of periosteum and marrow considerably lowers its vitality. Care must be taken, therefore, to prevent necrosis by limiting the removal of periosteum and endosteum to a distance of one centimeter. The procedure, furthermore, should be used only in healthy individuals, in an area of good nutrition, and under aseptic conditions. It should never be used when the resistance of the tissue is impaired by infection or circulatory disturbances (arteriosclerosis, diabetes). Failure to observe these precautions may result in the formation of a coronary sequestrum (Fig. 724). These cause prolonged suppuration until they are extruded or removed surgically and favor the proliferation of bone. They can be easily demonstrated with the x-ray.

When the supporting surface of a bone is naturally very small or gradually becomes pointed and conical, it lessens the stump's capacity for weight bearing. An attempt is made, therefore, to make the surface of the divided bone as large as possible and to counteract its change of form. Disarticulation ideally fulfills these conditions. The end of a divided shaft may be given some of the advantages of the disarticulation stump by an osteoplastic operation. The oldest and most popular osteoplastic methods of amputation are those of Pirogoff and Gritti. In Pirogoff's operation the posterior protuberance of the calcaneus is used; in Gritti's operation the anterior part of the patella with the attached skin covers the end of the bone (Fig. 725). A further advantage of these operations is that skin which is particularly resistant to pressure may be used in its natural relation to the adjacent bone

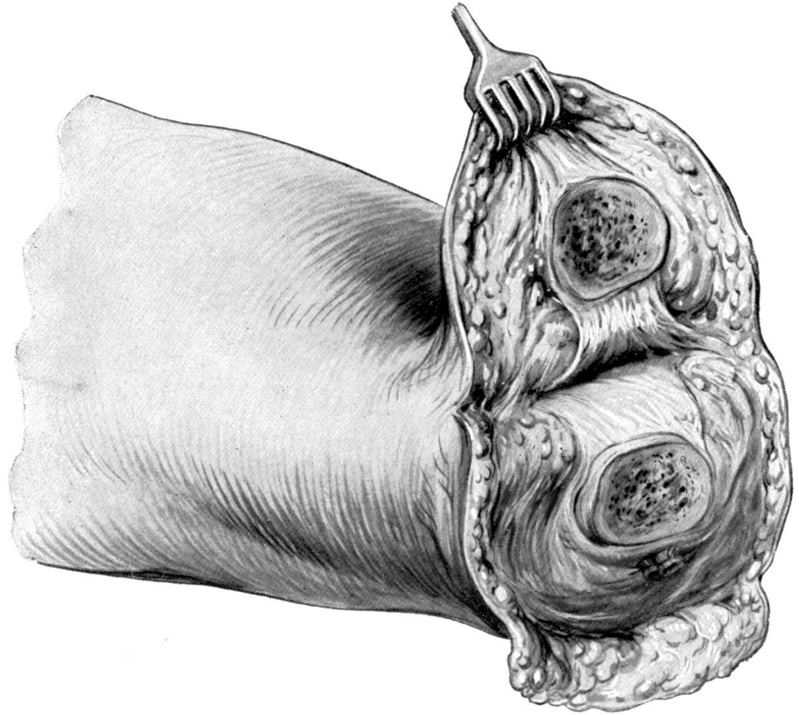

FIG. 725. Osteoplastic amputation of the thigh (Stokes-Gritti). The patella whose posterior surface has been sawed off is left in the anterior flap to cover the end of the femur.

without making a tissue cicatrix on the supporting surface. Sabanejeff's amputation of the femur is based upon the same principle. In this operation the osteoplastic flaps with the overlying skin are removed from the anterior surface of the proximal end of the tibia. Oehlecker's "step amputations" of the femur and the leg differ from Pirogoff's and Gritti's amputations only in being placed at higher levels. An advantage of Oehlecker's procedure, which proved excellent in amputation of infected limbs during the last war, lies in the fact that it is possible at first merely to form the osteoplastic flap and to put it in place only after the infection has subsided and the wound, which has been kept open for drainage, is ready to close. The original length of the flap affords sufficient covering even when it has considerably contracted.

The osteoplastic procedure, recommended by Bier, utilizes a bone flap which is pedunculated by its attached periosteum to cover the end of the divided tibia. The flap is taken from the anterior surface of the tibia below the site of amputation. In the Bier method the bone flap has no attachment to the overlying tissues. When I use the osteoplastic method in leg amputations I vary Bier's procedure slightly (Fig. 726). The bone and periosteal flap is left attached to the soft parts which form the anterior flap. In this way the nutrition of the bone is better maintained. Occasionally I use an

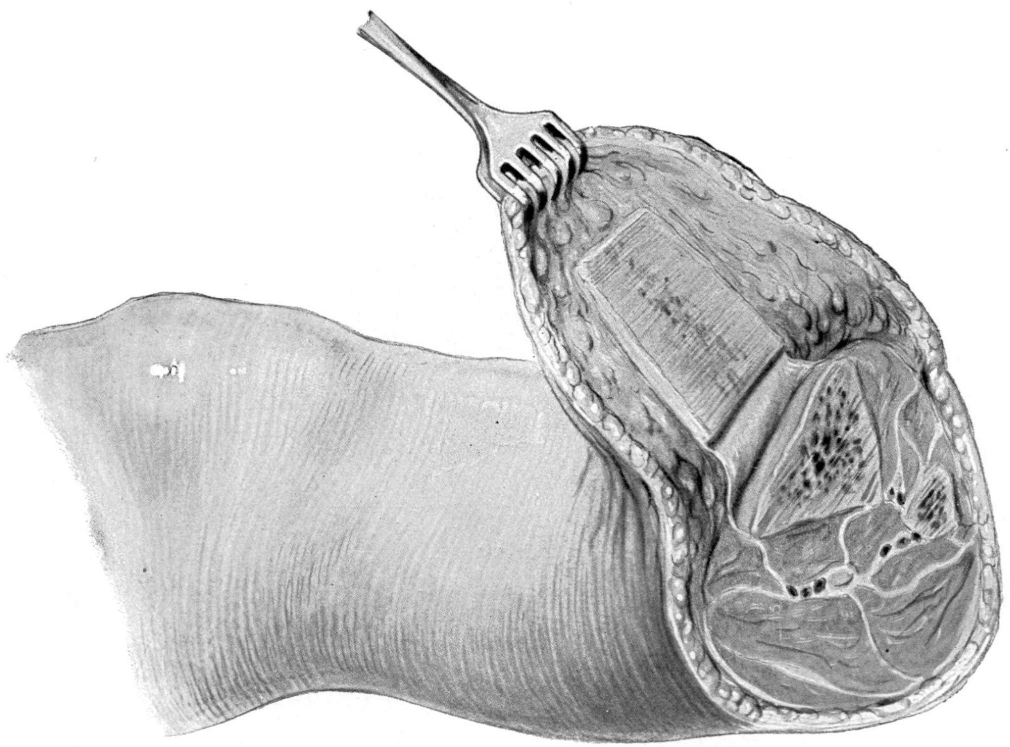

FIG. 726. Osteoplastic amputation of the leg. A small bone flap from the tibia is used to cover the ends of the tibia and fibula. It is not separated from the soft parts of the flap when this is elevated.

osteoperiosteal bone flap for a similar purpose. This method was previously described under cranial plastic operations (Hacker-Durante). The flap is formed by tangentially chiseling off a thin layer of bone with its overlying periosteum which is used to cover the end of the bone.

In the osteoplastic procedures described the bone flap does not always remain in position during healing but, because of mechanical influences, edema of the soft parts, or muscular and cicatricial traction it is frequently displaced, so that osseous union with the surface of the shaft in the proper position is far from constant. The result is that the new bony surface hoped for is not often obtained. This drawback, as well as that of the waste of material, is avoided by Kirschner's procedure of pegging the end of the amputated bone (Fig. 727). This consists in closing the medullary cavity of the shaft with a bone peg, taken from the section of limb removed, as for example, from the fibula. The amputation is completed without removing any periosteum. The bone peg, which must be of the same thickness and shape as the medullary cavity that is to be closed, is driven with a hammer into the cavity. It is advisable not to use too great force for this, in order to avoid splintering the compact bone. When the peg is firmly in place, the shaft is sawed off a few millimeters higher, to make the surface perfectly smooth.

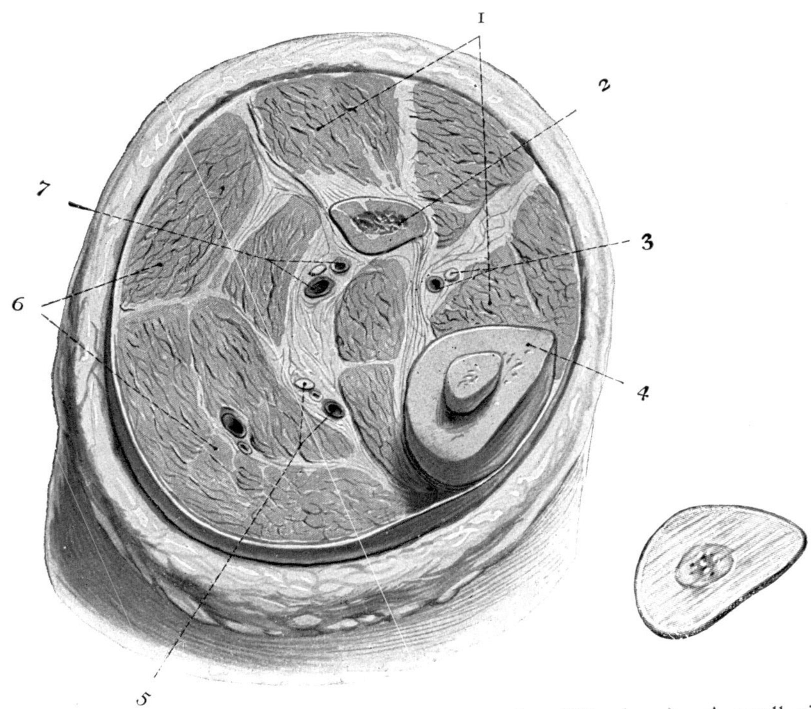

FIG. 727. Pegging the medullary cavity after amputation (Kirschner). A small piece of the resected fibula is inserted in the medullary canal of the tibia. The excess is sawed off again, so that the distal surface of the tibia is smooth. 1. Extensor muscles. 2. Fibula. 3. Deep peroneal nerve and ant. tibial artery. 4. Tibia. 5. Post. tibial vessels and tibial nerve. 6. Gastrocnemius muscles. 7. Peroneal vessels and superficial peroneal nerve.

Sauerbruch's plastic operation is the most radical in using the principle of osteoplasty. (This radical procedure has little value. I.S.R.) It replaces the femur and the excised anterior half of the soft parts of the thigh by the tibia rotated proximally at the knee through 180° and by the posterior half of the soft parts of the leg. The head of the tibia thus provides the weight-bearing surface of the stump and the malleolus lies in the acetabulum. This method may possibly be still better adapted for use in the arm in suitable cases.

Another plastic operation for covering the end of bone worth calling special attention to is Wilms' tendino-plastic amputation (Fig. 728). It is intended primarily for the amputation of the leg in the lower or middle part. The tendon of Achilles is divided as low as possible and turned back over the sawed surface of the tibia and fastened on its anterior surface. When the skin flaps used to cover the amputation wound are taken from the flexor side, the tendon is left attached to the overlying skin. Otherwise, the tendon is exposed and the skin flaps are made from whatever material is available. The quadriceps tendon may be used in a similar manner to cover the surface of the femur.

The same conditions must be present when an osteoplastic operation is done as for Bunge's aperiosteal resection (see page 624). These are favorable conditions for healing, absence of infection, of arteriosclerosis, and

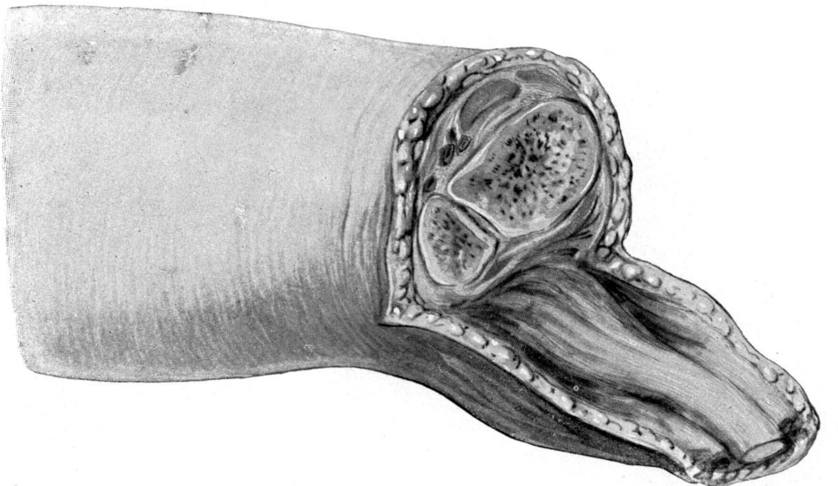

Fig. 728. Tendino-plastic amputation (Wilms). A long posterior flap which includes the Achilles tendon is used to cover the wound.

diabetes. Only Oehlecker's amputation has stood the test in the presence of infection.

E. CARE OF THE VESSELS

Protected by the artificial anemia induced by the tourniquet, the incised main vessels are first searched for in the wound according to their anatomical location. They are usually easily found between the proper muscles. The artery, vein, and as a rule the accompanying nerve are exposed individually far enough for each vessel to be grasped transversely with a hemostat (Fig. 729). They are then ligated with catgut. Silk is used only for ligating large arteries. From my experience, there is no objection to the ligation of the artery and vein together. Tying the vessel above a transversely placed hemostat insures that the ligature will surround the entire lumen of the vessel, and that it will lie proximal to the surface of the divided muscles. This lessens the danger of secondary hemorrhage in suppurating wounds. After the main vessels are ligated, other large vessels are found and ligated in the same way. The wound is then systematically searched for visible vessels which have been cut transversely, or for possible bleeding points which appear when pressure is made. These points are seized with hemostats and ligated with catgut. Most of the larger vessels supplying the muscles lie near the center of the transversely cut muscles.

The tourniquet should now be removed. Within a few seconds the large arteries begin pulsating, and a few moments later hemorrhage begins, which is partly parenchymatous and partly due to small arteries and veins that as yet have not been ligated. I consider the Vogel-Strauss procedure of first compressing the surface with gauze for some minutes after the removal of the tourniquet a waste of time. Instead of this, the bleeding vessels should be seized immediately in the open wound and ligated. Occasionally arterial bleeding does not begin for a few minutes, and these bleeding points should be watched for. It is a well proven rule not to consider the hemorrhage as

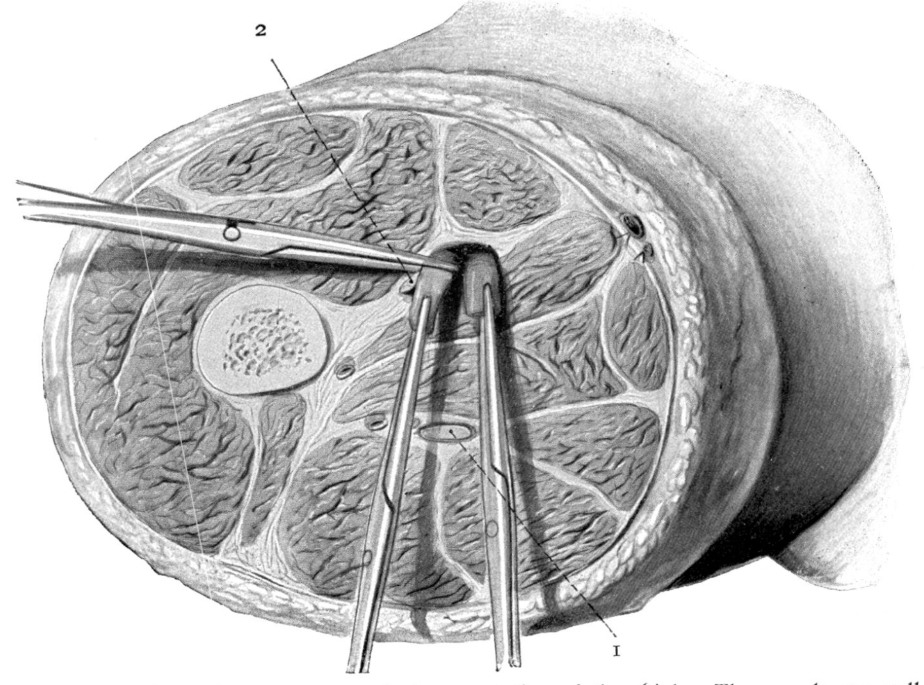

FIG. 729. Care of the great vessels in amputation of the thigh. The vessels are pulled out of the wound and hemostats are applied transversely. They are then doubly ligated. 1. Sciatic nerve. 2. Saphenous nerve.

ended before 5 minutes after the removal of the tourniquet. If an active parenchymatous hemorrhage does not occur after this time, if the muscles remain brownish and dry, and the pulsation of the ligated main artery is absent, as sometimes happens in amputations performed for circulatory disturbances, these indicate nutritional insufficiency of the amputation wound, and the question arises whether it would not be better to amputate higher in an area which is better nourished.

Careful hemostasis is a primary condition for undisturbed healing. Because there may be secondary oozing of blood and serum, even after scrupulous hemostasis, it is better to use drainage after the amputation of a very large extremity, even though asepsis has been maintained. One or two drains are placed in the corners of the line of suture for 24 to 48 hours (Fig. 721).

F. CARE OF THE NERVES

Pressure from the prosthesis may cause pain in any nerve of the stump. On the other hand, nerves caught in the cicatrix or those which develop neuromata may also cause pain even though they are not subjected to direct pressure. Since the nerves in the end of the stump are no longer of use, many of the painful amputation stumps can be avoided by a high resection of the major nerves of the part. The large nerve trunks are searched

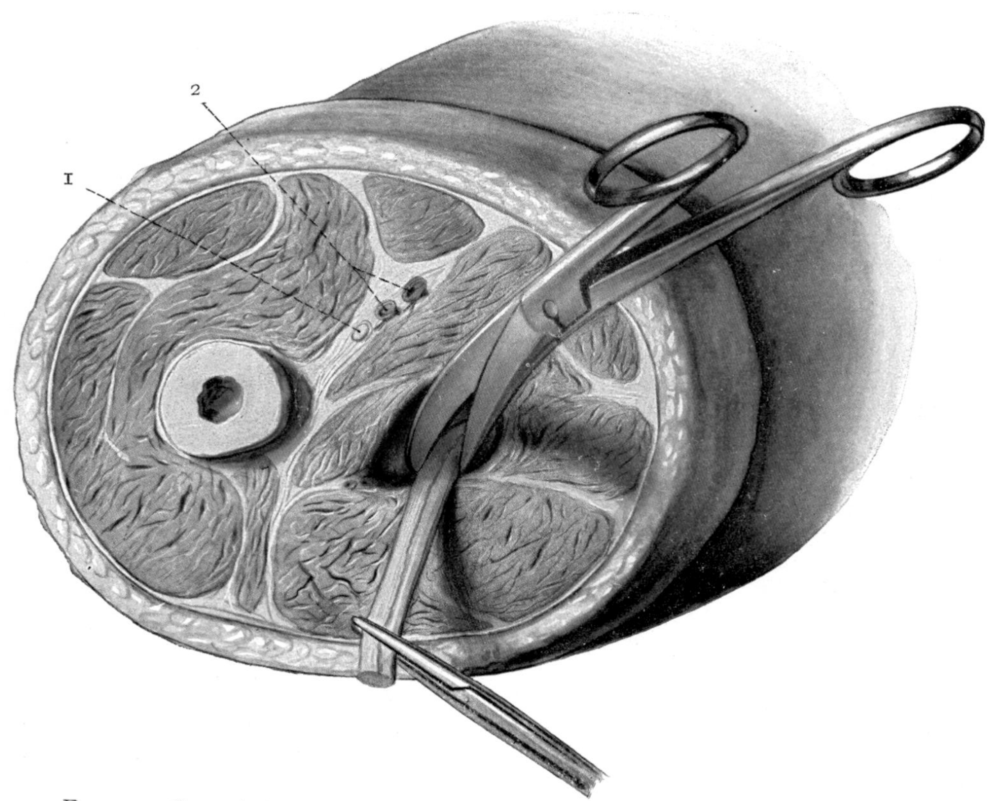

Fig. 730. Care of the nerves in an amputation of the thigh. The sciatic nerve is caught and pulled out of the wound. It is then divided as far proximally as possible. 1. Saphenous nerve, not yet resected. 2. Femoral vessels, ligated.

for, carefully exposed, followed up as far as possible by traction on the nerve and retraction of the muscles, and divided as high as possible. In particularly large nerves (sciatic) the important accompanying vessels should be exposed first and ligated with catgut. Lately, I have had excellent results after injecting 90 percent alcohol into the nerve proximal to the point of division.

Various procedures directed against the formation of amputation neuromata may be employed prophylactically, or they may be used subsequently when the occurrence of such a lesion shows the constitutional proclivity of the patient to it. The procedures considered in this connection are crushing, freezing, or the injection of 90 percent alcohol central to the point of incision, the use of a cautery instead of a knife for division of the nerve, and construction of a loop at the end of the nerve. The latter is described in Chapter VIII, D.

G. REAMPUTATIONS AND SECONDARY PLASTIC OPERATIONS

An amputation wound does not always heal spontaneously, nor does a sufficiently useful stump always follow healing. When conservative after-care does not obtain the desired results in such cases, secondary operations must ultimately be resorted to.

When the primary wound healing does not occur because of infection or necrosis of the flap, or when it is not desired, because of infection, as after

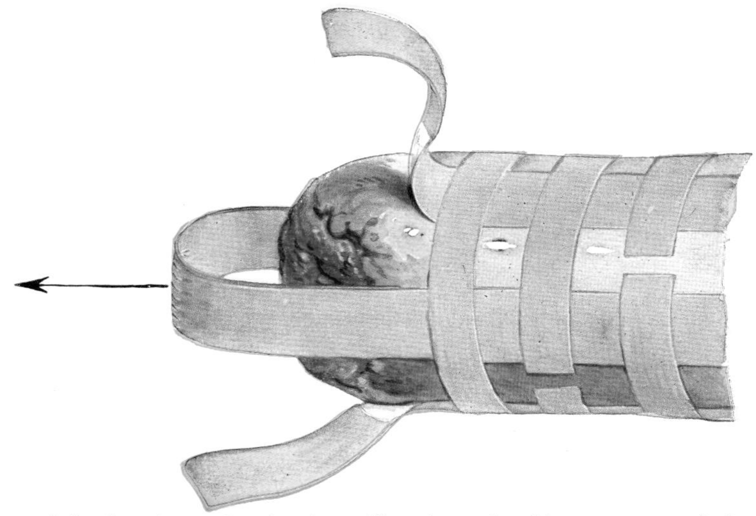

FIG. 731. Adhesive plaster dressing for pulling down the skin over a granulating stump.

the guillotine operation, the soft parts of the wound have a pronounced tendency to shrink and to retract proximally from the end of the bone. This tendency should be checked early by means of traction dressings. Four strips of adhesive plaster are applied to the skin in the longitudinal axis of the limb (Fig. 731), which are then fastened in place with adhesive plaster strips surrounding the limb transversely. Where the longitudinal strips are to lie over the dressings covering the wound, they are made non-adherent by pasting a bandage or another adhesive strip against them. The four adhesive strips are united in pairs distal to the wound margin and are connected by a cord passed over a pulley to a weight. Traction is in this way applied directly, while the patient is in bed. Similar traction may be obtained by using a stocking fastened to the stump with mastic.

As a rule, the traction dressing results in considerable diminution of the size of the wound, but not in its complete closure. Frequently an intractable ulcer remains in the region of the bone stump. When this occurs a choice must be made between a plastic operation to cover the skin defect, or reamputation. This is true when the tissues of the stump repeatedly break down, or when there is a very painful cutaneous scar on an otherwise healed amputation stump. If the scar is excised, the problem of covering the defect arises.

To cover the defect only healthy skin should be used. A pedunculated flap of skin and subcutaneous tissue is taken from the vicinity, or a flap with a temporary pedicle may be transferred from a distant site. Samter's bridge-flap (Fig. 732) is a good method of utilizing adjacent skin. A bilateral pedunculated flap is freed at the margin of the defect. It is drawn over the

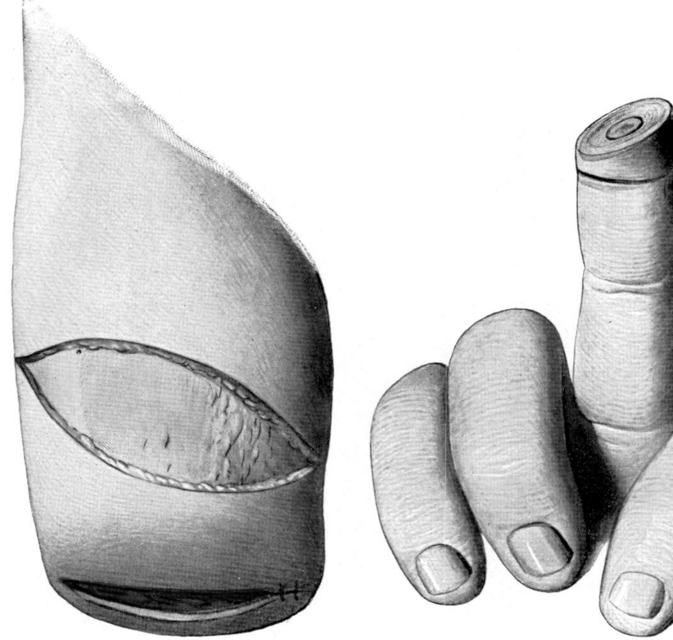

Fig. 732. Bridge-flap (Samter). An incision is made through the skin and subcutaneous tissue, well above the level of amputation. The flap is mobilized and brought down over the stump surface which has been prepared for secondary closure.

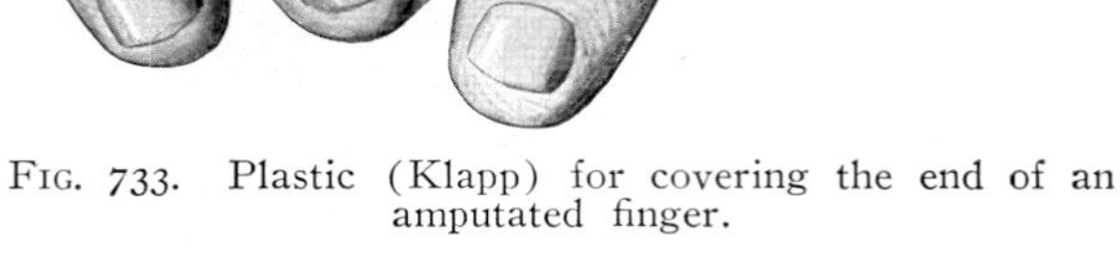

Fig. 733. Plastic (Klapp) for covering the end of an amputated finger.

defect and after removing the ulcer or scar tissue it is sutured in this new position. Klapp's sickle plastic (Fig. 733) is useful in closing defects on the ends of the fingers. Crescentic flaps are cut on the wound margin and pulled over the surface of the stump. The newly formed wound surfaces are drawn together or closed with Thiersch grafts.

In a flap temporarily pedunculated, the rules given in Chapter V, A, should be followed. Grafts for stumps of the leg are usually taken from the other leg and are pedunculated distally. Skin from the breast has been used to cover an ulcer on a stump of the thigh, the thigh being in extreme flexion at the hip joint. Skin from the breast and abdomen may be used for the arm. For the forearm and fingers, the scrotum and thigh may also be used. Pedunculated flaps, or even better, bridge-flaps may be transplanted, or the stump may be planted in a slit in the skin and separated later, with an attached portion of skin (Figs. 413 and 414).

Plastic procedures are difficult when excessively large flaps are transferred. The prospects are good only when the nutrition of the stump is good. A plastic operation involving a graft is contra-indicated in the presence of circulatory disturbances. Under such conditions either the end of the bone is resected, or an entirely new amputation of the limb is performed (reamputation). The end of the bone is best removed by the method described by Payr (Fig. 734). Through any scar tissue which may be present a transverse incision is made over the surface of the stump and extended for

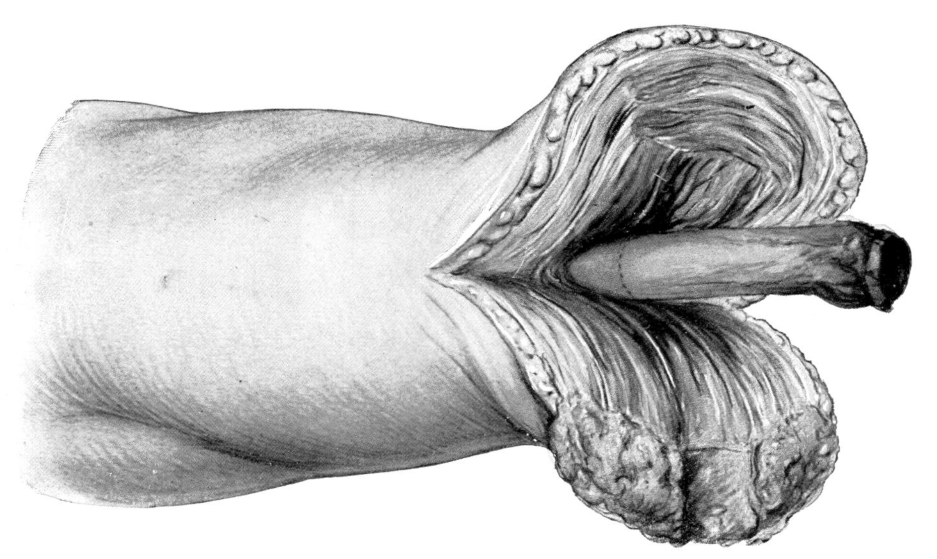

FIG. 734. Reamputation with double flaps. An anterior and a posterior flap are formed, freed from the bone, the edges of the wound are revised, and then closed over the resected bone.

some distance on both sides in the longitudinal axis of the limb. The two flaps thus formed are detached from the bone. The bone is exposed on all sides and resected. The margins of the flaps are revised and sutured together.

An obstinate fistula remaining in the area of the wound after amputation of a limb usually has its source in the depths of the wound. It may be caused by a ligature that has not been absorbed, or by disease of the bone, such as osteitis with or without the formation of a sequestrum, such as a coronary sequestrum (Fig. 724). In many cases the x-ray will clarify the nature of the disease, with or without filling the fistula with an opaque solution, or cautiously inserting a probe. If fishing for a thread or careful curetting does not bring results, the fistula should be split open or the bone exposed according to the procedure of Payr, and the focus removed.

Painful hypertrophies of the bone, or osteophytes, require resection of the bone or reamputation, which is to be preferred, because bone hypertrophies have a tendency to recur.

Painful neuromata (Fig. 736) either may be exposed, excised and the new end of the nerve handled according to the methods previously described, or the nerve trunk is exposed at the site of election proximal to the neuroma and its continuity interrupted by excising a piece of the nerve several centimeters long or by injecting 90 percent alcohol. Proximal interruption of the nerve has a double advantage, in that it removes at one stroke the pain produced by the amputation neuroma and by the cicatricial inclusion, and it insures against recurrence of the pain. Pain does not originate always in the larger nerve trunks, but more often springs from small cutaneous nerves. It

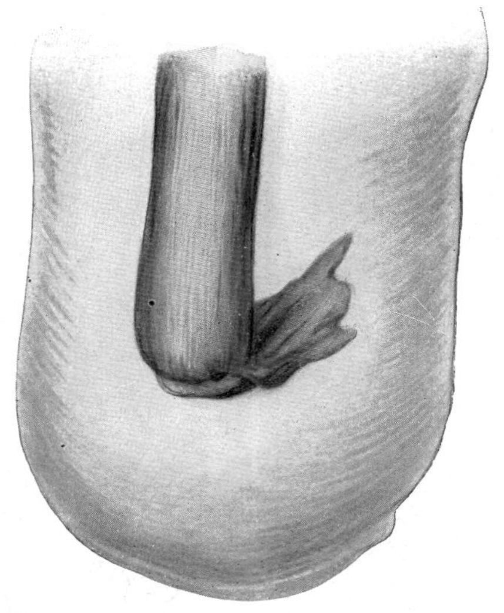

FIG. 735. Bone hypertrophy (osteophyte) on the bone stump of an amputated thigh.

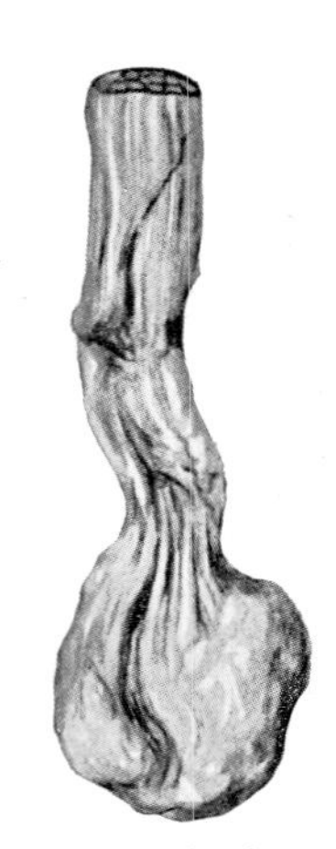

FIG. 736. Amputation neuroma of the sciatic nerve.

is the clinician's duty to clarify the situation, and the surgeon's task to search for and remove the offending structures.

H. AFTER-CARE OF THE STUMP

Even though a limb has been properly amputated and perhaps a secondary operation has been performed to improve the stump, there is no certainty that the stump will be a useful one. A further essential for obtaining the desired end is carefully directed and energetic after-care. Only when the after-care is recognized as of equal importance to the operation is a good functional result assured.

Every amputation of a section of a limb is associated with a disturbance of the equilibrium between the extensor and flexor muscles. For this reason, the adjacent joints show a pronounced tendency toward contracture with subsequent fibrous ankylosis, which affects the capacity for function of the stump disadvantageously. Efforts, therefore, must first be directed towards maintaining free mobility of the articulation, or articulations, of the remaining section of the extremity. If, at times, it is impossible to obtain free mobility, the limb should at least be placed in the position most favorable for the use of an artificial limb. Certain measures may be taken at the operation to avoid specific contractures, which tend to occur in certain joints, and muscular atrophy, by uniting the remaining flexor and extensor tendons over the end of the bone, or suturing certain tendons to suitable points on the bone, thus preventing bad position if ankylosis should occur. A few days after the operation the stump, which is elevated at first because of the danger of secondary hemorrhage, is fixed in such a position that the joint is partially bent by means of splints, sand bags, or traction, in a position that does not deviate far from the one most favorable to later use. Prolonged elevation of the thigh stump, still often used, is disposed to favor a disadvantageous contracture at the hip-joint, and in case of infection easily leads to the burrowing of pus in the muscle clefts (tubular abscess). If elevation of the operative area, as in the leg, can be combined with a dependent position of the distal section of the limb and with a favorable position of the joint, use may be made of this in acute infection.

Active or passive motion for the remaining part of the limb, should be instituted as soon as possible. This is permissible before the end of the

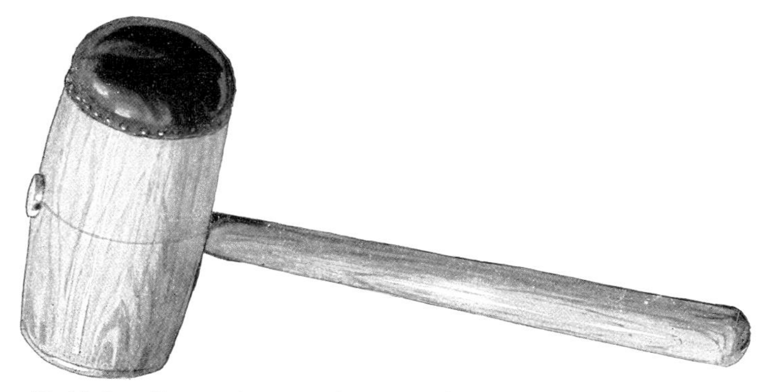

FIG. 737. Padded mallet, used to tap the supporting surface of an amputation stump.

first week. Even when attempts at active muscular exercise have no apparent results, they counteract the threatening atrophy. The exercises are increased as rapidly as possible during a regular exercise period and augmented by use of the pendulum apparatus. Massage, which should gradually become more vigorous, is an aid.

Hirsch's method for hardening the supporting surface is a deciding factor in increasing the capacity for weight-bearing. The old Greek saying is true in this relation: "The person who is not harassed, will not prosper." As soon as the wound has healed, or as soon as any infection which may have been present has subsided, attention is directed toward improving the weight-bearing capacity of the stump. In part this is done by the patient, and in part by the nurse, or masseur. Massage by patting or pounding is applied to the stump, first with the hand, later with a padded wooden mallet which is covered with felt or leather. The patient puts pressure on the stump as in walking, first in bed against a padded block of wood of the proper length (Fig. 738), later out of bed, while he props himself on the healthy leg with the aid of canes, and steps with the stump on rubber-sponge cushions, stools, chairs, or blocks of wood, corresponding in their height to the length of the stump (Fig. 739). The surface on which he puts his stump is at first covered with rubber cushions, felt, or leather, but later they are used without padding. In addition, the skin of the stump is hardened by frequent baths and alcohol rubs. Considerable resistance may have to be overcome in nervous and sensitive patients. The reward of indefatigable efforts is, as a rule, a stump capable of supporting a good load, and sometimes the entire weight.

An important question in the after-care is the time at which an artificial limb is to be fitted. From my experience the sooner this is done the better. Since the stump changes in shape and size in the first few months, it is necessary to use several temporary prostheses before the final one is made. The latter should fit perfectly. The temporary prostheses should if possible resemble the final prosthesis in their construction, but whether this ideal can

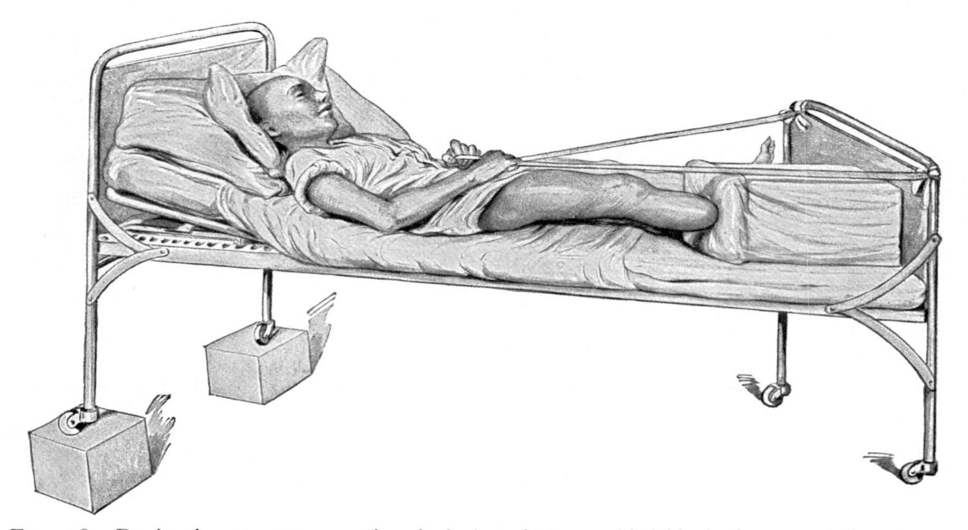

FIG. 738. Device for pressure exercises in bed against a padded block, for amputation stumps.

be fulfilled in practice depends upon the financial resources of the patient. One must frequently make concessions. With a clever mechanic the cost may be reduced to a minimum, since in the artificial limb only the inclosing basket is changed as the stump changes. The simplest form of substitute for an artificial leg is a peg with a plaster-cast basket fastened to the stump (Fig. 740). Fair results may be obtained with this method, especially if the important knee-joint can be supplied in amputations of the thigh.

The stump may undergo considerable change after many months, or even years, which should be taken into consideration in the fitting of the artificial limbs. The stumps have a tendency to become more and more conical, which is not only the result of progressive atrophy of the muscles and other soft parts, but also of the increasing atrophy of the bone, which now and then becomes quite tapered. As long as growth continues in children, the stump will continue to change.

The removal of a distal epiphysis has a very definite effect on the growth of the remainder of the extremity. In extremities where two bones have been divided, the ends remaining may grow unequally, for example, the tibia may outgrow the fibula. It may be necessary, when bone growth has ceased, to reoperate in order to improve the stump.

The best artificial limb is of little value to the patient if he is not systematically instructed in its use, and this can not be done by a lecture, but only by demonstration. He must be taught to use the prosthesis successfully for all the tasks of daily life. He must become skilful in its use. In most cases crutches should not be permitted in walking even at the beginning. The basket should fit the stump loosely and comfortably. I do not

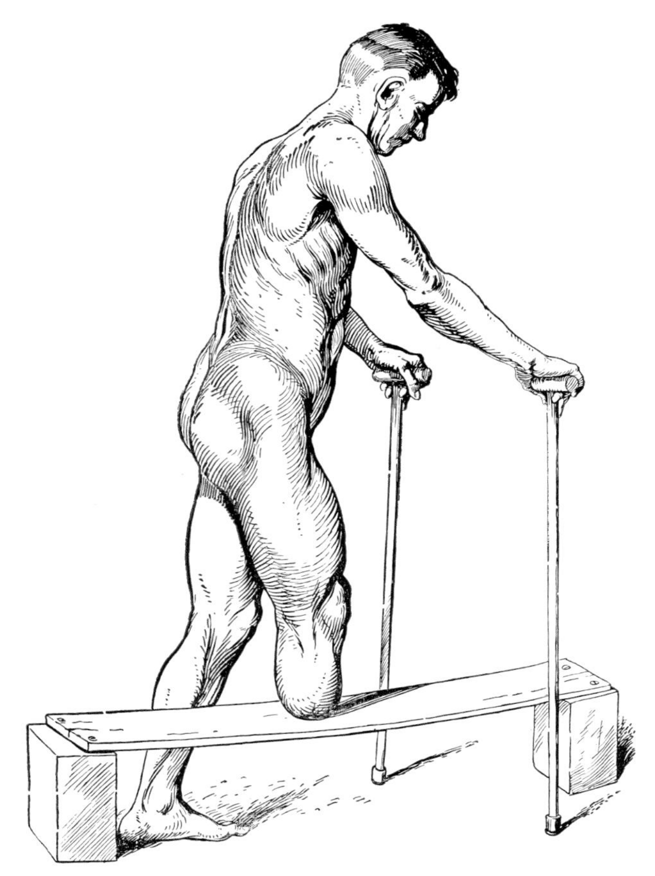

FIG. 739. Device for weight bearing exercises for amputation stumps. At first the bench is padded with rubber cushions of various thickness.

approve of bandaging the stump because through this muscular atrophy occurs, while every effort should be directed toward avoiding this.

I. KINEPLASTIC AMPUTATIONS

Vanghetti first devised and Ceci first put into practice the method of using the muscles remaining in the amputated stump for the voluntary movement of an artificial limb. Practical use of this idea was made during the war by Sauerbruch. He has shown that reliance on the continued conveyance of muscle force to the artificial limb can only be expected when the muscle which supplies the motive force (power pad) is perforated by a resistant tunnel (power canal). So that the canal of skin which traverses the muscle can withstand the constant pressure of the ivory pivot which transmits the force, it must consist of scar-free, well-nourished skin in all its thickness and must be large enough to be easily cleansed and to receive pegs of considerable size.

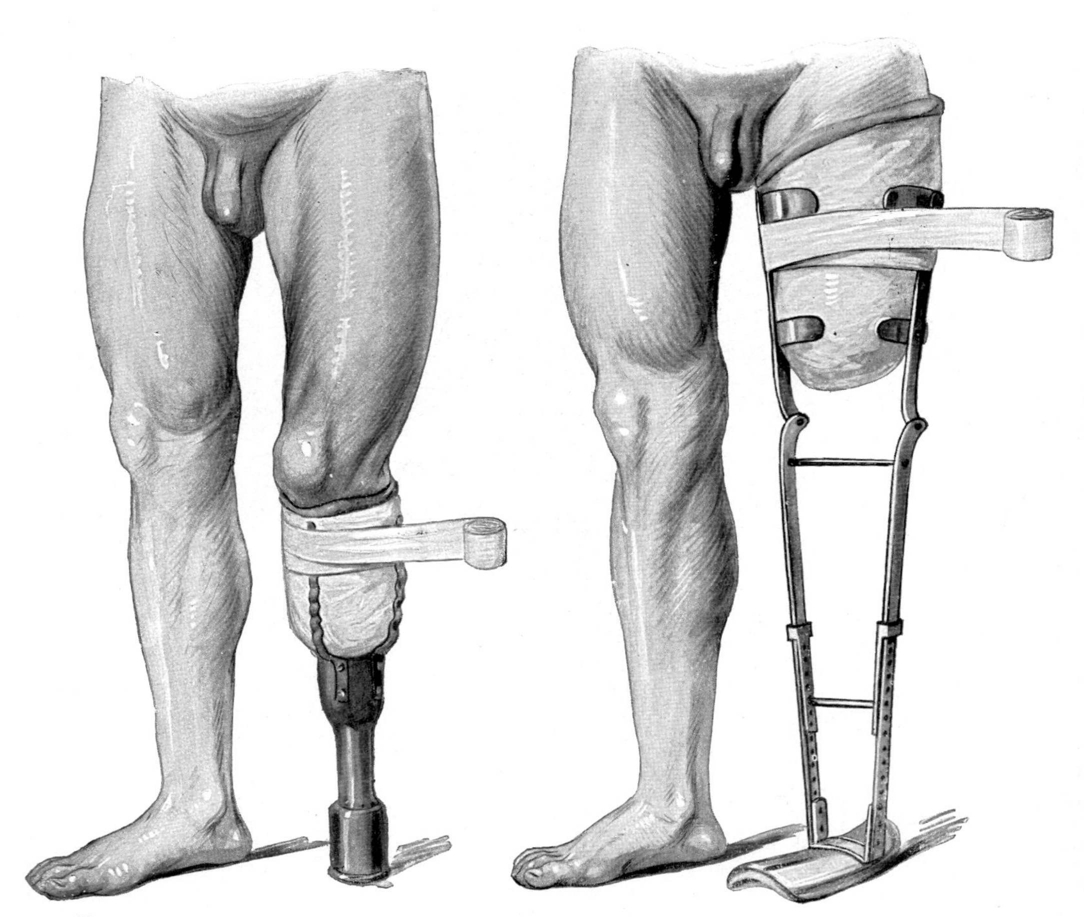

FIG. 740. Temporary prosthesis with plaster receptacle for the stump, after a leg amputation.

FIG. 741. Temporary prosthesis with plaster receptacle, after a thigh amputation.

Sauerbruch constructs the power canal, as a rule, out of the skin of the stump itself (Fig. 742) in the form of a pedunculated flap, which he sutures in tubular form, pulls through the canal made in the muscle of the stump and sutures to the skin of the opposite side. The skin tube may be taken from the skin of the chest in the form of a temporary pedunculated flap, if it is impossible to obtain skin from the stump.

Anschütz has observed in the graft pedunculated at one side only, repeated nutritional disturbances especially at the end of the skin tube, but which occasionally involved the entire tube. He therefore purposely uses bridge-flaps for the skin tunnel. Furthermore, Anschütz is positive that the most distal section of the muscle, that is close to the end of the stump, is not the most favorable site for the construction of a tunnel; that a canal placed rather at a considerable distance from the amputation scar has the advantage of better displacement and power development, because the muscle is free of scars and adhesions at this site. Anschütz outlines over the center of

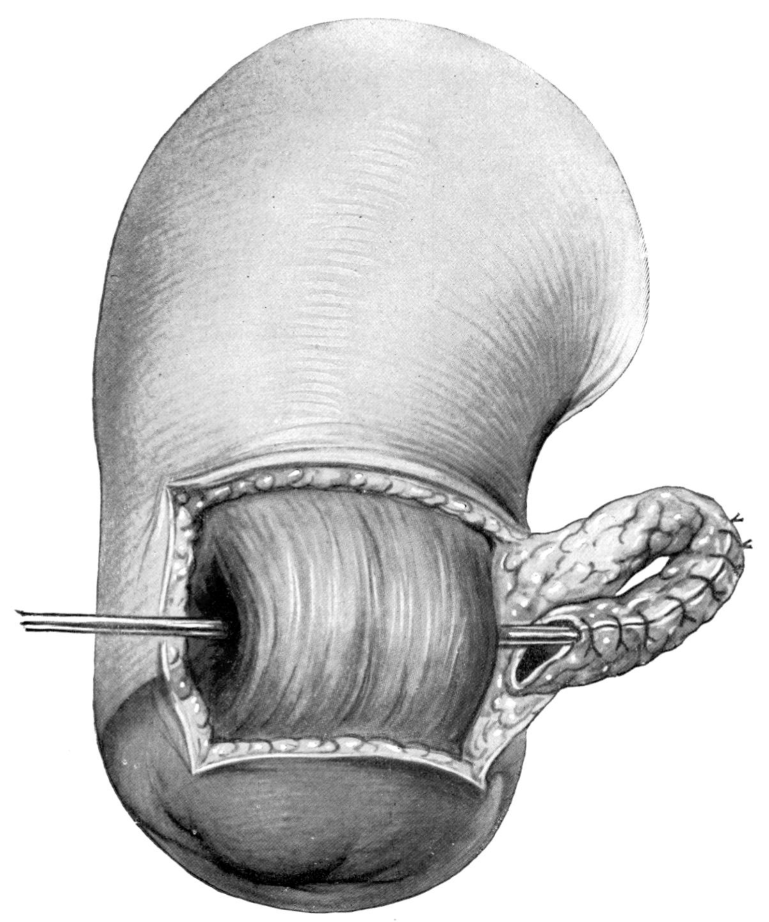

Fig. 742. Kineplastic arm stump with pedunculated skin tube (Sauerbruch). The skin tube is drawn through the distal section of the tunneled muscle.

the power-dispensing muscle a strip of skin about 5 cm. wide, extending over the entire width of the muscle and limited by two parallel transverse incisions (Fig. 743). He sutures this bridge together turning the epithelium inward, so as to construct a tube. He then completely divides the muscle lying underneath the skin tube as far distally as possible (Figs. 743, 744), splits the divided muscle parallel to its surface in the proximal direction for some distance, inserts the tunnel in the cleft of the muscle, and sutures the cleft together over the skin canal, after careful hemostasis. The skin tunnel thus passes through the center of the proximal portion of the transversely divided muscle, by means of which a particularly good source of power is provided. The two longitudinal sides of the rectangular skin defect are extended distally a few centimeters on each side (Fig. 744) and the rectangular skin flap

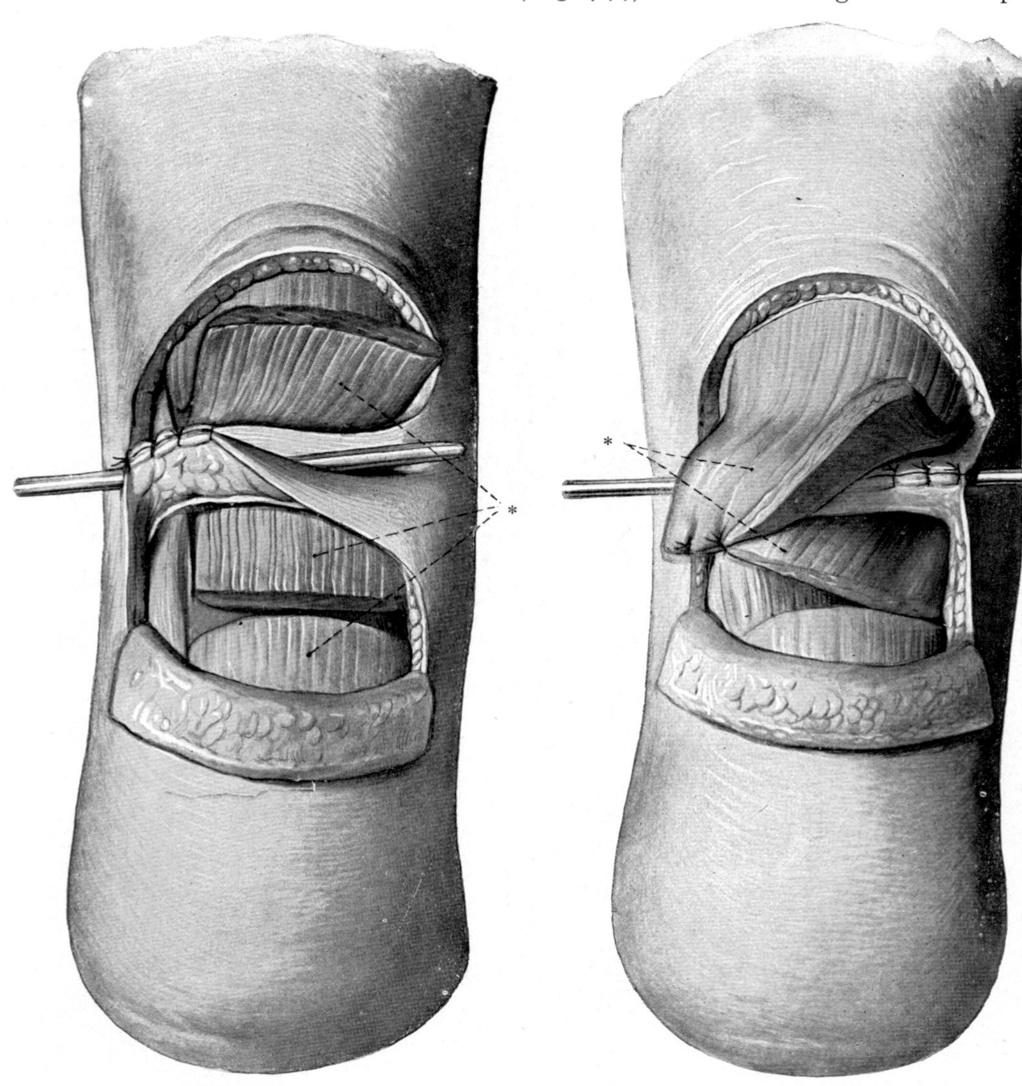

FIG. 743. Kineplastic arm stump with bilateral pedunculated skin tube (Anschütz). Formation of skin tube and splitting of muscle. * The skin tube is being formed in the split muscle.

FIG. 744. Kineplastic arm stump; continuation of previous illustration. * The superficial slit of the proximal part of the muscle is reunited so as to include the skin tube.

so circumscribed is detached from the base. In the subsequent suture of the proximal and distal skin margins (Fig. 745), the line of suture should lie somewhat proximal to the site of the canal so that the scar will be out of the way of injury. If the two transverse margins of skin can not be brought together, a transverse tension incision is made proximal to the site (Fig.

746). This defect is then covered with Thiersch grafts. If necessary, the wound may be closed by a skin flap from the thorax with a temporary pedicle.

Anschütz's tunnels may be used in the forearm as well as the arm. In the latter on the flexor side, the biceps is well adapted to this procedure;

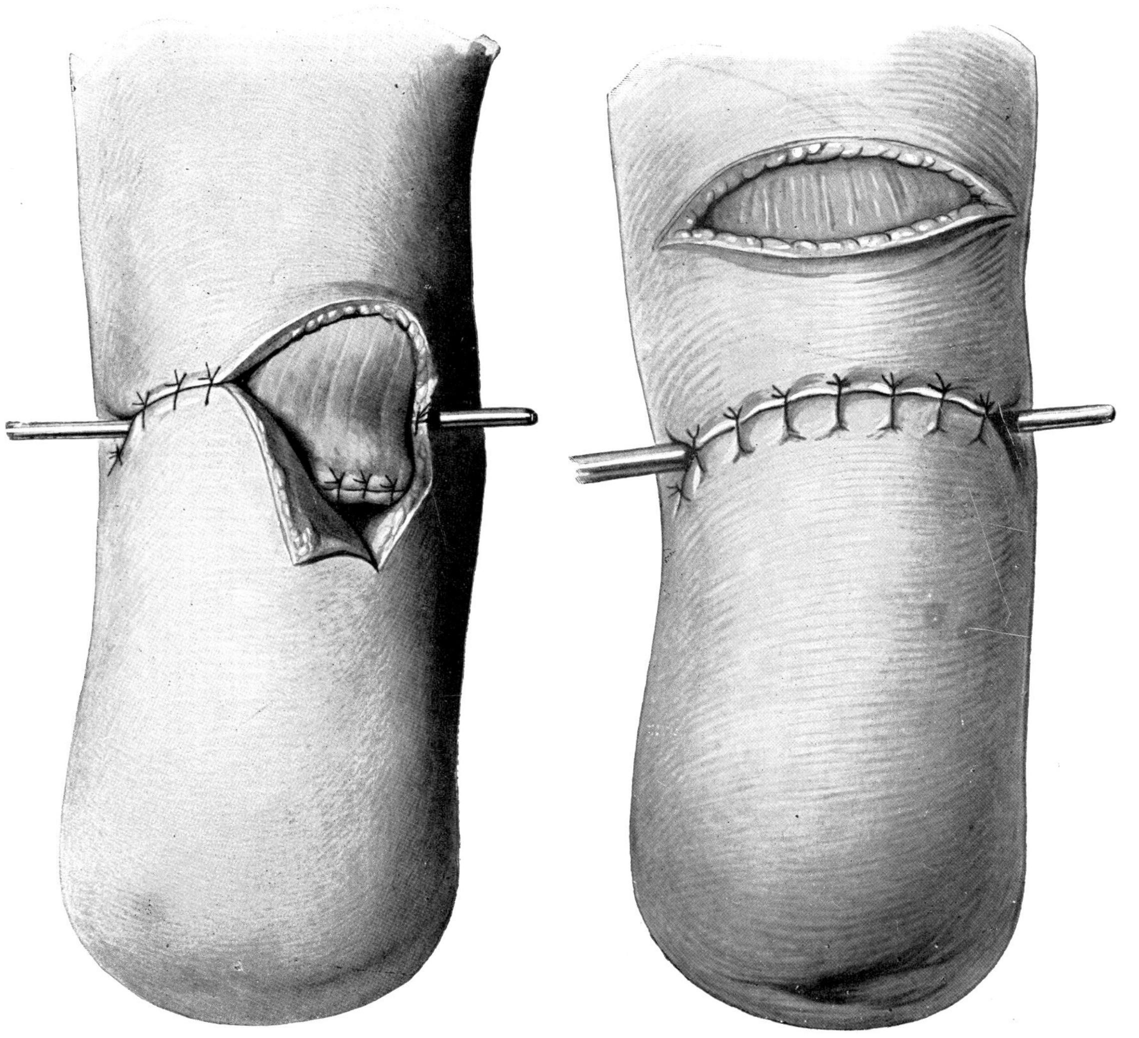

FIG. 745. Kineplastic arm stump, continuation of previous illustration. The skin is closed over the area of operation, by direct suture.

FIG. 746. Kineplastic arm stump, continuation of previous illustration. A proximal transverse tension incision may be required to unite the margins of the skin wound.

on the extensor side, the long head of the triceps is best used. If there are not sufficient muscles available on the arm stump, the canal may be placed through the pectoralis major.

The time between amputation and canalization of the muscles should be as short as possible, because the inactive muscles rapidly lose their power, elasticity and strength. In spite of this, muscles may be rendered useful for motion of the artificial limb years after the amputation, through energetic exercise. The formation of the skin tunnels must often be preceded by operations to free the muscles from scar tissue so that these may be used for power pads.

The kineplastic operation, of which only an outline has been given here, but which is described in detail in Sauerbruch's book on this subject, offers theoretically, without a doubt, an important therapeutic advance. Sauerbruch's cases show that practical results may be occasionally obtained. Horn, his assistant, has reported the end results of these cases. If other surgeons fail to obtain good results or only occasionally obtain these, it can not always be attributed to a faulty choice of stump material or to defective technic. I know from experience, that only a very few of those who have had an arm amputated feel the necessity for a complicated prosthesis in their calling and in everyday life. The one-armed person may help himself to an amazing degree within a short period of time, so that he learns rapidly to perform with the well arm, be it the right or the left, or the remainder of the amputated arm with or without a limb substitute, the usual requirements of daily life. He may learn to do delicate as well as rough work. The remainder of the cases are gratified by a prosthesis based on Carnes' principles, which also has a wide field of usefulness after the Sauerbruch operation. Most of the injured are satisfied with this condition and undertake with distrust and ill-will any additional operation involving new problems. A kineplastic operation may succeed only when the patient submits to a long period of treatment involving exercises before and after the operation, so as to win the necessary mastery of the individual muscles for complete control.

The construction of a skin tube in the muscles becomes, therefore, merely a small part of the entire treatment necessary in successful kineplasty. I think it is proper to employ this method only when the patient himself urges the operation, and when he is apprised of the sacrifice in time and energy required of him. From my experience and that of many other surgeons, these conditions are but seldom realized, but most often when both arms have been lost. The kineplastic amputation possesses thus far no great economic value.

Repeated attempts have been made to apply the kineplastic principle to the leg also, but with no success as yet.

Krukenberg suggested a special form of kineplastic amputation for the forearm, based upon entirely different principles. He forms a sort of claw from the radius and from the ulna, which are separated and made to oppose one another, a "lobster-claw," that can grasp as well as an artificial hand.

INDEX